Puzzling Cases of Epilepsy

Puzzling Cases of Epilepsy

Edited by

Dieter Schmidt and Steven C. Schachter

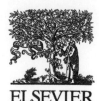

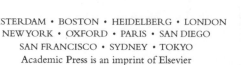

AMSTERDAM • BOSTON • HEIDELBERG • LONDON
NEW YORK • OXFORD • PARIS • SAN DIEGO
SAN FRANCISCO • SYDNEY • TOKYO
Academic Press is an imprint of Elsevier

Academic Press is an imprint of Elsevier
360 Park Avenue South, New York, NY 10010–1710
30 Corporate Drive, Suite 400, Burlington, MA 01803, USA
525 B Street, Suite 1900, San Diego, CA 92101-4495, USA
32 Jamestown Road, London NW1 7BY, UK
Radarweg 29, PO Box 211, 1000 AE Amsterdam, The Netherlands

Second edition **2008**

Library of Congress Cataloging-in-Publication Data
A catalog record for this book is available from the Library of Congress.

British Library Cataloguing in Publication Data
A catalogue record for this book is available from the British Library.

For information on all Academic Press publications
visit our web site at books.elsevier.com

Printed and bound in United States of America
08 09 10   10 9 8 7 6 5 4 3 2 1

ISBN: 978-0-12-374005-2

Contents

Preface   xxi

List of Contributors   xxiii

PART I

Diagnostic Puzzles and Uncertainties

1.   *A Young Woman with Mouth Jerking Provoked
         by Reading*   *3*
         Taoufik Alsaadi

2.   *Two Adult Patients with Infantile Spasms*   *6*
         Carol S Camfield and Peter R Camfield

3.   *An Infant with Partial Seizures and Infantile Spasms*   *10*
         Catherine Chiron and Nathalie Villeneuve

4.   *Epilepsia Partialis Continua versus Non-Epileptic
         Seizures*   *13*
         Alan B Ettinger

p0190   **5.** *Panic Attacks in a Woman with Frontal*
         Lobe Epilepsy   *20*

p0200   Thomas Grunwald, Martin Kurthen and Christian E Elger

p0210   **6.** *Frequent Night Terrors*   *24*

p0220   Cesare T Lombroso

p0230   **7.** *Genetic (Generalized) Epilepsy with Febrile*
         Seizures Plus   *29*

p0240   Ingrid E Scheffer

p0250   **8.** *A Visit to the Borderland of Neurology*
         and Psychiatry   *34*

p0260   Donald L Schomer

p0270   **9.** *A Case of Complex Partial Status Epilepticus* *38*

p0280   Alan R Towne

p0290   **10.** *Late-Onset Myoclonic Seizures in*
          Down's Syndrome   *42*

p0300   Hajo M Hamer, Jens C Möller, Susanne Knake,
         Wolfgang H Oertel and Felix Rosenow

p0310   **11.** *Fainting, Fear, and Pallor in a 22-Month-Old Girl*   *46*

p0320   Edwin Trevathan

p0330   **PART II**

Intriguing Causes and Circumstances

p0340   **12.** *Hyperactive Behavior and Attentional*
          Deficit in a 7-Year-Old Boy with Myoclonic Jerks   *51*

p0350   Johan Arends, Albert P Aldenkamp, and Biene Weber

13. *Temporal Lobe Epilepsy, Loss of Episodic Memory, and Depression in a 32-Year-Old Woman*   *56*

Christian G Bien

14. *Epileptic "Dreamy States" in a Young Man*   *61*

Warren T Blume

15. *Nocturnal Seizures in a Man with Coronary Disease*   *65*

P Barton Duell

16. *Non-convulsive Status Epilepticus and Frontal Lobe Seizures in a Patient with a Chromosome Abnormality*   *69*

Maurizio Elia

17. *An Unusual Cause of Nocturnal Attacks*   *73*

Donald W Gross, Eva Andermann, David C Reutens, Udaya Seneviratne, François Dubeau and Frederick Andermann

18. *Myoclonic Jerks in a Computer Specialist*   *76*

Dorotheé GA Kasteleijn-Nolst Trenité

19. *Their Previous Physicians had Told Them that They Should not Become Pregnant Because They have Epilepsy*   *80*

Barbara L Phillips, Ronald E Kramer and Kirsten A Bracht

20. *Status Epilepticus after a Long Day of White-Water Rafting in the Grand Canyon*   *85*

David M Labiner

21. *A Farmer Who Watched His Own Seizures*   *88*

Gerhard Luef

22. *The Borderland of Neurology and Cardiology*   *91*

Martha J Morrell

23. *A Man with Shoulder Twitching*   *95*

Erasmo A Passaro and Ahmad Beydoun

24. *The Girl with Visual Seizures Who wasn't Seeing*
Things – Transient Blindness in a Young Girl   *100*

Carl E Stafstrom

25. *A Young Man with Noise-Induced Partial Seizures*   *106*

Bettina Schmitz

26. *Non-convulsive Status Epilepticus in a Patient*
with Idiopathic Generalized Epilepsy   *112*

Eugen Trinka

27. *Pseudohypoglycemia Manifesting as Complex*
Partial Seizures in a Patient with
Type III Glycogen Storage Disease   *115*

P Barton Duell

PART III

Surprising Turns and Twists

28. *Recurrent Amnestic Episodes in a 62-Year-Old*
Diabetic Patient   *121*

Christine Adam, Claude Adam and Michel Baulac

29. *Attacks of Nausea and Palpitations in a Woman*
with Epilepsy   *126*

Jørgen Alving

30. *Absence Status Epilepticus in a 60-Year-Old Woman*   *131*

Gerhard Bauer

31. *Hemiplegia in a 76-Year-Old Woman with Status Epilepticus*   *135*

Susannne Aull-Watschinger, Paolo Gallmetzer and Christoph Baumgartner

32. *Persistence Pays Off*   *139*

Mark D Bej

33. *Drugs Did Not Work in a Little Girl with Absence Seizures*   *142*

David B Bettis

34. *"Alternative" Therapy for Partial Epilepsy – with a Twist*   *145*

Nadir E Bharucha and Thomas Kuruvilla

35. *A 19-Year-Old Man with Epilepsy, Aphasia, and Hemangioma of the Cranial Vault*   *148*

Paulo Rogério M de Bittencourt

36. *Severe Psychiatric Disorder in an 8-Year-Old Boy with Myoclonic–Astatic Seizures*   *152*

Césare Maria Cornaggia, Alessandra Mascarini and Guiseppe Gobbi

37. *A Girl with Two Epilepsy Syndromes*   *157*

Marie-José Penniello, Isabelle Jambaqué, Christine Bulteau, Perrine Plouin, Olivier Delalande and Olivier Dulac

38. *The Obvious Cause of Seizures May Not Be the Underlying Cause*   *163*

Keith R Edwards

p0870 **39.** *Absence Seizures in an Adult*   *165*
p0880   Edward Faught

p0890 **40.** *A Case Solved by Seizures During Sleep*   *168*
p0900   Jacqueline A French

p0910 **41.** *Alternative Psychosis in an Adolescent Girl?*   *171*
p0920   Andres M Kanner

p0930 **42.** *Exacerbation of Seizures in a Young Woman*   *174*
p0940   Pavel Klein

p0950 **43.** *Genetic Counseling in a Woman with a*
             Family History of Refractory Myoclonic Epilepsy   *178*
p0960   Dick Lindhout

p0970 **44.** *"Funny Jerks" Run in the Family*   *182*
p0980   Heinz-Joachim Meencke

p0990 **45.** *Side Effects That Imitate Seizures*   *184*
p1000   George Lee Morris III

p1010 **46.** *Epilepsy, Migraine, and Cerebral Calcifications*   *187*
p1020   Willy O Renier

p1030 **47.** *An Unusual Application of Epilepsy Surgery*   *191*
1040   Edward H Bertram and Jaideep Kapur

p1050 **48.** *All is Not What it Seems*   *194*
p1060   William E Rosenfeld and Susan M Lippmann

p1070 **49.** *A Patient Whose Epilepsy Diagnosis Changed*
             Three Times Over 20 Years   *197*
p1080   Masakazu Seino and Yushi Inoue

50. *If You Don't Succeed, Investigate* *202*

Michael R Sperling

51. *Should He or Shouldn't He? Is It Reasonable to Prescribe Carbamazepine after Lamotrigine-induced Stevens–Johnson Syndrome?* *206*

Fahmida Chowdhury and L Nashef

52. *The Value of Repeating Video–EEG Monitoring and the Importance of Concomitant ECG Tracings in the Evaluation of Changes in Seizure Semiology* *210*

Meriem K Bensalem-Owen and Toufic A Fakhoury

PART IV

Unforeseen Complications and Problems

53. *A 35-Year-Old Man with Poor Surgical Outcome after Temporal Lobe Surgery* *219*

Gus A Baker

54. *When More is Less* *222*

Carl W Bazil

55. *Change of Antiepileptic Drug Treatment for Fear of Side Effects in a 45-Year-Old Seizure-Free Patient* *226*

Elinor Ben-Menachem

56. *Personality and Mood Changes in a Teenager* *228*

Ahmad Beydoun, Ekrem Kutluay and Erasmo Passaro

57. *Monitoring Patients May Be More Important Than Their Laboratory Tests*   *233*

Jane Boggs

58 *Depression in a Student with Juvenile Myoclonic Epilepsy*   *237*

Enrique J Carrazana

59. *Osteomalacia in a Patient Treated with Multiple Anticonvulsants*   *241*

Joost PH Drenth, Gerlach FFM Pieters and Ad RMM Hermus

60. *Parkinsonism and Cognitive Decline in a 64-Year-Old Woman with Epilepsy*   *244*

Manuel Eglau, Peter Hopp and Hermann Stefan

61. *Problems in Managing Epilepsy during and after Pregnancy*   *247*

Cynthia L Harden

62. *Status Epilepticus in a Heavy Snorer*   *251*

Peter Höllinger, Christian W Hess and Claudio Bassetti

63. *A Boy with Epilepsy and Allergic Rhinitis*   *256*

Kazuie Iinuma and Hiroyuki Yokoyama

64. *Seizures and Behavior Disturbance in a Boy*   *259*

Sookyong Koh

65. *Abulia in a Seizure-Free Patient with Frontal Lobe Epilepsy*   *263*

Ennapadam S Krishnamoorthy and Michael R Trimble

66. *The Continuing Place of Phenobarbital*   *267*

Fumisuke Matsuo

67. *A Patient with Epilepsy Slips Down*
Some Attic Stairs   *270*

Rajesh C Sachdeo

68. *Bilateral Hip Fractures in a 43-Year-Old Woman*
with Epilepsy   *274*

Dieter Schmidt

69. *Picking a Wrong Antiepileptic Drug for a*
9-Year-Old Girl   *277*

Peter Uldall

70. *With Epilepsy You Never Know*   *282*

Walter van Emde Boas

PART V

Unexpected Solutions

71. *When Antiepileptic Drugs Fail in an Infant with*
Seizures, Consider Vitamin B6   *289*

Mary R Andriola

72. *A 12-Year-Old Boy with Daily Clonic Seizures* *292*

Eloy Elices and Santiago Arroyo

73. *A Child with Attention-Deficit Disorder, Autistic*
Features and Frequent Epileptiform
EEG Discharges   *296*

Frank MC Besag

p1590   **74.** *Complete Seizure Control in a 14-Year-Old Boy*
p1600   *after Temporal Lobectomy Failed*   *299*
                 Martin J Brodie

p1610   **75.** *Ictal Crying in a 32-Year-Old Woman*   *302*
p1620   Edward B Bromfield

p1630   **76.** *Healing Begins with Communicating the Diagnosis*   *306*
p1640   Orrin Devinsky

p1650   **77.** *An Unusual Case of Seizures and Violence*   *309*
p1660   Robert S Fisher

p1670   **78.** *Attacks of Generalized Shaking without Postictal*
                 Confusion   *313*
p1680   James S Grisolia

p1690   **79.** *Lennox–Gastaut Syndrome with Good Outcome*
                 Associated with Perisylvian Polymicrogyria   *316*
p1700   Marilisa M Guerreiro

p1710   **80.** *Temporal Lobe Resection in a Patient with Severe*
                 Psychiatric Problems   *319*
p1720   Reetta Kälviäinen

p1730   **81.** *An Open Mind Can Benefit the Patient*   *322*
p1740   Kaarkuzhali Babu Krishnamurthy

p1750   **82.** *An Unexpected Lesson*   *325*
p1760   Paul M Levisohn

p1770   **83.** *When Surgery Is Not Possible,*
                 All Hope Is Not Lost   *330*
p1780   Cassandra I Mateo and Brian Litt

84. *Sometimes Less Is More*   *334*

R Eugene Ramsay and Flavia Pryor

85. *Unexpected Benefit from an*
Old Antiepileptic Drug   *338*

Matti Sillanpää

86. *Status Epilepticus Responsive to Intravenous*
Immunoglobulin   *341*

Joseph I Sirven and Hoan Linh Banh

87. *Surgical Success in a Patient with*
Diffuse Brain Trauma   *346*

Brien J Smith

88. *Dietary Treatment of Seizures from a*
Hypothalamic Hamartoma   *350*

Vijay Maggio and James Wheless

89. *Can the Behavioral and Cognitive Effects of*
AEDs Be Predicted?   *354*

Kimford J Meador

90. *A Child with So-Called Nocturnal*
Paroxysmal Dystonia Whose Epilepsy Arose
from Orbital Cortex   *359*

Cesare T Lombroso

91. *The Night Mom Didn't Come Back*   *375*

Jane Boggs

92. *The EEG – Not the EEG Report – Makes the*
Difference   *379*

Jane Boggs

PART VI

Where Clinical Knowledge and
Preclinical Science Meet

93. *The Double-Hit Hypothesis:*
Is It Clinically Relevant?   387
Sookyong Koh and Kent Kelley

Comment: The Double-Hit Hypothesis: Is It
Clinically Relevant?   391
David Henshall

94. *Atypical Evolution in a Case of Benign*
Childhood Epilepsy with Centrotemporal
Spikes   396
Natalio Fejerman

Comment 1: Does Kindling in Humans
Occur? Comments Based on the Previous
Case Study   400
Dan McIntyre

Comment 2: Does Kindling in Humans Occur?
Comments Based on the Previous Case from a
Preclinical Perspective   403
Andreas Draguhn

95. *Does Status Epilepticus Represent a Different*
Pathophysiology than Epilepsy? A Patient
with Recurrent Status Epilepticus as the Single
Manifestation of Her Epilepsy   407
Christoph Baumgartner and Paolo Gallmetzer

Comment 1: Does Status Epilepticus Represent a Different Pathophysiology than Epilepsy? A Preclinical Perspective   *414*

Hana Kubova

Comment 2: Does Status Epilepticus Represent a Different Pathophysiology than Epilepsy? A Clinical Perspective   *417*

Gerhard Bauer and Eugen Trinka

96. *Why Do Some Patients Seem to Develop Tolerance to AEDs? Development of Antiepileptic Drug Tolerance in a Patient with Temporal Lobe Epilepsy*   *420*

Bassel Abou-Khalil

Comment 1: Why Do Some Patients Seem to Develop Tolerance to AEDs? A Preclinical Discussion   *423*

Wolfgang Löscher

Comment 2: How Can We Detect the Development of Tolerance (Loss of Effect) to AEDs in Patients with Epilepsy? A Clinical Discussion   *427*

Dieter Schmidt

97. *Why Is There a Similar Ceiling Effect for the Efficacy of Most If Not All Antiepileptic Drugs in Adult Epilepsy? Reaching the Ceiling or Hitting the Wall?*   *433*

Jane Boggs

p2240   *Comment 1: Why Is There a Similar Ceiling Effect for the Efficacy of Most If Not All Antiepileptic Drugs in Adult Epilepsy? A Clinical Perspective*   *437*

p2250   Rajiv Mohanraj and Martin J Brodie

p2220   *Comment 2: What Clinical Observations on the Epidemiology of Antiepileptic Drug Intractability Tell Us About the Mechanisms of Pharmacoresistance*   *441*

p2230   Michael A Rogawski

p2260   **98.**   *Difficult-to-Treat Idiopathic Generalized Epilepsy in a Young Woman*   *447*

p2270   Mar Carreño

p2280   *Comment 1: Can We Predict a Drug's Efficacy in a Specific Epilepsy Syndrome? A Preclinical Discussion.*   *451*

p2290   Emilio Perucca

p2300   *Comment 2: Bridging the Gap between Evidence-Based Medicine and Clinical Practice*   *454*

p2310   Jacqueline French

p2320   **99.**   *Psychogenic Non-Epileptic Seizures "Redux"*   *457*

p2330   Gregory Krauss

2340   *Comment 1: Is There a Neurobiological Basis to Stress-induced, Non-epileptic Behaviors that Mimic Seizures?*   *461*

p2350   Stephen C Heinrichs

Comment 2: Evidence for a Neurobiological Basis for Non-epileptic Seizures   *466*

Siddhartha S Nadkarni, Kenneth Alper and Orrin Devinsky

100.   *Why Does VNS Take So Long to Work?*   *470*

Paul Boon, Veerle De Herdt and Kristl Vonck

Comment 1: Commentary: Why Does VNS Take So Long to Work?   *473*

Steven Schachter

101.   *If at First You Don't Succeed …*   *478*

Andrew N Wilner

Comment 1: Why Antiepileptic Drugs Fail in Some Patients: A Preclinical Perspective   *481*

Heidrun Potschka

Comment 2: The Continuing Conundrum of Reversible Drug-resistant Epilepsy: A Clinical Perspective   *484*

Dieter Schmidt

102.   *Why Do Some Patients Have Seizures After Brain Surgery While Others Do Not?*   *489*

Christine Bower, David Millett and Jerome Engel Jr.

Comment 1: Why Do Some Patients Have Seizures After Brain Surgery While Others Do Not? A Comment on the Evidence   *494*

Samuel Wiebe

p2520   *Comment 2: Why Do Some Patients Have Seizures After Brain Surgery While Others Do Not? A Clinical Perspective*   *497*

p2530   József Janszky and Andras Fogarasi

p0090   **Index**   501

Preface to the second edition

The presentations and causes of epilepsy are so diverse and multifaceted that they impinge on virtually every aspect of modern medical science, from basic neuroscience to vocational rehabilitation. While a great number of excellent books have been written on various aspects of epilepsy, few have covered the individualized diagnostic and therapeutic challenges that clinicians must work through when evaluating and caring for patients with epilepsy. Indeed, the wide range of presentations and causes of epilepsy is well illustrated by puzzling cases that initially baffled epilepsy specialists – the experts – but from which important lessons were ultimately learned. That is the rationale for this book.

For this second edition, a number of experts have provided new case vignettes and others have contributed to a bench-and-bedside section in which they offer comments on individual cases from the perspectives of basic and clinical science.

We are grateful to all the contributors and to Elsevier for making the second edition possible. Most of all, we wish to thank the patients whose real-life experiences were the true inspiration for this book. Indeed, we learn most of what we know to be important as clinicians from our patients. Hopefully, this book will improve their care and raise scientific interest in solving the problems that they face every day from epilepsy.

Dieter Schmidt, MD, Berlin, Germany
Steven C. Schachter, MD, Boston, USA

List of Contributors

Numbers in Parenthesis indicate the pages on which the authors' contributions begin.

Bassel Abou-Khalil (420)
Department of Neurology
Vanderbilt University
A-0118 Medical Center North
Nashville, TN 37232-2551
USA

Christine Adam (121)
C/o Claude Adam
AP-HP, Epileptology Unit
Hôpital de La Pitié-Salpêtrière
Service de Neurologie 1
47-83 Bd de l'Hôpital
Paris Cedex 13, 75651
France

Claude Adam (121)
AP-HP, Epileptology Unit
Hôpital de La Pitié-Salpêtrière
Service de Neurologie 1
47-83 Bd de l'Hôpital
Paris Cedex 13, 75651
France

Albert P Aldenkamp (51)
Epilepsy Centre Kempenhaeghe
P.O. Box 61, Heeze, NL-5591 AB
The Netherlands

Kenneth Alper (466)
Comprehensive Epilepsy Center
NYU School of Medicine
403 East 34th Street, 4th Floor
New York, NY 10016
USA

Taoufik Alsaadi (3)
Department of Neurology
Sheikh Khalifah Medical Center
P.O. Box 51900
Abu Dhabi, 51900
UAE

Jørgen Alving (126)
Department of EEG and Epilepsy
  Monitoring
Danish Epilepsy Center
Dianalund, DK-4293
Denmark

Eva Andermann (73)
Montreal Neurological Institute
McGill University
3801 University Street, Rm 127
Montreal, QC H3A 2B4
Canada

Frederick Andermann (73)
Montreal Neurological Institute
McGill University
3801 University Street, Rm 127
Montreal, QC H3A 2B4
Canada

Mary R Andriola (289)
Department of Neurology
Stony Brook University
T12-20 Health Sciences Center
Stony Brook, NY 11794-8121
USA

Johan Arends (51)
Epilepsy Centre Kempenhaeghe
Sterkselseweg 65, Heeze, 5591 VE
The Netherlands

Santiago Arroyo (292)
C/Corb Mari 3 Esc1 3°B
Palma de Mallorca, Islas Baleares 08015
Spain

Susanne Aull-Watschinger (135)
Neurological University Clinic
Vienna General Hospital
Währinger Gürtel 18-20
Vienna 1090
Austria

Gus A Baker (219)
School of Clinical Science
University of Liverpool
Clinical Sciences Building
University Hospital Aintree
Liverpool, L69 3BX
UK

Hoan Linh Banh (341)
College of Pharmacy
Dalhousie University
5968 College Street
Halifax, NS B3H 3J5
Canada

Claudio Bassetti (251)
Neurologische Poliklinik
Universitätsspital,
  Frauenklinikstrasse 26
Zürich CH-8091
Switzerland

Gerhard Bauer (131, 417)
University Freiburg
Biology I, Hauptstrasse 1
Freiburg D-79104
Germany

Michel Baulac (121)
Hôpital de la Salpêtrière
Service deNeurologie, Epolepsie
47 Bld Hôpital
Paris 75013
France

Christoph Baumgartner (135, 407)
2nd Neurological Department
General Hospital Hietzing
Neurological Center Rosenhügel
Riedelgasse 5
A-1130 Vienna
Austria

Carl W Bazil (222)
The Neurological Institute
710 West 168th Street
New York, NY 10032
USA

Mark Bej (139)
Midwest Neuroscience Inc.
1 E. Main Street, Suite 200A
Norwalk, OH 44857-1512
USA

Elinor Ben-Menachem (226)
Institute of Clinical Neuroscience
Division of Neurology
Sahlgrenska Academy at Goteborg
  University
Goteborg 413 45
Sweden

Meriem K Bensalem-Owen (210)
Department of Neurology
KY Clinic, Rm L-007
Lexington, KY 40536-0284
USA

Edward H Bertram (191)
Department of Neurology
University of Virginia
P.O. Box 800394
Charlottesville, VA 22908-0394
USA

Frank MC Besag (296)
Twinwoods Health Resource Centre
Milton Road, Bedfordshire, MK41 6AT
UK

David B Bettis (142)
Pediatric Neurology of Idaho
Children's Specialty Center
100 East Idaho, Ste 201, Boise, ID 83712
USA

Ahmad Beydoun (95, 228)
American University of Beirut
Adult & Pediatric Epilepsy Program
P.O. Box 11-0236
Riad El-Solh/Beirut 1107 2020
Lebanon

Nadir E Bharucha (145)
Bombay Hospital and Medical Research
    Centre
12, Marine Lines, Mumbai 400 020
India

Christian G Bien (56)
Department of Epileptology
University of Bonn
Sigmund-Freud-Str., 25, Bonn, 53105
Germany

Warren T Blume (61)
London Health Sciences
    Centre – University Campus
339 Windermere Rd.
London, ON N6A 5A5
Canada

Jane Boggs (233, 379, 433)
Associate Professor of Neurology
Department of Neurology
Wake Forest University
P.O. Box 4111
Martinsville, VA 24115-4111
USA

Paul Boon (470)
Neurology Department
Ghent University Hospital
De Pintelaan 185, Block 3
Gent, Oost-Via, B-9000
Belgium

Christine Bower (489)
UCLA Department of Neurology
Seizure Disorder Center
710 Westwood Plaza, Suite 1-250
Los Angeles, CA 90095-1769
USA

Kirsten A Bracht (80)
Colorado Neurological Institute
Epilepsy Center, 701 E Hampden
    Avenue, Ste 530
Englewood, CO 80113
USA

Martin J Brodie (299, 437)
Epilepsy Unit
Western Infirmary
Glasgow, Scotland, G11 6NT
UK

Edward B Bromfield (302)
EEG Laboratory
Brigham and Women's Hospital
75 Francis Street
Boston, MA 02115
USA

Christine Bulteau (157)
Fondation Rothschild
Unité de neurochirurgie pédiatrique
25, rue Manin
Paris 75019
France

Carol S Camfield (6)
IWK Health Centre
5850/5980 University Avenue
P.O. Box 9700
Halifax, NS B3K 6R8
Canada

Peter R Camfield (6)
IWK Health Centre
5850/5980 University Avenue
P.O. Box 9700
Halifax, NS B3K 6R8
Canada

Enrique J Carrazana (237)
Neuroscience, Clinical Development and
    Medical Affairs
Novartis Pharmaceuticals
Building 403, Room 362, 59 Route 10
East Hanover, NJ 07936-1080
USA

Mar Carreño (447)
Epilepsy Unit
Department of Neurology
Hospital Clínic, c/Villarroel 170
Barcelona 08036
Spain

Catherine Chiron (10)
INSERM, U663, Paris, F-75015 France;
University Paris Descartes,
Faculty of Medicine, Paris, F-75005
France

Fahmida Chowdhury (206)
Department of Clinical Neuroscience
Institute of Psychiatry
King's College London
Box P041, De Crespigny Park
London, SE5 8AF
UK

Césare Maria Cornaggia (152)
Clinical Psychiatry
University of Milano Bicocca
V. Cadore 48, 20052 Monza, Milan
Italy

**Paulo Rogério M de
    Bittencourt (148)**
UNINEURO, Unidade de Neurologia
    Clinica
Rua Padre Anchieta 155
Curitiba, CEP 80.410-030, Paraná
Brazil

Veerle De Herdt (470)
Neurology Department
Ghent University Hospital
De Pintelaan 185, Gent B-9000
Belgium

Olivier Delalande (157)
Fondation Rothschild
Unité de neurochirurgie pédiatrique
25, rue Manin
Paris 75019
France

Orrin Devinsky (306, 466)
Neurology Epilepsy Center
NYU School of Medicine
Rivergate 403, East 34th Street, 4th Floor
New York, NY 10016
USA

Andreas Draguhn (403)
Institut für Physiologie und
    Pathophysiologie
Universität Heidelberg, Im Neuenheimer
    Feld 326
Heidelberg 69120
Germany

Joost PH Drenth (241)
Department of Medicine
Division of Gastroenterology and
    Hepatology
Radboud University Nijmegen Medical
    Center
P.O. Box 9101, Nijmegen, 6500 HB
The Netherlands

François Dubeau (73)
Department of Neurology and
    Neurosurgery
Montreal Neurological Institute and
    Hospital
3801 University Street, Ste 138
Montreal, QC H3A 2B4
Canada

P Barton Duell (65, 115)
Department of Medicine: Endocrinology,
    Diabetes and Clinical Nutrition
Oregon Health and Science University
3181 S.W. Sam Jackson Park Rd., L465
Portland, OR 97239
USA

Olivier Dulac (157)
Neuropaediatric Department
Hôpital Necker-Enfants Malades
149 rue de Sèvres
Paris 75015
France

Keith R Edwards (163)
Neurological Research Center
Southwestern Vermont Medical Center
140 Hospital Drive
Bennington, VT 05201
USA

Manuel Eglau (244)
Department of Neurology
University of Erlangen-Nurenberg
Schwabachanlage 6, Erlangen, D-91054
Germany

Christian E Elger (20)
Department of Epileptology
University of Bonn Medical Center
Sigmund-Freud-Str., 25
Bonn 53127
Germany

Maurizio Elia (69)
Department of Neurology
Oasi Institute for Research on Mental
    Retardation/Brain Aging
73 Via Conte Ruggero
Troina, EN 94018
Italy

Eloy Elices (292)
Global Therapeutic Area Head
CNS II, Eisai Medical Research, Inc.

Jerome Engel Jr. (489)
Jonathan Sinay Distinguished
    Professor, Neurology and
    Neurobiology
Chief, Division of Epilepsy and Clinical
    Neurophysiology
Director, Seizure Disorder Center
UCLA Reed Neurological Research
    Center
David Geffen School of Medicine
    at UCLA
710 Westwood Plaza, #1250
Los Angeles, CA 90095-1769
USA

Alan B Ettinger (13)
Department of Neurology – EEG Lab
Long Island Jewish Medical Center
270-05 76th Avenue
New Hyde Park, NY 11040
USA

Toufic A Fakhoury (210)
University of Kentucky
Dept of Neurology
KY Clinic Wing D Rm L44
740 S Limestone
Lexington, KY 40536-0284
USA

Edward Faught (165)
Epilepsy Center
University of Alabama
1719 6th Avenue S, CIRC 312
Birmingham, AL 35294-0021
USA

Natalio Fejerman (396)
Servicio de Neurologia
Hospital de Pediatria "Prof. Juan P.
    Garrahan"
Combate de los Pozos 1881
Buenos Aires, 1245
Argentina

Robert S Fisher (309)
Department of Neurology
Stanford University
Room A343 (mail), 300 Pasteur Drive
Stanford, CA 94305-5235
USA

Andras Fogarasi (497)
Epilepsy Center
Bethesda Children's Hospital
Bethesda Street 3, Budapest, H-1146
Hungary

Jacqueline A French (168, 454)
Comprehensive Epilepsy Center
NYU School of Medicine
403 East 34th Street, 4th Floor
New York, NY 10016
USA

Paolo Gallmetzer (135, 407)
2nd Neurological Department
General Hospital Hietzing
Neurological Center Rosenhügel
Riedelgasse 5
A-1130 Vienna
Austria

Giuseppe Gobbi (152)
Children Neurology Unit
Maggiore-Bellaria Hospital
Largo Nigrisoli 2, Bologna 40133
Italy

James S Grisolia (313)
4033 3rd Avenue # 410
San Diego, CA 92103
USA

Donald W Gross (73)
Health Sciences Centre
University of Alberta

2E3.19 Walter C Mackenzie
Edmonton, AB T6G 2B7
Canada

Thomas Grunwald (20)
Swiss Epilepsy Center
Bleulerstrasse 60, Zürich 8008
Switzerland

Marilisa M Guerreiro (316)
Department of Neurology
University of Campinas (Unicamp)
P.O. Box 6111
Campinas, SP 13083-970
Brazil

Hajo M Hamer (42)
Department of Neurology
Philipps-University Marburg
Rudolf-Bultmann-Str., 8
Marburg, D-35033
Germany

Cynthia L Harden (247)
Weill Medical College of Cornell
    University
525 East 68th Street, Rm K
New York, NY 10021
USA

Stephen C Heinrichs (461)
VA Medical Center, Research 151
    – Neuropharmacology
150 South Huntington Avenue
Boston, MA 02130
USA

David C Henshall (391)
Department of Physiology and Medical
    Physics
Royal College of Surgeons in Ireland
123 Street, Stephen's Green
Dublin 2
Ireland

Ad RMM Hermus (241)
University Medical Center Sint Radboud
471 Afd. Endocriene Ziekten,
    Postbus 9101
Nijmegen, 6500 HB
The Netherlands

Christian W Hess (251)
C/o Claudio Bassetti
Neurologische Poliklinik
Universitätsspital, Frauenklinikstrasse 26
Zürich, CH-8091
Switzerland

Peter Höllinger (251)
C/o Claudio Bassetti
Neurologische Poliklinik
Universitätsspital, Frauenklinikstrasse 26
Zürich, CH-8091
Switzerland

Peter Hopp (244)
Department of Neurology,
    Epilepsy Center, University
    of Erlangen-Nuremberg,
    Schwabachanlage 6
Erlangen, 91054
Germany

Kazuie Iinuma (256)
Ishinomaki Red Cross Hospital
71 Nishimichishita Hebita
Ishinomaki, Miyagi 986-8522
Japan

Yushi Inoue (197)
National Epilepsy Center
6-28 Urushiyama
Shizuoka 420-8688
Japan

Isabelle Jambaqué (157)
Université Paris Descartes
Institut de Psychologie, Boulogne
    Billancourt Cedex F-92100
Laboratoire Psychologie et Neurosciences
    Cognitives
CNRS FRE 2987, 71 Avenue Edouard
    Vaillant 92774
Boulogne Billancourt, 92100
France

József Janszky (497)
University of Pecs
Department of Neurology
Ret u. 2, Pecs, 7623
Hungary

Reetta Kälviäinen (319)
Kuopio Epilepsy Center
Kuopio University Hospital
POB 1777, Kuopio, 70211
Finland

Andres M Kanner (171)
Department of Neurological
  Sciences
Rush University Medical Center
1653W Congress Pkwy
Chicago, IL 60612-3833
USA

Jaideep Kapur (191)
Department of Neurology
University of Virginia
P.O. Box 800394
Charlottesville, VA 22908-0394
USA

**Dorotheé GA
  Kasteleijn-Nolst-Trenité (76)**
Department of Biomedical Genetics
University Medical Centre Utrecht
Postbus 85500, Utrecht, 3508 GA
The Netherlands

Kent Kelley (387)
Division of Neurology
Children's Memorial Hospital
Northwestern University
2300 Children's Plz, Box 51
Chicago, IL 60614
USA

Pavel Klein (174)
Mid-Atlantic Epilepsy and Sleep Center
LLC, 6410 Rockledge Dr, Ste 410
Bethesda, MD 20817
USA

Susanne Knake (42)
Department of Neurology
Philipps-University Marburg
Rudolf-Bultmann-Str.
8, Marburg, D-35033
Germany

Sookyong Koh (259, 387)
Division of Neurology
Children's Memorial Hospital
Northwestern University
2300 Children's Plz, Box 51
Chicago, IL 60614
USA

Ronald E Kramer (80)
Epilepsy Center
Colorado Neurological Institute
701 E Hampden Avenue, Ste 530
Englewood, CO 80113
USA

Gregory Krauss (457)
Department of Neurology
The Johns Hopkins Hospital
Meyer Building, Room 2-147, 600 N.
  Wolfe Street
Baltimore, MD 21287
USA

Ennapadam S Krishnamoorthy (263)
The Institute of Neurological Sciences
Voluntary Health Services
Taramani, Chennai 600 113
India

Kaarkuzhali Babu Krishnamurthy (322)
Beth Israel Deaconess Med Ctr
Neurology, KS-457, 330 Brookline Avenue
Boston, MA 02215
USA

Hana Kubova (414)
Department of Developmental Epileptology
Institute of Physiology
Academy of Sciences of the Czech Republic
Vídeská 1083, 142 20 Prague 4
Czech Republic

Martin Kurthen (20)
Swiss Epilepsy Center
Bleulerstrasse 60, Zürich, 8008
Switzerland

Thomas Kuruvilla (145)
Kusumagiri Mental Health Centre
Kakkanad, Cochin 682 030
Kerala, India

Ekrem Kutluay (228)
Department of Neurology
Medical College of Wisconsin
9200 W. Wisconsin Avenue
Milwaukee, WI 53226
USA

David M Labiner (85)
Department of Neurology
University of Arizona
1501 N. Campbell Avenue
P.O. Box 245023
Tucson, AZ 85724-5023
USA

Paul M Levisohn (325)
Department of Neurology
The Children's Hospital Denver
13123 E 16th Avenue
Aurora, CO 80045
USA

Dick Lindhout (178)
Department of Medical Genetics
University Medical Centre Utrecht
Box KC 04.084.02
Division of Biomedical Genetics
P.O. Box 85090
Utrecht, NL-3008 AB
The Netherlands

Susan M Lippmann (194)
The Comprehensive Epilepsy Care
Center for Children and Adults
222 S Woods Mill Rd., Ste 610N
Chesterfield, MO 63017
USA

Brian Litt (330)
Department of Neurology and
Bioengineering
University of Pennsylvania
3400 Spruce Street, HUP, 3 W Gates
Philadelphia, PA 19104-4283
USA

Cesare T Lombroso (24, 359)
319 Longwood Avenue
Boston, MA 02115
USA

Wolfgang Löscher (423)
Department of Pharmacology, Toxicology,
and Pharmacy
University of Veterinary Medicine
Hannover, Foundation
Bünteweg 17, Hannover D-30559
Germany

Gerhard Luef (88)
Universitätsklinik für Neurologie
Anichstrabe 35, Innsbruck, A-6020
Austria

Vijay Maggio (350)
Health Science Center
University of Tennessee
Le Bonheur Children's Medical Center
777 Washington Avenue, Suite 335
Memphis, TN 38105
USA

Alessandra Mascarini (152)
Clinical Psychiatry (SPDC)
San Gearado Hospital
Via Pergolesi 33, Monza (MI), 20052
Italy

Cassandra I Mateo (330)
2150 SE Salerno Rd., Ste 210
Stuart, FL 34997
USA

Fumisuke Matsuo (267)
Department of Neurology
University of Utah School of Medicine
30 N 1900 E RM 3R210
Salt Lake City, UT 84132
USA

Dan C McIntyre (400)
Department of Psychology
Institute of Neuroscience
Carleton University, 1125 Colonel
By Dr, Life Science Research Bldg
Ottawa, ON K1S 5B6
Canada

Kimford J Meador (354)
Department of Neurology
McKnight Brain Institute (L3-100)

University of Florida
100 South Newell Drive
P.O. Box 100236
Gainsville, FL 32610
USA

Heinz-Joachim Meencke (182)
Epilepsy Center Berlin-Brandenburg
Ev Krankenhaus Konigin
    Elisabeth Herzberge
Herzberge Str., 79, Berlin 10365
Germany

David Millett (489)
Department of Neurology
Rancho Los Amigos National
    Rehabilitation Center
Keck School of Medicine
University of Southern California
1510 San Pablo Street, HCC 643
Los Angeles, CA 90033
USA

Rajiv Mohanraj (437)
Department of Neurology
Hope Hospital, Stott Lane
Salford, Manchester, M6 8HD
UK

Jens C Möller (42)
Department of Neurology
Philipps-University Marburg
Rudolf-Bultmann-Str., 8
Marburg, D-35033
Germany

Martha J Morrell (91)
Stanford University
NeuroPace, Inc., 1375 Shorebird Way
Mountain View, CA 94043
USA

George Lee Morris III (184)
Regional Epilepsy Center
St. Luke's Medical Center
2801 W Kinnickinnic River
    Pkwy Ste 570
Milwaukee, WI 53215
USA

Siddhartha S Nadkarni (466)
NYU Comprehensive Epilepsy Center
403 East 34th Street, 4th Floor
New York, NY 10016
USA

Lina Nashef (206)
Neurology Department
King's College Hospital
Denmark Hill, London, SE5 9RS
UK

Wolfgang H Oertel (42)
Department of Neurology
Philipps-University Marburg
Rudolf-Bultmann-Str.
8, Marburg, D-35033
Germany

Erasmo A Passaro (95, 228)
Comprehensive Epilepsy Program
Bayfront Medical Center
601 7th Street South
St. Petersburg, FL 33701
USA

Marie-José Penniello (157)
Département de Pédiatrie
Centre Hospitalier et Universitaire de Caen
Avenue Côte de Nacre
Caen, 14033
France

Emilio Perucca (451)
Department of Internal Medicine and
    Therapeutics
Clinical Pharmacology Unit
University of Pavia
Piazza Botta 10, Pavia, 27100
Italy

Barbara L Phillips (80)
Epilepsy Center
Medical Director, Colorado Neurological
    Institute
701 E Hampden Avenue, Ste 530
Englewood, CO 80113
USA

Gerlach FFM Pieters (241)
University Medical Center
Sint Radboud, 471 Afd. Endocriene
  Ziekten
Postbus 9101, Nijmegen, 6500 HB
The Netherlands

Perrine Plouin (157)
Department of Clinical Neurophysiology
Hôpital Necker-Enfants Malades
149 rue de Sèvres, Paris 75015
France

Heidrum Potschka (481)
Institute of Pharmacology, Toxicology,
  and Pharmacy
Ludwig-Maximilians-University
  Munich
Koeniginstr. 16, Munich, 80539
Germany

Flavia Pryor (334)
International Comprehensive Epilepsy
  Center
University of Miami
410 Professional Arts Center
1150 N.W. 14th Street
Miami, FL 33136
USA

R Eugene Ramsay (334)
International Comprehensive Epilepsy
  Center
University of Miami
410 Professional Arts Center
1150 N.W. 14th Street
Miami, FL 33136
USA

Willy O Renier (187)
CWZ – Department of Neurology and
  Child Neurology
P.O. Box 9015, Nijmegen, NL-6500 GS
The Netherlands

David C Reutens (73)
Southern Clinical School
Monash University
Level 5, Block E, Clayton Rd
Clayton, Vic, Australia

Michael Rogawski (441)
University of California-Davis
4860 Y Street, Suite 3700
Sacramento, CA 95817
USA

William E Rosenfeld (194)
The Comprehensive Epilepsy Care
Center for Children and Adults
222 S Woods Mill Rd., Ste 610N
Chesterfield, MO 63017
USA

Felix Rosenow (42)
Department of Neurology
Philipps-University Marburg
Rudolf-Bultmann-Str., 8
Marburg, D-35033
Germany

Rajesh C Sachdeo (270)
10 Cliffview Ct.
Princeton Jct, NJ 08550
USA

Steven Schachter (473)
Beth Israel Deaconess Medical Center
330 Brookline Avenue, KS-478
Boston, MA 02215
USA

Ingrid E Scheffer (29)
Epilepsy Research Centre, Level 1
Neurosciences Building,
Heidelberg Repatriation Hospital
Austin Health, Heidelberg West, Vic 3081
Australia

Dieter Schmidt (274, 427, 484)
Epilepsy Research Group
Goethestr. 5, Berlin, D-14163
Germany

Bettina Schmitz (106)
Neurologische Klinik und
  Poliklinik
Charité – Campus Virchow Klinikum
Augustenburger Platz 1, Berlin 13353
Germany

30
80
50
60
70
80
30

Donald L Schomer (34)
Department of Neurology
Division of Epilepsy (EEG)
Beth Israel Deaconess Medical Center
330 Brookline Avenue
Boston, MA 02215
USA

40
50
60
70

Masakazu Seino (197)
National Epilepsy Center
6-28 Urushiyama, Shizuoka 420-8688
Japan

50

Udaya Seneviratne (73)
Consultant Neurologist
Department of Neuroscience
Monash Medical Centre
Clayton VIC 3168
Australia

00

80
90
20

Matti Sillanpää (338)
Departments of Public Health and Child
    Neurology
University of Turku
Kiinamyllynkatu 13, Turku 20520
Finland

00
10
20
30

030
040
050
060
070
080

Joseph I Sirven (341)
Department of Epilepsy and Neurology
Mayo Clinic Hospital
5777 E Mayo Blvd
Phoenix, AZ 85054
USA

090
100
110
120
130

150

Brien J Smith (346)
Neurology Department
Henry Ford Health Sciences Center
Henry Ford Hospital
2799 West Grand Blvd
Detroit, MI 48202
USA

170
180
190
200
210
220

Michael R Sperling (202)
Department of Neurology
Thomas Jefferson University
900 Walnut Street, Ste 200
Philadelphia, PA 19107
USA

Carl E Stafstrom (100)
Department of Neurology
University of Wisconsin
6000 Highland Avenue, Rm H6/528
Madison, WI 53792
USA

Hermann Stefan (244)
Department of Neurology
University of Erlangen-Nuremberg
Schwabachanlage 6, Erlangen 91054
Germany

Alan R Towne (38)
Department of Neurology
Virginia Commonwealth University
1101 East Marshall Street
Sanger Hall 6-013
P.O. Box 980599
Richmond, VA 23298-0599
USA

Edwin Trevathan (46)
National Center on Birth Defects and
    Developmental Disabilities, CDC
Mailstop E-87, Atlanta, GA 30333
USA

Michael R Trimble (263)
National Hospital for Neurology and
    Neurosurgery
Queen Square, London, WC1N 3BG
UK

Eugen Trinka (112, 417)
Clinical Department of Neurology
Innsbruck Medical University
Anichstrasse 35, Innsbruck, 6020
Austria

Peter Uldall (277)
Rigshospitalet, Neuropaediatric Clinic
    5003
Copenhagen Ø, DK-2100
Denmark

Walter van Emde Boas (282)
Department of EEG & EMU, Epilepsy
    Clinic Meer & Bosch

p7870

p8290
p8300
p8310
p8320
p8330

p8340

p8360
p8370
p8380
p8390

p8410

p8430

p8440

p8460
p8470

p8480
p8490

p8500
p8510
p8520
p8530
p8540

p8550
p8560

p8570
p8580

p8590
p8600

p8850 Stichting Epilepsie Instellingen Nederland
p8860 Achterweg 5, Heemstede, 2103 SW
p8870 The Netherlands
p8880

Nathalie Villeneuve (10)
p8890 Hospital Henri Gastaut
p8900 300 Boulevard Sainte Marguerite
p8670 Marseilles, 13006
p8680 France

p8690 **Kristl Vonck (470)**
p8700 Neurology Department
p8710 Ghent University Hospital
p8720 De Pintelaan 185, Block 3
Gent, Oost-Via, B-9000
p8740 Belgium

p8750 **Biene Weber (51)**
p8760 C/o Dr. Aldenkamp
p8770 Epilepsy Centre Kempenhaeghe
p8780 P.O. Box 61, Heeze, NL-5591 AB
p8790 The Netherlands

p8800 **James Wheless (350)**
p8810 Le Bonheur Children's Medical Center
p8820 University of Tennessee
p8830 777 Washington Ave Ste 335
Memphis, TN 38105
p8840 USA

Samuel Wiebe (494)   p8610
Division of Neurology   p8620
University of Calgary   p8630
Foothills Medical Centre,
1403 – 29 St NW   p8640
Calgary, AB T2N 2T9   p8650
Canada   p8660

Andrew N Wilner (478)   p8910
America Bldg, Ste 317   p8920
Goat Island, RI 02840   p8930
USA   p8940

Hiroyuki Yokoyama (256)   p8950
Faculty of Medicine   p8960
School of Nursing   p8970
Yamagata University   p8980
2-2-2 Iidanishi, Yamagata 980-9585   p8990
Japan   p9000

Index

A

Abdominal sensation, 322
Abdominal ultrasound, 244
Abrupt bradycardia-asystole, 377
Abscess, 228
Absence seizures, 132–134, 142–144, 197–201, 339
  in adults, 165–167
Absence status epilepticus, 131–134
Abulia, 263–265
ACLS. *See* Advanced cardiac life support (ACLS)
Activity-dependent intracellular acidification, 417
ADHD. *See* Attentional deficit hyperactive disorders (ADHD)
ADNFLE. *See* Autosomal dominant nocturnal frontal lobe epilepsy (ADNFLE)
Adrenocorticotropic hormone (ACTH), 6, 8
Adult epilepsy
  AED in, 437–439
  data review, 437–438
Adulthood, 392
Adult patients, infantile spasms, 6–9
Advanced cardiac life support (ACLS), 376
AED. *See* Antiepileptic drugs (AED)
AED-induced cognitive effects, 358
Affective disorders, 56–59
Alcohol abuse, 163–164
Allergic rhinitis, 256–258
  D-chlorpheniramine administration, 256
  diagnosis, 256
  outcome, 257
  treatment, 257
Allopregnanolone, 176
Alzheimer's disease, 323
Amantadine, absence seizures, 143

American Academy of Neurology, 248
American Clinical Neurophysiology Society, 382
Aminolevulinic acid dehydratase deficiency porphyria, 85–87
Amitriptyline, depression, 233
Amnesia, 319, 330
Amnestic episodes, diabetic patient, 121–124
Amygdalectomy, 320
Angioplasty, 307
Anovulatory menstrual cycles, 174–176
Anterior cingulate gyrus, frontal lobe epilepsy, 20–22
Anterior temporal lobectomy, post-operative seizure, 489–491
Anterograde amnesia, 302
Anticonvulsants, 242, 264
  influence of, 392
Antiendomysium, 242
Antiepileptic drugs (AED), tolerance, 420–422
  antiepileptic efficacy, loss of, 423–424
  detection of, 427–428
    clinical methods for, 430–431
    factors, 428–430
  group-response analysis, 425–426
Antiepileptic drugs (AED), 219, 320, 325, 338, 346, 354–358, 392
  cellular mechanisms, 441–442
  change of, 226–227
  drug resistance, 484–487
  efficacy prediction, 451–452
  failure of, 481–483
  intravenous, 408
  pharmacokinetics of, 481–482
  pharmacoresistance. *See* Pharmacoresistance
Antigliadin antibodies, 242
Anti-idiotype antibodies, 344

Aphasia, epilepsy with, 148–151
Apnea, 251
Aqueductal stenosis, 222
Arousal disorders, 359
Asperger syndrome, 297
Asphyxia, 319
Asymptomatic hyperammonemia, 235
Asystole, cardiac, 210–214
Attentional deficit, myoclonic jerks, 51–54
Attentional deficit hyperactive disorders
    (ADHD), myoclonic jerks, 51–54
Attention-deficit disorder, 297
Autistic feature, 297
Automated external defibrillators, 377
Autosomal dominant nocturnal frontal lobe
    epilepsy (ADNFLE), 365–366
Awakening epilepsy, 339

B
Babinski sign, 346
Barbiturate, 150–151
BCECTS. *See* Benign childhood epilepsy with
    centrotemporal spikes (BCECTS)
Behavioral disturbances
    epilepsy and, 152–156
Benign childhood epilepsy with centrotemporal
    spikes (BCECTS), 387, 391, 396–399
Benign focal epilepsies in childhood (BFEC), 398
Benzodiazepines (BZD), 251, 412, 423
    complex partial status epilepticus (CPSE), 40
    epilepsy with aphasia, 150–151
    hemiplegia, 136
BFEC. *See* Benign focal epilepsies in childhood
    (BFEC)
Bifrontal epilepsy, 226
Bilateral hip fracture, 274
Bilateral stereotaxic amygdalotomies, 310
Bilateral symmetric spike-and-wave discharges,
    338
Biopsy, 242
Blindness, transient, 100–104
Blood oxygen saturation, 361
Body mass index, 251
Bradycardia
    ictal, 93
    seizure of left temporal onset, 210–214
Bradykinesia, 244
Brain abscess, 96
Brain surgery
    anterior temporal lobectomy, 489–491
    cortical resection, 491–492
    MTLE, 494–495

    MTS, 495
    TLE-HS, 497–499
Brain trauma, 346–349
Breast cancer, 323
Bromides, 222
Bruising, 379

C
Cajal–Retzius cells, 403
Carbamazepine (CBZ), 362
    absence seizures in adults, 166
    after lamotrigine-induced Stevens-Johnson
        syndrome, 206–209
    bifrontal epilepsy, 227
    celiac disease with epilepsy, 188
    childhood occipital epilepsy, 102
    complex partial status epilepticus (CPSE), 39
    epilepsy with aphasia, 150
    infantile spasms, 7
    juvenile myoclonic epilepsy, 226
    left temporal lobe epilepsy, 47
    mesial temporal lobe epilepsy, 161
    monotherapy, 260, 297, 323
    night terrors, 26
    noise-induced partial seizures, 109
    right temporal lobe onset seizures, 93
    seizure disorder, 222
    visual seizures, 102
Carbonic anhydrase, 403
Cardiac rhythm, with seizures, 93
Cardiology, 91–94
Cardiopulmonary functions, 377
Cardiopulmonary resuscitation (CPR), 376
Catamenial partial epilepsy, 202–205
CBZ. *See* Carbamazepine (CBZ)
CD. *See* Cortical dysplasia (CD)
Celiac disease, 187–190
Cellular immune responses, 344
Cellular mechanisms, of AED, 441–442
Cellular pathophysiology, of SE, 414
Cerebral artery stroke, 274
Cerebral calcifications, 187–190
Cerebrospinal fluid (CSF), 342
    in hemiplegia, 135–136
    temporal lobe epilepsy, 122
Cerebrovascular disease, 233
Chevrie–Muller test, 159
Childhood epilepsy, 100–104, 190, 278
Children, parasomnias, 24–27
Chromosome abnormality, epilepsy associated
    with, 69–72
Chronic seizure disorder, 222–225

diagnosis, 223
   outcome, 223
   treatment, 223
   video EEG monitoring, 223
Cingulate epilepsy, 22
Cingulate gyrus, frontal lobe epilepsy, 20–22
Cingulotomy, 310
Cingulum, 310
Circuit of Papez, 310
Cisatracurium continuous infusion, 342
Citalopram, juvenile myoclonic epilepsy, 238
Clinical diagnosis of convulsive syncope, 314
Clinical trials, 454–455
   biased, 455–456
   population outcomes, 455
   tolerability and safety issues, 455
Clobazam
   epilepsia partialis continua, 292
   infantile spasms, 7
   noise-induced partial seizures, 109
Clonazepam
   absence seizures, 143
   after pregnancy, 248
   epilepsy with aphasia, 150
   frontal lobe onset seizures, 171
   panic disorder, 307
   porphyria, 86
Clopidogrel, coronary artery disease, 233
Cognitive disturbances
   epilepsy and, 152–156
Colostomy, 233, 234
Comatose state, 346
Complex partial seizures (CPS), 6–7, 8, 283
   AED tolerance, 420, 421–422
   frontal lobe, 168–170
   intracranial recording of initial part of, 21
   mesial temporal lobe epilepsy and, 161
   pseudohypoglycemia, 115–117
   side effects, 184–186
Complex partial status epilepticus (CPSE), 38–41
   clinical presentation, 235
Computed tomography (CT) scan, 229, 233,
   251, 259, 271, 282, 297
Computer specialist, myoclonic jerks in, 76–78
Concussion, 354
Confusional arousals, 24–27
Continuous positive airway pressure (CPAP), 252
Convulsion, generalized, 267, 282, 338
Coronary disease, nocturnal seizures in, 65–67
Corpus callosotomy, 352
Cortical dysplasia (CD), 318, 360
   right parietal focus, 191–193
   symptomatic partial epilepsy, 139–141
Cortical hyperexcitability, 404

Corticosteroids, 344
Corticotropin-releasing factor modulation,
   462–463
Counseling, genetic, 178–180
CPAP. *See* Continuous positive airway pressure
   (CPAP)
CPR. *See* Cardiopulmonary resuscitation
   (CPR)
Craniotomy, 228, 326
Cryptogenic epilepsies, 403
CSF. *See* Cerebrospinal fluid (CSF)
CT. *See* Computed tomography (CT)

D
D-chlorpheniramine, 256
Delusions. *See* Hallucinations
Depression, 56–59
   diagnosis of, 238–239
Depth electrode, 322, 369
Diabetes mellitus, 233
Diabetic patients, recurrent amnestic episodes
   in, 121–124
Diagnosis
   changing, 197–201
Dietary treatment, of seizures, 350
Diets, ketogenic, 352
Divalproex, 229
Double-hit hypothesis, of epileptogenesis,
   387–389, 391–393
Down's syndrome, myoclonic seizures in, 42–44
"Dreamy states", epileptic, 61–64
Dreifuss, Dr. Fritz, 375
Drug resistance, 484–487
   drug-related mechanisms, 487
   mechanism of, 485
   pharmacogenetics, 486–487
   remission of disease, 485–486
   surgery-related mechanisms, 487
Dysarthria, 316
Dysconjugate eye position, 346
Dysphasia, 219, 326
Dysphoria, prodromal symptoms of, 407

E
EEG, 320, 323, 331, 347, 379–383
   electrographic partial seizures, 228
   generalized spike–wave discharge, 223
   ictal, 410
   invasive, 409
   in PNES, 468
   video-telemetry, 334

Elderly patients, 121–124
Electrical status epilepticus during slow sleep
    (ESES), 398
Electrocorticography, 260, 303
Electrographic discharges, 360
Electrographic partial seizures, 228
Encephalitis, 342
Encephalomalacia, 229, 346
ENW. *See* Episodic nocturnal wanderings
    (ENW)
EPC. *See* Epilepsia partialis continua (EPC)
Epilepsia partialis continua (EPC), 13–17, 292
    left deltoid muscle, 95–98
Epileptic discharges, 93
Epileptiform discharges, 347, 351, 398
Epileptogenic antibodies, 344
Epileptogenic cortex, 352
Epileptogenicity, 348
Episodic memory loss, 56–59
Episodic neurological condition, 414
Episodic nocturnal wanderings (ENW), 365
Epworth Sleepiness Score, 251, 253
ESES. *See* Electrical status epilepticus during
    slow sleep (ESES)
Ethosuximide, 339
    absence seizures, 143
    absence seizures in adults, 166
    absence status epilepticus, 132
    ADHD, myoclonic seizures, 52
    nausea and palpitations, 128–129
Ethosuximide syrup, 279
Exacerbation, 174–176
Exanthema, generalized, 252

F
Facial grimacing, 350
Fainting, infantile, 46–48
Familial epileptic dyskinetic seizures, 367
Familial partial epilepsy with variable foci, 366
Fear, infantile, 46–48
Febrile convulsions, 338
Febrile illness, 290
Febrile seizures, 247
Febrile seizures plus (FS+), 31
    generalized epilepsy with, 29–32
Fejerman, Natalio, 400, 403
Felbamate
    absence seizures, 143
    myoclonic-astatic seizures, 154–155
Fetal hydantoin syndrome, 178–180
Fetus, 248
FLE. *See* Frontal lobe epilepsy (FLE)

Fluoxetine, depression, 263
Focal cortical dysplasia, 411
Focal motor seizures, 197–201
Focal status epilepticus, non-convulsive,
    135–138
Folate, pregnancy, 248
Folic acid
    progressive myoclonic epilepsy, 179
    seizure disorder, 222
Follicular stimulating hormone, 175
Fosphenytoin, 237
Frontal lobe epilepsy, 69–72, 171–173, 263, 336,
    360
    changing diagnosis, 197–201
    with complex partial and secondary
        generalized seizures, 88–90
    nonlesional, 418
    panic attacks, 20–22
    during sleep, 168–170
    startle-induced, 106–110
    tuberculous granuloma and, 145–147

G
GABA. *See* γ-aminobutyric acid (GABA)
GABAergic, 265, 416, 417
    inhibition, 404
GABA-induced network, 405
Gabapentin, 234, 335
    childhood occipital epilepsy, 102
    mesial temporal lobe epilepsy, 160
    monotherapy, 304
    night terrors, 26
Gadolinium enhancement, 341
γ-aminobutyric acid, 265
Gamma knife treatment, 353
Gastaut, H., 417
Gastaut-type idiopathic childhood occipital
    epilepsy, 100–104
Gastrointestinal complaints, 190
GCSE. *See* Generalized convulsive SE (GCSE)
Generalized convulsive SE (GCSE), 417
Generalized convulsive seizures, 336
Generalized epilepsy with febrile seizures plus
    (GEFS+), 29–32
Generalized tonic–clonic seizures (GTCS),
    112–114
Genetic counseling, 178–180
Genetic load, 393
Genetic studies, GEFS+, 29–30, 31
Gingival hyperplasia, 282
Glioma, 139–141
Gliosis, 192

Glutaminergic preponderance, 265
Gluten-free diet
  celiac disease with epilepsy, 188
Gluten-sensitive enteropathy, 242
Glycogen storage disease type III, 115–117
Grand mal, 233
GTCS. *See* Generalized tonic–clonic seizures
  (GTCS)

H
Hallucinations, 263
Hamartoma, 260
Head trauma, 163–164
Hemangioma, 148–151
Hemiparesis. *See* Hemiplegia
Hemiplegia, 274, 326, 346
  status epilepticus with, 135–138
  subdural hygroma, 135
Hippocampal abnormality, influence of, 392
Hippocampal atrophy, 348
  temporal lobe epilepsy, 121–124
Hippocampal injury, 392
Hippocampal malrotation, 391
Hippocampal pathology, 320
Hippocampal plasticity, 461–462
Hippocampal sclerosis, 57–59, 319, 323, 331
Hippocampal tumors, 58–59
Hippocampectomy, 320
Hippocampi, 310
Hippocampus, in temporal lobe epilepsy, 122–123
Hispanic, 248
Histamine H_1 antagonist, 256
Hydrocephalus. *See* Aqueductal stenosis
Hygroma, subdural, 135
Hyperactive behavior, myoclonic jerks, 51–54
Hyperammonemia, 235, 236, 245
Hyperandrogenism, 174–175
Hyperperfusion
  hemiplegia, 136
  noise-induced partial seizures, 107
Hyperperfusion, 362
  right temporal, 10–11
Hyperreflexia, 346
Hypersensitivity, 207–209
Hyperventilation, 237, 338
Hypoglycemia-induced seizures, 115–117
Hypogonadism, hypothalamic, 174–176
Hypomania, 231
Hypometabolism, 326
Hypothalamic hamartoma, 350
Hypothalamic hypogonadism, 174–176
Hypothyroidism, 251
Hypovitaminosis D, 243

Hypoxemia, nocturnal, 65–67
Hysteria. *See* Hypomania

I
Ictal bradycardia, 93
Ictal EEG, 409
Ictal hemiplegia, 135–138
Ictal pain, 192–193
Ictal SPECT, 325, 347
Ictal tachycardia, 93
Idiopathic generalized epilepsy, 252
  lamotrigine for, 113
  non-convulsive status epilepticus, 112–114
Infants
  fainting, 46–48
  fear, 46–48
  partial seizures in, 10–12
  spasms, 10–12
    adult patients, 6–9
Insomnia, 325
Insulin, 233
Interictal-ictal single-photon emission
    computed tomography (SPECT), 349
  EPC, 15
  right temporal hyperperfusion, 10–11, 12
Interictal psychosis, 320
Interictal SPECT, 347
Intracarotid amobarbital test, 303
Intracellular acidification, activity-dependent, 417
Intractable epilepsy, 88–90
Intravenous immunoglobulin (IVIG), 342
Intubation, 251
Invasive long-term monitoring, 25
IVIG. *See* Intravenous immunoglobulin (IVIG)

J
Jackson-Pratt drainage, 136
Juvenile myoclonic epilepsy (JME), 182–183,
    226, 237–239, 247, 447–449
  diagnosis, 237
  evidence-based treatment, 449
  examination, 237, 448
  outcome, 238
  with photosensitivity, 76–78
  treatment, 238

K
Ketogenic diets, 326, 352
  absence seizures, 143–144
Ketotifen, 256
Kinesiogenic dyskinesias, 370

L

Lamotrigine, 300, 302
  absence seizures in adults, 166
  GEFS+, 30
  for idiopathic generalized epilepsy, 113
  induced Stevens–Johnson syndrome, 206–209
  nausea and palpitations, 128–129
  night terrors, 26
  parkinsonism, 244
Landau-Kleffner syndrome, 157–162
Late-onset myoclonic epilepsy in Down's
    syndrome, 42–44
Left frontal abscess, 228–231
  diagnosis, 228
  EEG, 228
  outcome, 229–230
  treatment, 228, 229–230
Left frontal craniotomy, 228
Left frontal heterotopia, 323
Left hemiparesis, 326
Left temporal lobe epilepsy, 46–48, 388
Lennox-Gastaut syndrome, 8, 133, 316
Lesionectomy, 260
Levetiracetam monotherapy, 116, 229
Limb ataxia, 244
Limbic lobe, 63
Listlessness, prodromal symptoms of, 407
Liver
  enzymes, 342
  steatosis, 244
Lobectomy, 219, 303
Lobe heterotopia, 322
Long-term monitoring (LTM)
  invasive, 26
  scalp video-EEG for night terror episodes,
      24–26
Lorazepam, 228
  porphyria, 86
Lumbar puncture, 341
Luteinizing hormone, 174

M

Magnetic resonance imaging (MRI), 229, 247,
    260, 283, 289, 293, 316, 319, 322, 339,
    341, 349
Maximal electroshock (MES), 451
Medically refractory frontal lobe epilepsy, 412
Medically refractory partial seizures, 331, 347
Medically refractory seizures, 326
Menstrual cycles, anovulatory, 174–176
Menstrual exacerbations, 247
Mental retardation, 152–156

Mephenytoin, 222
Mesial temporal lobe epilepsy (MTLE), 320,
    494–495
  with mesial temporal sclerosis, 157–162
Mesial temporal sclerosis (MTS), 495
  mesial temporal lobe epilepsy with, 157–162
Methsuximide, absence seizures, 143
Midparahippocampal gyrus, 347
Migraine, 187–190
Mirtazapine, affective disorders, 57
Monoamine oxidase, 239
Monotherapy, 336
Mouse strains, 392
Mouth jerking, provoked by reading, 3–5
MRI. *See* Magnetic resonance imaging (MRI)
Multifocal partial epilepsy, 310
Multiple complex partial seizures, 228
Munchausen's syndrome, 194–196
Myocardial infarctions, 307
Myoclonic absence epilepsy, with developmental
    delay, 51–54
Myoclonic–astatic seizures
  psychiatric disorder with, 152–156
Myoclonic epilepsy
  in Down's syndrome, 42–44
  genetic counseling for refractory, 178–180
  juvenile, 182–183
Myoclonic jerks, 182–183
  attentional deficit, 51–54
  in computer specialist, 76–78
  hyperactive behavior, 51–54
Myoclonic twitching, generalized, 342
Myoglobinuria, 342

N

Nausea, 126–130
Neocortical kindling, 401
Neocortical onset, partial epilepsy of, 34–36
Nerve palsy, 219
Neuroimaging, 235, 263
  PNES, 467–468
Neurological sequelae, 228
Neurology, 91–94
Neuronal injury, 348
Neuronal synchronization, non-synaptic, 417
Neuropsychiatric syndromes, 265
Neuropsychological evaluations, 350
NFLE. *See* Nocturnal Frontal Lobe Epilepsy
    (NFLE)
Night seizures, 334
Night terrors, 24–27
Nitrazepam, infantile spasms, 6, 7

Nocturnal attacks, 73–75
Nocturnal epileptic dyskinesia, 367
Nocturnal Frontal Lobe Epilepsy (NFLE), 360
Nocturnal paroxysmal abnormal motor events, 359
Nocturnal paroxysmal dystonia (NPD), 73–75, 359
Nocturnal seizures, coronary disease, 65–67
Noise-induced partial seizures, 106–110
Non-convulsive status epilepticus, 69–72, 112–114, 135–138, 223, 228, 230
Non-epileptic seizures, 13–17
Nonlesional frontal lobe epilepsy, 418
Nonsynaptic neuronal synchronization, 417
Noradrenergic neurotransmission, 462
NPD. *See* Nocturnal paroxysmal dystonia (NPD)
Nystagmus, 311

O
Obscurations, visual, 100–104
Obstructive sleep apnea, 65–67, 252
Occipital epilepsy, 100–104
Olanzapine, 320
Oral diazepam, seizure disorder, 222, 223
Oral theophylline, asthma, 270
Orofacial automatisms, 319
Orthopedic evaluations, 306
Osteomalacia, 241–243
    diagnosis, 242
    laboratory testing, 241–242
    outcome, 242
    treatment, 242
Oxcarbazepine
    childhood occipital epilepsy, 102
    epilepsy with aphasia, 150
    visual seizures, 102

P
PA. *See* Paroxysmal arousals (PA)
Palm Desert Meeting on Epilepsy Surgery, 284
Palpitations, 126–130
Panayiotopoulos syndrome, 103
Panhypopituitarism, 352
Panic attacks, frontal lobe epilepsy, 20–22
Panic disorder, 307
Pansinusitis, 228
Papez loop, 63
Parahippocampal gyrus, 347
Paraldehyde, porphyria, 86
Paraneoplastic limbic encephalitis, 58–59

Parasomnias, 24–27, 359
Parkinsonism, 244–245
    diagnosis, 245
    laboratory studies, 244
    neurological examination, 244
    outcome, 245
    treatment, 245
Paroxysmal arousals (PA), 365
Paroxysmal behaviors, during sleep, 24–27
Paroxysmal dyskinesia, 360
Paroxysmal dystonia, nocturnal, 73–75
Partial epilepsy, 6–7, 8, 121–124, 145–147, 330, 348
    in adolescent female, 171–173
    catamenial, 202–205
    infantile, 10–12
    of left temporal lobe, 210–214
    of neocortical onset, 34–36
    noise-induced, 106–110
Pathophysiology, of SE, 417–418
Pentobarbital infusion, 342
Pentylenetetrazole (PTZ), 451
Performance IQ, 260
Perisylvian polymicrogyria, 316
Perisylvian syndrome, 318
PET. *See* Positron emission tomography (PET)
Petit mal, 334
P-glycoprotein, 443
    pharmacogenetic analysis, 482–483
Pharmacoresistance, 441–444
    target hypothesis, 442–443
    transporter hypothesis, 443
Phenobarbital, 234, 267–268
    absence status epilepticus, 132
    bifrontal epilepsy, 227
    frontal lobe epilepsy, 145–146
    juvenile myoclonic epilepsy, 226
    obstructive sleep apnea, 253
    right-sided clonic seizures, 7
Phenytoin, 228, 233, 339, 354, 380, 433
    EPC, 96
    frontal lobe epilepsy, 145–146
    hemiplegia, 136
    juvenile myoclonic epilepsy, 226
    nocturnal seizures, 66
    polycystic ovarian syndrome prophylaxis, 228
    status epilepticus, 164
Photosensitivity, 53
    juvenile myoclonic epilepsy with, 76–78
pH regulation, 405
Placebo, *vs.* AED, 454
Polycystic ovarian syndrome, 174–176
Polysomnography, 251, 306

Polyspike-wave complexes, 42, 43
Polytherapy, 356
Porphyria, aminolevulinic acid dehydratase deficiency, 85–87
Positron emission tomography (PET), 326
Postictal psychosis, 309
Postinfectious etiology, 342
Post-operative seizure, 489–493
    after anterior temporal lobectomy, 489–491
    cortical resection, 491–492
Post-traumatic epilepsy, 348
Post-traumatic neocortical temporal lobe epilepsy, 303
Pregnancy, 247–249
    diagnosis, 247
    epilepsy, 80–82
    examination, 247
    outcome, 248
    tonic–clonic seizures, generalized, 80–82
    treatment, 248
Prodromal symptoms
    of dysphoria, 407
    of listlessness, 407
Progesterone, anticonvulsant properties, 174–176
Progressive myoclonic epilepsy, 178–180
Pseudobulbar palsy, 317
Pseudohypoglycemia, 115–117
Pseudoseizures, 247
Psychiatric disorders, 152–156, 171–173, 358
Psychiatric support, 320
Psychogenic hypothesis, 360
Psychogenic non-epileptic seizures (PNES), 13–17, 457–460
    EEG in, 468
    examination, 458
    history, 466–467
    neuroimaging in, 467–468
    neuropsychological findings in, 468
    treatment, 458
Psychogenic pseudoseizures, 311
Psychomotor development, 316
Psychosis, 350
    in epilepsy, 171–173
    interictal, 320
Psychotherapy, 223, 239
Psychotropic effects, 355
Pyridoxine-dependent seizures, 290
Pyridoxine (Vit B$_6$), 290

R

Rapid eye movement (REM), 251
Rasmussen's encephalitis, 97, 294
Reading epilepsy (RE), 3–5

Rebound depolarization, 391
Reboxetine, 263
Refractory myoclonic epilepsy
    genetic counseling for, 178–180
    MRI negative, 206–209
REM. *See* Rapid eye movement (REM)
Renal functions, 342
Reproductive endocrine disorders, 174–176
Retrograde amnesia, 302
Right anterior temporal lobectomy, 219, 220
Right femoral fracture, 379
Right frontal lobectomy, 326
Right mesial temporal sclerosis, 219
Right parietal focus, 191–193
Right-sided clonic seizures, 7–8
Right-sided temporal lobe epilepsy, 22
Right temporal hyperperfusion, 10–11
Right temporal lobectomy, 323
Right temporal lobe epilepsy, 323
Right third nerve palsy, 219
Ring chromosome 20 syndrome (r20), 69–72
Risk factors, for cardiovascular disease, 379

S

Sclerosis, 57–59, 319, 323, 331
SCN1B mutations, 31
SE. *See* Status epilepticus (SE)
Secondary hyperparathyroidism, 242
Seizure semiology, change in, 210–214
Seizure exacerbation, 174–176
Seizure-terminating mechanisms, failure of, 412
Self-induction, 53
Semiology, 323, 349, 408
Serotonin reuptake inhibitors, 239
Sertraline, 233
    frontal lobe onset seizures, 172
Serum pyruvate, 341
Shoulder twitching, 95–98
Sildenafil, 263
Single-photon emission computed tomography (SPECT)
    EPC, 15
    ictal, 325, 347
    interictal, 347
    right temporal hyperperfusion, 10–11, 12
Skull fracture, 354
Sleep Apnea Scale of the Sleep Disorders Questionnaire (SA-SDQ) score, 67–68
SMA. *See* Supplementary motor area (SMA)
SPECT. *See* Single photon emission computed tomography (SPECT)
Spike-and-wave complexes, 338
Spina bifida, 248

Sporadic seizures, 391
Startle-induced frontal lobe epilepsy, 106–110
Status epilepticus (SE), 39, 407–412, 414–416,
      417–418
   absence, 131–134
   after white-water rafting, 85–87
   complex partial, 38–41
   GABA inhibition, 415
   hemiplegia in elderly female with, 135–138
   non-convulsive, 112–114
   non-convulsive focal, 135–138
   phenytoin, 164
   time-related pharmacoresistance, 415–416
Stereotaxic lesions, 311
Stevens–Johnson syndrome, 206–209
Stress-induced non-epileptic seizure, 461–464
   clinical practice, 463
   corticotropin-releasing factor modulation,
      462–463
   hippocampal plasticity, 461–462
   noradrenergic neurotransmission, 462
Subclinical rhythmic electrographic discharge of
      adults (SREDA), 67
Subdural electrodes, 303
Subdural grid electrodes, 326
Subdural hematoma, 270
Subdural hygroma, 135
Subnormal intelligence, 339
Substraction ictal single photon emission
      computed tomography, 229
Sudden unexplained death in epilepsy
      (SUDEP), 377
SUDEP. See Sudden unexplained death in
      epilepsy (SUDEP)
Sulthiame, 403
Supplementary motor area (SMA), 366
Supraventricular tachycardia, 194–196
Surgical resection
   infantile spasms, 11, 12
   left frontal lobe, 200
   right parietal focus, 192
Symptomatic focal epilepsy, 22
Symptomatic frontal lobe epilepsy, 283
Symptomatic generalized epilepsy, 352
Symptomatic localization-related epilepsy, 191–193
Symptomatic partial epilepsy, 139–141
Syndrome of familial epilepsy, 268

T
Tachycardia, 361
   ictal, 93
   supraventricular, 194–196
T-cells, in hypersensitivity reactions, 208–209

Temporal lobectomy, 323
Temporal lobe epilepsy, 56–59, 219, 238, 391
   AED tolerance in, 420–422
   hippocampal atrophy, 121–124
   mesial, 157–162
Temporal lobe epilepsy with hippocampal
      sclerosis (TLE–HS), 497–499
Temporal lobe resection, 319–321
Temporal lobe surgery, 219–221
   diagnosis, 219
   examination, 219
   outcome, 220
   overview, 219
   treatment, 220
Terfenadine, allergic rhinitis, 256
Tiagabine
   complex partial seizures, 185
   non-convulsive status epilepticus, 223
   seizure disorder, 222
Time-dependent pharmacoresistance, of SE,
      415–416
Titration, 342
TLE, temporal lobe epilepsy (TLE)
Todd's paresis, 137, 326
Tonic–clonic convulsion, 310
Tonic-clonic seizures, 202–205, 226, 228, 237,
      274, 339, 340, 341, 342, 350, 354, 408,
      433–435
   pregnancy, 80–82
Topiramate, 4, 234, 320, 335
   after pregnancy, 248
   bifrontal epilepsy, 227
   myoclonic seizures, 43
   seizure disorder, 222
Toxicity, warfarin, 194–196
Training, on EEG, 383
Transient blindness, 100–104
Transporter hypothesis, 443
Trauma, head, 163–164
Trigonum, 320
Tuberculous granuloma, 145–147
Tuberous sclerosis, 7, 8
Tumors, hippocampal, 58–59
Twitching, shoulder, 95–98

U
Uroneurologist, 263

V
Vagus nerve stimulation (VNS), 470–472
   clinical observation, 474–475
   clinical relevance, 474

Vagus nerve stimulation (VNS) (*Continued*)
    FDA approval, 474
    preclinical studies of, 473
    randomized trials, 474–475
Valproate, 227, 325, 339
    absence seizures in adults, 166
    childhood occipital epilepsy, 102
    encephalopathy, 245
    epilepsy with aphasia, 150
    frontal lobe onset seizures, 171
    GEFS+, 30
    in GTCS, 112
    hyperammonemia, 236
    juvenile myoclonic epilepsy, 226
    mesial temporal lobe epilepsy, 160
    monotherapy, 238
    with monotherapy for juvenile myoclonic
        epilepsy, 183
    myoclonic-astatic seizures, 154–155
    myoclonic seizures, 43
    parkinsonism, 244
    during pregnancy, 248
    progressive myoclonic epilepsy, 179
    Stevens–Johnson syndrome, 207
    tonic–clonic seizures, 203
Venlafaxine, affective disorders, 57
Ventricular shunt, 222
Verbal IQ, 260

Video-EEG monitoring, 222, 223, 226, 260,
    283, 294, 303, 325, 351, 360, 367, 388, 412
    change in seizure semiology, 210–214
Vigabatrin
    bifrontal epilepsy, 227
    infantile spasms, 7
    mesial temporal lobe epilepsy, 160
    seizure disorder, 222
    therapy, 227
Visual obscurations, 100–104
Visual seizures, 100–104
Visual stimuli, myoclonic jerks, 76–78
Vitamin D, 242, 243
VNS Therapy System™, 474
Vocational rehabilitation program, 323
Vomiting
    visual seizures, 103

W

Warfarin toxicity, 194–196
Welcome to Holland, 328

Z

Zolpidem, seizure disorder, 222
Zonisamide, 256

Diagnostic Puzzles and Uncertainties

A Young Woman with Mouth Jerking Provoked by Reading

Taoufik Alsaadi

HISTORY

A 20-year-old left-handed junior college student (who has a family history of left-handedness) reports episodes of jerking of her mouth that have been present since the age of 16 years. She was born at full term after a normal pregnancy and delivery. She experienced her first febrile convulsion at the age of 18 months. Convulsions persisted until she went to kindergarten. She then remained free of seizures until the episodes of mouth jerking that began when she was 16. Both her grandfather and her paternal great-aunt had seizures in adulthood.

These episodes of mouth jerking were mostly provoked by reading, especially reading aloud, but also by reading silently; rarely, they were triggered by conversational speech. Singing never triggered them. Spontaneous attacks did not occur. She has suffered a total of three of these convulsions since their onset. One of these occurred while she was hospitalized for video–electroencephalogram (EEG) monitoring.

The jerks responded poorly to carbamazepine, although generalized convulsions were prevented. Topiramate monotherapy at 100 mg twice a day controlled both the jerks and the convulsions.

EXAMINATION AND INVESTIGATIONS

Neurological examination, including mental status and language assessment, was normal. Her evaluation included admission for video–EEG monitoring. Several of her typical spells of mouth jerking were recorded: one attack progressed to a secondarily generalized seizure. This attack was associated with rhythmic spikes arising from the left central region (Figure 1.1).

Magnetic resonance imaging (MRI) scan of the brain with surface coils did not show any abnormalities.

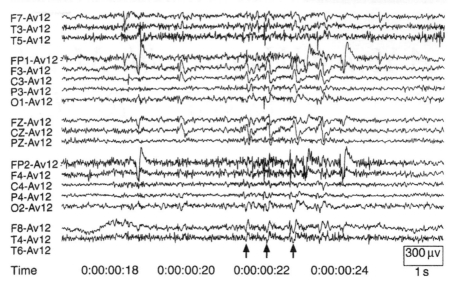

F7-Av12
T3-Av12
T5-Av12

FP1-Av12
F3-Av12
C3-Av12
P3-Av12
O1-Av12

FZ-Av12
CZ-Av12
PZ-Av12

FP2-Av12
F4-Av12
C4-Av12
P4-Av12
O2-Av12

F8-Av12
T4-Av12
T6-Av12

| 300 μv |

Time   0:00:00:18   0:00:00:20   0:00:00:22   0:00:00:24   1 s

f0010 FIGURE 1.1   Ictal EEG recording showing left central spikes (arrows) during the patient's typical "click".

s0030 ## DIAGNOSIS

p0060 Primary (inherited) reading epilepsy.

s0040 ## TREATMENT AND OUTCOME

p0070 Treatment with topiramate 100 mg twice a day was able to control her spells almost completely. She can now read well enough without having jerks. She has had no convulsions while talking.

p0080 The patient is currently engaged to be married and is planning to start a family in the near future. She was able to complete her college studies successfully and has now started to study to be a dental assistant.

s0050 ## COMMENTARY

s0060 ### Why did I choose this case?

p0090 First, this case and other cases of reflex epilepsy have long fascinated me. They are rare and offer tantalizing glimpses into the mechanism of epileptogenesis and the organization of cognitive function.

p0100 Second, reading epilepsy (RE) can go unrecognized for years since it can be easily mistaken for tics or hysterical seizures or for a primary language disorder if convulsions do not occur. Consequently, these patients may suffer psychosocial consequences for a long time before an accurate diagnosis is made.

Third, failure to recognize RE may result in unnecessary investigations and delay in initiating the appropriate treatment, since it can be successfully treated in most cases with anticonvulsants, especially valproate, clonazepam, or as was reported in the literature, with levetiracetam.[1–4]

What did I learn from this case?

This patient's RE was an inherited form of localization-related epilepsy that first manifests in early adolescence with mouth jerking or "clicking" that is provoked by reading for some time, but not by writing or thinking. It can be viewed as a form of a language-induced epilepsy, in which seizures are triggered by three modalities of linguistic tasks: reading, speaking, and writing.[4] Convulsions may occur if reading persists for a longer time.[5–8] This disorder should be distinguished from the secondary (symptomatic) form of RE by

- the lack of interictal EEG abnormalities;
- the lack of spontaneous seizures;
- a normal neurological examination; and
- a normal MRI study.

A positive family history of seizures or primary RE, or both, is another common feature of this disorder.[9,10] In some cases, but not all, jerks are associated with spikes, sharpened elements, and paroxysmal rhythmical delta activity over the dominant temporoparietal region. Moreover, recent work with fMRI suggests that RE is a focal epilepsy, but one in which subcortical structures are recruited during epileptiform discharges.[11]

Although spontaneous remission is unlikely, these cases respond well to anticonvulsant treatment, as suggested by previous studies in the literature.[1,2] In most cases, lifelong treatment is required.

REFERENCES

1. Saenz-Lope E, Herranz-Tannaro FJ, Masdeu JC. Primary reading epilepsy. *Epilepsia* 1985;**26**: 649–56.
2. Daly RF, Forster FM. Inheritance of reading epilepsy. *Neurology* 1975;**25**:1051–4.
3. Kasteleijn-Nolst Trenité DG, Hirsch E. Levetiracetam. Preliminary efficacy in generalized seizures. *Epileptic Disord* 2003;**5(suppl 1)**:S39–S44.
4. Valenti MP, Rudolf G, Carré S, et al. Language-induced epilepsy. Acquired stuttering, and idiopathic generalized epilepsy: Phenotypic study of one family. *Epilepsia* 2006;**47(4)**:766–72.
5. Login IS, Kolakovich TM. Successful treatment of primary reading epilepsy with clonazepam. *Ann Neurol* 1978;**4**:155–6.
6. Vanerzant C, Fitz R, Holmes G, et al. Treatment of primary reading epilepsy with valproic acid. *Arch Neurol* 1982;**39**:452–3.
7. Valenti MP, Tinuper P, Cerullo A, Carcangiu R, Marini C. Reading epilepsy in a patient with previous idiopathic focal epilepsy with centrotemporal spikes. *Epileptic Disord* 1999;**1**:167–71.
8. Pegna AJ, Picard F, Martory MD, et al. Semantically-triggered reading epilepsy: an experimental case study. *Cortex* 1999;**35**:101–11.
9. Yalcin AD, Forta H. Primary reading epilepsy. *Seizure* 1998;**7**:325–7.
10. Wolf P, Mayer T, Reker M. Reading epilepsy: report of five new cases and further considerations on the pathophysiology. *Seizure* 1998;**7**:271–9.
11. Archer JS, Briellmann RS, Syngeniotis A, Abbott DF, Jackson GD. Spike-triggered fMRI in reading epilepsy: involvement of left frontal cortex working memory area. *Neurology* 2003;**60**:415–21.

c0002

Two Adult Patients with
Infantile Spasms

Carol S Camfield and Peter R Camfield

s0010

HISTORY

p0010
The first patient is currently an 18-year-old woman who is moderately mentally hand-icapped and has two predominant seizure types – partial complex seizures and persistent infantile spasms.

p0020
She was born after a normal pregnancy to healthy, non-related parents with no family history of neurological problems. At 6 months of age she had a 4-day history of myoclonic seizures and flexor spasms occurring in clusters. Neurologic examination and development were normal for age. A routine electroencephalogram (EEG) showed typical hypsarrhythmia without focal features and a computed tomography (CT) scan was normal. A diagnosis of West syndrome was made and she was treated with adreno-corticotropic hormone (ACTH) (40 units intramuscularly) and nitrazepam (0.2 mg/kg twice daily) with an immediate, marked decrease in spasms and a normalization of the EEG over 3 weeks. However, occasional spasms continued for the next 6 weeks and ACTH was increased to 60 units/day for an additional 6 weeks. ACTH was discontinued at 8 months of age and nitrazepam at 10 months of age.

p0030
At the age of 21 months the patient's development was normal, however, she had "six strings of four to five spasms". With each spasm, her arms "shot up" and her head dropped forward for 2–5 s. She could remain standing during the spasms. Nitrazepam was restarted but was ineffective despite an increase in the dose to clinical toxicity. Valproate was added 2 weeks later. The runs of spasms decreased but did not stop.

p0040
About the same time she developed brief staring spells several times a day that were associated with speech interruption, odd facial expression, a small grunt, and occasional eye deviation to the right with clonic arm movements. ACTH 60 units/day was given for 5 weeks with a major decrease in the frequency of the spasms. The EEG was normal. Valproate was stopped and nitrazepam was continued. Over the next 5 months, strings of spasms recurred. Her development still seemed normal.

p0050
When the patient was 4 years old, Prof. Jean Aicardi paid a memorable visit to Halifax and felt that the patient had an "excellent" prognosis for intellectual development

with an emerging partial complex seizure disorder. Even the great ones are not always correct!

Starting at the age of 4½ years, carbamazepine was added for her complex partial seizures and her spasms continued with one "string" a day despite nitrazepam. She appeared disoriented during a string of spasms and briefly afterward. Sadly, her development plateaued, especially her speech.

The spasms continued, and at the age of 15 years, her complex partial seizures became more severe – she would wander aimlessly for up to 5 min during a complex partial seizure, which was obviously dangerous for her. A magnetic resonance imaging (MRI) scan was normal. Clobazam was ineffective and vigabatrin was of transient benefit. At the age of 18 years, vigabatrin was replaced with lamotrigine. Her spasms recurred with a remarkable string of spasms that lasted for 45 min. She continues treatment with vigabatrin plus carbamazepine.

The second patient is a 21-year-old woman who is mild to moderate mentally handicapped with tuberous sclerosis. On the second day of life she had right-sided clonic seizures that were treated with phenobarbital. Her neurologic and skin examinations were normal. The EEG showed a left central focal spike discharge.

Seizures persisted and were resistant to phenobarbital, carbamazepine, and phenytoin. At 6 months of age, she had a 1-week history of somnolence and loss of eye contact associated with the onset of typical infantile spasms. Spasms consisted of raising both arms and upward eye deviation for 1–2 s, with spasms repeating every 10–20 s for 5–10 min.

Her sibling and parents did not have a history of seizures or skin or retinal abnormalities.

The EEG showed a burst suppression pattern and hypsarrhythmia. For the first time, the typical hypopigmented macules of tuberous sclerosis were noted, but a CT scan (her first) was normal.

A diagnosis of West syndrome was made and she was treated with prednisone for 8 weeks, resulting in a more than 90% decrease in both the spasms and the brief right-sided focal seizures. Subsequently, the spasms disappeared, but the partial seizures gradually evolved into complex partial seizures and her EEG showed multifocal spike discharges.

At the age of 8 years, she began to have spasms again, and these have continued. She has 20–30 spasms in a series with one or two strings of spasms nearly every day. She is often incontinent during the string of spasms, which causes major restrictions in her social life. At the age of 18 years, she had her first and only generalized tonic–clonic seizure, which frightened her family more than any previous experience.

Over the years, treatment of her partial seizures and spasms has been ineffective; it has included phenobarbital, phenytoin, carbamazepine, prednisone, clonazepam, valproate, nitrazepam, the ketogenic diet, clobazam, felbamate (which produced a partial response with severe anorexia), vigabatrin, and lamotrigine.

Now, at the age of 21 years, her spasms occur daily with urination during the attacks. Her skin examination shows typical hypopigmented macules and adenoma sebaceum. Her CT scan shows multiple calcified tubers, but ultrasound of her kidneys is normal. Her EEG continues to show a multifocal spike pattern.

She works happily in a sheltered workshop and functions at the mild to moderate mentally handicapped level. Through Special Olympics she goes bowling and skating regularly.

s0020

COMMENTARY

p0170

Both patients illustrate that symptomatic and cryptogenic infantile spasms can persist into adulthood, apparently indefinitely. Experts in several recently published textbooks suggest that West syndrome is a disorder of infants only, which is true if persistent hypsarrhythmia is required for the diagnosis. Dulac, Plouin, and Schlumberger note that "hypsarrhythmia and therefore West syndrome is self-limited".[1] Indeed, the hypsarrhythmia stops but they do note that when West syndrome is followed by Lennox–Gastaut syndrome, "clusters of spasms persist in addition to the more characteristic seizures of Lennox–Gastaut". Jeavons and Livet do not mention persistence of spasms in their chapter on West syndrome in an authoritative book.[2]

s0030

What did we learn from these cases?

p0180

First, infantile spasms may reappear in adult life. Adults with spasms must be rare and we do not think that spasms begin *de novo* in adulthood – they always start before the age of 4 years. In both of these patients, the spasms began in the first year of life, stopped completely for several years during early childhood but then later returned. Both patients had persistent complex partial seizures; however, the parents immediately recognized when the spasms returned, although the EEG did not revert to hypsarrhythmia. When the spasms returned they were completely unresponsive to current treatment. At first glance, the spasms seem relatively trivial; however, the first patient was transiently confused after a string of spasms and the second patient was incontinent. These problems have serious consequences as to whether patients can be free from supervision, and an effective treatment would be welcome.

p0190

We conclude that our patients no longer continue to fulfill the criteria for West syndrome because of the evolution of the EEG; however, their problem is persistent spasms and it is a real problem. Spasms are not strictly age related.

p0200

The most effective treatment for infantile spasms is ACTH. The first patient had an excellent response to the first course of ACTH, but at the age of 2 years she had only a transient reduction in spasms. We have seen several other patients with spasms persisting into adulthood who also did not respond to repeated courses of ACTH.

p0210

Secondly, tuberous sclerosis may be difficult to diagnose in infants. The second patient had persistent partial seizures in the newborn period. We were very aware of the possibility of tuberous sclerosis and searched carefully for skin lesions, but there were not any. She was born in 1978 when CT scanning of the newborn was just beginning. The electromagnetic interference scan of the day was normal but did not have the resolution of our current spiral CT scans. Presumably an MRI scan would have shown tubers. However, we had to wait until the onset of spasms at 6 months of age before the typical depigmented ash-leaf spots of tuberous sclerosis were first seen.

p0220

Since then we have seen another newborn with partial seizures whose mother has definite tuberous sclerosis. Two child neurologists and a dermatologist searched with and without a Wood's lamp and could not find any skin lesions. When the patient was aged 12 months they suddenly "popped up"! The lesson is to keep looking if you suspect tuberous sclerosis.

How did these cases alter our approach to the care and treatment of our epilepsy patients?

In the follow-up of infantile spasms, we continue to ask about their reemergence. The spasms are relatively easily misdiagnosed in older people. The recognition of their intractability is depressing, but an important reality. Since our experience with these two cases, we are now aware of four other patients in our center and several more in other centers.

REFERENCES

1. Dulac O, Tuxtorn I. Infantile spasms and West syndrome. In: Roger J, Bureau M, Dravet C, Genton P, Tassinari CA, Wolf P. *Epileptic syndromes in infancy, childhood and adolescence*, 4th ed., John Libbey Eurotext, London, England, 2008;58–89.
2. Camfield PR, Camfield CS, Lortie A, Darwish HS. Infantile spasms in remission may re-emerge as intractable epileptic spasms. *Epilepsia* 2003;**44**:1592–5.

c0003

An Infant with Partial Seizures and Infantile Spasms

Catherine Chiron and Nathalie Villeneuve

s0010

HISTORY

p0010

A baby girl experienced infantile spasms with hypsarrhythmia at 6 months of age. Her pregnancy and psychomotor development were normal. Spasms were stopped by vigabatrin monotherapy and the hypsarrhythmia disappeared, but a right temporal focus of spikes persisted. A magnetic resonance imaging (MRI) scan was normal.

p0020

The child continued to develop satisfactorily until spasms recurred on vigabatrin at 12 months of age; these spasms were associated with partial seizures. The spasms were again rapidly controlled using hydrocortisone, but partial seizures persisted. They were stereotyped in semiology: the child hid her eyes with her right arm and cried for about 30 s, and then she recovered immediately. Ictal electroencephalogram (EEG) showed paroxysmal activity over the right hemisphere, but the onset could not be localized more precisely. The seizures were refractory to antiepileptic drugs (carbamazepine, valproate, benzodiazepines, phenytoin, lamotrigine and stiripentol) and to the ketogenic diet. She had between 5 and 10 seizures a day until she was 2½ years of age.

s0020

EXAMINATION AND INVESTIGATIONS

p0030

Neurological examination was normal except for moderate global mental retardation with predominant language dysfunction and hyperkinesia. A second MRI scan at age 2½ years was said to be normal. Ictal single-photon emission computed tomography (SPECT) scanning imaged a 20-s seizure with the semiology described above; this scan showed a focus of hyperperfusion in the right temporal pole, in contrast to right temporal hypoperfusion seen interictally (Figure 3.1). Further review of the MRI and comparison with subtraction interictal–ictal SPECT scans co-registered with MRI (see Figure 3.1) discovered an abnormal gyrus in the right temporal pole with a focal cortical dysplasia.

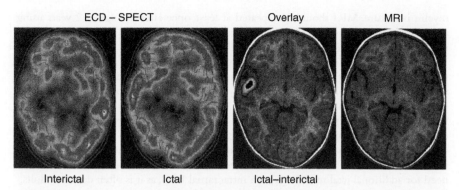

| ECD – SPECT | | Overlay | MRI |
| Interictal | Ictal | Ictal–interictal | |

FIGURE 3.1   From left to right, interictal SPECT showing a right temporal hypoperfusion, ictal SPECT showing a right temporal hyperperfusion, subtraction image (ictal–interictal) locating the ictal onset focus and MRI showing a subtle cortical abnormality in the right temporal pole, in a 2½-year-old girl presenting with refractory partial seizures. This focus corresponds to a dysplastic lesion, which has been discovered on MRI after analysis of the ictal SPECT (MRI had previously been interpreted as normal). After right temporal lobectomy limited to the pole, the child became seizure-free.

DIAGNOSIS

Infantile spasms (West Syndrome) and right temporal lobe epilepsy with a focal cortical dysplasia.

TREATMENT AND OUTCOME

The child underwent surgical resection of the right temporal pole without intracranial EEG recording. She has been seizure-free for 3 years and without antiepileptic drugs for 2 years. Language and behavior improved when she was aged 5 years, though she continues to have mild mental retardation.

COMMENTARY

Why did we choose this case?

We chose this case for three reasons. First, it shows that children with a focal lesion may have a generalized epilepsy. During the first year of life, infantile spasms with generalized seizures (epileptic spasms) and generalized EEG features between spasms (hypsarrhythmia) can be associated with partial seizures. This combination is quite frequent – a focal lesion is found in more than 50% of infantile spasms.

Secondly, such a lesion, although actively searched for on MRI, is often missed before the age of 2 years, owing to myelin immaturity. Among the causes of infantile spasms, focal cortical dysplasia may present with subtle MRI features limited to a lack of delineation of gray and white matter. These signs may not be present until myelin is mature. MRI should be repeated at least once after the age of 2 years using new sequences such as fluid attenuation inversion recovery (FLAIR), which appear to increase MRI sensitivity in infants.

p0080   Thirdly, focal surgical resection can be successfully performed in very young children. Whereas spasms are usually easily controlled in focal cortical dysplasia, partial seizures are known to be highly refractory to medical treatment. Presurgical investigations in young children should involve the same procedures as in adults, namely video–EEG monitoring of seizures, MRI, neuropsychological evaluation, and functional imaging, if possible. In the present case, ictal SPECT had a great impact on our decision to proceed with surgery. The excellent concordance between ictal semiology, ictal SPECT and the lesion on MRI allowed us to perform the resection without the need for additional ictal recordings with intracranial EEG, as it is often done in adults.

s0070   ## What did we learn from this case and how did it alter our approach to the care and treatment of our epilepsy patients?

p0090   Two particular aspects of this case impressed us and have modified our approach to our patients. First, the interictal EEG focus – right temporal spikes – was noticed from the beginning of the story and proved to be a key point. It represented the only focal sign and was present for many months. In retrospect, this finding was highly relevant. We have to be aware of such subtle and peculiar features.

p0100   Secondly, ictal SPECT was a crucial component of the presurgical examination, although the patient's seizures were short and we had some difficulty identifying them clinically. Because the parents were able to recognize the onset of every seizure, their presence when ictal SPECT was performed was the most important reason for the success of this examination.

FURTHER READING

Chugani HT, Shields WD, Shewmon DA, Olson DM, Phelps ME, Peacock WJ. Infantile spasms: I. PET identifies focal cortical dysgenesis in cryptogenic cases for surgical treatment. *Ann Neurol* 1990;**27**:406–13.

Dulac O, Chugani H, Dalla-Bernadina B (eds). *Infantile spasms and West syndrome*. WB Saunders: London, 1994.

Chiron C, Vera P, Kaminska A, *et al*. Single-photon emission computed tomography: ictal perfusion in childhood epilepsies. *Brain Dev* 1999;**100**:1–3.

Epilepsia Partialis Continua versus Non-Epileptic Seizures

Alan B Ettinger

HISTORY

A 42-year-old right-handed male was evaluated for episodes of twitching movements of the right hand that began 2 weeks earlier. He had a 3-year history of bipolar disorder, which was well controlled on valproate 1500 mg/day. He was moderately overweight and had a history of sleep apnea treated with continuous positive air pressure (CPAP).

The episodes were stereotypic, beginning with numbness of the left hand and arm and a flushed feeling in his face. This was followed by uncontrollable twitching movements of the right hand. The episodes lasted from 10 min to 4 h and occurred at an average of four times a week. Lorazepam 2 mg/kg intravenously had been administered at another hospital during a prolonged episode but had no effect. All episodes occurred while the patient was awake and there were no precipitants such as sleep deprivation.

Previous diagnostic testing included normal magnetic resonance imaging, EEG, complete blood count, and blood chemistry as well as a negative Lyme titer.

EXAMINATION AND INVESTIGATIONS

Video–EEG monitoring revealed stereotyped sensorimotor episodes beginning with a sensation of numbness in the left hand and in the neck and face. Subsequently, right-sided flexion–extension movements occurred. These movements involved the second, third, fourth, and fifth digits at the metacarpophalyngeal joints or the entire hand. The movements were usually arrhythmic but were sometimes rhythmic at 1–3 Hz. Movements would intermittently stop for several seconds. The episodes lasted 7–10 min and did not occur during sleep.

The episodes stopped briefly when the patient's attention was diverted while performing a left upper extremity task. There was no weakness during or between episodes. The patient appeared to be in no emotional distress during the episodes and would speak calmly to examiners. One episode that began 6h before a second admission to our unit was terminated immediately with a placebo "antidote" administered intravenously. During the episodes, there was no change on EEG. An ictal single-photon emission computed tomography (SPECT) scan revealed no perfusion abnormalities.

s0030   ## DIAGNOSIS

p0060   Psychogenic non-epileptic seizures (PNESs).

s0040   ## TREATMENT AND OUTCOME

p0070   The patient initially accepted the diagnosis of non-epileptic seizures but subsequently expressed skepticism and sought a second opinion because of persistent episodes.

s0050   ## COMMENTARY

p0080   Epilepsia partialis continua (EPC) is a relatively rare form of seizure that is characterized by localized, prolonged myoclonic jerking.[1] This disorder can affect most muscle groups, especially in the distal limbs.[2] Among different cases of EPC, motor activity varies in distribution, rate, rhythm, and intensity.[1,2] EPC may lack a visually detectable scalp EEG correlate.[2,3]

p0090   PNESs resemble epileptic seizures but result from psychological factors, not from central nervous system dysfunction.[4,5] Although the medical literature usually focuses on cases with bilateral motor activity and unresponsiveness,[6–8] PNESs are also associated with focal muscle activity and preserved responsiveness. In such cases, differentiating partial motor seizures from non-epileptic seizures can be very challenging.

s0060   ### What did I learn from this case?

p0100   This case demonstrated to me the difficulties in distinguishing PNESs with prolonged focal motor activity from EPC, as well as the potential hazards of misdiagnosis.

p0110   Several features helped distinguish this case from true EPC. The appearance of the movements suggested a potential psychogenic origin. Movements varied between episodes, on one occasion with flexion–extension movements at the metacarpophalangeal joints and at other times with flexion–extension movements at the wrist.

p0120   A psychogenic mechanism was further supported by the transient abolition of movements when the face or contralateral extremity was engaged in an effortful task. This probably occurred because of the patient's inability to coordinate simultaneous movements on a functional basis. A similar finding has emerged in studies of posthypnotic suggestion. Task interference occurs when subjects receive a posthypnotic suggestion to search for one number and are asked to search for another number in a series of digits.[9] Thus, although posthypnotic suggestion and conversion symptoms are executed without conscious awareness, they tap the same attentional networks that are used to execute conscious tasks. Although inhibition or activation of movements related to EPC may occur with voluntary motor tasks or sensory stimulation of the affected limb,[10,11] this patient and two others I have seen demonstrated abolition of activity when they performed tasks using other parts of the body. Eliciting and abolishing typical episodes with normal saline and suggestion provide very strong support for the diagnosis of non-epileptic seizures.

Most patients with EPC demonstrate varying degrees of peri-ictal muscle weakness. This patient had no paresis immediately before, during, or between episodes.[1,2,11–13] Furthermore, his calm demeanor – he appeared undisturbed by the events – also suggested non-epileptic seizure, although this was a less definitive sign.

The failure to see hyperperfusion on ictal SPECT scan also suggests non-epileptic seizure. Notably, some have argued that sufficiently vigorous motor activity could theoretically bring about at least a small degree of hyperperfusion, although there are few cases reporting this possibility.[14] The sensitivity of ictal SPECT scanning in EPC is unknown, however several reports suggest that SPECT scanning is sensitive and can reveal hyperperfusion even in the absence of EEG changes.[15,16]

Our patient had no demonstrable etiology for EPC despite vigorous blood testing and neuroimaging. While the number of idiopathic cases of EPC is unknown, most reports of EPC describe readily identified causes such as metabolic,[17] inflammatory,[18] infectious,[19–21] vascular,[2] neoplastic,[12] and other structural[22] etiologies. Although one of my patients had a history of seizures, the other two showed no evidence of neurological or metabolic disturbance.

A number of features demonstrated in this case were not helpful in distinguishing PNESs from EPC. For example, the arrhythmic movements did not prove their functional nature, since EPC movements are often arrhythmic.[2] The failure to demonstrate episodes during sleep does not exclude EPC since it can diminish or stop during sleep.[2] A history of bipolar disorder was also not helpful since psychiatric disturbances are common in epilepsy including depression[23] and anxiety,[24] and even bipolar symptoms.[25] Finally, the failure of these episodes to respond to antiepileptic drugs did not exclude EPC, since the response to antiepileptic drugs, including intravenous benzodiazepines, is often limited in some forms of EPC.[2]

Other techniques can help distinguish EPC from non-epileptic seizure. Supplemental scalp electrodes near the sensory–motor strip may enhance the identification of changes on EEG during the episodes. Other electrophysiological techniques, including demonstration of giant somatosensory evoked potentials[26,27] and isolated spikes preceding myoclonic jerks on back-averaged EEG,[3,27] can also help to diagnose EPC.

How did this case alter my approach to the care and treatment of my patients with epilepsy?

I have learned to recognize the possibility of non-epileptic events resembling EPC by the presence of the following features:

- variability in the areas of motor activity in the same patient;
- distribution and spread of motor activity without a neuroanatomic basis;
- transient abolition of movements with distraction (e.g. when other body parts are engaged in effortful tasks);
- eliciting and abolishing typical episodes with suggestive techniques;

u0050   • absence of motor weakness during or in between episodes;
u0060   • absence of EEG correlate of motor activity; and
u0070   • absence of hyperperfusion on ictal SPECT scan.

p0260   This case has also motivated me to keep abreast of the clinical signs reported in the current neurology literature that help the clinician distinguish the wide varieties of PNESs from epileptic seizures. A summary of the broader distinction between epileptic and PNESs is summarized in Table 4.1.

t0010   TABLE 4.1   Clinical Semiology of Epileptic versus Psychogenic Non-epileptic Seizures

Sign	Epileptic	PNES	References
Ictal heart rate	Increased in both convulsive and non-convulsive	Not as high in convulsive and unchanged in non-convulsive	[28]
Eye closure during motor phase of seizure	Most open eyes	Most close eyes during event; sustained, forceful eye closure with active opposition could occur in episodes of unresponsiveness	[29]
Non-physiologic eye movements	Uncommon	Downward eye deviation to side head is turned on	[30]
Pelvic thrusting	Common especially in frontal lobe epilepsy, less often in temporal lobe; more likely retropelvic	Common, usually forward thrusting	[8, 31, 32]
Weeping	Very uncommon	More common	[33]
Laughter	May occur in gelastic epilepsy	Uncommon	[34]
Weeping	Less common	May occur	[33, 35]
Post-event nose rubbing or cough	Can occur	Not described	[36]
Ictal stuttering	Uncommon	Can occur	[37]
Vocalization during tonic–clonic phase	Very uncommon	May occur	[38]
Duration of convulsive-like events	Frontal lobe seizures are brief; the major convulsive activity even of generalized status epilepticus tends to be less than 2 min	Often longer, usually minutes to >1 h	[7, 39]
Nature of movements	Quick tonic posturing in frontal lobe seizures	Very variable with waxing and waning, stop and start, changing over minutes	[8, 40]
If convulsive-like events:	More of a defined progression of motor activity	Asynchronous out-of-phase non-physiologic and in multiple directions, may have side to side head movements, opisthotonic-like movements	[7]

(Continued)

TABLE 4.1   Continued   t0010

Sign	Epileptic	PNES	References
Prolonged ictal atonia	Very rare	May occur	[41]
Arising from sleep	More common	Uncommon; may be in a non-physiologic pseudo-sleep	[42, 43, 40]
Ictal injury	More common	May occur; in up to 50%	[44]
Tongue biting	More common, usually lateral tongue	Less common; more likely lip or tip of tongue; may be more common by history than through objective documentation	[29]
Frequency after video–EEG diagnosis compared to prior to admission	No change	Reduced	[45]
Duration	May exceed 10–15 min	Usually <2 min	[46]
Pathological reflexes	May have positive Babinski with decreased papillary reactivity to light	Retention of normal reflexes	[47]
Occurring in presence of witness	No relation	More likely	[46]
Induced or aborted by placebo/suggestion	Uncommon	More common	[46]
Incontinence	Common in convulsive seizures	May be reported, less likely to be objectively documented	[48]
Lack of cyanosis	Rare in major convulsive events	Common	[38]
Rapid reorientation after major movements of seizure	Uncommon except in specific seizure types like frontal lobe seizures	Common	[42, 49]

REFERENCES

1. Watanabe K, Kuroiwa Y, Toyokura Y. Epilepsia partialis continua. Epileptogenic focus in motor cortex and its participation in transcortical reflexes. *Arch Neurol* 1984;**41**:1040–4.
2. Thomas JE, Reagan TJ, Klass DW. Epilepsia partialis continua. *Arch Neurol* 1977;**34**:266–75.
3. Hallett M, Chadwick D, Marsden CD. Cortical reflex myoclonus. *Neurology* 1979;**29**:309–18.
4. Ozkara C, Dreiffus FE. Differential diagnosis in pseudoepileptic seizures. *Epilepsia* 1993;**34**:294–8.
5. Bazil CW, Kothari M, Luciano D, et al. Provocation of nonepileptic seizures by suggestion in a general seizure population. *Epilepsia* 1994;**34**:768–70.
6. Gulick TA, Spinks IP, King DW. Pseudoseizures: ictal phenomena. *Neurology* 1982;**32**:24–30.
7. Gumnit RJ, Gates JR. Psychogenic seizures. *Epilepsia* 1986;**27(suppl 2)**:S124–S129.
8. Gates JR, Ramani V, Whalen S, et al. Ictal characteristics of pseudoseizures. *Arch Neurol* 1985;**42**: 1183–7.

9. Kihlstrom JF. The cognitive unconscious. *Science* 1987;**237**:1445–52.

10. Wieser HG, Graf HP, Bernoulli C, Siegfried J. Quantitative analysis of intracerebral recordings in epilepsia partialis continua. *Electroencephalogr Clin Neurophysiol* 1977;**44**:14–22.

11. Hefter H, Witte OW, Reiners K, Niedermeyer E, Freund H-J. High frequency bursting during rapid finger movements in an unusual case of epilepsia partialis continua. *Electromyogr Clinc Neurophysiol* 1994;**34**:95–103.

12. Botez MI, Brossard L. Epilepsia partialis continua with well-defined subcortical frontal tumor. *Epilepsia* 1974;**15**:39–43.

13. Juul-Jension P, Denny-Brown D. Epilepsia partialis continua. *Arch Neurol* 1966;**15**:563–78.

14. Biraben A, Taussig D, Bernard AM, et al. Video-EEG and ictal SPECT in three patients with both epileptic and non-epileptic seizures. *Epileptic Disord* 1999;**1**:51–5.

15. Katz A, Spencer S. The role of ictal SPECT in the diagnosis of psychogenic seizures. *Epilepsia* 1992;**33**:53.

16. Sztriha L, Pavics L, Ambrus E. Epilepsia partialis continua: follow-up with 99mTc-HMPAO-SPECT. *Neuropediatrics* 1994;**25**:250–4.

17. Singh BM, Strobos RJ. Epilepsia partialis continua associated with nonketotic hyperglycemia: clinical and biochemical profile of 21 patients. *Ann Neurol* 1980;**8**:155–60.

18. Gray F, Serdaru M, Baron H. Chronic localized encephalitis (Rasmussen's) in an adult with epilepsia partialis continua. *J Neurol Neurosurg Psychiatry* 1987;**50**:747–51.

19. Komsuoglu SS, Liman O, Gurkan H. Epilepsia partialis continua following pertussis infection. *Clin Electroencephalogr* 1985;**16**:45–7.

20. Piatt JH, Hwang PA, Armstrong DC. Chronic focal encephalitis (Rasmussen syndrome): six cases. *Epilepsia* 1988;**29**:268–79.

21. Chalk CH, McManis PG, Cascino GD. Cryptococcal meningitis manifesting as epilepsia partialis continua of the abdomen. *Mayo Clin Proc* 1991;**66**:926–9.

22. Andermann F. Epilepsia partialis continua and other seizures arising from the precentral gyrus: high incidence in patients with Rasmussen syndrome and neuronal migration disorders. *Brain Dev* 1992;**14**:338–9.

23. Ettinger AB, Reed M, Cramer J. Epilepsy Impact Project Group. Depression and co-morbidity in community-based patients with epilepsy or asthma. *Neurology* 2004;**63**:1008–14.

24. Harden CL, Goldstein MA, Ettinger AB. Anxiety disorders in epilepsy. In: Ettinger AB, Kanner AM, eds. *Psychiatric issues in epilepsy: a practical guide to diagnosis and treatment*, 2nd ed. Philadelphia: Lippincott Williams & Wilkins, 2007: 248–63.

25. Ettinger AB, Reed ML, Goldberg JF, Hirschfeld RMA. Prevalence of bipolar symptoms in epilepsy vs other chronic health disorders. *Neurology* 2005;**65**:535–40.

26. Chauvel P, Liegeois-Chauvel C, Marquis P, Bancaud J. Distinction between the myoclonus-related potential and the epileptic spike in epilepsia partialis continua. *Electroencephalogr Clin Neurophysiol* 1986;**64**:304–7.

27. Cowan JMA, Rothwell JC, Wise RJS, Marsden CD. Electrophysiological and positron emission studies in a patient with cortical myoclonus, epilepsia partialis continua and motor epilepsy. *J Neurol Neurosurg Psychiatry* 1986;**49**:796–807.

28. Opherk C, Hirsch LJ. Ictal heart rate differentiates epileptic from non-epileptic seizures. *Neurology* 2002;**58**:636–8.

29. DeToledo JC, Ramsay RE. Patterns of involvement of facial muscles during epileptic and nonepileptic events: review of 654 events. *Neurology* 1996;**47**:621–5.

30. Henry JA, Woodruff GH. A diagnostic sign in states of apparent unconsciousness. *Lancet* 1978;**2**:920–1.

31. Geyer JD, Payne TA, Drury I. The value of pelvic thrusting in the diagnosis of seizures and pseudoseizures. *Neurology* 2000;**54**:227–9.

32. Saygi S, Katz A, Marks DA, Spencer SS. Frontal lobe partial seizures and psychogenic seizures: comparison of clinical and ictal characteristics. *Neurology* 1992;**42**:1274–7.

33. Bergen D, Ristanovic R. Weeping is a common element during psychogenic nonepileptic seizures. *Arch Neurol* 1993;**50**:1059–60.

34. Gumpert J, Hansotia P, Upton A. Gelastic epilepsy. *J Neurol Neurosurg Psychiatry* 1986;**33**:479–83.
35. Flügel D, Bauer J, Kaseborn U, Burr W, Elger CE. Closed eyes during a seizure indicate psychogenic etiology: a study with suggestive seizure provocation. *J Epilepsy* 1996;**9**:165–9.
36. Wennberg R. Postictal coughing and noserubbing coexist in temporal lobe epilepsy. *Neurology* 2001;**56**:133–4.
37. Vossler DG, Haltiner AM, Schepp SK, *et al.* Ictal stuttering: a sign suggestive of psychogenic nonepileptic seizures. *Neurology* 2004;**63**:516–9.
38. James MR, Marshall H, Carew-McColl M. Pulse oximetry during apparent tonic-clonic seizures. *Lancet* 1991;**337**:394–5.
39. Reuber M, Elger CE. Psychogenic nonepileptic seizures: review and update. *Epilepsy Behav* 2003;**4**:205–16.
40. Jobst BC, Williamson PD. Frontal lobe seizures. *Psychiatr Clin North Am* 2005;**28**:635–51, 648–9.
41. Leis AA, Ross MA, Summers AK. Psychogenic seizures: ictal characteristics and diagnostic pitfalls. *Neurology* 1992;**42**:95–9.
42. Kanner AM, Morris HH, Luders H, *et al.* Supplementary motor seizures mimicking pseudoseizures: some clinical differences. *Neurology* 1990;**40**:1404–7.
43. Benbadis SR, Lancman ME, King LM, *et al.* Preictal pseudosleep: a new finding in psychogenic seizures. *Neurology* 1996;**47**:63–7.
44. de Timary P, Fouchet P, Sylin M, *et al.* Non-epileptic seizures: delayed diagnosis in patients presenting with electroencephalographic (EEG) or clinical signs of epileptic seizures. *Seizure* 2002;**11**:193–7.
45. Ettinger AB, Devinsky O, Weisbrot DM, Goyal A, Ramakrishna R. A comprehensive profile of clinical, psychiatric and psychosocial characteristics of patients with psychogenic non-epileptic seizures. *Epilepsia* 1999;**40**:1292–8.
46. Bhatia MS. Pseudoseizures. *Indian Pediatr* 2004;**41**:673–9.
47. Scheepers B, Budd S, Curry S, Gregory S, Elson S. Non-epileptic attack disorder: a clinical audit. *Seizure* 1994;**3**:129–34.
48. Ettinger AB, Dhoon A, Weisbrot DM, Devinsky O. Predictive factors for outcome of non-epileptic seizures after diagnosis. *J Neuropsychiatry Clin Neurosci* 1999;**11**:458–63.
49. Williamson PD, Jobst BC. Frontal lobe epilepsy. *Adv Neurol* 2000;**84**:215–42.

c0005

Panic Attacks in a Woman with Frontal Lobe Epilepsy

Thomas Grunwald, Martin Kurthen and Christian E Elger

s0010

HISTORY

p0010
A 32-year-old woman presented with frequent simple and complex partial seizures since the age of 22. Often she would suffer from attacks of intense panic, which were frequently followed by *déjà-vu* experiences or by a poorly localized tingling sensation in the body. During these episodes she would normally tremble and utter short phrases such as, "Oh, no" or "Oh, God". These symptoms sometimes preceded a partial or complete loss of consciousness during which the patient would verbalize recurring syllables ("a ta ta ta ta"). She then would display perseverative movements that resembled body-rocking or complex actions that sometimes had an aggressive quality. For instance, we recorded seizures during which she tore off the electrode cap and pulled the mattress off her bed.

p0020
These seizures had never been controlled despite treatment with carbamazepine, phenytoin, lamotrigine, and clonazepam in monotherapy and in combination. The patient had graduated from extended elementary school and had begun training to be a nurse. However, she had to abandon her plans because of frequent seizures. When she was admitted for presurgical evaluation she was unemployed and single.

s0020

EXAMINATION AND INVESTIGATION

p0030
On admission, the patient's neurological and psychiatric examinations were normal. Neuropsychological tests revealed prominent non-verbal memory deficits. Scalp EEG recordings showed an interictal right temporal sharp wave focus. Ictal recordings, which were initially obscured by muscle artifacts, were characterized by theta-wave activity over the right temporal lobe. Magnetic resonance imaging (MRI) scans were negative but positron emission tomography demonstrated right temporal hypometabolism consistent with the localization of hyperperfusion during an ictal single photon emission computed tomography examination.

Puzzling Cases of Epilepsy

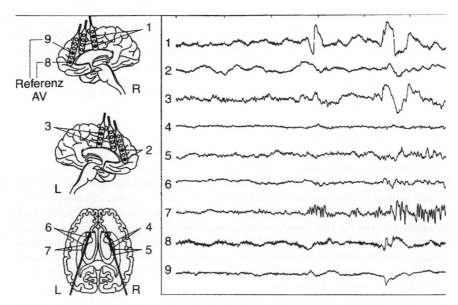

FIGURE 5.1   Intracranial recording of the initial part of a complex partial seizure. Channel 8 shows low amplitude fast activity in the anterior cingulate gyrus before and during a fast spread of seizure activity to the left hippocampus (channel 7) and right hippocampus (channel 5).

Four seizures were recorded invasively using bilateral basal and lateral temporal as well as interhemispheric subdural strip electrodes and hippocampal depth electrodes. All seizures started with characteristic low amplitude fast activity within the right anterior cingulate gyrus (Figure 5.1).

DIAGNOSIS

Cryptogenic frontal lobe epilepsy with simple and complex partial cingulate seizures.

TREATMENT AND OUTCOME

An anterior mesial frontal resection, which included the anterior half of the right superior frontal gyrus and the right anterior cingulate gyrus, was performed. This procedure resulted in complete seizure control. Postoperative histopathological examinations revealed a glioneural hamartoma within the anterior cingulate gyrus.

Because the patient has now been seizure-free for 24 months, we have started to taper her carbamazepine and lamotrigine.

COMMENTARY

This case demonstrates the importance of seizure semiology. During the presurgical evaluation of our patient, the results from non-invasive electrophysiological and functional imaging studies all pointed to the seizures originating within the right temporal lobe. In addition, our patient experienced auras with fear and *déjà-vu* and exhibited non-verbal memory deficits. These symptoms can also be associated with right-sided temporal lobe epilepsy. The only clue that the seizures arose from the anterior cingulate gyrus was the motor and hypermotor (complex movement) signs, which had a somewhat aggressive quality. This single clinical observation necessitated the use of interhemispheric subdural strip electrodes and, eventually, permitted the localization of the primary epileptogenic area.

Secondly, this case shows that morphological lesions causing symptomatic focal epilepsy can remain undetected by MRI scans. This is important because the correlation between structural lesions and the prognosis of epilepsy surgery is well known, especially in patients with seizures of extratemporal origin. Although 60–80% of patients with lesional focal epilepsy become seizure-free postoperatively, outcome in non-lesional patients is often less successful. Our case indicates, however, that clearly localizing signs and findings may be related to a minor lesion that can be demonstrated histopathologically but that may have been too small to be detected by MRI. In such cases, invasive recordings are warranted and necessary to prove the localization of focal seizure onset. However, if localizing signs and findings cannot be obtained, it seems advisable to postpone further invasive studies until improved imaging techniques may justify the implantation of electrodes.

What did we learn from this case?

The anterior cingulate gyrus maintains massive interconnections, both with the limbic system and with the frontal, temporal, and parietal neocortex. Therefore, cingulate seizures can have different possible propagation pathways, which may be responsible for the variability of their expression as seizures. Thus patients suffering from cingulate epilepsy can present with findings that are normally associated with epileptogenic foci in different areas of the brain. Ictal symptoms may include, for instance, somatosensory feelings, absence-like arrest, fear, vocalizations, and verbalizations as well as complex (hypermotor) movements. Moreover, electrostimulation of this area in humans can elicit both movements and feelings of anxiety while in non-human primates it can also elicit vocalizations indicative of alarm or separation anxiety. Thus, the anterior cingulate gyrus may subserve the association of complex behavior with adequate emotional qualities and vice versa. However, its pathological activation can also elicit one without the other because cingulate gelastic seizures are characterized by laughter without the subjective feeling of mirth. Because this structure seems to be capable of mediating neocortical and limbic functions, it is an important target of neuropsychological research on cognitive processes in both healthy volunteers and patients with psychopathological disorders.

This case suggests that there may be other patients with cingulate epilepsy in whom all the findings point to a temporal lobe origin. Therefore, if results from non-invasive examinations are consistent with temporal lobe epilepsy but are not backed by MRI studies, the search for another possible seizure focus should continue and should always include the anterior cingulate gyrus.

FURTHER READING

Devinsky O, Morrell M, Vogt BA. Contributions of anterior cingulate gyrus to behavior. *Brain* 1995; **118**:279–306.

Grunwald Th, Kurthen M, Elger CE. Predicting surgical outcome in epilepsy: how good are we? In: Schmidt D, Schachter SC, eds. *Epilepsy: problem solving in clinical practice.* London: Martin Dunitz, 2000: 399–410.

Jurgens U. Vocal communications in primates. In: Kesner RP, Olton DS, eds. *Neurobiology of comparative cognition.* Hillsdale, NJ: Erlbaum, 1990: 51–76.

Mazars G. Criteria for identifying cingulate epilepsies. *Epilepsia* 1970;**11**:41–7.

So KN. Mesial frontal epilepsy. *Epilepsia* 1998;**39(suppl 4)**:49–61.

von Cramon D, Jurgens U. The anterior cingulate cortex and the phonatory control in monkey and man. *Neurosci Biobehav Rev* 1983;**7**:423–5.

Williamson PD, Spencer DD, Spencer SS, Novelly RA, Mattson RH. Complex partial seizures of frontal lobe origin. *Ann Neurol* 1985;**18**:497–504.

c0006

Frequent Night Terrors*

Cesare T Lombroso

s0010

HISTORY

p0010

A 6-year-old boy was referred because of nightly events thought to be nightmares. These events had started when he was 4 years old and had progressively increased until they happened several times a night. They adversely affected his daytime performance and caused stress in the family.

p0020

No benefit had been obtained from benzodiazepines or counseling with a behavioral therapist familiar with sleep disorders. His past medical history was unremarkable. There was some relevant family background: a sibling, an aunt, and a cousin had suffered from febrile convulsions, the cousin later developing non-febrile seizures.

s0020

EXAMINATION AND INVESTIGATIONS

p0030

The patient had normal general and neurological examinations. Metabolic screening and scalp EEGs were normal. He was admitted for scalp video-EEG long-term monitoring (LTM). Several stereotypical events were captured, all occurring at night. He would awaken from quiet, non-rapid eye movements (non-REM) sleep, sit up looking frightened and seeking and grabbing his mother, and fleetingly exhibit dystonic posturing of his flexed left arm. There were also several bouts of a dry cough without drooling. The events lasted less than 1 min, after which he quickly returned to sleep. Similar episodes recurred between four and eight times during the night. In the morning he had some vague recollection of the events and specifically stated that he had awoken because of "fear and a feeling in my throat".

p0040

The accompanying ictal EEG showed an arousal pattern out of non-REM sleep and, amidst muscle artifacts, some bilateral frontal low-voltage theta activity. An ictal

---

*Case published in part (*Epilepsia* 2000; **41**:1221–6).

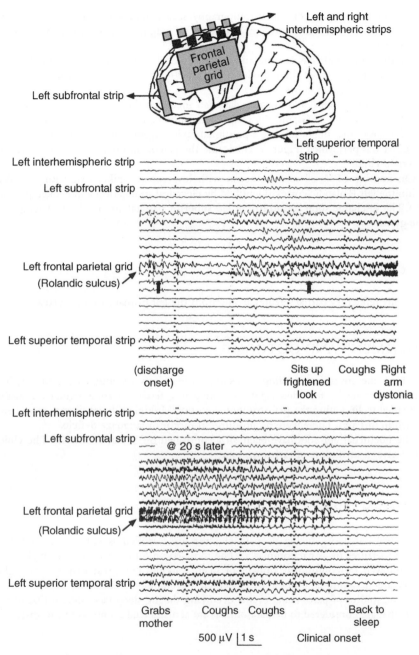

FIGURE 6.1   The placement of grids and strips (top) and a portion of the many ictal EEGs accompanying the events (bottom) recorded on invasive long-term monitoring.

single-photon emission computed tomography scan demonstrated an area of hyper-perfusion within the left frontotemporal lobes. A magnetic resonance imaging scan was normal.

p0050   Another trial with clonazepam did not help. Carbamazepine at top blood levels reduced the frequency of the episodes by about 30–40%. Trials with lamotrigine and gabapentin caused skin rashes.

p0060   At this point, clinical and imaging data had increased the suspicion of an epileptic disorder but routine EEGs and the scalp LTM had failed to demonstrate interictal or ictal discharges that might localize a presumed epileptogenic focus. Therefore, an invasive LTM was performed (Figure 6.1) because the parents insisted that "all be done" to help their child.

p0070   On invasive LTM, all seizures began with low-voltage spikes originating focally within the left Rolandic cortex (identified by electrical stimulation and evoked potentials). The discharge soon spread to the left superior parietal and to the first temporal lobe gyrus.

DIAGNOSIS

p0080   Medically refractory partial seizures arising from the left primary motor cortex.

TREATMENT AND OUTCOME

p0090   Based on the invasive recordings, resective surgery was recommended. At surgery, electrocorticography recorded vigorous spiking in a restricted zone, which was again confirmed to lie within the primary motor cortex. Multiple subpial slicings were performed in this area. There were no postsurgical motor or language deficits.

p0100   The nocturnal episodes have been 90% controlled on 5-year follow-up. The child still receives a small dose of carbamazepine.

COMMENTARY

p0110   Paroxysmal behaviors during sleep in children are classified as either sleep-induced epileptic seizures or as parasomnias.[1–3] The most common parasomnias are night terrors, followed by confusional arousals or sleep walking. The great majority of night terrors are parasomnias caused by a benign developmental disorder of arousal.[1–3] However, studies of paroxysmal events occurring during sleep have shown that some events that are considered to be parasomnias are actually ictal events, as in this case.[4,5]

What did I learn from this case and how did it alter my approach to the care and treatment of my epilepsy patients?

p0130   My evaluation of this patient and investigations of several other children with atypical, frequent night terrors show that it is reasonable to consider epileptic events in

TABLE 6.1   Main Features Suggesting an Ictal Origin for Episodes
Mimicking the Common Night Terrors or Confusional Arousals

	N.T.	C.A.	E.N.T.
Familial incidence	Yes	±Yes	?
Non-REM onset	Yes early	Yes anytime	Yes
Nightly events	Usually once	Usually once	Several
Intense fear	Yes	No	Yes
Stereotypy	No	No	Yes
Hallucinations	Probably	No	No
Duration	>4–5 min	Variable 1–5 min	<2 min
Responsiveness	No	±	Yes
Dystonia	No	No	Yes
Autonomic signs	No	No	Yes
Amnesia	Yes	±	No

N.T., night terrors; C.A., confusional arousals; E.N.T., epileptic night terrors.

the differential diagnosis. The main features that suggest an ictal origin for episodes mimicking the common night terrors or confusional arousals are listed in Table 6.1. Perhaps one important clue is the dystonic or tonic posturing of one or more limbs, although this may occur only fleetingly. Subtle posturing might suggest other types of frontal lobe epilepsy, such as those arising from the supplementary motor areas[6–8] or a so-called nocturnal paroxysmal dystonia, also once considered to be a parasomnia.[1,4,5] These seizures, and some other types of partial epilepsy arising from frontal lobe cortex, differ significantly from the ictal nocturnal events described in children who are thought to suffer from night terrors.[5,6,9]

How frequently are "night terrors" actually seizures? From my study alone it is impossible to estimate the frequency of ictal events masquerading as parasomnias and, specifically, the frequency of those mimicking night terrors or confusional arousals. My referred population is evidently strongly biased toward those children who do not respond favorably to the use of benzodiazepines or behavioral counseling and who exhibit multiple episodes during their sleep. It is very probable that the great majority of the common night terrors are not epileptic in origin. The few that are seizures can be suspected only from careful histories, adequate LTM investigation, and the other parameters listed in Table 6.1, and they represent another example of the kaleidoscopic group of distinct clinical phenotypes from epileptogenic foci within the frontal lobes.

REFERENCES

1. Thorpy MJ. Classification and nomenclature of the sleep disorders. In: Thorpy MJ, ed. *Sleep disorders.* New York, NY: Marcel Dekker, 1990:155–78.
2. Broughton RJ. Sleep disorders: disorders of arousal? *Science* 1968;**159**:1070–8.
3. Guilleminault C, Silvestri R. Disorders of arousal and epilepsy following sleep. In: Sterman MB, Shouse MN, Passuants P, eds. *Sleep and epilepsy.* New York, NY: Academy Press, 1982:513–31.

4. Lugaresi E, Cirignotta F, Montagna P. Nocturnal paroxysmal dystonia. *J Neurol Neurosurg Psychiatry* 1986;**49**:375–80.

5. Lombroso CT. Nocturnal paroxysmal dystonia due to a subfrontal cortical dysplasia. *Epileptic Disord* 2000;**2**:15–20.

6. Penfield W, Welch K. The supplementary motor area of the cerebral cortex. *Arch Neurol Psychiatr* 1951;**66**:289–317.

7. Wieser HG, Swartz BE, Delgado-Escueta AV, *et al.* Differentiating frontal lobe seizures from temporal lobe seizures. In: Chauvel P, Delgado-Escueta AV, *et al*, eds. *Advances in neurology*, 57. New York, NY: Raven, 1992:272–4.

8. Williamson PD, Van Hess PC, Wieser HG. Surgically remediable extratemporal syndromes. In: Engel J Jr, ed. *Surgical treatment of the epilepsies*, 2nd ed. New York, NY: Raven, 1993:68–73.

9. Scheffer IE, Bhatia KP, Lopes Cendes I, *et al.* Autosomal dominant nocturnal frontal lobe epilepsy: a distinctive clinical disorder. *Brain* 1995;**118**:61–73.

10. Vigevano F, Fusco L. Hypnic tonic postural seizures in healthy children provide evidence for a partial epileptic syndrome of frontal lobe origin. *Epilepsia* 1993;**39**:110–9.

Genetic (Generalized) Epilepsy with Febrile Seizures Plus

Ingrid E Scheffer

HISTORY

A 5½-year-old girl presented in January 2001 with recent onset of generalized tonic–clonic, absence, and atonic seizures. Her first afebrile generalized tonic–clonic seizure (GTCS) occurred 4 months earlier and lasted 90 s. There was no aura apparent nor any focal features. She had three further brief afebrile GTCS over the ensuing 4 months.

Atonic drop attacks began 2 months prior to presentation. Her eyelids fluttered briefly, she crumpled forwards or backward and lost awareness for only a second. She sustained facial injuries with these attacks. Brief absence seizures also occurred on two occasions. These consisted of staring for 1–5 s without eyelid fluttering or automatisms.

She had not had myoclonus, tonic seizures or febrile seizures. Perinatal history and developmental history were normal. She was right-handed and developmentally normal.

The family history was significant (Figure 7.1). The patient is the elder of two daughters to unrelated Australian parents. There is no family history of epilepsy on the mother's side but there is an extensive family history of seizures on the father's side, although the father himself had not had seizures.

EXAMINATION AND INVESTIGATIONS

General and neurological examinations were normal. There were no neurocutaneous stigmata or dysmorphic features.

Routine EEG showed three irregular generalized polyspike–wave discharges during hyperventilation. Intermittent photic stimulation did not evoke epileptiform abnormalities. MRI brain scan performed later, at 12 years for persistent headache, was normal.

Molecular genetic analysis showed the same single-stranded conformational analysis band shift as the c.387C→G mutation in the β-1 subunit gene of the neuronal sodium channel (*SCN1B*) that had been found in the wider family. Sequencing of other family members had confirmed this band shift as c.387C→G.[1]

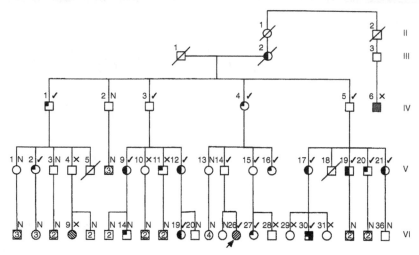

f0010   FIGURE 7.1   Pedigree of an Australian GEFS+ family showing the presence of the C121W mutation in SCNIB. The arrow denotes the patient described here. √, *SCNIB*(C121W) mutation; ×, negative for mutation; N, not tested; ▢, febrile seizures (FS); ▮, febrile seizures plus (FS⁺); ◼, FS and partial
epilepsy; ▨, neonatal, febrile and partial seizures; ▧, GTCS; ▩, GTCS, absences and atonic seizures;
▱, deceased; ☐, unaffected male; O, unaffected female; O, mixed gender; II–VI, denotes generations.

s0030   ## DIAGNOSIS

p0080   Familial epilepsy syndrome of generalized epilepsy with febrile seizures plus (GEFS+)
with the patient's phenotype comprising generalized tonic–clonic, atonic, and absence
seizures.

s0040   ## TREATMENT AND OUTCOME

p0090   The patient was commenced on valproate but her attacks were not fully controlled on
38 mg/kg per day. She had a further cluster of seizures in December 2000, including
unusual attacks with bilateral facial clonic activity with limp limbs; these attacks required
rectal diazepam after 5 min. Higher doses of valproate were tried without full seizure
control, so lamotrigine was added. Seizure freedom was established by October 2001
on a combination of valproate, lamotrigine, and clobazam. Side effects included tremor
and fatigue; tremor was likely to be exacerbated by combination valproate–lamotrigine
therapy. Despite these side effects, she was excelling at school in the first grade.

p0100   The patient was seizure-free from 7 years until 11 years on a combination of valproate and lamotrigine, clobazam was weaned. She experienced three GTCS from 11 years
of age. Concerns about her learning were just emerging and audiological assessment
showed a major auditory processing difficulty. Neuropsychological evaluation is underway.

s0050   ## COMMENTARY

p0110   This patient has one of the more severe phenotypes in the GEFS+ spectrum, which
we originally described in 1997.[2] GEFS+ is a familial epilepsy syndrome characterized

by phenotypic heterogeneity.[3] GEFS+ can be diagnosed in a family where at least two individuals have phenotypes falling within the GEFS+ spectrum. The most common phenotype in GEFS+ is classical febrile seizures, followed by febrile seizures plus (FS+). FS+ applies when a child has febrile seizures that extend past the usual accepted maximum age limit of 6 years, and/or has afebrile GTCSs. The phenotypes in the moderately severe part of the GEFS+ spectrum include febrile seizures or FS+ with other types of generalized seizures such as atonic, myoclonic or absence seizures and also partial seizures.[4–7] At the severe end of the GEFS+ spectrum, the epileptic encephalopathies of myoclonic–astatic epilepsy of Doose and Dravet syndrome may occur.[3,8] The absence seizures may differ from those typically seen in childhood absence epilepsy as they may be infrequent in GEFS+, but this is not always the case. Many patients with GEFS+ have normal routine EEG studies but some have generalized spike–wave activity.

Molecular genetic studies of GEFS+ have shown that mutations of two different neuronal sodium channel subunits and a GABA$_A$ receptor subunit are found in a minority of families. Initially a mutation was found in *SCN1B* in a large Tasmanian family.[9] Subsequently, mutations were found in the α-1 subunit gene (*SCN1A*) that encodes the pore-forming subunit of the ion channel.[10,11] Mutations were also identified in the gamma 2 subunit gene of the GABA$_A$ receptor (*GABRG2*) in families with GEFS+.[12–14]

There are now seven families with GEFS+ with *SCN1B* mutations.[1,4,9,12,13,15] This patient's family is the second family in which a *SCN1B* mutation was reported.[1] The extended family contained 19 members with seizures, including 16 with typical GEFS+ phenotypes. The mutation (c.387C→G) in *SCN1B*, found in this family and in the original Tasmanian family, changes a conserved cysteine residue to tryptophan (C121W), disrupting a putative disulphide bridge that maintains an extracellular immunoglobulin-like fold.[1,9] Functional studies of the sodium channel comprising the mutant β-1 subunit with a wild-type alpha subunit in *Xenopus laevis* oocytes were consistent with a loss of function.

The patient and her father both carry this mutation and the patient's phenotype can be regarded as one of the moderately severe phenotypes of the GEFS+ spectrum. The patient's course has been relatively mild for this end of the GEFS+ spectrum but learning issues are now emerging which is not surprising. The majority of patients with GEFS+ have a good prognosis but some continue to have refractory epilepsy.

GEFS+ was recognized through large autosomal-dominant families but even in these families, there is evidence of other genes modifying the phenotype. Other genes are likely to explain why one family member has febrile seizures while another has Dravet syndrome. GEFS+ usually follows complex inheritance where many genes are involved. This is especially likely in small families, which are more common in clinical practice, where only a few individuals are affected. In families with complex inheritance, there has been considerable effort placed in trying to find susceptibility genes. Initial reports of variants of the delta subunit gene of the GABA$_A$ receptor *GABRD* and the calcium channel subunit gene *CACNA1H* suggest they may be susceptibility alleles for GEFS+.[16–18]

Why did I choose this case?

I chose this case because it demonstrates the clinical relevance of GEFS+. This patient shows that the clinical diagnosis can be made on the basis of the electroclinical presentation in the setting of a significant family history. A key to making the diagnosis lies in obtaining further details about the family history so that the genetic context of the patient's epilepsy can be understood.

p0170   This case is important in demonstrating the spectrum of the more severe phenotypes of GEFS+. This patient may be broadly considered as having myoclonic–astatic epilepsy presenting without febrile seizures with a relatively good outcome. Myoclonic–astatic epilepsy is known for its variable prognosis with some cases having an excellent outcome.[19]

s0070   ## What did I learn from this case?

p0180   This case once again emphasizes how genetic epilepsies that follow autosomal-dominant inheritance, as GEFS+ does in this patient's family, result in further family members becoming affected over time. Genetic epilepsies are not always benign and easily controlled, nor do they always resolve spontaneously.

p0190   Many cases of GEFS+ follow complex inheritance (where multiple genes and environmental factors play a part), so that the family history will not always be as striking as in this child. Nevertheless, the nature of seizure disorders in a few other family members may be a valuable clue to the etiology and diagnosis. Importantly, bilineal inheritance of seizure disorders is not uncommon and suggests that the patient is at risk of inheriting more than one epilepsy gene.

s0080   ## ACKNOWLEDGEMENTS

p0200   The author is indebted to the patient and her family for participating in her research.

REFERENCES

1. Wallace R, Scheffer IE, Parasivam G, et al. Generalized epilepsy with febrile seizures plus: mutation of the sodium channel subunit SCN1B. *Neurology* 2002;**58(9)**:1426–9.
2. Scheffer IE, Berkovic SF. Generalized epilepsy with febrile seizures plus. A genetic disorder with heterogeneous clinical phenotypes. *Brain* 1997;**120**:479–90.
3. Singh R, Scheffer IE, Crossland K, Berkovic SF. Generalized epilepsy with febrile seizures plus: a common, childhood onset, genetic epilepsy syndrome. *Ann Neurol* 1999;**45(1)**:75–81.
4. Scheffer IE, Harkin LA, Grinton BE, et al. Temporal lobe epilepsy and GEFS+ phenotypes associated with SCN1B mutations. *Brain* 2007;**57(12)**:265–72.
5. Abou-Khalil B, Ge Q, Desai R, et al. Partial and generalized epilepsy with febrile seizures plus and a novel SCN1A mutation. *Neurology* 2001;**57(12)**:265–72.
6. Ito M, Nagafuji H, Okazawa, et al. Autosomal dominant epilepsy with febrile seizures plus with missense mutations of the (Na+)-channel alpha 1 subunit gene, SCN1A. *Epilepsy Res* 2002;**48(1–2)**:15–23.
7. Baulac S, Gourfinkel-An I, Picard F, et al. A second locus for familial generalized epilepsy with febrile seizures plus maps to chromosome 2q21–q33. *Am J Hum Genet* 1999;**65**:1078–85.
8. Singh R, Andermann E, Whitehouse WP, et al. Severe myoclonic epilepsy of infancy: extended spectrum of GEFS+? *Epilepsia* 2001;**42(7)**:837–44.
9. Wallace R, Wang DW, Singh R, et al. Febrile seizures and generalized epilepsy associated with a mutation in the Na+ channel beta1 subunit gene SCN1B. *Nat Genet* 1998;**19(4)**:366–70.
10. Escayg A, MacDonald BT, Meisler MH, et al. Mutations of SCN1A, encoding a neuronal sodium channel, in two families with GEFS+ 2. *Nat Genet* 2000;**24(4)**:343–5.

11. Wallace R, Scheffer IE, Barnett S, *et al*. Neuronal sodium-channel alpha1-subunit mutations in generalized epilepsy with febrile seizures plus. *Am J Hum Genet* 2001;**68(4)**:859–65.

12. Baulac S, Huberfeld G, Gourfinkel-An I, *et al*. First genetic evidence of GABA(A) receptor dysfunction in epilepsy: a mutation in the gamma2-subunit gene. *Nat Genet* 2001;**28(1)**:46–8.

13. Wallace R, Marini C, Petrou S, *et al*. Mutant GABA(A) receptor gamma2-subunit in childhood absence epilepsy and febrile seizures. *Nat Genet* 2001;**28(1)**:49–52.

14. Harkin LA, Bowser DN, Dibbens LM, *et al*. Truncation of the GABA(A)-receptor gamma2 subunit in a family with generalized epilepsy with febrile seizures plus. *Am J Hum Genet* 2002;**70(2)**:530–6.

15. Audenaert D, Claes L, Ceulemans B, Löfgren A, Van Broeckhoven C, De Jonghe P. A deletion in SCN1B is associated with febrile seizures and early-onset absence epilepsy. *Neurology* 2003;**61(6)**:854–6.

16. Dibbens LM, Feng HJ, Richards MC, *et al*. GABRD encoding a protein for extra- or perisynaptic GABAA receptors is a susceptibility locus for generalized epilepsies. *Hum Mol Genet* 2004;**13(13)**:1315–9.

17. Heron SE, Phillips HA, Mulley JC, *et al*. Genetic variation of CACNA1H in idiopathic generalized epilepsy. *Ann Neurol* 2004;**55(4)**:595–6.

18. Heron SE, Khosravani H, Varela D, *et al*. Extended spectrum of idiopathic generalized epilepsies associated with CACNA1H functional variants. *Ann Neurol* 2007;**17**. (Epub 14 August 2007.)

19. Doose H. Myoclonic-astatic epilepsy. *Epilepsy Res* 1992;**suppl 6**:163–8.

c0008

A Visit to the Borderland of Neurology and Psychiatry

Donald L Schomer

s0010

HISTORY

p0010
Mrs. N was 52 years old in 1980 when I first met her. She was referred by her psychiatrist for an opinion about her behavior.

p0020
In 1963 she was admitted to a psychiatric facility for profound depression after the birth of her fifth child. She had a previous history of depression but was now thought to be acutely psychotic. She failed to respond to multiple antidepressants but subsequently responded to electroconvulsive therapy. She required long-term use of both antidepressants and antipsychotics.

p0030
In 1974 she was driving a car that was involved in an accident, and she struck her head on the windshield. Between 6 and 8 months later she began experiencing complex visual hallucinations. She would suddenly see six German soldiers stacked in a triangular formation one on top of two on top of three. They wore Kaiser Willhelm helmets, reminiscent of World War I, and occasionally spoke to her in muffled tones telling her to harm herself. These were interpreted as command hallucinations. She was committed to a locked psychiatric unit for several years.

p0040
In 1977 she was struck in the head by another inpatient and rendered unconscious for several days. She suffered a subarachnoid hemorrhage. A few months later, she began having a second type of complex visual hallucination. This time the image was of an elderly woman sitting in a rocking chair that reminded her of a painting by Grandma Moses. She felt that this woman was a premonition of her own future. The woman rocked back and forth while several small rat-like animals chewed at her fingers, which were dangling to the side of the chair. Mrs. N would get comfort only by cutting herself with a sharp object when these hallucinations were present. The frequency of their occurrence steadily increased over the years to the point where they happened several times daily.

p0050
The referring psychiatrist had first met Mrs. N in 1979. The history that he had obtained revealed that the patient saw these images only in her left visual field. An EEG was performed (the first EEG in her now long medical–psychiatric history), and

this showed frequent right parietal and temporal interictal spikes. He treated her initially with phenytoin, but she developed a rash after 1 day. She was switched to carbamazepine, which she tolerated. She remained without hallucinations for the next 6 months, the longest symptom-free period in 5 years. The hallucinations then started to recur, prompting the referral to me.

EXAMINATION AND INVESTIGATIONS

My examination revealed a pleasant, engaging woman who was knowledgeable about current events and told me several humorous stories about her interactions with her congressman, which I was later able to confirm as being accurate. She had mild left arm drift and posturing, slight left-sided hyper-reflexia and absent Babinski responses. Of note, she had normal visual fields and intact higher level cognitive sensory functions. She was found to have a small nodular contrast-enhancing abnormality in the right parietotemporo-occipital junction on computed tomography scanning. Her EEG confirmed the previously described abnormalities.

DIAGNOSIS

Recurrent simple partial seizures coming from the right parietotemporal region, secondary to a probable arteriovenous malformation.

TREATMENT AND OUTCOME

My initial treatment was with medication. First, the carbamazepine was raised to maximum tolerated levels, which produced some improvement. Phenytoin was re-introduced and she tolerated it without developing a rash. She went for many years with very few seizures. Her evaluation for the "lesion" revealed a probable old arteriovenous malformation that had been obliterated by the hemorrhage that followed the physical attack she had suffered several years earlier.

After about 7 years of good seizure control, the seizures again gradually increased in frequency until she was experiencing them every 1–2 days. There had been no significant change in other medication except that conjugated estrogen had been added about 4 years earlier to treat menopausal symptoms.

She then underwent a surgical approach. Intraoperatively, with electrodes over the exposed right lateral temporoparietofrontal neocortex and with acute depth electrodes in the right anterior hippocampus and amygdala, she experienced a seizure. Coincident with the appearance of the German soldiers, she had sustained seizure activity posterior to a scarred-appearing area at the junction of the right posterior superior temporal gyrus and the inferior parietal junction. She felt fear and the desire to injure herself at the same time that the discharge spread to the deeper structures in the temporal lobe. The pathology revealed an old occluded arteriovenous malformation on the surface, as well as hippocampal sclerosis.

Postoperatively, she did well for a number of years until she slipped on the ice and suffered an acute intracerebral hemorrhage that left her with a left hemiparesis and hemianopia. Several years later, she developed acute leukemia and died of its complications in 1997.

COMMENTARY

This unfortunate woman had symptoms of partial epilepsy of a neocortical onset that went unrecognized for many years. She was treated with multiple drugs that were targeted at alleviating symptoms without really treating the underlying disorder. She underwent numerous electroconvulsive therapy sessions that may have contributed to her overall state of intractability. All the while she harbored an undiagnosed arteriovenous malformation that declared itself following an assault.[1]

What did I learn from this case?

The following lessons were evident to me:

- The history is perhaps the most important clinical tool that we have available.[2] When in doubt, retake the history. There were many clues in this case that the events were convulsive in origin. The symptoms were paroxysmal in origin, not related to environmental triggers. Their appearances were stereotypic. Her interpersonal skills were normal, not typical of a psychotic person. The EEG and clinical responses to antiseizure medication supported the diagnosis.
- Partial seizures may have a progressive pattern without evidence for an underlying progressive lesion.[3] In her case, perhaps the use of unopposed estrogen played a role in the progressive nature of her epilepsy.[4,5]
- The appearance of a rash following the initiation of high doses of phenytoin does not always preclude its potential long-term use.[6,7]
- Epilepsy surgery is not the exclusive domain of the young – Mrs. N responded well to the surgical approach until she was injured in an accident. If she had been diagnosed earlier and treated aggressively, I am convinced she would have had a more benign course.[8]
- Dual pathology may play a significant role in the development of intractability.[9] Improved brain imaging allows us to diagnose dual pathology earlier and should be considered whenever neocortical-onset seizures that later take on a clinical picture of temporolimbic epilepsy are recognized.
- Did her years of exposure to a variety of antidepressants, antipsychotics, and AEDs predispose her to her final illness – acute leukemia?[10]

How did this case alter my approach to the care and treatment of my epilepsy patients?

For the reasons noted above, I teach the importance of the history to my residents and fellows. I am cautious about the use of unopposed estrogen when there is the history of symptom progression after the introduction of estrogen therapy. I weigh the pros and cons of aggressive medical–surgical treatment in all my patients. Finally, my group uses newer noninvasive technology at an early stage in an attempt to improve our understanding of the pathological basis for epilepsy.

REFERENCES

1. LeBlanc R, Feindel W, Ethier R. Epilepsy from cerebral arteriovenous malformations. *Can J Neurol Sci* 1983;**10**:91–5.
2. Schomer DL, O'Connor M, Spiers P, Seeck M, Bear D, Mesulam MM. Temporal limbic epilepsy and behavior. In: Mesulam MM, ed. *Behavioral neurology*. London: Oxford University Press, 2000.
3. Elwes RDC, Johnson AL, Reynolds EH. The course of untreated epilepsy. *Lancet* 1988;**297**:948–50.
4. Logothitis J, Harner R, Morrell F, Torres F. The role of estrogens in catamenial exacerbation of epilepsy. *Neurology* 1959;**9**:352–60.
5. Herzog A, Seibel MM, Schomer DL, Vaitukaitis JL, Geschwind N. Reproductive endocrine disorders in women with partial seizures of temporal lobe origin. *Arch Neurol* 1986;**43**:341–6.
6. Kimball OP, Horan TN. The use of Dilantin in the treatment of epilepsy. *Ann Intern Med* 1939;**13**:787–93.
7. Wilson JT, Hojer B, Tomson G. High incidence of concentration dependent skin reactions in children treated with phenytoin. *BMJ* 1978;**1**:1583–6.
8. Elwes RDC, Reynolds EH. First seizure in adult life. *Lancet* 1988;**ii**:36.
9. Levesque MF, Nakasoto N, Vinters HV, Babb TL. Surgical treatment of limbic epilepsy associated with extra hippocampal lesions: the problem of dual pathology. *J Neurosurg* 1991;**75**:354–70.
10. White S, McLean A, Howland C. Anticonvulsant drugs and cancer: a cohort study in patients with severe epilepsy. *Lancet* 1979;**ii**:458–61.

c0009

A Case of Complex Partial Status Epilepticus

Alan R Towne

s0010

HISTORY

p0010

The patient is a 56-year-old man who was admitted to the hospital for bizarre behavior. He had a history of hypertension and hypercholesterolemia, which had been diagnosed approximately 15 years ago. Six years before admission he experienced a cerebral infarct in the distribution of the left middle cerebral artery distribution, and he had mild residual right hemiparesis. Approximately 1 year after this he was noted to have episodes of staring followed by confusion that lasted for approximately 15 min. A neurological evaluation at that time demonstrated left temporal spike discharges emanating maximally from the T3 electrode, with minimal temporal slowing. A diagnosis of complex partial seizures was made and the patient was started on carbamazepine and had no further seizures after attaining a dose of 1200 mg/day.

p0020

On the day of admission the patient was found wandering in the street by another pedestrian. He was taken to the closest emergency department.

s0020

EXAMINATION AND INVESTIGATIONS

p0030

In the emergency department, the patient was found to be confused and unable to answer simple questions. He was slightly lethargic and oriented to name only. One-step commands were performed with difficulty. General physical examination, including vital signs, was unremarkable. Neurological examination revealed right hemiparesis. Laboratory tests including complete blood count, serum electrolytes, magnesium, and toxicology screen were normal. Computed tomography (CT) scanning of the head revealed an old left middle cerebral artery infarct without acute changes. The carbamazepine level was 3 μg/ml.

p0040

The patient was kept in the emergency department for continued observation. He was noted to have changes in mentation ranging from mild impairment of consciousness

38

to almost complete unresponsiveness, during which he would not respond to simple questions. Past medical history was unobtainable and the patient had no identification on his person. Because no previous medical information was available, the working diagnosis by the emergency room staff was drug or toxin exposure or a psychiatric, encephalopathic or cerebrovascular etiology.

Neurological and psychiatric consultations were obtained. As part of his workup, the neurology consultant ordered an EEG, which demonstrated rhythmic left posterior temporal sharp activity with intermittent spread to the right hemisphere. This activity was continuous with the frequency of the ictal discharges ranging from 0.5 to 6 Hz.

DIAGNOSIS

Complex partial status epilepticus (CPSE) associated with low carbamazepine levels.

TREATMENT AND OUTCOME

On the basis of the EEG findings, the patient was given 5 mg lorazepam by slow intravenous push followed by 1000 mg of fosphenytoin.

Fifteen minutes after the injection of lorazepam the patient was noted to be slightly lethargic but able to follow simple one-step commands. The EEG demonstrated cessation of the continuous seizure activity. However, the left hemispheric slowing remained. The patient was able to give his full name and the fact that he had discontinued taking his carbamazepine approximately 3 days before admission.

The importance of compliance with antiepileptic medication was stressed to the patient, and he has had no further seizures. He was told not to make any changes to his regimen unless this was discussed with his neurologist.

COMMENTARY

This case illustrates some important points pertinent to the diagnosis and management of CPSE. As in this patient, 30–50% of patients with CPSE have a history of seizures before developing CPSE.[1] In those adult patients who develop CPSE without an antecedent history, CPSE occurs most commonly in association with symptomatic neurological disease such as herpes simplex encephalitis or cerebral infarction. In patients with a history of epilepsy, precipitating factors include recent infection and inadequate anticonvulsant levels. A possible precipitant of status epilepticus (SE) in this patient may have been the low carbamazepine level. CPSE has also been reported after cerebral angiography and can be associated with thrombotic thrombocytopenic purpura. Other precipitants include alcohol withdrawal, drug overdose, myelography, tumor, and certain medications (e.g. cephalosporins).

The incidence of CPSE is difficult to assess because the paucity of clinical symptoms may not raise a suspicion of possible SE and because there are few population-based studies. A population-based study carried out in Richmond, Virginia, USA, revealed that CPSE represented approximately 5% of the total number of convulsive and non-convulsive episodes and 35% of non-convulsive episodes.[2] Other studies have demonstrated that CPSE accounts for 10–40% of all cases of non-convulsive SE.[1,3] The elderly population represents an even greater challenge in diagnosis as the clinical manifestations may be subtle, consisting of prolonged confusion, unusual behavior, minor motor manifestations, aphasia or coma.[4]

p0120   CPSE is defined as 30 min or more of discrete or continuous partial seizures without full recovery of consciousness. The characteristic clinical manifestation is impairment of consciousness, which can vary from mild alteration of mentation to complete unresponsiveness. CPSE may also be characterized by a cyclic pattern in which phases of unresponsiveness alternate with partially responsive phases. During the periods of partial responsiveness, automatisms, and abnormal speech patterns may be present. During the unresponsive phase, complete speech arrest usually occurs, occasionally accompanied by stereotyped automatisms.[5,6]

p0130   The clinical manifestations of CPSE are varied and may be difficult to differentiate from generalized non-convulsive SE. The accompanying behavior can range from confusion to bizarre or psychotic-type behavior. Lateralizing or localizing neurological deficits (e.g. aphasia, ictal paresis) may also be seen. Although the duration of CPSE is usually between 30 min and several hours, recent reports have described examples of CPSE lasting for months, indicating that prolonged fugue states can be caused by CPSE.

p0140   CPSE should be suspected in any patient who is being evaluated for confusion or unresponsiveness. Other conditions that may be confused with CPSE include absence SE, prolonged post ictal states, psychiatric syndromes (such as somatoform disorder and psychosis), and cerebral circulation disorders, including transient ischemic attacks, and stroke with delirium. Other conditions such as encephalopathies, migraine, and transient global amnesia also need to be considered in the differential diagnosis.

p0150   To prevent serious morbidity and mortality, CPSE must be promptly diagnosed and treated. Among patients with convulsive SE, mortality ranges from 10% to 40% depending on the etiology, the duration of SE and the response to treatment. Recent studies have indicated that CPSE is also associated with increased morbidity and mortality.[7] Identification of CPSE may be delayed in patients who are comatose or who do not present with clinical manifestations that suggest ongoing seizure activity. Thus, EEG confirmation is mandatory to make the diagnosis for this condition. Recent studies of SE in comatose patients reveal that approximately 10% of these patients are in electrographic SE despite the fact that the patient may not demonstrate obvious clinical activity or may demonstrate only subtle clinical manifestations. Thus, patients who have persistent alterations of mental status should be evaluated immediately by EEG.[7,8]

p0160   Diagnostic evaluation of patients with CPSE should also include studies to identify the etiology of the event. These studies include laboratory tests to investigate the possibility of metabolic disorders, infections, toxic exposure, and withdrawal conditions. Neuroimaging studies such as CT or magnetic resonance imaging scanning can reveal abnormalities that may be diagnostic. Although not usually performed, ictal single-photon emission CT scanning can also provide information about the localization of the seizure, especially in atypical cases.

p0170   The treatment of CPSE is similar to that of generalized convulsive SE.[9] However, since the patient may not be obtunded during the seizures, the physician may not want to use large quantities of sedating anticonvulsants. Benzodiazepines, such as diazepam, lorazepam or midazolam, are usually used as first-line choices. A benzodiazepine is generally followed by intravenous fosphenytoin or other intravenous anticonvulsants.

What did I learn from this case?

This case illustrates that the diagnosis of complex partial seizures is not always obvious. In cases such as this, patients may not be able to give an adequate history, and previous records may not be readily available. This condition may be mistaken for a drug-related disorder or a psychiatric disorder. I realized that I would have missed this diagnosis if the patient had not undergone EEG monitoring to document the presence of ongoing seizure activity.

How did this case alter my approach to the care and treatment of my epilepsy patients?

I have become more sensitized in entertaining the diagnosis of non-convulsive SE in patients who are comatose. This applies both to patients in the emergency department and to patients in the intensive care unit. EEG seizure activity may be present even in the absence of any obvious clinical seizure activity.

REFERENCES

1. Towne AR, Waterhouse EJ. Rational diagnosis of subtle and non-convulsive status epilepticus. In: Schmidt D, Schachter SC, eds. *Epilepsy: problem solving in clinical practice*. London: Martin Dunitz, 2007:79–93.
2. DeLorenzo RJ, Hauser WA, Towne AR, *et al*. A prospective population-based epidemiologic study of status epilepticus in Richmond, Virginia. *Neurology* 1996;**46**:1029–35.
3. Krumholz A, Sung GY, Fisher RS, Barry E, Bergey GK, Grattan LM. Complex partial status epilepticus accompanied by serious morbidity and mortality. *Neurology* 1995;**45**:1499–504.
4. Towne AR. Epidemiology and outcomes of status epilepticus in the elderly. In: Ramsay RE, Cloyd JC, Kelly KM, Leppik IE, Perucca E, eds. *International review of neurobiology*. San Diego, CA: Elsevier Inc, 2007:111–27.
5. Williamson PD. Complex partial status epilepticus. In: Engel J Jr, Pedley TA, eds. *Epilepsy: a comprehensive textbook*. Philadelphia, PA: Lippincott–Raven, 1997:618–723.
6. Treiman D, Delgado-Escueta A. Complex partial status epilepticus. In: Delgado-Escueta A, Wasterlain C, Treiman D, *et al*, eds. *Status epilepticus*, 34. NY: Raven, 1983:69–81.
7. Towne AR, Waterhouse EJ, Boggs JG, Garnett LK, Brown AJ, Smith JR Jr, DeLorenzo RJ. Prevalence of nonconvulsive status epilepticus in comatose patients. *Neurology* 2000;**54**:340.
8. Towne AR, Waterhouse EJ, Boggs JG, Garnett LK, Brown AJ, DeLorenzo RJ. Prevalence of nonconvulsive status epilepticus in comatose patients. *Neurology* 2000;**54**:340–5.
9. Treiman DM. Effective treatment for status epilepticus. In: Schmidt D, Schachter SC, eds. *Epilepsy: problem solving in clinical practice*. London: Martin Dunitz, 2000:253–65.

c00010

Late-Onset Myoclonic Seizures in Down's Syndrome

Hajo M Hamer, Jens C Möller, Susanne Knake,
Wolfgang H Oertel and Felix Rosenow

s0010

HISTORY

p0010

A 55-year-old man with Down's syndrome was admitted to our hospital after a generalized myoclonic–tonic seizure. Approximately 3 years before admission, myoclonic jerks (particularly of the upper extremities) had started. These usually occurred in the morning and could be improved by administration of valproate (1800 mg/day). The dose was reduced because of daytime somnolence, and this reduction coincided with the occurrence of the first generalized myoclonic–tonic seizure, as described by a witness. Due to aggressive behavior during the addition of lamotrigine, the medical regimen was not closely followed, and additional generalized myoclonic–tonic seizures occurred.

s0020

EXAMINATION AND INVESTIGATIONS

p0020

Apart from increased muscle tone and gait disturbance, physical examination did not reveal any significant neurological abnormalities. A mini-mental state examination yielded a score of 1 point. A computed tomography scan revealed cortical atrophy; magnetic resonance imaging was not possible because of non-compliance on the part of the patient. The clinical diagnosis of Down's syndrome was confirmed by cytogenetical analysis.

p0030

An EEG was recorded when serum valproate levels were below detection threshold that showed generalized continuous slowing and generalized polyspike–wave complexes (Figure 10.1). The details of the myoclonic seizures, which were preceded by generalized polyspikes on the EEG, have been described elsewhere.[1]

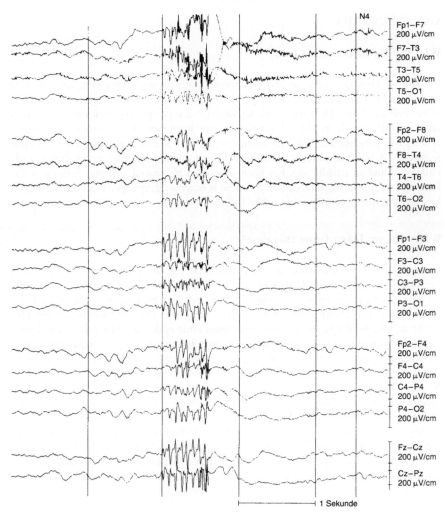

FIGURE 10.1   EEG showing generalized continuous slowing and generalized polyspike–wave complexes.

DIAGNOSIS

Late-onset myoclonic epilepsy in Down's syndrome.

TREATMENT AND OUTCOME

On a low dose of valproate (900 mg/day), the patient's generalized myoclonic–tonic seizures were finally controlled but his myoclonic jerks increased over the subsequent months. Therefore, topiramate (100 mg/day) was introduced, which led to significant and sustained improvement.

s0050   ## COMMENTARY

s0060   ### Why did we choose this case?

p0060   Epilepsy in Down's syndrome becomes more common with advancing age, affecting more than 46% of patients over the age of 50 years (compared with approximately 9% of patients aged over 18 years).[2–4] So far, descriptions of epilepsy with onset during or after the fifth decade in Down's syndrome have been rare, but reports have included at least two patients who have myoclonic seizures as well as generalized tonic–clonic seizures.[5,6] A bimodal onset of seizures in Down's syndrome, with peaks during early childhood and in middle age, has been described by several authors.[7,8] Because the longevity of subjects with Down's syndrome is increasing, epilepsy with late onset will be encountered more frequently in the future.[9]

s0070   ### What did we learn from this case?

p0070   Epilepsy in Down's syndrome that is characterized by seizure onset after the fourth decade may comprise myoclonic jerks and occasional generalized tonic–clonic seizures associated with progressive dementia.[5,6,10] We therefore propose that late-onset myoclonic epilepsy in Down's syndrome (as characterized in this case) should be included in the differential diagnosis of adult-onset myoclonic epilepsies. The time-locked association of polyspike–wave complexes preceding the myoclonus in our patient[1] and in the patient reported by Genton and Paglia[5] allows it to be classified as a primary generalized epileptic myoclonus. Late-onset myoclonic epilepsy in Down's syndrome may be successfully controlled by valproate and topiramate. However, topiramate must be used with particular caution in patients with Down's syndrome since it carries a risk of cognitive side effects.

p0080   Myoclonus is also found in the majority of Alzheimer's disease patients with epilepsy.[11] Since the accumulation of β-amyloid has been found both in patients with Alzheimer's disease and in aging Down's syndrome patients with dementia,[12] a common pathogenesis of dementia and myoclonic epilepsy in elderly Down's syndrome patients and patients with Alzheimer's disease appears possible.[13,14]

s0080   ### How much did this case alter our approach to the care and treatment of our epilepsy patients?

p0090   Late-onset epilepsy in elderly, demented Down's syndrome patients is characterized by myoclonus, occasional generalized tonic–clonic seizures or generalized myoclonic–tonic seizures, generalized epileptiform discharges on the EEG, and slow progression. Myoclonus in this syndrome can probably be classified as primary generalized epileptic myoclonus. Late-onset myoclonic epilepsy in Down's syndrome should be included in the differential diagnosis of adult-onset myoclonic epilepsies.

REFERENCES

1. Möller JC, Hamer HM, Oertel WH, Rosenow F. Late-onset myoclonic epilepsy in Down's syndrome (LOMEDS). Seizure 2001;10:303–6.

2. Veall RM. The prevalence of epilepsy among mongols related to age. *J Ment Deficiency Res* 1974;**18**:99–106.
3. Tangye SR. The EEG and incidence of epilepsy in Down's syndrome. *J Ment Deficiency Res* 1979;**23**:17–24.
4. McVicker RW, Shanks OE, McClelland RJ. Prevalence and associated features of epilepsy in adults with Down's syndrome. *Br J Psychiatry* 1994;**164**:528–32.
5. Genton P, Paglia G. Epilepsie myoclonique sénile? Myoclonies epileptiques d'apparition tardive dans le syndrome de Down. *Epilepsies* 1994;**1**:5–11.
6. Li LM, O'Donoghue MF, Sander JW. Myoclonic epilepsy of late onset in trisomy 21. *Arq Neuropsiquiatr* 1995;**53**:792–4.
7. Pueschel SM, Louis S, McKnight P. Seizure disorders in Down syndrome. *Arch Neurol* 1991;**48**:318–20.
8. Prasher VP. Epilepsy and associated effects on adaptive behaviour in Down's syndrome. *Seizure* 1995;**4**:53–6.
9. Baird PA, Sadovnick AD. Life expectancy in Down syndrome adults. *Lancet* 1988;**2**:1354–6.
10. Evenhuis HM. The natural history of dementia in Down's syndrome. *Arch Neurol* 1990;**47**:263–7.
11. Hauser WA, Morris ML, Heston LL, Anderson VE. Seizures and myoclonus in patients with Alzheimer's disease. *Neurology* 1986;**36**:1226–30.
12. Petronis A. Alzheimer's dementia and Down syndrome: from meiosis to dementia. *Exp Neurol* 1999;**158**:403–13.
13. Collacott RA. Epilepsy and associated effects on adaptive behaviour in Down's syndrome. *J Intellect Disability Res* 1993;**37**:153–60.
14. De Simone R, Daquin G, Genton P. Senile myoclonic epilepsy in Down syndrome: a video and EEG presentation of two cases. *Epileptic Disord* 2006;**8**:223–7.

c00011

Fainting, Fear, and Pallor in a 22-Month-Old Girl*

Edwin Trevathan

s0010

HISTORY

p0010

JH, an otherwise normal 22-month-old girl, was brought to her pediatrician's office after a "fainting spell." JH was playing after breakfast when she ran to her mother, grabbed her mother's dress, appeared pale, and then lost consciousness. After JH collapsed to the floor she slept for about 10 min before awaking in her usual state of health. Her examination and development were normal. The pediatrician considered a diagnosis of cardiac arrhythmia (such as paroxysmal atrial tachycardia) as well as gastroesophageal (GE) reflux, and ordered an electrocardiograph (ECG) and an esophageal pH probe, both of which were normal. The mother was reassured and the child was placed on thickened feeds for presumed gastroesophageal reflux.

p0020

Two weeks later, JH was playing with her dolls on the family kitchen floor. As JH was singing a children's song, the mother reported that she suddenly stopped singing and was noted to appear afraid and look pale before running to grab her mother's skirt and "fainting." The child was taken to the local emergency room, where she had a normal examination, a normal ECG, a normal chest X-ray, and normal routine blood tests. As the emergency room physician was leaving the room JH had her third spell – this time witnessed by a pediatric emergency room specialist. The look of sudden panic or fear was time-locked with the sudden pale appearance and staring straight ahead and also with cessation of normal play activities. The child had subtle lip pursing movements and her hands were held at the mid-line as she "tapped her thumbs together." The physician noted that her pupils were dilated and that she seemed unable to respond to his questioning. Her pulse rate, previously 90 beats/min, was noted to be 130 beats/min and regular during the spell. After about 90 s (which the mother described as "about 5 min"), the child fell asleep. She awoke 10 min later in her usual state of health. However, the emergency room physician noted that she had mild right central facial weakness upon awakening and that she did not speak for 30 min after waking from the spell; thereafter, she returned to her usual behavior with fluent, intact language.

*This article represents the views of the author, and does not necessarily represent the position of the Centers for Disease Control and Prevention (CDC).

EXAMINATION AND INVESTIGATIONS

I was consulted in the emergency room and noted that the patient's physical examination was normal, with the exception of a very subtle facial asymmetry – slightly less facial movement of the right face when speaking. The mother's account was reviewed in detail. All three spells were witnessed by the mother and were noted to be stereotypical. The spells were all heralded by a sudden look of fear with sudden loss of normal color of the facial skin, cessation of play, staring, and subtle (but stereotypic) hand movements. An electroencephalogram (EEG) performed within a few hours demonstrated left temporal theta waves, without epileptiform activity. The diagnosis of complex partial seizures of probable left temporal origin was made, and JH was started on carbamazepine (CBZ). A magnetic resonance imaging scan of the brain demonstrated thickening of the cortex within the left temporal lobe, with a significant reduction in white matter volume in the left temporal lobe compared with the same area on the right. The right hippocampus was very small, with very high signal on T2-weighted imaging.

After 7 months of freedom from seizures on CBZ, the seizures recurred. These seizures now occurred in clusters several times a week, and on rare occasions they were associated with secondary generalization. The seizures failed to respond to CBZ, phenytoin, valproate, lamotrigine, topiramate, and clonazepam in maximum tolerated doses. Video–EEG monitoring demonstrated that all interictal spikes and ictal onsets came from the left temporal lobe. A modified left temporal lobectomy with complete resection of the dysplastic cortex was performed, with cessation of seizures and freedom from seizures for more than 3 years of follow-up. The pathology was consistent with focal cortical dysplasia.

DIAGNOSIS

Left temporal lobe epilepsy.

COMMENTARY

Both the manifestations and the pathology associated with temporal lobe seizures are different in children from adults. The semiology of JH's seizures, like other young children with temporal lobe seizures, was primarily remarkable for a look of fear, cessation of normal play activities and pallor. The typical oral and hand automatisms usually seen among adults with mesial temporal lobe epilepsy are often not seen or are so subtle in children that they are not noticed or reported by parents and non-physician observers.[1]

Obtaining an EEG within 24 h of the spell[1] may increase the diagnostic yield of an EEG, but the most important diagnostic feature is the history. The manifestations of temporal lobe seizures in children are sometimes unrecognized by pediatricians and adult neurologists alike. Stereotypic spells of staring and pallor, with a look of fear or with associated clinging behavior (or both), associated with an alteration in consciousness and sleep, are manifestations of complex partial seizures of temporal lobe origin in children.[2]

Physicians who manage children with partial seizures should realize that failure of the seizures to respond to the first drug increases the likelihood that the child will develop intractable seizures. Failure to respond to three drugs used appropriately for partial seizures is predictive of intractability, and early referral to a pediatric epilepsy surgery center can improve the child's long-term outcome.[3]

REFERENCES

1. Bourgeois BF. Temporal lobe epilepsy in infants and children. *Brain Dev* 1998;**20**:135–41.
2. King MA, Newton MR, Jackson GD, *et al*. Epileptology of the first-seizure presentation: a clinical, electroencephalographic, and magnetic resonance imaging study of 300 consecutive patients. *Lancet* 1998;**352**:1007–11.
3. Kwan P, Brodie MJ. Early identification of refractory epilepsy. *N Engl J Med* 2000;**342**:314–19.

PART II

Intriguing Causes and Circumstances

Hyperactive Behavior and Attentional Deficit in a 7-Year-Old Boy with Myoclonic Jerks

Johan Arends, Albert P Aldenkamp and Biene Weber

HISTORY

A 7-year-old boy was referred to our child neurological program for learning disabilities with complaints about hyperactive behavior, attention deficit, lack of concentration, and unexplained fluctuations in school performance. Moreover, short periods (lasting some seconds) of sudden change of alertness were reported; the change in alertness was accompanied by loss of cognitive function. These short episodes occurred both at school and at home, mostly when the boy was watching television or playing computer games. There was no amnesia for these events or change of facial color, but sometimes there were stereotyped movements. Most of these events were interpreted as symptoms of the attention-deficit hyperactivity disorder (ADHD) and the movements were interpreted as "tics."

Hyperactive behavior had started at a very young age and did not respond to treatment (e.g. with methylphenidate). After starting in regular education, the boy had been referred to special education because of the hyperactive behavior, combined with conduct disorders. Psychomotor development was normal, although language development was delayed.

EXAMINATION AND INVESTIGATIONS

Neurological examination was normal. The patient was right-handed.

EEG showed normal background activity with frequent multifocal (poly)spike-waves (occurring six times in each 10 s). These waves were sometimes localized frontally and at other times they were generalized. During the recording, eight short seizures combined with epileptiform discharges were observed; these occurred only when the patient was watching television and they were accompanied by jerks. There was no specific photosensitivity to light stimuli, but there may have been sensitivity to specific patterns (e.g. the red colors on the television screen).

Neuropsychological investigation showed subnormal intelligence (Wechsler full-scale intelligence quotient (IQ) was 56), with corresponding verbal and performance scores (verbal IQ was 62 and performance IQ was 54). Beery tests for psychomotor development showed a psychomotor delay of about 3 years, a delay in language development, and symptoms of ADHD (especially attentional deficits and hyperactive behavior) and conduct disorders. There was evidence that the ADHD was a secondary symptom. During several periods, the sudden drops in alertness were observed. After such episodes, the symptoms of ADHD increased.

EEG combined with neuropsychological assessment showed frequent multifocal epileptiform discharges of sharp waves, spike-waves, and polyspike-waves. During this period, frequent myoclonic jerks were observed (74 jerks in a recording that lasted 30 min). These jerks especially involved the shoulders (the left and right shoulders independently) with hypertonia. In addition there were infrequent absence seizures (four were recorded in half an hour). The myoclonic jerks were most pronounced when the patient was watching television, but they were also present during absence seizures when he was not watching television. The myoclonic absences interfered significantly with cognitive function such that the patient did not react to questions during the myoclonic seizure and did not remember being questioned after the seizure. Simultaneously with these seizures the EEG showed generalized discharges with spike-waves and polyspike-waves over a period of 5–13 s; sometimes there also was localized activity of frontal origin. In addition, photosensitivity for patterns and bright colors was established. This was accompanied by self-induction. The patient reported feeling a pleasant sensation in his head during the seizures. Figure 12.1 shows a sample of the EEG discharges during the myoclonic absence seizures.

Magnetic resonance imaging scanning showed no abnormalities.

DIAGNOSIS

Myoclonic absence epilepsy[1] with developmental delay and secondary ADHD symptoms with conduct disorders.

TREATMENT AND OUTCOME

Some anti-epileptic drugs (e.g. carbamazepine, phenytoin, vigabatrin, gabapentin) may increase the frequency or severity of these seizures. About 50% of patients respond favorably to valproate, ethosuximide, or lamotrigine, either in monotherapy or in combination.[2] However, treatment should be initiated carefully, since high doses of these drugs can also lead to an increase in seizure frequency, probably through the alteration of vigilance.

In this patient, treatment was initiated with ethosuximide 250 mg twice daily using 62.5 mg/ml syrup; however, the syrup was changed to tablets after poor drug compliance and the dose was increased to 750 mg/day. At this dose the patient was reported to be slow and tired, and seizure frequency increased. After the dose was lowered to 500 mg/day, his seizure frequency decreased. Because we considered the ADHD symptoms

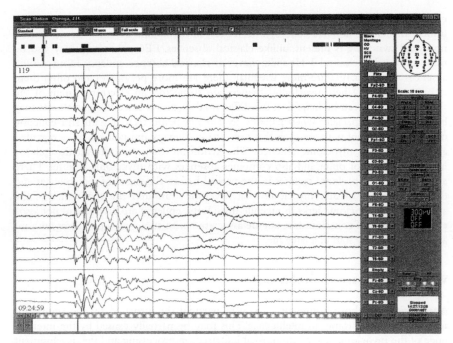

FIGURE 12.1   Ictal EEG during a myoclonic absence seizure.

to be secondary, no pharmacological treatment for ADHD was started. To assist the patient's parents, practical counseling was provided in the home, especially focused on improving the family's strategies for coping with the epilepsy and the bad behavior and on implementing strategies to improve drug compliance. A behavior modification program was also started to reduce self-induction. About 1½ years after starting this combined treatment strategy, the patient was considered almost seizure-free.

COMMENTARY

Why did we choose this case?

Although it is documented that the syndrome of myoclonic absence epilepsy is associated with mental retardation (in 45% of patients at onset of the epilepsy, with a further 25% developing mental retardation during the course of the disease),[3] our case illustrates that the myoclonic jerks can also interfere with cognitive function and thus cause state-dependent cognitive impairment in addition to the trait-dependent impairments caused by the syndrome. Although photosensitivity is described as a rare comorbid symptom, seizures may be precipitated by light stimulation. In this case, self-induction was also present. This may contribute to the intractability in some cases and therefore compliance should be carefully monitored. Family counseling may be needed as in this case.

The differential diagnosis of myoclonic absence epilepsy may be difficult. For example, when there is a myoclonic component, the differential diagnosis may involve childhood or juvenile absence epilepsies; these, however, rarely affect the upper limbs (unlike myoclonic absence epilepsy). Moreover, in myoclonic absence seizures almost no eyelid twitching is present, unlike classical absences. EEG recordings may also be misinterpreted as classical 3-Hz spike-waves of classical absence epilepsy. In myoclonic absences the discharges are more irregular, there are more polyspikes and often there is an asymmetry. When myoclonic absences are suspected, an electromyogram of the shoulder muscles can be helpful in the differential diagnosis since the myoclonias may be very subtle, especially when patients are already being treated with anti-epileptic drugs. Every patient with absences that prove to be therapy resistant has to be regarded as suffering from myoclonic absences. The syndrome of myoclonic–astatic epilepsy has a similar age of onset and also combines absences with myoclonic seizures. There are, however, tonic–clonic seizures in the period before the onset of the absences and drop attacks, and massive myoclonus that develops soon after the appearance of the absences. The myoclonic jerks in juvenile myoclonic epilepsy are briefer, and not associated with loss of consciousness, but are associated with tonic–clonic seizures without absences, and they start at a later age.

What did we learn from this case?

Apart from the above comments, we were particularly surprised by the significant impact of the syndrome on intelligence. This may be partially caused by the interference of the myoclonic jerks with normal information processing and the development of ADHD as a secondary symptom. In particular, the cognitive effects of the myoclonic jerks may be substantial because of the high frequency of seizures.

Moreover, in this specific case the seizures may be confused with behavioral symptoms during longer periods – at the time of referral, all this boy's symptoms had been erroneously interpreted as being due to ADHD or as being repetitive tics.

Although the syndrome of myoclonic absence epilepsy is often associated with developmental delay, this is too often seen as an untreatable trait-factor. State-dependent factors such as high seizure frequency and conduct disorders should be vigorously treated. This may result in a normal or only slightly delayed development.

In a recent study, 7 of 14 patients with myoclonic absence epilepsy showed evidence of a chromosome abnormality syndrome (trisomy 12 p and Angelman syndrome).[4] In this patient no chromosomal investigations were performed. This should be done in patients with more than one seizure type, early-onset seizures, or severe developmental delay.

REFERENCES

1. Tassinari CA, Lyagoubi S, Santos V, et al. Etude des décharges de pointes ondes chez l'homme. II. Les aspects cliniques et electroencephalographiques des absences myocloniques. Rev Neurol. 1969;121:379–83.
2. Perucca E, Gram L, Avanzini G, Dulac O. Antiepileptic drugs as a cause of worsening of seizures. Epilepsia 1998;39:5–17.
3. Dulac O, Kaminska A. Intractable myoclonic absences. In: Schmidt D, Schachter SC, eds. Epilepsy: problem solving in clinical practice. London: Martin Dunitz, 2000: 361–4.
4. Elia M, Guerrini R, Musumeci SA, Bonanni P, Gambardella A, Aguglia U. Myoclonic absence-like seizures and chromosome abnormality syndromes. Epilepsia 1998;39:660–3.

FURTHER READING

Aldenkamp AP, Overweg-Plandsoen WCG, Arends J. An open nonrandomized clinical comparative study evaluating the effect of epilepsy on learning. *J Child Neurol* 1999;**14**:795–801.

Overweg-Plandsoen WCG, Van Bronswijk JC, Arends J, Aldenkamp AP. The effect of epileptiform discharges and difficult-to-detect seizures on cognitive function. *Epilepsia* 1999;**40(suppl 2)**:100–1.

Aldenkamp AP, Arends J. The relative influence of epileptic EEG discharges, short nonconvulsive seizures and type of epilepsy on cognitive function. *Epilepsia* 2004;**45**:54–63.

Aldenkamp AP, Arends J. Effects of epileptiform EEG discharges on cognitive function: Is the concept of "transient cognitive impairment" still valid? *Epilepsy Behav* 2004;**5(S1)**:25–34.

c00013

Temporal Lobe Epilepsy, Loss of Episodic Memory, and Depression in a 32-Year-Old Woman

Christian G Bien

s0010

HISTORY

p0010

This previously healthy woman, a smoker for more than 10 years (one pack per day), experienced her first seizure (tonic–clonic) at the age of 32 years. She did not have a history of epilepsy-related central nervous system (CNS) disorders such as febrile seizures, head trauma or CNS infection. Subsequently, she developed complex partial seizures, with features suggesting an origin in the dominant temporal lobe, at a frequency of three a day. Several anticonvulsive drug regimens (valproate, valproate plus phenytoin, lamotrigine) did not control the seizures. In parallel to the epilepsy, the patient developed severe loss of episodic memory and mood lability with a predominance of depression and – later on – verbal aggression.

s0020

EXAMINATION AND INVESTIGATIONS

p0020

The patient was admitted to the Epilepsy Center of the University of Bonn, Germany, 9 months after her initial seizure. Physical examination revealed no focal neurological deficits. She had severe affective abnormalities, consisting of major depression with lability of mood. Neuropsychological testing revealed verbal and visual memory deficits.

p0030

A magnetic resonance imaging (MRI) scan showed left-sided hippocampal volume loss with increased T2 signal, indicating hippocampal sclerosis. Interictal EEG revealed bilateral anterior temporal epileptiform discharges (sharp waves, sharp-and-slow waves). Recordings of five habitual seizures showed a uniform left temporal onset of rhythmic theta activity with spread to the contralateral temporal lobe contacts

Puzzling Cases of Epilepsy

within 6–20 s. Positron emission tomography scanning revealed left temporal hypermetabolism. Ictal single-photon emission computed tomography scanning showed left temporal hyperperfusion. A search for neoplasia, including serum testing for autoantibodies associated with paraneoplastic neurological syndromes, was negative. There were no abnormal values in standard tests of the cerebrospinal fluid, including an extensive serological search for neurotropic infectious agents.

DIAGNOSIS

Temporal lobe epilepsy with complex partial and secondarily generalized tonic–clonic seizures, memory loss, and organic affective syndrome presumed to be due to limbic encephalitis.

TREATMENT AND OUTCOME

Owing to the severe memory deficits, resective epilepsy surgery was initially withheld. Several drug regimens failed to control the seizures. The patient's affective disorder was treated with mirtazapine and later with mirtazapine plus citalopram.

On the basis of the suspected diagnosis of a chronic encephalitic origin of the left temporomedial damage (non-paraneoplastic limbic encephalitis), immunosuppressive therapy was started 10 months after the first seizure. The patient received prednisolone 100 mg/day for 1 month. After this, the daily dose was reduced by 10 mg/month.

The patient became seizure-free for 3 months, but her memory function did not change and the affective abnormalities increased – suicidal tendencies as well as aggressive behavior were noted. A change of the antidepressant drug therapy to venlafaxine led to an improvement. However, the psychic abnormalities were still unbearable for the patient and her family. Since these problems were in part attributed to the high-dose corticosteroid treatment, prednisolone was tapered down.

The seizures recurred. A Wada test indicated left hemispheric language dominance. A left-sided amygdalohippocampectomy was offered to the patient, but she and her family were thoroughly informed about the risk of a further decline of her verbal memory performance. The patient wished to be operated on, and 17 months after her first seizure, the procedure was performed.

Histopathological investigation of the hippocampal specimen obtained during epilepsy surgery revealed segmental neuronal loss and astrogliosis (hippocampal sclerosis) and perivascular and parenchymatous inflammatory infiltrates consisting of T lymphocytes (Figure 13.1).

Eleven months after surgery, the patient was seizure-free apart from three complex partial seizures, which had occurred when the patient had not regularly taken her antiepileptic medication (lamotrigine 400 mg/day postoperatively). A renewed search for neoplasia was initiated.

COMMENTARY

The case illustrates that mediotemporal lobe epilepsy with hippocampal sclerosis may rarely present as an adult-onset disease on the basis of chronic limbic encephalitis.

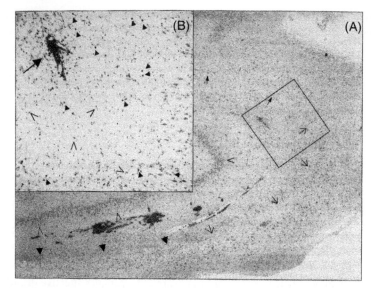

FIGURE 13.1   (A) Hippocampus. Arrowheads: sector cornu ammonis (CA) 1, which is almost completely devoid of neurons. Arrows with wide angle: cornu ammonis 2, with neurons largely preserved. Arrows with filled head: cornu ammonis 3, with almost no neurons preserved. Open angles: dentate gyrus, preserved. Hematoxyline and eosin; original magnification ×25. (B) Detail of (A) (box). Large arrow: vessel and perivascular space containing numerous lymphocytes. Arrowheads: parenchymatous lymphocytes. Open angles: microglial cells. Immunohistochemical staining for leukocyte common antigen (CD45), slight counterstaining with hemalum; original magnification ×100.

Limbic encephalitis is usually associated with a neoplasia and is then known as paraneoplastic limbic encephalitis. However, cases without neoplasia have been identified in a cohort of patients undergoing presurgical evaluation (non-paraneoplastic limbic encephalitis). Limbic encephalitis should be included in the differential diagnosis of temporal lobe epilepsy that is not typical for the "classical" syndrome of temporal lobe epilepsy with medial sclerosis. Such cases are characterized by a subacute onset of pharmacoresistant temporal lobe seizures, affective abnormalities, severe memory loss, and limbic lesions on the MRI scan. A malignant condition, usually a small cell lung cancer in the presence of characteristic autoantibodies, needs to be excluded. Long-term follow-up in cases of suspected paraneoplastic limbic encephalitis is mandatory because the neurological syndrome may begin more than 2 years before the detection of the underlying tumor.

What did I learn from this case?

Even though the condition can be securely diagnosed only on the basis of a histological examination, clinical data and neuroradiological findings may suggest the diagnosis. Treatment of these pharmacoresistant syndromes is difficult, because not only the seizures but also the severe memory deficits and the affective disorder need to be accounted for when a regimen is planned. In cases of paraneoplastic limbic encephalitis, treatment of the underlying neoplasm is the most effective therapy. In patients with non-paraneoplastic limbic encephalitis, high-dose immunosuppression can be performed in addition to anticonvulsive and antidepressant pharmacotherapy. Patients with non-paraneoplastic limbic encephalitis (and paraneoplastic limbic encephalitis alike) usually present with bilateral mediotemporal lesions. However, unilateral cases may occur, as shown by the patient presented here. For patients with non-paraneoplastic limbic encephalitis who have unilateral lesions, resective temporal lobe surgery should be considered. The patient presented here became almost seizure-free after amygdalohippocampectomy.

What I have learned from this type of patient during the last 6 years?

Since 2001, when the first edition of this volume was prepared, some new pieces of information have become available on patients like the one presented here. Based on the published data on this syndrome, our group recently proposed formal diagnostic criteria for limbic encephalitis. According to these criteria, the diagnosis of limbic encephalitis is confirmed in this patient.[1]

Regarding the particular constellation of adult-onset temporal lobe epilepsy with hippocampal sclerosis as the morphological substrate, more data have become available recently. In a retrospective study, we showed that in half of the patients with this syndrome limbic encephalitis was definitely or possibly the underlying cause.[2]

Sub-syndromal classification of limbic encephalitides is more refined today than in 2001. Antibodies against voltage-gated potassium channels have been identified as defining a usually non-paraneoplastic form of limbic encephalitis with a mostly good response to immunotherapy.[3,4] Most recently, a group of female patients in the age range 14–44 years characterized by an immune-mediated CNS disease associated with ovarian teratomata and "hippocampal neuropil" antibodies directed against subunits of the N-methyl-D-aspartate (NMDA) receptor has been described. Most of the patients had signs and symptoms suggesting involvement of wider brain areas than just of its temporomedial portion. Nevertheless, tumor search in patients with (suspected) limbic encephalitis should probably include a thorough gynecological examination including transvaginal ultrasound examination.[5,6]

REFERENCES

1. Bien CG, Elger CE. Limbic encephalitis: a cause of temporal lobe epilepsy with onset in adult life. *Epilepsy Behav* 2007;**10**:529–38.
2. Bien CG, Urbach H, Schramm J, et al. Limbic encephalitis as a precipitating event in adult-onset temporal lobe epilepsy. *Neurology* 2007;**69**:1236–44.
3. Vincent A, Buckley C, Schott JM, et al. Potassium channel antibody-associated encephalopathy: a potentially immunotherapy-responsive form of limbic encephalitis. *Brain* 2004;**127**:701–12.
4. Thieben MJ, Lennon VA, Boeve BF, Aksamit AJ, Keegan M, Vernino S. Potentially reversible autoimmune limbic encephalitis with neuronal potassium channel antibody. *Neurology* 2004;**62**:1177–82.
5. Bataller L, Kleopa KA, Wu GF, Rossi JE, Rosenfeld MR, Dalmau J. Autoimmune limbic encephalitis in 39 patients: immunophenotypes and outcomes. *J Neurol Neurosurg Psychiatry* 2007;**78**:381–5.
6. Dalmau J, Tüzün E, Wu HY, et al. Paraneoplastic anti-N-methyl-D-aspartate receptor encephalitis associated with ovarian teratoma. *Ann Neurol* 2007;**61**:25–36.

FURTHER READING

Bien CG, Schulze-Bonhage A, Deckert M, *et al*. Limbic encephalitis not associated with neoplasm as a cause of temporal lobe epilepsy. *Neurology* 2000;**55**:1823–8.

Gultekin SH, Rosenfeld MR, Voltz R, Eichen J, Posner JB, Dalmau J. Paraneoplastic limbic encephalitis: neurological symptoms, immunological findings and tumour association in 50 patients. *Brain* 2000;**123**:1481–94.

Epileptic "Dreamy States" in a Young Man

Warren T Blume

HISTORY

A 20-year-old left-handed, right-footed, right-eyed and previously neurologically healthy man began to have focal and generalized seizures without known cause at the age of 15.

The focal seizures began as a "dreamy state," otherwise described as an unreal faint feeling or as a cephalic sensation followed by nausea and occasionally euphoria. The patient denied loss of awareness but stared straight ahead without oroalimentary or manual automatisms. He emerged gradually without postictal dysphasia or other Todd's phenomenon. These attacks had become more frequent over the years and were occurring about 35 times a month and clustering up to 17 a day.

Fear, olfactory or gustatory sensations, motor phenomena, interictal language or speech impairment, and other experiential phenomena did not accompany these attacks.

About 20 generalized tonic–clonic (grand mal) seizures had occurred over the past 6 months, occasionally in sequences of up to 10–15 min in length.

The central nervous system functional enquiry was clear – his memory and judgment were subjectively intact although he found that the medications had slowed his ability to react.

The neurological history was also clear – febrile seizures, meningitis, encephalitis or major head injury had not occurred.

EXAMINATION AND INVESTIGATIONS

The neurological examination was normal. Visual fields, pupils, and fundi were normal. There was no focal motor deficit, and his gait and coordination were normal. Neuropsychological testing revealed no abnormalities. Memory was normal.

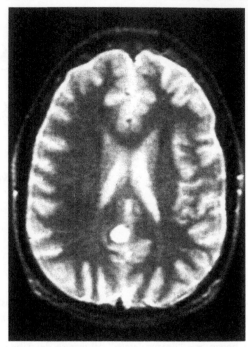

f0010   FIGURE 14.1   Discrete right mesial parietal lesion on magnetic resonance imaging scan.

0080   His awake and sleep interictal electroencephalogram (EEG) was normal. A single clinical seizure was associated with 6-Hz rhythmic waves at Fz, Cz, C4, and F4 with spread to P4 and also involving F8 but with only slight involvement of M2, M1, and elsewhere. Therefore, the seizure appeared to have a parasagittal origin with greater involvement of the right side. Nausea was the only clinical symptom of this attack.

p0090   A small, approximately circular mass lesion in the mesial aspect of the right parietal region was identified on magnetic resonance imaging without contrast enhancement (Figure 14.1).

p0100   A habitual seizure was recorded by subdural EEG, revealing onset in the right posterior cingulate area (Figure 14.2).

p0110   Histological examination of the completely resected focal right mesial parietal lesion disclosed a dysembryoplastic neuroepithelial tumor.

DIAGNOSIS

p0120   Partial seizures secondary to a dysembryoplastic neuroepithelial tumor.

TREATMENT AND OUTCOME

p0130   No seizures have occurred since the right posterior cingulate lesion was resected.

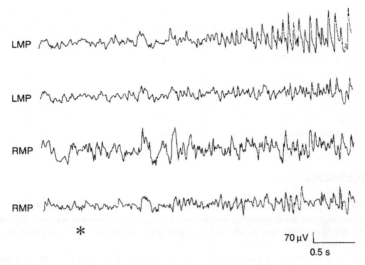

FIGURE 14.2   Right subdurally recorded clinical seizure beginning in third channel (*) as irregularly sequential spikes spreading first ipsilaterally (fourth channel) and then contralaterally (first, then second channel) and becoming maximally expressed on left. LMP, left mesial parietal (cingulate gyrus); RMP, right mesial parietal (cingulate gyrus).

COMMENTARY

The limbic lobe comprises a ring of phylogenetically primitive cortex, including the cingulate gyrus, the parahippocampal gyrus (which is the anterior–inferior extension of the cingulate gyrus), and the hippocampal formation. The hippocampus connects with the anterior thalamic nuclei via the fornix and the mamillothalamic tract. The posterior cingulate receives afferents from the anterior thalamic nuclei, thus completing the Papez loop.[1] The posterior cingulate gyrus receives much more abundant afferents from the orbital frontal cortex, the parahippocampal gyrus, the dorsolateral frontal lobe, and the parietal lobe than the anterior cingulate gyrus does. The posterior cingulate gyrus sends efferents to the hippocampus via the entorhinal cortex.

Reports describing semiology of seizures arising from the cingulate gyrus are few and often contain limited detail. Phenomena described include fear, aggressive verbalizations, staring, gestural automatisms, asymmetric tonic events, ocular and cephalic version, and autonomic phenomena involving the respiratory, cardiovascular, and digestive systems. Some of these phenomena probably represent spread of the ictus to adjacent motor regions and even to other parts of the limbic system.[2–4]

What did I learn from this case?

Although the majority of seizures with experiential and epigastric phenomena arise from the temporal lobe, a minority of such attacks may involve other portions of the limbic system, which may have explained the symptomatology here. No clinical feature would specify the mesial parietal region as an origin for such attacks, but the very prominent tendency for generalized tonic–clonic seizures raises the possibility of a parasagittal focus. Limbic seizures that arise from one or both temporal lobes would probably be associated with interictal temporal spikes on at least one EEG, while neuropsychological testing would usually disclose a verbal or non-verbal memory impairment.[5]

p0170   Normal findings from these examinations would raise the possibility of an extratemporal origin for these seizures, including the cingulate gyrus or the orbital frontal area. Ictal propagation of posterior cingulate seizures to the supplementary sensory–motor areas could produce diffuse or unilateral sensory phenomena and progression to asymmetrical postural seizures.[6,7] However, such phenomena did not appear in this patient.

REFERENCES

1. Papez JW. A proposed mechanism of emotion. *Arch Neurol Psychiatry* 1937;**38**:725–43.
2. Mazars G. Cingulate gyrus epileptogenic foci as an origin for generalized seizures. In: Gastaut H, Jasper H, Bancaud J, Waltregny A, eds. *The physiopathogenesis of the epilepsies*. Springfield, IL: Charles C Thomas, 1969: 186–9.
3. Bancaud J, Talairach J. Clinical semiology of frontal lobe seizures. In: Chauvel AV, Delgado-Escueta AV, *et al*, eds. *Advances in neurology*, vol 57. New York: Raven, 1992: 3–58.
4. Williamson PD. Frontal lobe seizures. Problems of diagnosis and classification. In: Chauvel P, Delgado-Escueta AV, Halgren E, Bancaud J, eds. *Advances in neurology*, vol 57. New York: Raven, 1992: 289–309.
5. Jones-Gotman M, Harnadek M, Kubu CS. Neuropsychological assessment for temporal lobe epilepsy surgery. *Can J Neurol Sci* 2000;**27**(**suppl 1**):S39–S43.
6. Tukel K, Jasper H. The electroencephalogram in parasagittal lesions. *Electroencephalogr Clin Neurophysiol* 1952;**4**:481–94.
7. Penfield W, Jasper H. *Epilepsy and the functional anatomy of the human brain*. Boston: Little, Brown, 1954: 94.

Nocturnal Seizures in a Man with Coronary Disease

P Barton Duell

HISTORY

A 69-year-old man experienced three episodes of generalized tonic–clonic seizures that occurred at 3.00 or 4.00 AM, during sleep. The seizures were observed by his wife. His mental status after each seizure was consistent with a postictal state.

He had a history of stable asymptomatic coronary artery disease, combined hyperlipidemia, treated hypothyroidism, and an increased body mass index of $31 \, kg/m^2$. He had undergone coronary artery bypass surgery at the age of 62 but had no history of myocardial infarction. He subsequently had percutaneous coronary angioplasty three times between the ages of 67 and 68. He had been a non-smoker for 30 years. He rarely consumed alcoholic beverages.

His mother, father, and paternal grandfather had died from cerebrovascular accidents at the ages of 94, 79, and 80, respectively. He had no personal or family history of seizures, but he had sustained mild head trauma without loss of consciousness 1½ years previously.

His medications were niacin (500 mg three times a day orally), aminosalicylic acid (81 mg/day orally), and desiccated porcine thyroid gland (1.5 grains [90 mg]/day orally).

EXAMINATION AND INVESTIGATIONS

His neurological examination was unremarkable and non-focal. The results of brain computerized tomography and brain magnetic resonance imaging were normal. A cardiovascular evaluation did not reveal evidence of myocardial ischemia or cardiac arrhythmias.

He was subsequently found to have nocturnal hypoxemia caused by obstructive sleep apnea, which was ameliorated by treatment with continuous positive airway pressure (CPAP) during sleep.

s0030

DIAGNOSIS

p0070

Generalized tonic–clonic seizures precipitated by nocturnal hypoxemia caused by obstructive sleep apnea.

s0040

TREATMENT AND OUTCOME

p0080

He was initially treated with phenytoin 400 mg/day in divided doses for control of seizures. CPAP used at night alleviated the episodic hypoxemia. He remained seizure-free for 1 year after discontinuation of phenytoin until he traveled to an altitude of about 2100 m and slept without using his CPAP machine (the altitude at home was about 100 m). After that single seizure, he had no additional seizures during the subsequent 12 years.

s0050

COMMENTARY

p0090

I chose this case for several reasons. First, the new onset of seizures in a 69-year-old man with coronary atherosclerosis is often attributable to causes such as cerebrovascular disease, cardiac arrhythmias, hypotension, embolic phenomena, metabolic abnormalities, and intracranial tumors or other intracranial pathology.[1] Despite the increased prevalence of obstructive sleep apnea among overweight patients, this diagnosis is often not considered in patients with seizure disorders. Moreover, patients are not always able to characterize the timing of their seizures well enough to delineate a purely nocturnal pattern of occurrence.

p0100

Second, although the patient's previous mild head trauma could have caused brain injury that resulted in the development of an epileptogenic focus, such pathology alone was insufficient to explain his seizures. It is plausible that an epileptogenic focus was unmasked by hypoxemia resulting from obstructive sleep apnea.

p0110

Third, because the patient had only a limited number of seizures, it was not initially apparent that his seizures always occurred nocturnally during the middle of sleep. This observation narrowed the differential diagnosis and led to the diagnosis of obstructive sleep apnea.

s0060

What did I learn from this case?

p0120

Obstructive sleep apnea is an under-diagnosed condition that is associated with severe health consequences. Although this diagnosis is sometimes suggested by a characteristic constellation of symptoms, many of the symptoms are non-specific and easily disregarded by patients and their health-care providers. In some cases, seizures are the presenting sign of sleep apnea,[2–4] as in this patient. A prospective study of 283 adult epilepsy patients identified obstructive sleep apnea in 15.4% of males and 5.4% of females.[5] Patients with epilepsy and obstructive sleep apnea were older, more frequently male, sleepier, experienced onset of seizures at a later age, and had higher body weight compared to subjects with epilepsy only.[5] Another prospective study of 39 candidates for epilepsy surgery identified obstructive sleep apnea in 33% of patients.[6] Affected patients were more likely to be older, male, have a higher Sleep Apnea Scale of the Sleep Disorders Questionnaire (SA-SDQ) score, and were more likely to have seizures during sleep.[6] Thus, obstructive sleep apnea appears to be common in epilepsy patients, particularly among older overweight men with seizures during sleep, as characterized by the patient in this case report.

Treatment of sleep apnea in children[7] and adults[8] with epilepsy has been shown to improve seizure control, as predicted. In one study of three adults and one child with obstructive sleep apnea, treatment with CPAP for 8 weeks was associated with at least a 45% reduction in seizure frequency.[9] In another study of seven patients treated for sleep apnea, three patients became seizure-free and one experienced a 95% reduction in seizures, but three had <50% improvement in seizure frequency while taking the same antiseizure medications.[10]

Polysomnography testing also has been shown to identify previously unrecognized nocturnal seizures in some patients,[8] but it is important to be aware that subclinical rhythmic electrographic discharge of adults (SREDA) can be observed as an uncommon non-seizure finding during all stages of sleep (including rapid eye movement [REM] sleep).[11] In addition, patients with a seizure disorder may experience an increase in the frequency of seizures if they develop obstructive sleep apnea,[12] a situation that could occur as a consequence of marked weight gain.[13] In one retrospective study, 21 of 27 patients (78%) with epilepsy experienced a clear increase in seizure frequency after the onset of obstructive sleep apnea.[14] The SA-SDQ, a 12-item validated measure of sleep-related breathing disorders, can be a useful screening tool for identifying obstructive sleep apnea in some patients with seizure disorders,[6] but the sensitivity of 75–80% and specificity of 65–67% are suboptimal.[15] Excessive daytime sleepiness was more prevalent in 26 children with seizure disorders compared to matched controls (OR for daytime sleepiness 15.3) and was associated with a 38.5% prevalence of sleep-disordered breathing (assessed with the Pediatric Sleep Questionnaire [PSQ] and Pediatric Daytime Sleepiness Scale [PDSS]).[16]

Patients who present with sleep apnea appear to have an increased risk of seizures. The results of a retrospective study from Prague suggest that 19 (4%) of 480 adult patients with sleep apnea had experienced at least two seizures in adulthood.[17] The mean age of the 19 patients at the time of the initial seizure was 48 ± 16 years; their mean body mass index was 32 ± 10 kg/m^2. Despite the limitations of this study, the results suggested that patients with sleep apnea may have a higher prevalence of seizures than the general population, which has been estimated to be 0.5–1.0% in Minnesota, USA.[18]

In summary, hypoxemia resulting from sleep apnea can precipitate seizures or exacerbate an underlying seizure disorder. Thus, it may be useful to consider the possibility of sleep apnea in patients who are being evaluated for seizures, particularly among those in whom seizures occur exclusively during sleep. Obstructive sleep apnea is also more common among epilepsy patients who are older, male, overweight, and have a later age of onset of seizures. In addition, patients who are being treated for sleep apnea and nocturnal hypoxemia, but who are not known to have a seizure disorder, may warrant careful assessment and monitoring for the possibility of hypoxemia-induced seizure activity.

REFERENCES

1. Stephen LJ, Brodie MJ. Epilepsy in elderly people. *Lancet* 2000;**355**:1441–6.
2. McNamara ME. Detection of sleep apnea during standard ambulatory cassette EEG recording for seizures: two case reports. *Clin Electroencephalogr* 1990;**21**:168–9.

3. Bradley TD, Shapiro CM. ABC of sleep disorders. Unexpected presentations of sleep apnoea: use of CPAP in treatment. *BMJ* 1993;**306**:1260–2.

4. Yanaihara T, Yokoba M, Kubota M, *et al.* Recurrent pulmonary edema associated with obstructive sleep apnea syndrome. *Nihon Kokyuki Gakkai Zasshi* 2006;**44(11)**:812–16.

5. Manni R, Terzaghi M, Arbasino C, Sartori I, Salimberti CA, Tartara A. Obstructive sleep apnea in a clinical series of adult epilepsy patients: frequency and features of the comorbidity. *Epilepsia* 2003;**44(6)**:836–40.

6. Malow BA, Levy K, Maturen K, Bowes R. Obstructive sleep apnea is common in medically refractory epilepsy patients. *Neurology* 2000;**55(7)**:1002–7.

7. Koh S, Ward SL, Lin M, Chen LS. Sleep apnea treatment improves seizure control in children with neurodevelopmental disorders. *Pediatr Neurol* 2000;**22**:36–9.

8. Malow BA, Fromes GA, Aldrich MS. Usefulness of polysomnography in epilepsy patients. *Neurology* 1997;**48(5)**:1389–94.

9. Malow BA, Weatherwax KJ, Chervin RD, *et al.* Identification and treatment of obstructive sleep apnea in adults and children with epilepsy: a prospective pilot study. *Sleep Medicine* 2003;**4(6)**:509–15.

10. Vaughn BV, D'Cruz OF, Beach R, Messenheimer JA. Improvement of epileptic seizure control with treatment of obstructive sleep apnoea. *Seizure* 1996;**5(1)**:73–8.

11. Fleming WE, Avidan A, Malow BA. Subclinical rhythmic electrographic discharge of adults (SREDA) in REM sleep. *Sleep Medicine* 2004;**5(1)**:77–81.

12. Bazil CW. Sleep and epilepsy. *Curr Opin Neurol* 2000;**13(2)**:171–5.

13. Lambert MV, Bird JM. Obstructive sleep apnoea following rapid weight gain secondary to treatment with vigabatrin (Sabril). *Seizure* 1997;**6**:233–5.

14. Hollinger P, Khatami R, Gugger M, Hess CW, Bassetti CL. Epilepsy and obstructive sleep apnea. *European Neurology* 2006;**55(2)**:74–9.

15. Weatherwax KJ, Lin X, Marzec ML, Malow BA. Obstructive sleep apnea in epilepsy patients: the Sleep Apnea scale of the Sleep Disorders Questionnaire (SA-SDQ) is a useful screening instrument for obstructive sleep apnea in a disease-specific population. *Sleep Medicine* 2003;**4(6)**:517–21.

16. Maganti R, Hausman N, Koehn M, Sandok E, Glurich I, Mukesh BN. Excessive daytime sleepiness and sleep complaints among children with epilepsy. *Epilepsy Behav* 2006;**8(1)**:272–7.

17. Sonka K, Juklickova M, Pretl M, Dostalova S, Horinek D, Nevsimalova S. Seizures in sleep apnea patients: occurrence and time distribution. *Sb Lek* 2000;**101**:229–32.

18. Hauser WA, Annegers JF, Kurland JF. Incidence of epilepsy and unprovoked seizures in Rochester, Minnesota. *Epilepsia* 1993;**34**:453–68.

FURTHER READING

Duell PB. Role of sleep apnoea in epilepsy in elderly people. *Lancet* 2000;**356**:162. [A brief synopsis of this case was previously published in this paper.]

16

Non-convulsive Status Epilepticus and Frontal Lobe Seizures in a Patient with a Chromosome Abnormality

Maurizio Elia

HISTORY

The patient is a 27-year-old man who developed normally until his first seizure at 3 years of age. Initially, his seizures were characterized by myoclonic jerks of the upper limbs. The seizures increased in frequency until they occurred many times a day during infancy. Over time the seizures changed and began to include impaired consciousness, pallor, abdominal pain, the expression of fear, mydriasis, motor automatisms, and complex visual hallucinations. They often had a long duration and occurred in clusters. Other seizures were characterized by a staring gaze, diffuse hypertonia, and clonic jerks of the upper limbs.

Polytherapy with phenobarbital, carbamazepine, valproate, and phenytoin had little effect.

When the patient came to my attention, there were behavioral disturbances with frequent and sudden outbursts of rage. Daily episodes of non-convulsive status epilepticus occurred out of wakefulness, characterized by clouding of consciousness, unresponsiveness to stimuli, crying or expression of terror, gestures, and verbal automatisms. He was also having several partial seizures at night that were characteristic of seizures of frontal lobe onset.

The patient was born at term and delivery was uneventful. His mother suffered from epilepsy and took antiepileptic drugs during pregnancy.

EXAMINATION AND INVESTIGATIONS

No gross dysmorphic features were evident. Neurological examination showed only a subtle postural tremor of the hands.

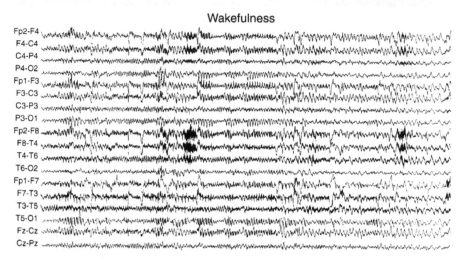

f0010   FIGURE 16.1   EEG recording during non-convulsive status epilepticus showing quasi-continuous diffuse slow spike-and-wave complexes and slow waves, which are sometimes intermixed with brief runs of 4–5 Hz spike-and-wave complexes.

p0060   A magnetic resonance imaging (MRI) scan of the brain was normal. Evaluation with the Wechsler Adult Intelligence Scale revealed mild mental retardation (full-scale IQ 64, verbal IQ 60, performance IQ 73). Interictal EEG was characterized by long sequences of slow spike-and-wave complexes that were more prominent over the frontal regions of both hemispheres. During non-convulsive status epilepticus, diffuse slow spike-and-wave complexes and slow waves were quasi-continuous and sometimes intermixed with brief runs of 4–5 Hz spike-and-wave complexes (Figure 16.1). Ictal EEG showed an initially diffuse low-voltage fast activity, which was more evident over the frontal leads, followed by a short burst of rhythmic spike-and-wave complexes and then by pseudoperiodic runs of slow waves for many seconds. The recruiting rhythm was accompanied by a tonic contraction of deltoid muscles.

p0070   The patient's karyotype showed 46, XY/46, XY, r(20) (p13q13.3) 90% mosaic.

s0030   # DIAGNOSIS

p0080   Non-convulsive status epilepticus and frontal lobe seizures due to ring chromosome 20 [r(20)] syndrome.

s0040   # TREATMENT AND OUTCOME

p0090   Treatment with phenytoin 300 mg/day, lamotrigine 200 mg/day, felbamate 2100 mg/day, and vigabatrin 3000 mg/day in different combinations did not control the episodes of status epilepticus or the partial seizures.

COMMENTARY

In recent years, several chromosomal syndromes have been identified that seem to show a peculiar clinical and EEG picture, such as Angelman syndrome, fragile X syndrome, Miller–Dieker syndrome, and Wolf–Hirschhorn syndrome. However, on very few other occasions have seizures and EEG characteristics been described in detail, which would be necessary to define an electroclinical phenotype and eventually to classify the epilepsy syndrome. Furthermore, it is conceivable that other chromosomal abnormalities would manifest a specific electroclinical picture that could help the epileptologist to choose the genetic analysis to be carried out as well as helping to identify specific genes that influence the process of epileptogenesis.

This case fully confirms that r(20) syndrome represents a new model of a symptomatic partial epilepsy, which certainly deserves to be included in a future classification of epileptic syndromes and diseases.

What did I learn from this case?

This case aroused my interest for several reasons. The r(20) syndrome has been reported in more than 50 cases, mostly sporadic or mosaic. Patients with r(20) syndrome present with mental retardation of varying degree and no gross dysmorphic features apart from rare heart or urogenital anomalies. An assessment of all reported cases has revealed that the ratio of mosaicism is significantly associated with age at seizure onset, intelligence quotient and malformation, but not with the response of epilepsy to drug treatment.

Seizures are present in 90% of cases and are invariably intractable. They begin at between 1 month and 21 years of age and are mostly complex partial seizures or partial seizures with secondary generalization, sometimes with a frontal pattern, sometimes induced by emotions or by playing video games.

Some patients with r(20) syndrome responding to vagus nerve stimulation have been reported.

The r(20) syndrome represents a newly described and peculiar combination of clinical findings and seizure patterns, including – mostly in adolescents and adults – episodes of non-convulsive status epilepticus that often herald the onset of seizures and that occur in many cases with a daily or weekly frequency, lasting 10–50 min. It should be emphasized that some ictal manifestations, such as those observed in this case, could be misdiagnosed as behavioral changes. Interictal EEG shows slow waves, spikes, sharp waves, or spike-and-wave complexes over the frontal regions. The ictal EEG is characterized by long runs of slow waves intermixed with high-voltage spikes, which are diffusely prominent over the frontal regions and changing in frequency during the discharges. Moreover, bursts of 5-Hz theta-waves, sometimes without apparent clinical manifestations, have been reported in r(20) syndrome. MRI evidence of frontal lobe dysplasias has been sporadically reported. Furthermore, a PET study showed that [18F]fluoro-l-DOPA uptake was significantly decreased bilaterally in the putamen and in the caudate nucleus of 14 patients with r(20) syndrome.

The pathophysiology of epilepsy in r(20) syndrome is not clearly understood, although it is known that the gene for autosomal-dominant nocturnal frontal epilepsy (CHRNA4) maps at the 20q13.2–q13.3 region. Other candidate genes, in the same region, are KCNQ2 gene related with familial benign neonatal convulsions and the melanocortin receptor gene (MC3R), which could be involved in the circadian pattern of epileptiform activity in r(20) syndrome. No mutations or deletions of these genes have been found until now in r(20) syndrome.

p0170   I think that routine cytogenetic studies should be performed in all patients who present with this clinical picture, particularly in the absence of clear malformations on MRI.

FURTHER READING

Augustijn PB, Parra J, Wouters CH, Joosten P, Lindhout D, van Emde Boas W. Ring chromosome 20 epilepsy syndrome in children: electroclinical features. *Neurology* 2001;**57**:1108–11.

Biraben A, Semah F, Ribeiro MJ, Douaud G, Remy P, Depaulis A. PET evidence for a role of the basal ganglia in patients with ring chromosome 20 epilepsy. *Neurology* 2004;**63**:73–7.

Canevini MP, Sgro V, Zuffardi O, *et al.* Chromosome 20 ring: a chromosomal disorder associated with a particular electroclinical pattern. *Epilepsia* 1998;**39**:942–51.

Inoue Y, Fujiwara T, Matsuda K, *et al.* Ring chromosome 20 and nonconvulsive status epilepticus: a new epileptic syndrome. *Brain* 1997;**120**:939–53.

Petit J, Roubertie A, Inoue Y, Genton P. Non-convulsive status in the ring chromosome 20 syndrome: a video illustration of 3 cases. *Epileptic Disord* 1999;**1**:237–41.

Ville D, Kaminska A, Bahi-Buisson N, Biraben A, Plouin P, Telvi L, Dulac O, Chiron C. Early pattern of epilepsy in the ring chromosome 20 syndrome. *Epilepsia* 2006;**47**:543–9.

17

An Unusual Cause of Nocturnal Attacks

Donald W Gross, Eva Andermann, David C Reutens, Udaya
Seneviratne, François Dubeau and Frederick Andermann

HISTORY

A 32-year-old right-handed man developed nocturnal attacks at the age of 6 months. These attacks were brief and associated with stiffening of the limbs without loss of consciousness. A diagnosis of nocturnal paroxysmal dystonia was entertained. Despite multiple trials of antiepileptic drugs, the attacks continued in clusters of 10–20 per night with several weeks between bouts.

EXAMINATION AND INVESTIGATIONS, TREATMENT AND OUTCOME

Neurological examination, interictal EEG and magnetic resonance imaging (MRI) were normal. Because of the uncertainty of the diagnosis, the patient had prolonged video–EEG monitoring. A total of 46 seizures with stereotyped clinical manifestations were recorded. The seizures started with facial movements and were sometimes associated with a groan. The patient would then sit up from sleep, stiffen and flex his upper limbs, and become apneic. Most attacks lasted less than 30 s, and longer attacks were associated with perioral cyanosis. During the seizures he retained awareness, and on some occasions he was able to respond to questioning. The postictal period was brief and there was no postictal slowing.

On reduced doses of antiepileptic drugs, the patient had two flurries of over 50 attacks a night, each bout being associated with a single generalized tonic–clonic seizure. During both these episodes, he required intubation and mechanical ventilation and developed a transient hypoxic encephalopathy.

After each flurry the seizures stopped spontaneously, but because of the dramatic history, carbamazepine 1000 mg/day and phenytoin 200 mg/day were continued.

p0050   Six years after the episode of status epilepticus, his nearly 4-year-old daughter developed similar nocturnal attacks. They were also associated with respiratory distress and tonic posturing, and they also occurred in clusters. Sleep EEG was normal. After the introduction of carbamazepine 200 mg/day she had a few attacks and then became seizure-free.

s0030   ## DIAGNOSIS

p0060   Autosomal dominant nocturnal frontal lobe epilepsy (ADNFLE).

s0040   ## COMMENTARY

p0070   ADNFLE is being increasingly diagnosed. Patients have normal MRI scans and often do not show interictal or ictal EEG abnormalities. Carbamazepine appears to be the most effective antiepileptic drug, but up to 30% could be refractory to treatment.[1,2]

p0080   We report an apparently sporadic case that for many years had presented a problem in diagnosis. The familial nature of this patient's epilepsy became apparent only when his younger daughter developed identical nocturnal attacks. Both had clusters of stereotyped nocturnal seizures with tonic posturing and respiratory distress.

p0090   The clinical syndrome in this family was that initially described as sporadic paroxysmal nocturnal dystonia.[3,4] Subsequent studies have established this to be a focal epilepsy of frontal lobe origin.[5] Seizures tend to occur during non-REM sleep, particularly stage 2 sleep. In addition to tonic and hyperkinetic seizures, paroxysmal arousals and nocturnal wandering have been described as different manifestations of nocturnal frontal lobe epilepsy.[6] A clue to the epileptic nature of the disorder in the father was the occurrence of a generalized tonic–clonic seizure during a flurry of attacks.

p0100   Another interesting finding is the striking remission in the father, which has also been previously reported.[7] In this patient a spontaneous remission is suspected, but owing to the severity of the previous symptoms, it has not been possible to withdraw the anticonvulsants.

p0110   Previously reported families have shown autosomal-dominant inheritance of the disorder.[4,5] It is possible that the proband in this family had a spontaneous mutation of the responsible gene; however, some of the previous families have been reported to have a low penetrance. The mutation could have occurred in a recent ancestor with lack of expression, or there may have been a failure of recognition of the syndrome in previous generations.[5]

p0120   Currently there are three genes known to be associated with ADNFLE. CHRNA4, CHRNB2, and CHRNA2 genes encode alpha-4, beta-2, and alpha-2 subunits of the neuronal nicotinic acetylcholine receptor, respectively. Mutations of these genes are considered to be the underlying cause of this syndrome. A possible aetio-pathogenic role of corticotrophin-releasing hormone gene in this condition has been suggested recently.[8] A missense mutation of the nicotinic acetylcholine receptor on chromosome 20q13.2–13.3 has been previously reported in two families with ADNFLE,[9] which was not found in this family. Some families demonstrate complete penetrance, whereas others show reduced penetrance (29–87%).[6] More recently there has been a suggestion of genetic heterogeneity in familial frontal lobe epilepsy.[10,11]

What did we learn from this case?

As the proband of this family presented as a sporadic case, it is possible that other sporadic cases may also prove to be familial, highlighting the importance of considering the diagnosis in apparently sporadic patients with frontal lobe epilepsy who do not have a demonstrable structural lesion.

REFERENCES

1. Provini F, Plazzi G, Tinuper P, et al. Nocturnal frontal lobe epilepsy: a clinical and polygraphic overview of 100 consecutive cases. Brain 1999;**122**:1017–31.
2. Oldani A, Zucconi M, Asselta R, et al. Autosomal dominant nocturnal frontal lobe epilepsy: a video-polysomnographic and genetic appraisal of 40 patients and delineation of the epileptic syndrome. Brain 1998;**121**:205–23.
3. Lugaresi E, Cirignotta F, Montagna P. Nocturnal paroxysmal dystonia. J Neurol Neurosurg Psychiatry 1986;**49**:375–80.
4. Lee BI, Lesser RP, Pippenger CE, et al. Familial paroxysmal hypnogenic dystonia. Neurology 1985;**35**:1357–60.
5. Scheffer IE, Bhatia KP, Lopes-Cendes I, et al. Autosomal dominant nocturnal frontal lobe epilepsy: a distinctive clinical disorder. Brain 1995;**118**:61–73.
6. Combi R, Dalpra L, Tenchini ML, Ferini-Strambi L. Autosomal dominant nocturnal frontal lobe epilepsy: a critical overview. J Neurol 2004;**251**:923–34.
7. Reutens DC, Andermann F, Olivier A, Andermann E, Dubeau F. Unusual features of supplementary sensorimotor area epilepsy: cyclic pattern, unusual sensory aura, startle sensitivity, anoxic encephalopathy, and spontaneous remission. In: Lüders HO, ed. Advances in neurology, vol 70. Philadelphia: Lippincott–Raven, 1996: 293–300.
8. Combi R, Dalpra L, Ferini-Strambi L, Tenchini ML. Frontal lobe epilepsy and mutations of the corticotropin-releasing hormone gene. Ann Neurol 2005;**58**:899–904.
9. Steinlein OK, Mulley JC, Propping P, et al. A missense mutation in the neuronal nicotinic acetylcholine receptor alpha 4 subunit is associated with autosomal dominant nocturnal frontal lobe epilepsy. Nature Genet 1995;**11**:201–3.
10. Berkovic SF, Scheffer JE. Genetics of human partial epilepsy. Curr Opin Neurol 1997;**10**:110–4.
11. DeMarco EV, Gambardella A, Annesi F, et al. Further evidence of genetic heterogeneity in families with autosomal dominant nocturnal frontal lobe epilepsy. Epilepsy Res 2007;**74**:70–3.

c00018

Myoclonic Jerks in a Computer Specialist

Dorotheé GA Kasteleijn-Nolst Trenité

s0010

HISTORY

p0010
A 32-year-old man was referred for evaluation of myoclonic jerks and dizziness while working in front of a computer. He owned his own computer firm.

p0020
He had experienced myoclonic jerks of the arms from the age of 8 years. These jerks generally occurred 1 min after he got out of bed and lasted from a few minutes to several hours. As a boy, he was noted to "spill his milk" and sometimes his legs "gave way." The myoclonic jerks occurred with or without loss of consciousness. Sleep deprivation, and more especially, stressful situations such as examinations, provoked seizures.

p0030
On his 16th birthday he had his first tonic–clonic seizure while driving his new motorcycle to school; according to his parents the road was "shiny." Within a period of 3 weeks, another two tonic–clonic seizures occurred without an aura. Treatment with valproate changed the seizure pattern. For the past 7 years he has had no more tonic–clonic seizures. However, myoclonic jerks and dizziness have continued to occur once in a while, such as shortly after wakening, but mainly when he works in front of a computer screen, particularly a bad quality black and white screen or a screen with a frequency of less than 70 Hz, regardless of color. He prefers to work with a gray background, without bright colors or pictures with colors and high contrast, such as a combination of yellow and blue. Furthermore, fast movements on the screen have caused dizziness.

p0040
Seizures have never occurred in front of a television set; in general, he avoids watching television but if he does, he keeps a distance between him and the set.

p0050
In addition, he has had myoclonic jerks triggered by malfunctioning fluorescent lighting. Other visual stimuli, such as sunlight through trees or on water, or black and white striped patterns (closing blinds, escalators) have never caused myoclonic jerks. Sailing is his hobby and he has never had seizures while doing this. Neither has driving been a problem – however, he nearly always wears dark brown sunglasses.

p0060
His current medication is valproate 2300 mg/day (the serum valproate concentration is 114 mg/l).

His family history is positive for epilepsy in his grandfather and uncle on his father's side. No further description is available.

EXAMINATION AND INVESTIGATIONS

On investigation, no neurological abnormalities were found and intelligence was normal. A computed tomography scan was normal. An EEG showed alpha activity, which was intermingled with sharp components; the alpha activity increased after hyperventilation. There were no spontaneous epileptiform discharges. Photic stimulation with flash frequencies between 2 and 60 Hz in the conditions eye closure, eyes closed, and eyes open was performed; pattern stimulation with black and white striped patterns was tested; and the patient was asked to watch a 50-Hz television showing various programs. Finally, a 70-Hz computer screen with scrolling text and graphic elements was used.

Generalized epileptiform discharges, which were maximal over the occipito-temporal areas, were recorded with photic stimulation at 30 and 40 Hz during eye closure; these discharges were associated with consistent dizziness. Epileptiform discharges, which were confined to the occipital area, occurred during photic stimulation at 23, 25, 30 and 50 Hz during eye closure, during photic stimulation at 25–40 Hz with eyes closed, and at a distance of 50 cm from the 50-Hz television set, which displayed a computer game, a flashing black and white video clip, and an advertisement. Dizziness was again noted. The pattern on the 70-Hz computer monitor did not evoke abnormalities.

DIAGNOSIS

Juvenile myoclonic epilepsy with photosensitivity, and sensitivity for specific visual stimuli.

TREATMENT AND OUTCOME

At work, the patient started to use only a 135-Hz monitor and his complaints of dizziness and jerks disappeared. His morning jerks continued.

COMMENTARY

This case shows that a history of dizziness and jerks, eyelid myoclonia, or loss of consciousness should be taken seriously. As in this case, most patients note myoclonia or dizziness during diffuse or generalized epileptiform discharges evoked by photic stimulation or other visual stimuli such as television (only classical absence seizures are not noticed by the patients themselves). This is very useful knowledge for patients. They can find out what visual stimuli in daily life cause risks. By closing one eye or switching off the television or computer screen as soon as signs and symptoms occur, they can reduce the risk of having a tonic–clonic seizure, unless they are extremely photo-sensitive and not taking anti-epileptic medication.

Another reason I chose this case is that this patient had a combination of sponta-neous seizures, typical for juvenile myoclonic epilepsy, and a clear history of photo-sensitive epilepsy. Although it is known that 30% of patients with juvenile myoclonic epilepsy show a photoparoxysmal response in their EEG, a history of visually induced seizures is often lacking. This could result from difficulty in discriminating between seizures that occur spontaneously and seizures that are visually induced, or from lack of knowledge about the possibility of provocation of seizures by television, sunlight, or visual patterns.

Finally, this case shows how patients can learn to avoid certain situations; this patient restricted his proximity to a television screen and wore dark sunglasses while driving or sailing.

What did I learn from this case?

I learnt that patients can be sensitive to very specific visual stimuli. This patient had a history of computer-induced seizures but not television-induced seizures, which to my knowledge was very unlikely. He had myoclonic jerks caused by malfunction-ing fluorescent lighting but never had seizures elicited by sunlight on water or sun-light through trees. This apparent inconsistency in clinical history proved to be in line with the EEG investigations in which all kinds of visual stimuli were used to provoke photosensitivity.

This case also taught me that even with a very high dosage of valproate (2300 mg/day), a reaction to visual stimuli was still present. The tonic–clonic seizures disappeared but the myoclonic jerks (both the spontaneous jerks and the visually induced jerks) did not change with valproate therapy.

ACKNOWLEDGEMENT

I would like to thank P Voskuil, neurologist from the Hans Berger Clinic in Breda, Holland, for refer-ring this patient to me. I am also grateful to the EEG technician, E Dekker (SEIN).

The author was supported by an FP6 program 2005-Marie Curie Excellence grant 024224.

FURTHER READING

Harding GFA, Jeavons PM. *Photosensitive epilepsy*. London: Heinemann, 1994.

Kasteleijn-Nolst Trenité DGA, Pinto D, Hirsch E, Takahashi T. Photosensitivity, visually induced seizures and epileptic syndromes. In: Roger J, Bureau M, Dravet Ch, Genton P, Tassinari CA, Wolf P, eds. *Epileptic syndromes in infancy, childhood and adolescence*, 4th ed. UK: John Libbey & Co, 2005: 395–420. Chapter 26.

Piccioli M, Vigevano F, Buttinelli V, Kasteleijn-Nolst Trenité DGA. Do videogames evoke different types of epileptic seizures? *Epilepsy Behav* 2005;**7**(**3**):524–30.

Ricci S, Vigevano F, Manfredi M, Kasteleijn-Nolst Trenite DGA. Epilepsy provoked by television and video games: safety of 100 Hz screens. *Neurology* 1998;**50**:790–3.

Ricci S, Vigevano F. The effect of video-game software in video-game epilepsy. *Epilepsia* 1999; **40(suppl 4)**:31–7.

Wilkins AJ, Darby CE, Binnie CD, Stefensson SB, Jeavons PM, Harding GFA. Television epilepsy: the role of pattern. *Electroencephalogr Clin Neurophysiol* 1979;**47**:163–71.

Wilkins AJ. *Visual stress*. Oxford: Oxford University Press, 1995.

c00019

Their Previous Physicians had Told Them that They Should not Become Pregnant Because They have Epilepsy

Barbara L Phillips, Ronald E Kramer and Kirsten A Bracht

s0010

HISTORY

p0010
The first case involves a 39-year-old right-handed woman who presented for evaluation of uncontrolled seizures. Seizure onset had been at the age of 10, when she had presented with a generalized tonic–clonic convulsion. She was placed on medication at that time but her seizures continued.

p0020
Her seizures were described as generalized tonic–clonic convulsions. They occur approximately once a year. In addition, the patient has seizures that are thought to be possible complex partial seizures. These are characterized as a change in mental status with a behavioral arrest, followed by eye fluttering and some subtle picking motions of the upper extremities. These seizures last less than 30 s. They tend to occur in clusters that last for 1–2 h, and they occur on a monthly basis.

p0030
The seizures were thought to be related to menstrual periods but she was unable to document any such correlation on seizure logs. Sleep deprivation did exacerbate the patient's tonic–clonic seizures.

p0040
The patient had a history of a vascular headache disorder, which was quiescent. She was gravida 0, para 0. She was a high school graduate who was attending a business school to become a court reporter. She denied tobacco or alcohol use. A maternal first cousin suffered from recurrent generalized tonic–clonic seizures. Her brother had suffered one generalized tonic–clonic seizure but was not being treated. Her mother had a history of migraine headaches.

p0050
Her previous physicians had told her that she should not become pregnant because she has epilepsy.

p0060
The second case also involves a 39-year-old right-handed woman, who presented with two unprovoked generalized tonic–clonic seizures at the age of 37. She had been

Puzzling Cases of Epilepsy

placed on valproate after her second seizure and remained seizure-free on valproate monotherapy.

Her past medical history was notable for two episodes of deep vein thromboses in the left lower extremity, at the ages of 23 and 37, which had been treated with aspirin. Coagulopathy workup had been negative. The patient had a 2-year history of a vascular headache disorder. While on valproate she remained free of headaches.

The patient was a gravida 2, para 1 female at presentation. She had a 7-year-old daughter who was alive and well. She was a college graduate working as an accountant. Her family history revealed a migraine headache disorder in her mother. Coronary artery disease had occurred in a brother at the age of 46 and in her father at the age of 51.

The patient had recently been told by her referring physicians that because she now had a seizure disorder and was on seizure medications she could not get pregnant.

EXAMINATIONS AND INVESTIGATIONS

In the first patient, the neurological examination was unremarkable. A previous computed tomography scan and EEG were reported as normal. The patient had a magnetic resonance imaging (MRI) scan, which was also normal. Video–EEG monitoring demonstrated generalized spike–wave discharges interictally as well as in association with her clinical events.

In the second patient, the neurological examination was also unremarkable. MRI showed non-specific white matter changes consistent with small vessel disease that was felt to be mildly excessive for her age. Routine sleep-deprived EEG showed a bilateral, intermittent frontotemporal dysrhythmia, maximal over the left frontotemporal region.

DIAGNOSES

The first patient was diagnosed with primary generalized epilepsy characterized by primary generalized tonic–clonic seizures and atypical absence seizures.

The second patient was diagnosed with seizure disorder secondary to small vessel disease of the brain. It was unclear whether chronic epilepsy existed in the patient and needed treatment.

TREATMENTS AND OUTCOMES

The first patient had been previously maintained on a four-drug regimen: carbamazepine 800 mg/day, acetazolamide 200 mg/day, ethosuximide 500 mg/day, and phenobarbital 60 mg/day.

After our diagnosis had been established, medication simplification and switches were attempted. Side effects occurred with valproate monotherapy and then with felbamate monotherapy. Monotherapy with lamotrigine and with topiramate were each unsuccessful because of lack of seizure control. The patient was maintained on a regimen of lamotrigine 500 mg/day and topiramate 200 mg/day. She did not suffer any further generalized tonic–clonic seizures and her atypical absence clusters were reduced to occasional isolated seizures every few weeks.

p0160   After her first evaluation and visit, issues of epilepsy and pregnancy were discussed. The patient was told about her options and placed on supplemental folic acid. Once the patient had been stabilized on a combination of lamotrigine and topiramate, she became pregnant. Amniocentesis and ultrasound performed at 18 weeks gestation were normal and no complications or malformations were expected according to the obstetrician in the high-risk obstetrical clinic.

p0170   The second patient was told that she was a candidate for medication withdrawal since she had remained seizure-free for over 2 years and her diagnosis was somewhat in doubt. She had been maintained on valproate monotherapy 1250 mg/day with levels running approximately 40 μg/ml. Because of her concerns regarding recurrent seizures, this was continued and she was placed on supplemental folic acid.

p0180   On follow-up, she became pregnant with twins. She remained seizure-free during the pregnancy on her baseline dose of valproate. During the end of her first trimester she suffered another deep venous thrombosis in her left lower extremity and was placed on heparin for the remainder of her pregnancy. Repetitive ultrasounds were all normal and no complications were anticipated by the obstetrical staff.

p0190   Both women completed their pregnancies successfully by C-sections without complication. The babies had normal examinations and obtained normal developmental milestones on time. No subsequent developmental problems with the children have been reported to the authors since these cases were first reported.

s0050   ## COMMENTARY

p0200   The first patient presented had seizures that were uncontrolled with polypharmacy. The second patient had significant systemic disease and seizures that were controlled with monotherapy. Both women had been explicitly instructed by previous physicians not to have children because they had epilepsy. They were following these instructions when they arrived at our epilepsy center, although they both wished to become pregnant. After several counseling sessions, they chose to become pregnant in full understanding and acceptance of the risks involved.

p0210   The majority of pregnancies in women with epilepsy proceed without complications. There are, of course, increased risks to both mother and child. Some of these risks extend beyond the pregnancy itself in regard to long-term effects of drug exposure in utero or potential drug exposure to the baby if breast feeding is a consideration by the mother. Historically, there have been prejudices against any person with epilepsy becoming pregnant and there were laws in the USA to regulate fertility and marriage as late as the 1980s.[1]

p0220   An increase in seizure frequency during pregnancy occurs in only 20–30% of patients.[2,3] This increase may reflect altered metabolism or altered pharmacokinetics of antiepileptic drugs during pregnancy. Non-compliance is an important issue to address. Women with seizures have an increased risk of obstetrical complications, including anemia, hyperemesis gravidarum, preeclampsia, premature labor, and abruptio placentae from trauma.[4]

p0230   Blood levels of AEDs can be significantly altered during pregnancy for both physiologic (i.e. pharmacokinetic) and social (i.e. non-compliance with oral intake) reasons. Take, for example, the recent findings regarding lamotrigine. Pregnancy is known to increase the clearance of lamotrigine by at least >65% and, in some reports, up to

300% between conception and the second and third trimesters.[5,6] Baseline blood level of lamotrigine should be done during pregnancy planning. Levels should be monitored, especially in the first two trimesters, when dose increases are frequently needed.[6] Soon after delivery, lamotrigine clearance returns to baseline and the dose must be rapidly reduced to the prepregnancy amount to avoid drug toxicity.

Congenital malformations are more frequent in the offspring of women with epilepsy and risks are further enhanced by antiepileptic drugs. Minor and major anomalies can occur up to three times more often in women with epilepsy, with risks increasing almost exponentially as the number of drugs increases.[7] Although fetal exposure is usually an unavoidable risk, drug withdrawals before conception should always be considered in women whose seizures have been controlled for a reasonably long period of time, usually greater than 2 years, or in whom the diagnosis is suspect. Prolonged EEG testing with ambulatory or video–EEG equipment may aid in the decision to withdraw medication or not.

Prenatal counseling is the most critical aspect in managing women of child-bearing potential. Physicians should follow published guidelines.[3,7] The goals of these guidelines are:

- to obtain patient compliance with a proactive treatment plan;
- to minimize drug burden;
- to maximize seizure control;
- to monitor fetal development with the patient's goals in mind; and
- to communicate frequently and often with the obstetrical team prior to delivery.

What did we learn from these cases?

Even today, older approaches and historic biases in regard to epilepsy and pregnancy still exist in the medical community. Some physicians may feel the need to provide guidance that absolutely guarantees a good outcome – a goal that is, of course, impossible to achieve. Physicians may also feel pressured to make decisions that are really best left to the patient and her partner in regard to the issues that surround epilepsy and pregnancy.

How did these cases alter our approach to the care and treatment of our epilepsy patients?

Similar cases and issues come up frequently in our epilepsy clinic. As a result, we now discuss family planning issues at the very first visit with all women of child-bearing potential. A separate visit is set aside solely to discuss the issues of pregnancy and epilepsy. Such an approach is especially needed in today's medical environment in which time pressures for clinicians keep increasing.

We now understand that there are never any absolute right or wrong answers about epilepsy and pregnancy. The physician's roles are to provide education, statistics, and a risk–benefit analysis that helps the patient make decisions, then to implement the safest and most medically sound treatment plan with the patient's goals in mind. It is up to the patient to make an informed decision. Some patients may require a more active level of leadership from the physician, but we believe that most patients and couples can integrate this medical information in the context of their own life choices.

REFERENCES

1. Engel J Jr. Psychosocial management. In: Engel J Jr, ed. *Seizures and epilepsy*. Philadelphia: FA Davis, 1989: 475–90.
2. Cantrell DC, Riela SJ, Ramus R, Riela AR. Epilepsy and pregnancy: a study of seizure frequency and patient demographics. *Epilepsia* 1997;**38(suppl 8)**:231.
3. Morrell MJ. Guidelines for the care of women with epilepsy. *Neurology* 1998;**51(suppl 4)**:517–21.
4. Foldvary N. Treatment of epilepsy during pregnancy. In: Wyllie E, ed. *The treatment of epilepsy: principles and practice*, 3rd ed. Baltimore: Williams and Wilkins, 2001: 769–86.
5. Tran TA, Leppik IE, Blesi K, Sathanandan ST, Remmel R. Lamotrigine clearance during pregnancy. *Neurology* 2002;**59(2)**:251–5.
6. Tomson T, Battino D. Pharmacokinetics and therapeutic drug monitoring of newer antiepileptic drugs during pregnancy and the puerperium. *Clin Pharmacokinet* 2007;**46(3)**:209–9.
7. Delgado-Escueta AV, Janz D. Consensus guidelines: preconception counseling, management, and care of the pregnant woman with epilepsy. *Neurology* 1992;**42(suppl 5)**:149–60.

Status Epilepticus after a Long Day of White-Water Rafting in the Grand Canyon

David M Labiner

HISTORY

The patient was a 31-year-old woman who was vacationing in Arizona. After a long day of white-water rafting on the Colorado River in the Grand Canyon, she developed her first-ever seizures. They were described by a paramedic that witnessed them as being generalized tonic–clonic events that were associated with aspiration. She was taken to the closest hospital and treated with phenytoin and phenobarbital. After an initial improvement, she developed status epilepticus and was transferred to my facility. She was treated with pentobarbital for her status epilepticus and her seizures were controlled, but attempts to decrease the barbiturates caused further partial seizures with secondary generalization characterized by focal motor activity as well as generalized convulsive activity. Attempts to use both carbamazepine and valproate were not successful, owing to a marked increase in hepatic enzymes.

Family history was notable for psychiatric disease in two brothers.

EXAMINATION AND INVESTIGATIONS

The patient was intubated and on a ventilator. There were no focal neurological findings. Neuroimaging studies were negative. When the barbiturates were reduced, the EEG was compatible with status epilepticus, with multifocal epileptiform features.

Extensive evaluation of serum, spinal fluid, and urine were initially unrevealing. After approximately 90 days, a diagnosis of aminolevulinic acid dehydratase deficiency porphyria was made by red blood cell enzyme analysis.

DIAGNOSIS

Status epilepticus associated with aminolevulinic acid dehydratase deficiency porphyria.

85

s0040   TREATMENT AND OUTCOME

p0060   Once the diagnosis of porphyria was made, the patient was tapered off barbiturates and switched to intravenous lorazepam and then to oral clonazepam. She awoke from the prolonged drug-induced coma and was discharged from the hospital on clonazepam. However, she complained of memory problems and intermittent confusion as well as seizures. The seizures were characterized as periods of behavioral arrest and staring associated with automatisms, followed by up to 30 min of confusion. These events were felt to be consistent with complex partial seizures occurring up to 15 times a day.

p0070   Because of its cognitive side effects, the dose of clonazepam was slowly reduced. The patient was readmitted to the hospital with convulsive status epilepticus that was treated with lorazepam and paraldehyde. She was started on gabapentin 300 mg/day and her dose was rapidly increased to 900 mg/day. The patient had no further convulsive activity once the gabapentin was initiated. Her dose was further increased in increments of no greater than 300 mg twice a week. Seizure control was significantly improved at 1800 mg/day with no significant side effects. At higher doses, the patient had significant side effects, particularly somnolence and confusion.

p0080   The patient remained under adequate control for the next 9 months, when she developed pneumonia in the setting of an exacerbation of her porphyria and subsequently died. Her death was unrelated to seizures or the use of gabapentin.

s0050   COMMENTARY

p0090   This case represented an unusual case of partial epilepsy caused by a metabolic disorder. Seizures are not a major manifestation of the porphyrias, and the diagnosis was not made for 3 months despite appropriate screening 2 weeks after the onset of her symptoms. Porphyria syndromes are inherited in an autosomal–dominant fashion except for congenital erythropoietic porphyria, which is autosomal recessive. Although the abnormalities are present from birth, the symptoms typically do not appear until after puberty. The syndromes are characterized by acute attacks separated by latent periods. The primary neurological and psychological manifestations of the disorder are peripheral neuropathy, weakness, paresis, sensory abnormalities, respiratory paralysis, seizures, hyporeflexia, cranial nerve palsies, behavioral changes, irritability or anxiety, hallucinations, and depression.

p0100   Seizures associated with porphyria can be especially difficult to treat because many of the commonly used antiepileptic drugs can cause exacerbations of the syndrome. This phenomenon has been well documented for the barbiturates, phenytoin, and carbamazepine. Benzodiazepines, valproate, and even bromides have been advocated for treating seizures associated with porphyria.

s0060   **What did I learn from this case? How did this case alter my approach to the care and treatment of my epilepsy patients?**

p0110   Often we do not consider metabolic etiologies as a major cause of partial seizures and therefore miss the diagnosis of the underlying etiology. Apart from reacquainting myself with the diagnosis and features of porphyria, I realized that some of the treatments that were given to this patient (barbiturates and phenytoin) probably caused an exacerbation of her underlying disorder. Moreover, the nature of the disease often requires persistence and repeated testing to establish the diagnosis.

Additionally, gabapentin was not yet available in the USA nor was it known to be safe in treating seizures related to porphyria. Because of the desperate situation of this patient, we sought and obtained compassionate use of this drug based on what was known at the time about its lack of hepatic metabolism. We correctly reasoned that it would be safe to try gabapentin in this patient, and it turned out to be effective. Not only did we learn that gabapentin was a good anticonvulsant, we were able to use it as monotherapy to control this patient's seizures.

FURTHER READING

Desnick RJ. The porphyrias. In: Isselbacher KJ, Braunwald E, Wilson JD, Martin JB, Fauci AS, Kasper DL, eds. *Harrison's principles of internal medicine*. New York: McGraw-Hill, 1994: 2073–9.

Krauss GL, Simmons-O'Brien E, Campbell M. Successful treatment of seizures and porphyria with gabapentin. *Neurology* 1995;**45**:594–5.

Labiner DM, Ahern GL, Kolb MA, Johnson DS, Vengrow MI. Gabapentin is both safe and effective in treating seizures associated with porphyria. *Epilepsia* 1994;**35(suppl 8)**:53.

Reynolds NC Jr., Miska RM. Safety of anticonvulsants in hepatic porphyrias. *Neurology* 1981; **31**:480–4.

c00021

A Farmer Who Watched His Own Seizures

Gerhard Luef

s0010

HISTORY

p0010

The patient was a 37-year-old man with a history of epilepsy since the age of 3. Two different seizure types were described – episodes of altered consciousness and abnormal behavior, and transient loss of consciousness associated with tonic posturing and clonic limb movements and sometimes with loss of bladder control and lacerations of the tongue.

p0020

There was no family history of seizures. Pregnancy and delivery were normal; however, he had low birth weight and needed to be observed in an incubator. Developmental milestones in the first 3 years were unremarkable.

p0030

The patient had been treated with a number of different antiepileptic drugs including phenytoin, carbamazepine, valproate, primidone, vigabatrin, and topiramate, either alone or in combination, but he still had uncontrolled seizures. On a combination of topiramate 600 mg/day and phenytoin 350 mg/day (giving serum levels for phenytoin of 18.5 μg/ml and for topiramate of 6.9 μg/ml), his seizure severity was markedly reduced, but he still suffered from between about 7 and 10 complex partial seizures a month. The combination did, however, render him free of generalized tonic–clonic seizures.

p0040

The major problem for this patient, a farmer with poor educational background, was that he could not find a wife because of his seizures. After 8 months on stable dosages and plasma concentrations, he underwent a presurgical evaluation.

s0020

EXAMINATION AND INVESTIGATIONS

p0050

Clinical examination revealed no pathological findings. Neuropsychological examination found verbal and visual memory deficits and cognitive deficits. Several EEGs demonstrated diffuse slowing and intermittent theta-wave activity in the left fronto-temporal region. Magnetic resonance imaging scanning demonstrated gliosis in the left posterior cruz.

p0060

After withdrawal of his antiepileptic drugs, two seizures were recorded with video–EEG monitoring. The first event occurred while the patient was lying in bed. There were chewing automatisms followed by complex fine motor automatisms and dystonic posturing of the right arm and left leg, vocalization, and arrhythmic head movements. There was no response to an examining nurse and consciousness was impaired. The second event started from a sitting position and was similar to the first with automatisms, but this one was followed by a tonic–clonic seizure. Both seizures started with left frontal theta rhythm, followed by slowing in the left temporal region and ending with diffuse slowing.

DIAGNOSIS

Frontal lobe epilepsy with complex partial and secondary generalized seizures.

TREATMENT AND OUTCOME

Since medical treatment did not achieve complete seizure control, I recommended a presurgical evaluation. During 1 week of video–EEG monitoring, we recorded only two seizures and so monitoring was continued for another week. The patient was discharged on the same antiepileptic drug combination – topiramate and phenytoin – and a new date for epilepsy monitoring was set in 6 months.

During a lecture to students, he was asked if he would like to see the two seizures that had been recorded by video–EEG monitoring. He agreed. He was deeply impressed by seeing his own seizures and did not stop talking about his seizures over the next few days.

During a follow-up appointment 3 months after being sent home from the hospital, he reported having had six observed seizures in the first 3 weeks after discharge, with freedom from seizures since then. He went another 3 months without a seizure, and so the scheduled admission for repeat video–EEG monitoring was canceled.

He was last seen in November 2000 (3 years later) on the original combination of 600 mg topiramate and 350 mg phenytoin, and he was satisfied because his seizures had been completely eliminated.

COMMENTARY

Intractability is not an absolute phenomenon. Some patients are inadequately treated. Other patients who are labeled with chronic epilepsy do not in fact have epilepsy (e.g. some have pseudoseizures). As in this case, a small fraction of patients with intractable epilepsy will be rendered seizure-free by adjunctive therapy such as vagus nerve stimulation, EEG biofeedback, transcranial magnetic stimulation, or self-control techniques.

More than 50% of patients with seizures preceded by auras reported they were able to avoid complex partial seizures or secondary generalization by engaging in special behaviors.[1] These are very individual methods such as complex motoric manœuvres, relaxation techniques, and sensory stimulation (e.g. smell). Self-assertion might be another such method, as I believe occurred in this case.

What did I learn from this case?

Epilepsies are a heterogeneous group of disorders. The prognosis depends more on the etiology of the seizures and the clinical background of the patient than on the seizures or the treatment prescribed. Psychosocial aspects of the disorder frequently have the most far-reaching implications for the patient and family, and this should be borne in mind when planning comprehensive management.

Present-day pharmacological and neurosurgical options offer more solutions for our patients than ever before. However, it is the information about the various aspects of epilepsy that we provide patients which helps them the most in achieving optimal seizure control. In this case, the information that made the greatest difference was having the patient watch the video–EEG recording.

This case taught me that patients undergoing a presurgical evaluation should always be offered the opportunity of watching their own seizures. In my experience, patients respond in one of two ways. Some deny that they have seizures, but most others are impressed by the experience, and some of them might have a therapeutic benefit, as in this case.

REFERENCE

1. Wolf P. Aura interruption: how does it become curative? In: Wolf P, ed. *Epileptic seizures and syndromes: with some of their theoretical implications.* London: J Libbey, 1994: 667–73.

The Borderland of Neurology and Cardiology

Martha J Morrell

HISTORY

FH is a 35-year-old right-handed woman entrepreneur who presented because of recent episodes of altered awareness. She had an unremarkable past medical history until 5 months before presentation, when the first episode occurred. She and her husband were dining out when she suddenly developed nausea and a headache. Although she had consumed one or two glasses of wine, she did not feel intoxicated. She requested that they leave and, while walking through the parking lot, became dizzy and diaphoretic. Her husband helped her to the car. While they were driving home, she became limp and pale and did not respond to her husband's voice or touch for at least 4 min. He called for emergency help and was met by an ambulance on the way home.

She was transported to a nearby hospital where she appeared groggy but oriented. Blood pressure and heart rate were normal, as was an electrocardiogram (ECG). She quickly returned to normal and was released home. She recalls nothing from the time she left the restaurant until she was in the emergency room.

The second episode occurred 2 weeks before her presentation. Her husband returned from an early Saturday morning errand and found her lying on the bathroom floor. She was confused and slow to respond, and said repeatedly, "I really feel sick" and "my head really, really hurts." There were no signs of trauma. The patient recalled being in the bedroom and did not know how she had got to the bathroom, which was on the other side of the house. As her husband helped her up, she vomited and was incontinent of urine.

She was taken by ambulance to her community hospital. For approximately 6 h she appeared confused. In the hospital, they noted that her tongue was bitten. Blood pressure and heart rate were unremarkable and an ECG was normal. A head computed tomography scan was negative. She returned home and fell deeply asleep for several hours. When she awoke, she remembered nothing of the event or the hospital evaluation.

Past medical history was remarkable for a 1-year history of bifrontal headaches with nausea. She had a syncopal episode in 1990 on a train, when she had become diaphoretic, complained, "I am not feeling well" and lost awareness. Her husband put p0060 her head down and she returned to normal within 1 min. She had no risk factors for epilepsy. She took no medications or recreational drugs.

Review of systems revealed episodes of mild light-headedness associated with menses. She recalled several nights of intense dreams, diaphoresis, and disrupted sleep over the past year.

p0070 Family history was negative for epilepsy, although her 55-year-old mother had a history of syncope and hypoglycemia, as well as headaches. Her father, two brothers, one sister, and an 18-month-old son were all in good health.

s0020 ## EXAMINATION AND INVESTIGATIONS

p0080 General and neurological examinations were unremarkable. A brain magnetic resonance imaging scan was normal, as was an ECG and awake and sleeping EEG. A tilt table test was normal.

p0090 In the midst of this evaluation, the patient had a third and fourth event. Both were preceded by nausea, an intense feeling of illness, diaphoresis, and pallor. The third occurred while at the hairdresser. She appeared groggy but conscious for 20 min and then returned to baseline. The fourth episode occurred at dinner. She was groggy and confused for 20 min, even though her husband lay her down on the floor and elevated her legs. While in this position, she stiffened and had a generalized tonic–clonic seizure with tongue biting and incontinence. She was taken by ambulance to her local emergency room, received phenytoin intravenously, and was admitted for 3 days. No further episodes occurred. Both ECG and EEG were normal, as were thyroid function tests and a glucose tolerance test. The patient declined her cardiologist's recommendation to have a cardiac pacemaker installed.

p0100 Three days later, she was taken off phenytoin and admitted for 5 days of continuous video–EEG monitoring with simultaneous ECG monitoring. No events occurred and no ECG or EEG abnormalities were detected. A second tilt table test was positive because of a typical event and significant bradycardia induced with isoproterenol.

s0030 ## INITIAL DIAGNOSIS, TREATMENT, AND OUTCOME

p0110 The patient was diagnosed with cardiogenic syncope. After obtaining a second and third cardiology consultation, she had a cardiac pacemaker implanted.

p0120 Eight months after the initial presentation, the patient's husband called and reported that she had perimenstrual episodes of confusion and memory loss.

p0130 Blood pressure (taken several times by him) was 110–120/50–60 mmHg each time and heart rate was 65–80 beats per minute. He was very concerned because of 2 days of repeated episodes of confusion and poor responsiveness with continuous profound memory impairment.

p0140 She was admitted to the hospital, where examination was remarkable for psychomotor retardation and amnesia. An EEG showed rhythmic right temporal delta activity. The patient and the EEG cleared with intravenous lorazepam, although she remained amnestic for events over 4 days. The pacemaker was interrogated and was functioning normally but was being repeatedly activated for heart rates less than 65 beats per minute.

SECOND DIAGNOSIS, TREATMENT, AND OUTCOME

The patient was diagnosed with right temporal lobe onset seizures and treated with carbamazepine. She continues to have one or two brief episodes at menses every two to four menstrual cycles. She has declined to change her medication regimen. The pacemaker is in place and working.

COMMENTARY

This patient has localization-related epilepsy of right anterior temporal lobe origin that causes cardiac rhythm disturbance. Her presentation was most consistent with decreased cerebral perfusion pressure leading to an alteration in consciousness and, on several instances, generalized tonic–clonic seizures. The diagnosis was difficult to make because of the unusual presentation and because sophisticated EEG and cardiac diagnostic testing were initially negative. Persistence paid off and a final diagnosis was ultimately achieved.

Cardiac rhythm changes are common with seizures. Nearly 40% of patients with medically intractable localization-related epilepsy display cardiac rhythm or repolarization abnormalities during or immediately after seizures recorded with continuous monitoring with ECG and EEG.[1] These cardiac rhythm and conduction abnormalities are seen more often in generalized tonic–clonic seizures than in complex partial seizures.

Ictal tachycardia is the most typical ictal cardiac rhythm disturbance. In one study of 92 seizures in 41 patients,[2] 82.5% developed ictal tachycardia. Changes in heart rate occurred before the onset of EEG seizure in 76.1% of seizures. Early tachycardia was more common in seizures of temporal lobe onset.

Ictal bradycardia is less common but not unusual; 3.3% of persons monitored during seizures with continuous video–EEG monitoring showed bradycardia just before or during the seizure.[2]

This patient had an ictal bradycardia syndrome that led to vasovagal syncope and a syncopal convulsion. This syndrome is seen most often in people with temporal lobe epilepsy.[3] Whether these cardiac rhythm disturbances increase the risk of sudden unexplained death is not known. However, given the potentially catastrophic consequences of this abnormality of cardiac rhythm, it seems prudent to implant a cardiac pacemaker, in addition to providing antiepileptic drugs.

Epileptic discharges may alter cardioregulatory regions of the brain, including the limbic cortex and hypothalamus. These autonomic changes may present as simple partial seizures or may occur without obvious ictal manifestations. Therefore, autonomic simple partial seizures can be difficult to diagnose.

Another interesting feature of this case is the catamenial pattern to her seizures. Between one-third and one-half of women with epilepsy have catamenial seizure patterns.[4] Cardiac events that display cyclical patterns associated with menstruation may represent autonomic seizures, and epilepsy should be considered in the differential diagnosis.

What did I learn from this case?

This case reinforced my appreciation of the importance of entertaining a broad differential diagnosis whenever a patient presents with paroxysmal episodes of altered consciousness. It may be very difficult to establish a definitive diagnosis in these cases. For this woman, the diagnosis could not be made definitely until the cardiac rhythm abnormality was controlled. The EEG changes induced by the cerebral hypoperfusion would most likely have obscured an ictal pattern. Therefore, re-evaluation with video–EEG monitoring after the pacemaker was implanted was appropriate.

s0070

How did this case alter my approach to the care and treatment of my epilepsy patients?

p0250

I believe that dual therapy – treatment of the seizures and the cardiac rhythm disturbance – is appropriate for seizures with autonomic features. For this patient, the after-effects of seizures included days of amnesia. This frightened her and affected her work performance, which required excellent recall of intricate financial dealings. My impression was that the prolonged amnesia was a consequence of the cerebral hypoperfusion rather than the ictal discharge itself. Since seizures in at least 30% of patients with localization-related epilepsy are not completely controlled with antiepileptic drugs, I think it is wise to provide prophylactic treatment for bradycardia in order to lessen the postictal symptoms. Although this approach is speculative, I believe that a patient like this is also at higher risk of sudden unexplained death and that the pacemaker provides a degree of protection.

REFERENCES

1. Nei M, Ho RT, Sperling MR. EKG abnormalities during partial seizures in refractory epilepsy. *Epilepsia* 2000;**41**:542–8.
2. Schernthaner C, Lindinger G, Potselberger K, *et al.* Autonomic epilepsy: the influence of epileptic discharges on heart rate and rhythm. *Wien Klin Wochenschr* 1999;**111**:392–401.
3. Reeves AL, Nollet KE, Klass DW, Sharbrough FW, So EL. The ictal bradycardia syndrome. *Epilepsia* 1996;**37**:983–7.
4. Morrell MJ. Epilepsy in women: the science of why it is special. *Neurology* 1999;**53**(suppl 1):S42–S48.

A Man with Shoulder Twitching

Erasmo A Passaro and Ahmad Beydoun

HISTORY

A 52-year-old left-handed man presented to the emergency room because of near-continuous twitching of his left shoulder. This shoulder twitching was irregular in frequency, lasted several minutes at a time, and waxed and waned in intensity. The twitching ceased when he was asleep and decreased in intensity when he was distracted.

With detailed questioning, the neurology house officer learned that the patient had intermittent twitching of his left calf muscle while gardening 5 days earlier. The following day, this twitching spread to his left quadriceps muscle and his abdominal muscles. He and his wife visited a local emergency room, at which time the twitching involved the entire left side of his body. He was placed on clonazepam and was scheduled for an outpatient neurology appointment. The report of the non-contrast brain computed tomography (CT) scan from the local emergency room was unremarkable except for a questionable right parietal hypodensity on a single slice. He denied loss of awareness, motor weakness or sensory changes with these events.

The past medical history was unremarkable. There was no recent history of head trauma, fever, or headache. There were no risk factors for stroke except for a history of heavy cigarette smoking, and no past history of transient ischemic attack or cerebral infarction. There was no history of alcohol or drug abuse. He had never experienced a similar type of event in the past.

His social history revealed that he had been happily married for several years and had a multiple pack-year smoking history. He had recently retired from the local fire department after several years of service.

EXAMINATION AND INVESTIGATIONS

The patient was afebrile with normal vital signs. Both his general physical examination and his neurological examination, which included normal strength and symmetric deep tendon reflexes, were unremarkable. The observed left shoulder twitching caused his proximal arm to move in an irregular manner. There was no clonic twitching in the proximal or distal arm or hand. The left shoulder twitching ceased when he was asleep or distracted. The twitching increased if he was asked to move his left arm voluntarily. The intensity of the twitching was variable. Suspecting that the events might be non-epileptic, the neurology house officer applied a saline patch to the patient's shoulder and the twitching appeared to subside. Interestingly, he was not significantly distressed about the twitching, although his wife was visibly upset.

p0060   A 21-channel digital EEG was performed. The left shoulder twitching was recorded. The EEG showed electromyographical artifact that correlated with the shoulder twitching; however, no significant change in the EEG activity from baseline was noted. Although this EEG was normal, he was admitted for video–EEG long-term monitoring because of the history earlier in the week of twitching in his calf with subsequent involvement of his left hemibody. Futhermore, the CT scan report of an equivocal hypodensity in the right parietal region raised further suspicion that these events might be epileptic in origin.

p0070   While he was monitored with video–EEG, his head was kept stationary to reduce movement artifact and to increase the possibility of identifying an EEG correlate. Furthermore, to facilitate the identification of an EEG correlate in the central region, the EEG was reformatted with a montage consisting of a longitudinal bipolar chain over the parasagittal region and transverse bipolar chains across the frontal, central, and parietal regions. The EEG sensitivity was increased to 5 µV/mm and the high-frequency filter was reduced to 15 Hz. With these maneuvers, a sharp wave was observed with maximal negativity at the right central electrode and the vertex electrode. This discharge occurred a few milliseconds before each left shoulder twitch.

s0030   ## DIAGNOSIS

p0080   Epilepsia partialis continua (EPC) involving the left deltoid muscle.

s0040   ## TREATMENT AND OUTCOME

p0090   The EPC persisted despite a phenytoin level of 18 µg/ml. A magnetic resonance imaging (MRI) scan with gadolinium enhancement revealed a large ring-enhancing lesion involving the high convexity of the right parietal lobe with significant surrounding edema. Twenty-four hours later, the patient developed progressive left hemiparesis over several hours. A repeat brain MRI showed that the lesion had doubled in size.

p0100   On the basis of this rapid increase in the size of the lesion, a brain abscess was suspected, and the patient was brought to the operating room for right parietal craniotomy and needle aspiration of the lesion. Neuropathology confirmed the presence of a brain abscess. He was placed on intravenous antibiotics for several weeks. Several months later, in follow-up, he had a mild decrease in the fine motor skills of his left hand that made it difficult for him to play the guitar. He has had no further seizures since his surgery.

s0050   ## COMMENTARY

p0110   The unusual features of this patient's left shoulder twitching raised the possibility that this event was non-epileptic in origin. In particular, the twitching was irregular and frequent but intermittent; it disappeared in sleep and decreased with distraction or when a sensory stimulus was applied to the shoulder.

EPC is a rare type of localization-related motor epilepsy; it is defined as spontaneous regular or irregular clonic twitching of cerebral cortical origin, sometimes aggravated by action or sensory stimuli, that is confined to one part of the body and that continues for a period of hours, days, or weeks.[1] Occasionally, it is characterized by tonic contraction of the distal hand or arm, sometimes with superimposed clonic tremulousness. EPC was initially described by the Russian neurologist Kojewnikow in children with the Russian spring–summer tick-borne viral encephalitis. EPC can arise from primary motor or sensory cortex, premotor cortex, or supplementary sensorimotor cortex.[2]

EPC may present with unusual features. For example, EPC may be reduced or disappear in sleep[3] and increase with movement. The muscle twitches are sometimes irregular and can vary in intensity. Approximately one patient in three has the entire side of the body involved. However, a single part of the body may be involved, such as the hand or fingers (or both) or, less commonly, proximal muscles, such as the deltoid, pectoralis, triceps muscle,[3] abdominal muscles,[4] the face,[5] or the tongue.[6] In some patients, when multiple muscles are involved, asynchrony of muscle twitching can be present. Occasionally, dystonic[7] or choreiform[8] movements can be observed. These unusual features often confound the diagnosis and sometimes suggest a movement disorder or a psychogenic etiology.

Furthermore, the routine EEG during these events does not show an epileptiform correlate in over half of cases.[9] An EEG correlate is not observed because a large area of cortical neurons need to be firing synchronously for the amplitude of the EEG activity to be large enough for a scalp EEG correlate to be observed.[10] Often an EEG correlate is obtained only with EEG back-averaging techniques. In some cases, the jerks can be induced with transcranial magnetic stimulation.[7]

In children, the most common cause of EPC is Rasmussen's encephalitis.[7] In adults, the most common etiologies include a cerebral infarct, a neoplasm, or acute infection.[7,10] It is less commonly seen in focal cortical dysplasia,[11] infectious mass lesion (especially tuberculosis[12]), and non-ketotic hyperglycemia.[13] Rarely, EPC is caused by neurotoxicity arising from penicillin, azlocillin, or cephotaxime in high doses, diagnostic use of metrizamide,[10] cat scratch disease,[14] a ketotic hyperglycemia,[15] or adult onset Rasmussen's encephalitis.[16] EPC due to anti-Hu associated paraneoplastic encephalomyelitis[17] or autoimmune thyroiditis[18] have also been reported.

EPC is usually refractory to antiepileptic drugs. When EPC is refractory to medications and a structural etiology is present, neurosurgical removal[19] is most effective but may result in a fixed motor deficit.[10]

What did I learn from this case?

EPC may present with irregular clonic twitching of a single muscle group, which may be irregular in frequency and vary in intensity. In addition, the twitching may be reduced in sleep, aggravated by movement or, occasionally, improved by a sensory stimulus. Furthermore, sometimes a patient's unique emotional reaction to an illness, which in this case was indifference, may incorrectly suggest a psychogenic etiology.

Since many cases do not show an EEG correlate, an alternate diagnosis might be incorrectly considered. Maneuvers to eliminate movement artifact that obscure the recording and digital EEG reformatting are necessary to increase the yield of routine EEG. In cases where the routine EEG shows no epileptiform correlate and an epileptic process is being considered, EEG back-averaging may be helpful. Neuroimaging to exclude a structural cause should be performed. In cases where a structural lesion is not present (i.e. early encephalitis process), ictal SPECT, functional MRI,[5,20] or diffusion weighted MRI[21,22] can be helpful for localization and diagnostic confirmation when necessary.

s0070

How did this case alter my approach to the care and treatment of my epilepsy patients?

p0190

Seizures may have unusual manifestations that can mimic non-epileptic conditions such as movement disorders and psychogenic seizures. A clinician must always keep an open mind and take a meticulous history from the patient and family about the description, onset, and evolution of the event. For example, in this case the earlier history of Jacksonian spread raised the suspicion of epileptic seizures. In addition, careful correlation of clinical behavior with the EEG, montage reformatting, and maneuvers to reduce movement artifact were necessary to increase the yield of non-invasive ictal EEG.

REFERENCES

1. Obeso JA, Rothwell JC, Marsden CD. The spectrum of cortical myoclonus from focal reflex jerks to spontaneous motor epilepsy. *Brain* 1985;**108**:193–224.
2. Young GB, Blume WT. Periodic lateralized frontal epileptiform discharges with ipsilateral epilepsia partialis continua. *Epilepsia* 2007;**48**:597–8.
3. Thomas JE, Reagan TJ, Klass DW. Epilepsia partialis continua: a review of 32 cases. *Arch Neurol* 1977;**34**:266–75.
4. Fernandez-Torre JL, Calleja J, Pascual J, Galdos P, DePablos C, Berciano J. Epilepsia partialis continua of the abdominal muscles: a detailed electrophysiologic study of a case. *Mov Disord* 2004;**19**:1375–8.
5. Espay AJ, Schmithorst VJ, Szaflarski JP. Chronic isolated hemi-facial spasm as a manifestation of epilepsia partialis continua. *Epilepsy Behav* 2007;**12**:332–6.
6. Vukadinovic Z, Hole MK, Markand ON, Batt BH, Sokol DK. Lingual epilepsia partialis continua in a girl. *Epileptic Disord* 2007;**9**:323–6.
9. Cockerell C, Rothwell J, Thompson PD, Marsden CD, Shorvon SD. Clinical and physiologic features of epilepsia partialis continua: cases ascertained in the UK. *Brain* 1996;**119**:393–407.
7. Zyss J, Xie-Brustolin J, Ryvlin P, Peysson S, Beschet A, Sappey-Mariner D, Hermier M, Thobois S. Epilepsia partialis continua with dystonic hand movement in a patient with a malformation of cortical development. *Mov Disord* 2007;**22**:1703–96.
8. Kankirawatana P, Dure LS 4th, Bebin EM. Chorea as a manifestation of epilepsia partialis continua in a child. *Pediatr Neurol* 2004;**31**:126–9.
10. Biraben A, Chauvel P. Epilepsia partialis continua. In: Engel J Jr, Pedley TA, eds. *Epilepsy: a comprehensive textbook.* Philadelphia: Lippincott-Raven, 1997: 2447–53.
11. Kuznicky R, Berkovic S, Andermann F, Melanson D, Olivier A, Robitaille Y. Focal cortical myoclonus and rolandic cortical dysplasia: clarification by magnetic resonance imaging. *Ann Neurol* 1988;**23**:317–25.
12. Juul-Jensen P, Denny-Brown D. Epilepsia partialis continua. *Arch Neurol* 1966;**15**:563–78.
13. Singh BM, Strobos RJ. Epilepsia partialis continua associated with non-ketotic hyperglycemia: clinical and biochemical profile of 21 patients. *Ann Neurol* 1980;**8**:155–60.

14. Nowakowski GS, Katz A. Epilepsia partialis continua as an atypical presentation of cat scratch disease in a young adult. *Neurology* 2002;**59**:1815–6.

15. Placidi F, Floris R, Bozzao A, Romigi A, *et al.* Ketotic hyperglycemia and epilepsia partialis continua. *Neurology* 2001;**57**:534–7.

16. Villani F, Pincherle A, Antozzi C, *et al.* Adult onset Rasmussen's encephalitis: anatomical-electrographic-clinical features of 7 Italian cases. *Epilepsia* 2006;**47(suppl 5)**:41–6.

17. Shavit YB, Graus F, Probst A, Rene R, Steck AJ. Epilepsia partialis continua: a new manifestation of anti-Hu associated paraneoplastic encephalomyelitis. *Ann Neurol* 1999;**45**:255–8.

18. Aydin-Ozemir Z, Tuzun E, Baykan B, *et al.* Autoimmune thyroid encephalopathy presenting with epilepsia partialis continua. *Clin EEG Neurosci* 2006;**37**:204–9.

19. Ng YT, Kerrigam JF, Rekate HL. Neurosurgical treatment of status epilepticus. *J Neurosurg* 2006;**105(5 suppl)**:378–81.

20. Jackson GD, Connelly A. Cross JH. Functional magnetic resonance imaging of focal seizures. *Neurology* 1994;**44**:850–6.

21. Huang CW, Hsieh YJ, Pai MC, Tsai JJ, Huang CC. Non-ketotic hyperglycemia-related epilepsia partialis continua with ictal unilateral parietal hyperperfusion. *Epilepsia* 2005;**46**:1843–4.

22. Senn P, Lovblad KO, Zutter D, *et al.* Changes on diffusion weighted MRI with focal motor status epilepticus. *Neuroradiology* 2003;**45**:246–9.

The Girl with Visual Seizures Who wasn't Seeing Things – Transient Blindness in a Young Girl

Carl E Stafstrom

s0010   ## HISTORY

p0010   Lauren, a 10-year-old girl, presented with a several month history of episodes that she described as follows: "I see floating colored dots. Then my eyes cross and I suddenly can't see – I just see black in both eyes" (Figure 24.1). "I get real scared when things go blank. I feel like I'm in La-La Land."

p0020   The first spell occurred a few days after her dog was killed by a car. She had about 30 or 35 spells over the 3 months before presentation at the clinic; each spell was identical. The spells lasted from 30 to 60 s and she recovered quickly, but they were often followed by an occipital or retro-orbital throbbing headache, and occasionally by nausea and vomiting. Witnesses confirmed that Lauren is lucid during a spell – she can reply to questions and follow instructions. She recalls each spell clearly afterward ("My mind was playing tic-tac-toe"). Witnesses also describe her eyes "darting back and forth rapidly" during a spell and Lauren describes "shaky vision." Spells seem to be more frequent when she is outside in the sun, looking out of a window or watching television.

p0030   Lauren is a healthy, normally developing girl. Pregnancy, labor, and delivery were uneventful. She reached all developmental milestones on time and she is a good student. She is active in dance. Her mother recently divorced and remarried. There is no family history of epilepsy or migraine.

p0040   Past evaluations included a normal brain magnetic resonance imaging (MRI) scan and a routine electroencephalogram (EEG). Previous physicians concluded that Lauren suffered from a combination of migraine and depression, with psychosomatic spells related to post-traumatic stress (resulting from her parents' divorce and the death of her beloved pet).

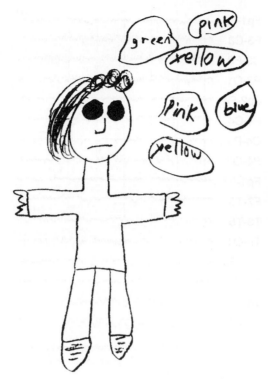

FIGURE 24.1   The patient's diagram of her spells of visual obscurations. The child was asked, "Please draw a picture of what it is like to have one of your spells." Her first subjective symptom was of colored spots floating in her left visual field. A few seconds later, vision in both eyes became obscured (note the blackened eyes).

EXAMINATION AND INVESTIGATIONS

Lauren was a delightful, articulate girl with age-appropriate cognitive skills. Her general physical and detailed neurological examinations were normal. She became tearful when discussing the recent death of her dog. When asked to draw a picture describing her symptoms during a spell, she produced the drawing shown in Figure 24.1.

The routine EEG (see Figure 24.2) showed frequent right occipital spike–wave and polyspike discharges, single or in trains up to 1.5 s, with amplitudes up to 200 μV. The posterior dominant rhythm was slightly slower on the right. During the EEG, Lauren fortuitously had one of her typical spells. She suddenly announced, "I'm having one," whereupon right-beating nystagmus was seen for the next 15 s. During the spell she counted to 15 but could not count fingers; she followed an instruction to stick out her tongue and was able to state her name and age correctly. She recalled a spoken phrase afterward. Fifty seconds after the onset, she announced, "It's over." On EEG, the episode began with a burst of polyspike–wave activity in the right posterior quadrant. This evolved into diffuse low-voltage fast activity that increased in amplitude, becoming 8–10 Hz spike-waves, maximal in the right posterior region. After 30 s, the spikes dissipated and were replaced by diffuse slowing that was maximal in the right occipital area.

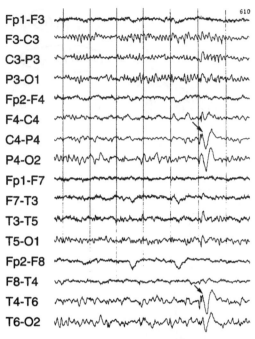

f0020 FIGURE 24.2   Interictal EEG recording (awake, eyes closed) showing right occipital high-voltage spike–wave complexes (arrows), superimposed on right posterior slowing.

s0030
DIAGNOSIS

p0070
Gastaut-type idiopathic childhood occipital epilepsy, or Gastaut-type benign childhood epilepsy with occipital paroxysms (BCEOP).[1] This syndrome was previously called BCEOP[2] or late-onset benign occipital seizures.[3,4]

s0040
TREATMENT AND OUTCOME

p0080
Lauren was initially treated with valproic acid. Her spells subsided promptly, but returned several months later and did not respond to increasing doses. She was switched to carbamazepine with excellent results until a few breakthrough seizures prompted the addition of gabapentin. On this regimen she remained seizure-free for 4 years, but then seizures with an identical semiology returned. Treatment was initiated with oxcarbazepine, on which she remained for 2 years. Lauren is now off all antiepileptic drugs. She is now 20 years old, married, and has a healthy infant daughter.

s0050
COMMENTARY

p0090
This patient presented with brief, stereotypic episodes of visual obscuration with mild confusion but preserved awareness. Her seizures are therefore complex partial in type.

The clinical symptomatology and interictal and ictal electrographic localization suggest a right occipital origin. Her normal development and neurologic status and the lack of any lesion on brain MRI scan suggest an idiopathic etiology.

Lauren's initial complaints were considered by several physicians to be psychological in nature on the basis of their onset after significant psychosocial stressors (parental divorce, death of pet) and her dramatic self-reports (e.g. "I'm going blind again!"). Indeed, many patients with seizures, particularly complex partial seizures, present with vague complaints or behaviors that are considered psychogenic until further detailed history and investigations establish the correct diagnosis.

Other practitioners suggested that Lauren had migraines, a plausible diagnosis given her transient visual loss followed by throbbing headache and nausea. However, several features in this case suggested that epilepsy should have been included in the differential diagnosis. Lauren's spells were stereotyped and frequent. Each episode was brief, with visual symptoms lasting less than 1 min and the headache persisting for only a few minutes. There is no family history of migraine, which lessens but does not exclude the possibility of migraine.

The benign occipital epilepsies of childhood are idiopathic, localization-related age-specific epilepsy syndromes.[1,2,5] Several varieties exist, based on age of onset, daytime versus nighttime occurrence and subtleties of symptoms.[3,4,6,7] The spectrum includes Panayiotopolous syndrome and Gastaut-type BCEOP.[1,8,9] Recent classification schemes and clinical research distinguish the two syndromes as distinct. Panayiotopolous syndrome occurs in younger children (usually 3–8 years) and includes nocturnal occurrence, prominent ictal vomiting, and other autonomic dysfunction, and only rare description of visual hallucinations.[3,10] Gastaut-type BCEOP, however, begins later (mean onset 8 years), and seizures usually occur during the day without vomiting and with frequent visual symptoms.[5]

Given Lauren's age and clinical features, she best fits the late-onset form of benign occipital epilepsy of childhood, Gastaut-type BCEOP. Clinical symptoms of this syndrome vary widely[5,9,11,12] and typical features may include elementary visual hallucinations, blindness, head or eye deviation, alteration of consciousness, generalized or hemiclonic seizures, and postictal headache; nausea or vomiting occur in some cases but not as commonly as in Panayiotopoulos syndrome. Ictal episodes in Gastaut-type BCEOP are brief, usually shorter than 1–2 min, and occur several times per day. Interictal electrophysiological investigations reveal high-amplitude sharps or spike-waves in the occipital or posterotemporal regions, usually suppressed by eye opening. Treatment with carbamazepine or clobazam is often successful. At least 60% of children remit spontaneously by their late teenage years[4] but seizure recurrence is common, as occurred in Lauren's case.[8] Gastaut-type BCEOP likely forms part of a "seizure susceptibility syndrome" spectrum that includes Panayiotopoulos syndrome, Rolandic epilepsy, and perhaps febrile seizures. This spectrum encompasses syndromes with region-specific cortical hyperexcitability that varies with age and might have a common genetic basis.

What did I learn from this case?

The examining physician should not be biased by prior medical evaluations and should bear in mind that epilepsies present with a wide variety of clinical manifestations, including subtle alterations of mental status and what might seem like "hysterical" symptoms. We should pay particular attention to a child's own description of the symptoms. Although several authors have commented that a child's lack of verbal sophistication, especially at young ages, may make an accurate diagnostic assessment difficult,[3,7] with concerted effort one can often obtain a wealth of information from the child. Indeed, children's artistic impressions of their seizures correlate closely with the clinically determined seizure type and offer insights into the child's self-image.[13]

p0150   In this case, previous physicians either considered Lauren's symptoms to be psychogenically based, given the proximate psychosocial stressors, or else lumped her symptoms into migraine. Although it is important to consider the psychosocial factors that may contribute to a child's symptoms, ictal details should be carefully sorted out before assuming causality. The aura of migraine typically consists of scotomata, scintillations, or visual obscurations. Occipital seizures more commonly present as transient colored circular patterns, as seen in this child's drawing (see Figure 24.1); zig-zag and achromatic patterns are distinctly unusual.[3,14] It is also important to rule out symptomatic causes of occipital epilepsy and to recognize that the proportion of cases of benign occipital epilepsy among children with occipital spikes is small.[15]

s0070   ## How did this case alter my approach to the care and treatment of my epilepsy patients?

p0160   I try to pay close attention to the child's own description, both verbal and pictoral, of his or her event. Having the child illustrate his or her symptoms by drawing a picture is a very useful adjunctive diagnostic approach.[13] This technique is simple, involves no expense and is particularly useful in younger children who cannot articulate their symptoms well. Lauren's dramatic and insightful depiction of her initial visual symptoms (colored spots) supports the diagnosis and her illustration is very similar to those drawn by much older patients with this syndrome.[3,4]

p0170   This case also emphasizes the importance of EEG evaluation of spells of uncertain etiology. Although we were extremely fortunate to obtain an ictal recording of Lauren's spell during a routine EEG, which clinched the diagnosis, such serendipity occurs rarely. Hospital-based or ambulatory EEG monitoring (preferably with video) should enhance our yield of diagnosing the wide variety of spells that occur in children.

REFERENCES

1. Engel J Jr. A proposed diagnostic scheme for people with epileptic seizures and epilepsy: report of the ILAE task force on classification and terminology. *Epilepsia* 2001;**42**:796–803.
2. Commission on Classification and Terminology of the International League against Epilepsy. Proposal for revised classification of epilepsies and epilepsy syndromes. *Epilepsia* 1989;**30**:389–99.
3. Panayiotopoulos C. Elementary visual hallucinations, blindness, and headache in idiopathic occipital epilepsy: differentiation from migraine. *J Neurol Neurosurg Psychiatr* 1999;**66**:536–40.
4. Panayiotopoulos C. Benign childhood partial seizures and related epileptic syndromes. London: John Libbey & Company, Ltd, 1999.
5. Gastaut H. A new type of epilepsy: benign partial epilepsy of childhood with occipital spike-waves. *Clin Electroencephalogr* 1982;**13**:13–22.
6. Ferrie C, Beaumanoir A, Guerrini R, *et al.* Early-onset benign occipital seizure susceptibility syndrome. *Epilepsia* 1997;**38**:285–93.

7. Andermann F, Zifkin B. The benign occipital epilepsies of childhood: an overview of the idiopathic syndromes and of the relationship to migraine. *Epilepsia* 1998;**39(suppl 4)**:S9–S23.

8. Ferrie C, Caraballo R, Covanis A, *et al.* Panayiotopoulos syndrome: a consensus view. *Dev Med Child Neurol* 2006;**48**:236–40.

9. Chahine LM, Mikati MA. Benign pediatric localization-related epilepsies: II. Syndromes in childhood. *Epileptic Disord* 2006;**8**:243–58.

10. Covanis A. Panayiotopoulos syndrome: a benign childhood autonomic epilepsy frequently imitating encephalitis, syncope, migraine, sleep disorder, or gastroenteritis. *Pediatrics* 2006;**118**:1237–43.

11. Maher J, Ronen G, Ogunyemi A, Goulden K. Occipital paroxysmal discharges suppressed by eye opening: variability in clinical and seizure manifestations in childhood. *Epilepsia* 1995;**36**:52–7.

12. van den Hout B, van der Meij W, Wienke G, *et al.* Seizure semiology of occipital lobe epilepsy of children. *Epilepsia* 1997;**38**:1188–91.

13. Stafstrom CE, Havlena J. Seizure drawings: insight into the self-image of children with epilepsy. *Epilepsy Behav* 2003;**4**:43–56.

14. Panayiotopoulos C. Visual phenomena and headache in occipital epilepsy: a review, a systematic study and differentiation from migraine. *Epileptic Disord* 1999;**1**:205–16.

15. Libenson M, Caravale B, Prasad A. Clinical correlations of occipital epileptiform discharges in children. *Neurology* 1999;**53**:265–9.

c00025

A Young Man with Noise-Induced Partial Seizures

Bettina Schmitz

s0010

HISTORY

p0010 A 34-year-old Turkish man started having seizures at the age of 16. Most of his seizures were induced by unexpected noises, like the opening of a door or the ringing of a bell. These acoustic triggers could be relatively subtle, such as the sound induced by the clumsy handling of cutlery by the patient himself. Seizures occurred exclusively when the patient was awake and increased in frequency over the years.

p0020 When he was first seen in my clinic in 1988 he was 22 years old and was having up to 10 seizures every day. He had been treated by a number of neurologists, all of whom had diagnosed psychogenic seizures. Drug treatments had included tranquilizers, neuroleptic drugs, and antidepressants, but none of these therapies had a significant effect on the frequency of his seizures.

p0030 The patient was born in Turkey. Pregnancy and delivery were described as normal, but he had delayed development of motor and verbal skills. He had been a moderate scholar and finished school at the age of 16, the same year his seizures first started.

p0040 He was married and had a 2-year-old healthy child but had been out of work since the age of 18 on account of his seizures. He lived with his family. Owing to the frequency of his seizures, which often caused the patient to fall and had produced multiple injuries in the past, he was looked after in a highly protective manner.

s0020

EXAMINATION AND INVESTIGATIONS

p0050 Neurological examination revealed a hypotrophy of the right arm and leg and a mild right-sided central hemiparesis.

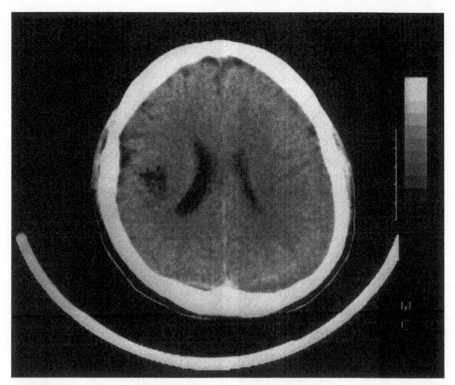

FIGURE 25.1   CT scan demonstrating a left-sided porencephalic lesion and ipsilateral hemispheric hypotrophy.

Cranial computed tomography (CT) scanning showed a left frontoparietal hypodense region suggestive of infarction and ipsilateral hemispheric atrophy (Figure 25.1). These findings were confirmed on magnetic resonance imaging. HMPAO (=99 mTc, hexamethyl propyleneamine oxime) single photon emission CT scanning showed the extensive area of hypoperfusion in the left hemisphere, most marked in the frontoparietal region and hypoperfusion in the contralateral right cerebellum.

Interictal electroencephalograms (EEGs) were normal except for a mild slowing in the left frontocentral region. Five seizures were recorded during video-telemetry. Seizures were all induced by an unexpected acoustic stimulus (Figure 25.2). The seizures started with a startle reaction, followed by tonic posturing with symmetrical extension of arms and legs, accompanied by a loud, undulating, high-pitched vocalization. This was followed by rhythmic pelvic movements, a rolling of the body and frenetic, thrashing movements of all limbs. There was also enuresis associated with long seizures. There was no postictal confusion – the patient was immediately able to act and speak, and he claimed to be aware of everything that happened during the seizure. Seizure duration was always less than 1 min. The duration and severity of seizures were inconstant; however, the sequence of motor elements was highly stereotypic. Ictal surface EEGs were unrevealing beyond movement artifacts.

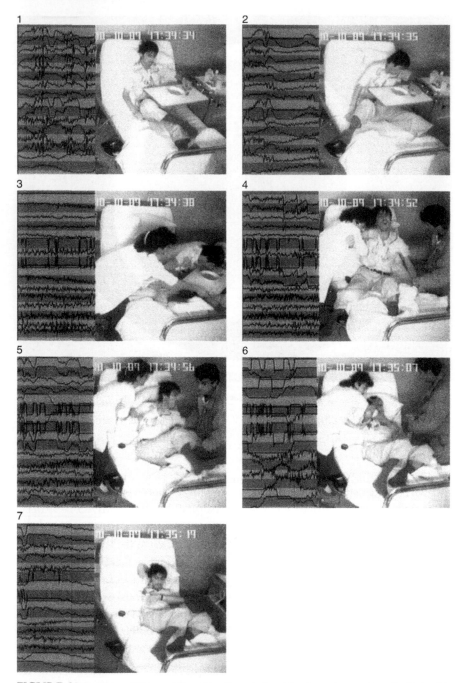

FIGURE 25.2   Video–EEG recording of a seizure induced by the patient accidentally hitting his plate with his cutlery (1, 2). There is an initial tonic phase with vocalization (3), followed by hypermotor automatisms (4, 5), sudden cessation of movements, (6) and immediate reorientation (7). The duration of seizure was 40 s. The EEG includes artifacts.

DIAGNOSIS

Symptomatic frontal lobe epilepsy with startle-induced tonic and hypermotor seizures secondary to perinatal brain damage with left frontoparietal infarction.

TREATMENT AND OUTCOME

After I had first seen this patient in 1988 and made the diagnosis of epilepsy, he was put on carbamazepine monotherapy, which reduced the frequency and severity of his seizures for only a short period. He then was put on add-on propranolol 40 mg/day with mild benefit. Following the introduction of clobazam, seizure frequency was markedly reduced, and after a gradual increase to 80 mg/day he became seizure-free. Since then, seizures have recurred only twice, the first time during a period of fever, the second time in relation to non-compliance. He has slowly stopped his comedication and is now on monotherapy with clobazam 40 mg/day, which has slowly been decreased over the past 12 years. He is back at work, is seizure-free, and has no side effects from his medication.

COMMENTARY

This patient is a typical case of startle-induced frontal lobe epilepsy. Startle-induced seizures were classified among the reflex epilepsies by Alajouanine and Gastaut in 1955.[1] The most common trigger is a sudden auditory stimulus. Onset is in the first 20 years of life. Startle epilepsy occurs almost exclusively in patients with brain lesions, which usually date back to the prenatal or perinatal period. In most cases lesions are unilateral and consist of porencephalic cysts or local atrophy. Many patients have hemiparesis and some degree of mental retardation. Seizures start with an abrupt startle reaction followed by a tonic phase. Both cortical and subcortical structures may be involved in the pathophysiology of startle-induced seizures. It has been postulated that the startle response triggers an epileptogenic region, which in turn activates an epileptogenic region that may be located near the supplementary motor cortex.[2]

Response to conventional drug treatment is poor. The best results have been reported with a combination of carbamazepine and benzodiazepines.[3]

The first modern report of a series of patients with frontal lobe seizures that had been carefully studied with intracranial electrodes appeared in 1985.[4] Subsequent reports confirmed the existence of this peculiar type of seizure disorder with prominent motor automatisms, and three major subtypes have now been well defined.[5] Many neurologists were unfamiliar with frontal lobe epilepsies and, because of the often bizarre and expressive seizure phenomena, frontal lobe seizures (also called pseudopseudoseizures) were often misdiagnosed as pseudoseizures until the late 1980s.

What did I learn from this case?

In one's first year of training one learns from every patient. This case taught me a number of lessons.

p0140   First, this patient had a disorder that I had never heard of in medical school. It was exciting to learn that, although his syndrome is rare, there had been a number of then recent studies that showed he was not at all unique but a rather typical case. Thus, I learned that in medicine we may still discover distinct syndromes provided we look for typical patterns.

p0150   Second, it is a good example of the challenge in making the diagnosis of epileptic seizures versus psychogenic seizures. My immediate impression had been that his seizures were not organic because they looked very dramatic and they were always triggered by an external stimulus. Startle epilepsy is an example of a seizure disorder in which psychological and organic mechanisms are closely intertwined, because seizures are triggered by a psychophysiological reflex mechanism. I was also misled by the fact that the patient's consciousness was preserved throughout the seizure. The fact that these frontal hypermotor automatisms can occur with intact consciousness shows that the brain still has lessons to teach us about clinical–anatomical relationships.

p0160   Third, although for pragmatic reasons it might be preferable to have a limited number of antiepileptic drugs, there are always patients who may profit from one of the old or second-line drugs and who respond differently from the majority of patients. This patient did not develop cognitive problems and did not develop tolerance when treated with clobazam. These side effects have caused many epileptologists to exclude clobazam completely from their drug repertoire.

p0170   Fourth, even patients with difficult-to-treat seizures that seem desperate do not justify therapeutic nihilism. Severe epilepsy leads to behavioral problems and social difficulties, as in this case. His marriage was threatened by his disabling seizure disorder and a regular job seemed impossible, owing to cultural reasons as well as to the realistic risks of frequent motor seizures. However, social development may normalize after seizure control. It happened in this case because the patient's role was not fixed and adjusted to his seizure disorder when he was successfully treated.

s0070   ## How much did this case alter my approach to the care and treatment of my epilepsy patients?

p0180   This patient was one of my first telemetry cases in my first year of work in a specialized epilepsy unit. Back then I witnessed discussions about the then-novel concept of frontal lobe epilepsies and can remember senior epileptologists admitting that they had falsely diagnosed cases in the past as psychogenic seizures. (Dieter Janz referred to a patient of his with nocturnal hypermotor seizures as the "werewolf-man" who, in retrospect, had had typical nocturnal frontal lobe seizures.)

p0190   I hope that this case contributed to my self-criticism with respect to the firmness of my clinical diagnoses. More generally, this case is a good example of the fact that it is always justified to keep an open mind about what is claimed to be medical fact and about the opinions of authorities, because these "facts" and opinions obviously can be wrong. I hope that cases like this one have made me a more tolerant teacher – especially when young doctors in my courses do not simply accept my "epileptological wisdom" but request evidence, which I am often not able to provide.

p0200   Certainly, each time this patient visits my clinic, which he does once a year with one of his children, he nourishes and renews my endurance and optimism when planning and modulating treatment strategies for patients with complicated epilepsies.

REFERENCES

1. Alajouanine A, Gastaut H. La syncinésie-sursaut et l'épilepsie-sursaut à déclanchement sensoriel ou sensitif inopiné. *Rev Neurol* 1955;**93**:29–41.
2. Tassinari CA, Rubboli G, Michelucci R. Reflex epilepsies. In: Dam M, Gram L, eds. *Comprehensive epileptology*. New York: Raven Press, 1990: 233–46.
3. Sáenz-Lope E, Herranz-Tanarro FJ, Masdeu JC, Chacon Pena JR. Hyperekplexia: a syndrome of pathological startle responses. *Ann Neurol* 1984;**15**:36–41.
4. Williamson PD, Spencer DD, Spencer SS, Novelly RA, Mattson RH. Complex partial seizures of frontal lobe origin. *Ann Neurol* 1985;**18**:497–504.
5. Williamson PD, Engel J, Munari C. Anatomic classification of localization-related epilepsies. In: Engel J, Pedley TA, eds. *Epilepsy: a comprehensive textbook*. Philadelphia: Lippincott-Raven, 1997: 2405–16.

Non-convulsive Status Epilepticus in a Patient with Idiopathic Generalized Epilepsy

Eugen Trinka

HISTORY

A 50-year-old otherwise healthy woman had a history of generalized tonic–clonic seizures (GTCS) since she was 19 years old. At that time, a computed tomography scan of the brain, her neurological examination, and her family history were all unremarkable. The EEG showed generalized spike–wave discharges, and a diagnosis of idiopathic generalized epilepsy with GTCS was made. Valproate was introduced and her seizures were well controlled with a daily dose of 1800 mg.

After the onset of intolerable tremor, valproate was discontinued slowly and lamotrigine was gradually introduced, with an increase in dose of 25 mg every second week up to 400 mg/day (serum concentration 7.26 mg/l).

She tolerated the medication well without any side effects but the characteristics of her seizures changed. In addition to her usual GTCS, she developed frequent episodes of impaired cognition, disturbed behavior, and myoclonic jerks that affected her arms and face, lasted for 2–6 h and sometimes evolved into a GTCS. These episodes occurred approximately every 2 weeks. Clobazam was added, up to 30 mg/day, without success. The patient was admitted to our hospital in a confusional state with psychomotor slowing, slight myoclonias, and disturbed behavior.

EXAMINATION AND INVESTIGATIONS

On neurological examination the patient was confused and only partly responsive. There were slight myoclonias in her face and arms. The EEG showed continuous generalized spike–wave activity and generalized fast polyspike activity. A magnetic resonance imaging scan of the brain was normal.

DIAGNOSIS

Non-convulsive status epilepticus caused by iatrogenic exacerbation of idiopathic generalized epilepsy.

TREATMENT AND OUTCOME

Intravenously administered lorazepam (4 mg) stopped these episodes and normalized the EEG. Lamotrigine was stopped and topiramate was slowly introduced (with a 25 mg increase in dose per week). Repeated EEGs were normal and the patient was seizure-free. Unfortunately, she developed intolerable psychomotor slowing and speech problems that led to discontinuation of topiramate.

Primidone was started and titrated to 750 mg/day without any side effects. Her seizures remained well controlled for the next 6 months and the EEG was normal.

COMMENTARY

I chose this case, first, because it shows that even after a long course of good seizure control, severe worsening may occur if there are any precipitating factors – in this case a change of medication from valproate to lamotrigine.

Lamotrigine is often used in the treatment of idiopathic generalized epilepsy. Its efficacy is well documented in open-label studies and in one double-blind placebo-controlled study. However, it is not clear which patients will respond promptly and which patients will not be controlled with this drug. There are some reports of seizure aggravation with lamotrigine, although the mechanisms and the incidence are not well known. Whether the seizure aggravation was due to the introduction of lamotrigine or to discontinuation of valproate remains unclear in this case.

Secondly, this case demonstrates that careful monitoring of clinical symptoms, seizure frequency, and the EEG is helpful in determining the cause of aggravation or worsening of seizures when an effective antiepileptic drug is being discontinued and another drug is being introduced.

What did I learn from this case?

Apart from the seizure aggravation during the discontinuation of valproate and the introduction of lamotrigine, I was impressed by the change in seizure type. The patient had previously suffered from GTCS. After the introduction of lamotrigine the patient experienced frequent episodes of confusion and myoclonic jerks in her face and arms, resembling non-convulsive status epilepticus. The EEG showed runs of polyspikes followed by slow spike–waves. The seizure semiology was previously not experienced by the patient and closely corresponds to Oller-Daurella's "tonic-automatic crises." The seizure type was completely suppressed by topiramate, although at the price of side effects. Primidone was introduced with success. It seems curious to me that although there are many new antiepileptic drugs, there are at least some patients who end up with older drugs after failure or side effects with the newer ones.

FURTHER READING

Buchanan N. The use of lamotrigine in juvenile myoclonic epilepsy. *Seizure* 1996;**5**:149–51.

Buoni S, Grosso S, Fois A. Lamotrigine in typical absence epilepsy. *Brain Dev* 1999;**21**:303–6.

Catania S, Cross H, deSousa C, Boyd S. Paradoxical reaction to lamotrigine in a child with benign focal epilepsy of childhood with centrotemporal spikes. *Epilepsia* 1999;**40**:1657–60.

Frank M, Enlow T, Holmes G, *et al.* Lamictal (lamotrigine) monotherapy for typical absence seizures in children. *Epilepsia* 1999;**40**:973–9.

Gericke CA, Pickard F, deSaint-Martin A, *et al.* Efficacy of lamotrigine in idiopathic generalized epilepsy syndromes: a video–EEG-controlled, open study. *Epileptic Disord* 1999;**1**:159–65.

Guerrini R, Dravet C, Genton P, *et al.* Lamotrigine and seizure aggravation in severe myoclonic epilepsy. *Epilepsia* 1998;**39**:508–12.

Guerrini R, Belmonte A, Parmeggiani L, Perucca E. Myoclonic status epilepticus following high-dosage lamotrigine therapy. *Brain Dev* 1999;**21**:420–4.

Oller-Daurella L. Tonic-automatic crises: clinical and EEG description. Discussion of their place in the epileptic crises classification and their representation in different potentials. *Arch Neurobiol [Madrid]* 1970;**33**:303–16.

Pseudohypoglycemia Manifesting as Complex Partial Seizures in a Patient with Type III Glycogen Storage Disease

P Barton Duell

HISTORY

A 32-year-old man with type III glycogen storage disease was referred because of spells suspected to be caused by hypoglycemia. During the preceding 12–14 years he had experienced clusters of stereotypical spells occurring on 4–6 consecutive days every 3–4 months. Each cluster started with a single spell on the first day followed by increasingly frequent spells, occurring up to 12 times daily on the last day of the cluster. The spells occurred during wakefulness and sleep and were described by the patient as "dizzy headrushes" that sometimes were triggered by a thought or seeing a familiar object. During the spells he feels dizzy, sometimes near-syncopal, often hot and sweaty, sometimes cold, and occasionally has palpitations. He has no dyspnea or chest discomfort. Spells witnessed by his family were described as follows: he freezes in position, stares straight ahead, is unresponsive to questions, repetitively smacks his lips, has slight tremulousness, and stiffens his arms, all of which last for a total duration of 30–60 s. He subsequently appears confused and groggy for 15 min after the event, but feels fatigued and somewhat disoriented for the rest of the day. The spells are unaffected by eating. He has no urinary incontinence, tongue biting, or headaches.

He had no history of birth trauma, febrile seizures, meningitis or encephalitis, head trauma, or family history of seizures. He had hepatomegaly as an infant and was diagnosed with type III glycogen storage disease at the age of 18 months on the basis of a liver biopsy. Aside from hepatomegaly during infancy, the type III glycogen storage disease has been asymptomatic. His older sister also has type III glycogen storage disease, but she does not have spells. He occasionally takes ibuprofen. He smokes cigarettes, but rarely consumes beer.

EXAMINATION AND INVESTIGATIONS

Vital signs were repeatedly normal. His cardiac and neurologic examinations were normal. A non-fasting serum glucose concentration obtained shortly after a spell was 112 mg/dl. Another post-spell serum glucose concentration was 88 mg/dl. Other laboratory test results, including hepatic transaminase measurements, were normal. Magnetic resonance imaging (MRI) of his brain demonstrated focal gliosis along the left lateral ventricle, but no cortical abnormalities. The results of a routine awake and asleep electroencephalogram (EEG) were normal.

DIAGNOSIS

1. Complex partial seizures
2. Pseudohypoglycemia
3. Asymptomatic type III glycogen storage disease.

TREATMENT AND OUTCOME

He was initially treated with levetiracetam at a dosage titrated up to 500 mg po BID. After 5 months of no seizures, the patient reduced his dosage of levetiracetam to 250 mg po BID. He has remained free of seizures for an additional 7 months.

COMMENTARY

This case is interesting for several reasons. First, the diagnosis of type III glycogen storage disease distracted his other physicians from the diagnosis of seizures. Since glycogen storage diseases can be associated with hypoglycemia[1,2], there was an initial concern that this patient's infrequent spells were episodes of hypoglycemia. However, a careful history, coupled with an awareness that his glycogen storage disease was asymptomatic, led to the diagnosis of a seizure disorder. Hypoglycemia-induced seizures are common in untreated children with several types of glycogen storage disease, but this is a rare manifestation in adults. Although some forms of glycogen storage disease are sometimes associated with non-hypoglycemic seizures (e.g. types V[3] and VII[4]), this is not a typical feature in adults with type III glycogen storage disease. Second, despite the prior concerns about the possibility of hypoglycemia, the patient did not meet the criteria for hypoglycemic spells. Although some of his symptoms were potentially compatible with hypoglycemia, he had no biochemical evidence of hypoglycemia associated with spells, his symptoms were unaffected by eating, and his spells were too sudden in onset and too brief to be attributable to hypoglycemia.

What did I learn from this case?

Establishing the diagnosis of partial seizures is often a diagnostic challenge for physicians, particularly when the seizures occur infrequently. A careful history is essential for establishing the possibility of partial seizures, but patients often are unable to provide sufficient details. Additional history obtained from family members and friends can provide a more complete description of the spells, as it did in this case.

Since hypoglycemia can cause a myriad of symptoms, and type III glycogen storage disease can be associated with hypoglycemia, it was initially appropriate to consider this diagnosis. In addition, the patient's description of the spells was potentially compatible with hypoglycemia. However, the diagnosis of true hypoglycemia requires satisfaction of Whipple's triad:[5]

1. Symptoms compatible with hypoglycemia
2. Biochemical evidence of hypoglycemia at the time of symptoms
3. Symptoms that resolve after resolution of hypoglycemia.

Although some of his symptoms were suggestive of hypoglycemia, the rapidity of onset and resolution over minutes was incompatible with hypoglycemia. Thus, he did not meet any of the three criteria for establishing a diagnosis of hypoglycemia. Moreover, a more complete description of the spells by his family members was most compatible with complex partial seizures.

Glycogen storage diseases are uncommon (<1 in 20,000 births) inborn errors of glycogen metabolism that are caused by mutations in various genes involved in glycogen synthesis, degradation, or regulation.[6,7] There are more than a dozen types that are defined on the basis of the mutant gene and affected tissues, which are primarily the liver and muscles. The age of onset varies from birth to adulthood. Hepatic defects in glycogen metabolism may be manifested as hepatomegaly or hypoglycemia, whereas defects in the muscle may be associated with exercise intolerance, weakness, fatigue, and muscle cramps. Type III glycogen storage disease (also known as glycogen debrancher deficiency, amyloglucosidase deficiency, Cori disease, Forbes disease, and limit dextrinosis) can affect the liver and/or muscles depending on the tissue distribution and type of defect in the debranching enzyme, amyloglucosidase.[8] This patient had only hepatomegaly in infancy that resolved later in life.

Although we often strive to identify a unifying diagnosis that accounts for all facets of a patient's condition, and we sometimes doubt a conclusion that a patient has two or three diagnoses, this patient did not have a single unifying diagnosis. The correct diagnosis was not established until possibilities other than a potentially unifying diagnosis of type III glycogen storage disease were considered. Fortunately, he has done well after initiating anti-seizure medication.

REFERENCES

1. Talente GM, Coleman RA, Alter C, et al. Glycogen storage disease in adults. *Ann Int Med* 1994; **120**:218–26.
2. Goldberg T, Slonim AE. Nutritional therapy for hepatic glycogen storage diseases. *J Am Diet Assoc* 1993;**93**:1423–30.
3. Walker AR, Tschetter K, Matsuo F, Flanigan KM. McArdle's disease presenting as recurrent cryptogenic renal failure due to occult seizures. *Muscle Nerve* 2003;**28**:640–3.

4. Al-Hassnan ZN, Al-Budhaim M, Al-Owain M, Lach B, Al-Dhalaan H. Muscle phosphofructokinase deficiency with neonatal seizures and nonprogressive course. *J Child Neurol* 2007;**22**:106–8.
5. Whipple AE. The surgical therapy of hyperinsulinism. *J Int Chir* 1938;**3**:237–76.
6. Shin YS. Glycogen storage disease: clinical, biochemical, and molecular heterogeneity. *Semin Pediatr Neurol* 2006;**13**:115–20.
7. Ozen H. Glycogen storage diseases: new perspectives. *World J Gastroenterol* 2007;**13**:2541–53.
8. Lucchiari S, Fogh I, Prelle A, Parini R. Clinical and genetic variability of glycogen storage disease type IIIa: seven novel AGL gene mutations in the Mediterranean area. *Am J Med Genet* 2002;**109**:183–90.

Surprising Turns and Twists

Recurrent Amnestic Episodes in a 62-Year-Old Diabetic Patient

Christine Adam, Claude Adam and Michel Baulac

HISTORY

In December 1996, after a recent diagnosis of type 2 diabetes, a 62-year-old right-handed man began to experience episodes resembling "transient global amnesia," lasting 15 min to 1 h. The episodes started on waking, with the loss of ability to plan his activities, accompanied by a series of questions about what he had done the previous day, accompanied by a feeling of perplexity. Otherwise his behavior seemed normal. There were no automatisms or other motor signs. He was not able to recall any details of the amnesic episode.

EXAMINATION AND INVESTIGATIONS

Two electroencephalograms (EEGs) showed ictal discharges from the right frontotemporal region, but a subsequent 24-h ambulatory EEG was normal. Magnetic resonance imaging (MRI) scanning of the brain showed right hippocampal atrophy with a high T2 signal.

The patient received valproate for 2 months, and he seemed to improve during that time. Meanwhile, his diabetes worsened, blood glucose levels fluctuating between 0.5 and 3.5 g/l were noted and insulin was started. He continued to have both hypoglycemic episodes as well as marked hyperglycemic episodes. The amnestic episode was thought to be caused by transient hypoglycemia at that time, which could not be confirmed later with concomitant measurements.

The patient was seen in our hospital in May 1997 for evaluation of a few further similar episodes. A first EEG captured some slow spikes as well as a "subclinical" right temporal lobe seizure on a later, standard EEG whose interpretation was uncertain. Nonetheless, vigabatrin was added to valproate. The amnestic episodes were infrequent during the following 6 months (occurring about once every 2 months), and they happened during periods of normal or high blood glucose levels.

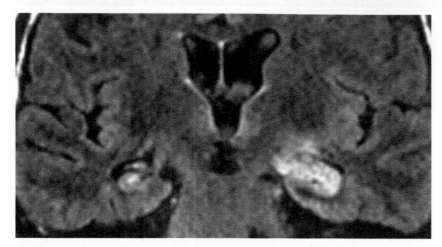

FIGURE 28.1   MRI coronal image of a FLAIR sequence, perpendicular to the long axis of hippocampus, at day 11 of an amnestic simple partial status epilepticus. The left hippocampus is swollen and hyperintense. The atrophy of the right hippocampus is known and seems stable since the beginning of the epilepsy.

In October 1997, the events shortened to a few minutes but increased dramatically in frequency, leading to a quasi-permanent amnestic state in which both anterograde and retrograde memories were affected. The patient was able to retain only very small amounts of information. He complained of gait trouble, behavioral changes, and a mild temporal-spatial disorientation. EEGs established a definite diagnosis of simple partial status epilepticus, showing temporal lobe seizures on both sides independently (but predominantly on the left). Up to three events in 30 min were recorded. Each seizure remained largely confined to one temporal lobe, although they would propagate mildly to neighboring regions without any further clinical symptomatology. There was no evidence of impairment of consciousness. On admission the cerebrospinal fluid (CSF) was found to contain 0.4 g/l of protein, normal cell count, and normal glucose levels (the patient was hyperglycemic at that time). Interferon-α was undetectable. The CSF remained normal 3 days and 1 week later. Herpes simplex virus-1 antibodies and the polymerase chain reaction were negative in the CSF. Other laboratory tests (including virology, bacteriology, autoimmunity and inflammatory, and paraneoplastic markers) were negative.

The seizures remained very active for 2 weeks despite clonazepam followed by intravenous phenytoin, together with high doses of oral antiepileptic drugs in combination (valproate, phenytoin, vigabatrin, and clonazepam). Over the next 2 weeks the seizures disappeared, as shown by EEG monitoring. A brain MRI at day 11 of admission showed a swollen and T2-hyperintense left amygdalo-hippocampal complex with an unchanged right hippocampus (Figure 28.1). Despite the resolution of the status epilepticus, the amnestic and behavioral symptoms regressed slightly and partially during the 2 months of hospitalization. A series of brain MRIs showed: at day 42 of arrival, decreased swelling on the left side; 3 months later, disappearance of swelling and evolution into a notable hippocampal atrophy on the left side and an increase of right hippocampal atrophy (Figure 28.2). The latest MRI (November 1998) confirmed bilateral hippocampal atrophy.

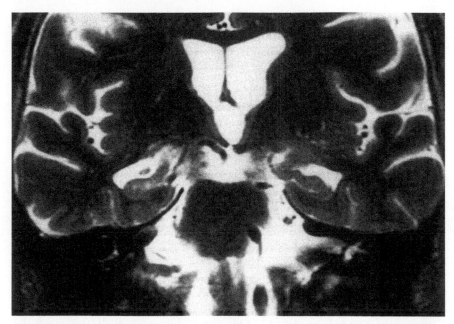

FIGURE 28.2   Coronal slice of a T2-weighted MRI scan perpendicular to the long axis of hippo-campus, 5 months after the occurrence of an amnestic simple partial status epilepticus. The left hippo-campus is dramatically atrophic and the right hippocampus (originally affected) also showed a notable loss of volume.

The clinical evolution was poor, with persistent anterograde amnesia, spatial-temporal disorientation, and behavioral disorders with disinhibition and joviality.

DIAGNOSIS

Temporal lobe epilepsy with simple partial status epilepticus and subsequent hippocampal atrophy.

COMMENTARY

Why did we choose this case?

There are three reasons why we chose this case. First, it is well known that the epileptic origin of amnestic episodes may be difficult to recognize, especially in older patients.[1,2] In our observation, these episodes were initially misdiagnosed for hypoglycemias, owing to the existence of difficult-to-treat diabetes. These manifestations were quite different from those of typical medial temporal lobe epilepsy (MTLE)[3] despite the presence of unequivocal hippocampal sclerosis on the first MRI scan. MTLE with hippocampal sclerosis is known to begin at about 9 years of age with a large range of age of onset, but an onset at the age of 62 seems exceptional, and a purely amnestic symptomatology at disease onset and such a pejorative evolution was never reported before.

Moreover status epilepticus is exceptional in classical MTLE. Our patient is much closer to the clinical entity reported under the term "transient epileptic amnesia," which is defined by specific characteristics – onset in middle or old age, amnestic seizures lasting for a few minutes to an hour and occurring on waking, and sometimes simple partial status epilepticus of very long duration (lasting days).[1,2] The mechanisms of prolonged amnesia are only hypothetical and could be of post-ictal origin.[1,4] In this entity, Lee et al.[5] have reported a transient MRI abnormality, but no evidence of hippocampal damage has been described until now.

Alternatively, the MRI evolution in our case evokes partly what is observed in limbic encephalitis.[6] However, the right hippocampal atrophy of our patient was already present at the beginning of his epilepsy and no blood or CSF abnormalities were found.

What did we learn from this case?

We learnt that a new kind of epileptic event could create acute hippocampal damage. Previously, three types of events have been incriminated: early (most often febrile) convulsions;[7–9] rarely generalized or focal tonic–clonic status epilepticus[10] and even a single, brief tonic–clonic seizure.[11] Our case of hippocampal damage seems the first one to be associated with simple partial status epilepticus. We found no definite argument in favor of other underlying mechanisms such as a meningoencephalitis or anoxic–ischemic factors of systemic origin. This might indicate that very focal epileptic activity is able to be deleterious *per se*.

Hippocampal damage as a consequence of epileptic activity has generally been reported early in life, in young children[7–9] or in children, adolescents or young adults[10,11] and after single epileptic events. Our case is remarkable in that it occurred in an older adult and after repeated seizures over several weeks. This long duration was probably important in the development of this seizure-induced hippocampal damage. By contrast, the adult case reported by Jackson et al.[11] experienced only a short tonic–clonic seizure, but this was combined with severe respiratory disorders.

REFERENCES

1. Gallassi R. Epileptic amnesic syndrome: an update and further considerations. *Epilepsia* 2006;**47(suppl 2)**:S103–S105.
2. Zeman AZJ, Boniface SJ, Hodges JR. Transient epileptic amnesia: a description of the clinical and neuropsychological features in 10 cases and a review of the literature. *J Neurol Neurosurg Psychiatr* 1998;**64**:435–43.
3. French JA, Williamson PD, Thadani VM, et al. Characteristics of medial temporal lobe epilepsy: I. Results of history and physical examination. *Ann Neurol* 1993;**34**:774–80.
5. Lee BI, Lee BC, Hwang YM, et al. Prolonged ictal amnesia with transient focal abnormalities on magnetic resonance imaging. *Epilepsia* 1992;**33**:1042–6.
4. Maheu G, Adam C, Hazemann P, Baulac M, Samson S. A case of post-ictal transient anterograde and retrograde amnesia. *Epilepsia* 2004;**45**:1459–60.
6. Bien CG, Urbach H, Schramm J, et al. Limbic encephalitis as a precipitating event in adult-onset temporal lobe epilepsy. *Neurology* 2007;**69**:1236–447.

7. Nohria V, Lee N, Tien RD, *et al*. Magnetic resonance imaging evidence of hippocampal sclerosis in progression: a case report. *Epilepsia* 1994;**35**:1332–6.
8. Perez ER, Maeder P, Villemure KM, *et al*. Acquired hippocampal damage after temporal lobe seizures in 2 infants. *Ann Neurol* 2000;**48**:384–7.
9. Van Landingham KE, Heinz ER, Cavazos JE, Lewis DV. Magnetic resonance imaging evidence of hippocampal injury after prolonged focal febrile convulsions. *Ann Neurol* 1998;**43**:413–26.
10. Tien RD, Felsberg GJ. The hippocampus in status epilepticus: demonstration of a signal intensity and morphological changes with sequential fast spin-echo MR imaging. *Radiology* 1995;**194**: 249–56.
11. Jackson GD, Chambers BR, Berkovic SF. Hippocampal sclerosis: development in adult life. *Dev Neurosci* 1999;**21**:207–14.

Attacks of Nausea and Palpitations in a Woman with Epilepsy

Jørgen Alving

HISTORY

The patient was a 28-year-old woman referred for evaluation of seizures. Her seizures had begun when she was 12 years with generalized tonic–clonic seizures and, allegedly, psychomotor seizures that were not further described. Seizures usually occurred just after awakening.

She was initially treated with carbamazepine and then with phenytoin, but treatment was changed to valproate because of side effects and insufficient seizure control. Valproate was reasonably effective, but because of unacceptable weight gain, her treatment was changed to a combination of lamotrigine and vigabatrin.

At the time of the referral, she was having approximately one seizure a month. She gave the following descriptions of her seizures: "nausea, palpitations, and an urge to urinate or defecate, sometimes ending in a generalized convulsion", and "difficulty concentrating and understanding others, talking 'gibberish', and a strong urge to urinate, lasting 15–20 minutes".

Her family history was positive for unspecified epilepsy in an aunt and a cousin. Her birth, developmental milestones, and school performance were unremarkable, and there was no previous neurological illness.

EXAMINATION AND INVESTIGATIONS

Her neurological examination, including mental status examination, was normal. The initial EEG showed generalized paroxysmal abnormalities, and the brain magnetic resonance imaging scan was normal.

She was admitted to the hospital for EEG monitoring. A routine EEG, including a sleep EEG, was normal. A 96-h ambulatory eight-channel cassette-EEG (while she was on 2000 mg vigabatrin and 300 mg lamotrigine per day) showed no abnormality despite two episodes with nausea.

During a second admission, she had a cluster of the seizures described above. Video–EEG recording showed innumerable generalized bursts of 4–6 Hz spike–polyspike-waves (Figure 29.1), each burst lasting 1–2 s and accompanied by a slight lapse of consciousness and upward deviation of the eyes with blinking, but no clonic movements in the extremities. Over a 2-h period, the paroxysmal bursts became more intense and frequent, finally terminating in a generalized tonic–clonic seizure, initiated by massive clonic movements in her face.

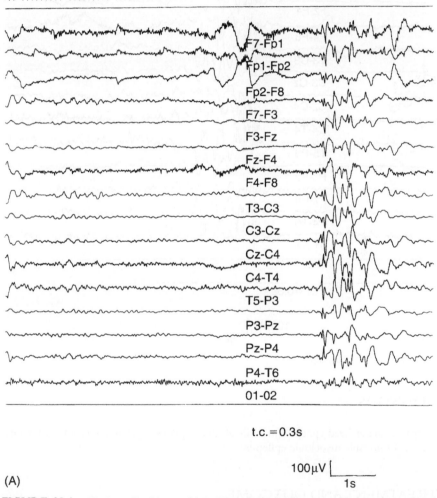

(A)

FIGURE 29.1   (A) Generalized burst of 3.5–6 Hz spike/polyspike-wave, with very minor clinical phenomena, occurring 20 min. before a tonic–clonic seizure. (B) Generalized burst of more pronounced polyspike-wave, with more marked clinical features (upward eye deviation), occurring 1 min. before a tonic–clonic seizure. (C) Generalized burst of polyspike-wave, with clinical features as in (B), occurring after a short generalized flattening and immediately followed by a generalized tonic–clonic seizure.

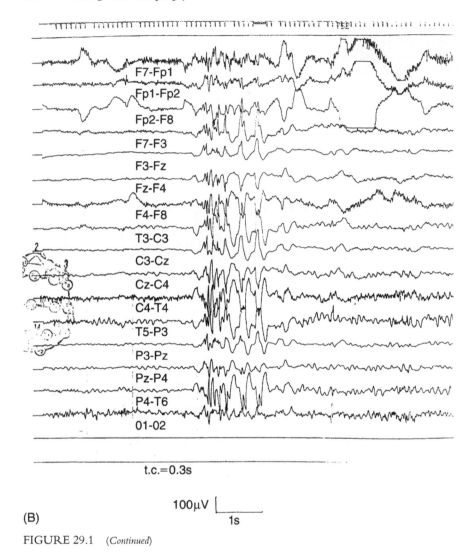

t.c.=0.3s

100μV

1s

(B)

FIGURE 29.1   (*Continued*)

DIAGNOSIS

Idiopathic generalized epilepsy (juvenile absence epilepsy, cycloleptic type), with some features of juvenile myoclonic epilepsy.

TREATMENT AND OUTCOME

After the video–EEG, valproate was re-instituted, and ethosuximide was subsequently added, with much improved seizure control. Because of recurrent problems with weight gain, valproate was replaced by lamotrigine. During a 2-year follow-up, on a combination

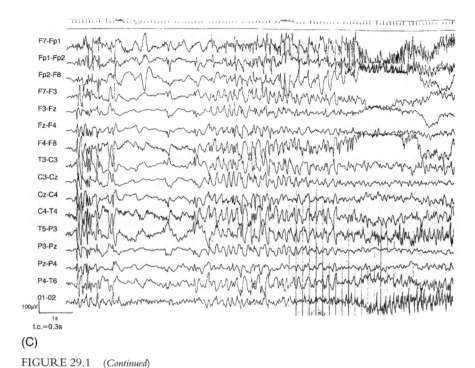

(C)

FIGURE 29.1   *(Continued)*

of lamotrigine 600 mg/day and ethosuximide 1000 mg/day, she has had only one generalized tonic–clonic seizure and two episodes with clustered absences.

COMMENTARY

This patient's aura-like phenomena with strong autonomic components had obviously been misinterpreted as evidence of focal seizures. Furthermore, several normal EEGs despite prolonged monitoring made a diagnosis of idiopathic generalized epilepsy less likely, until a rather short but intensive session of video–EEG monitoring together with the history (including the age at onset) led to the correct classification of her seizure types and epilepsy syndrome.

The paradoxical exacerbation of generalized seizures with vigabatrin and carbamazepine is well known, but there is no evidence in this case to suggest that vigabatrin was responsible for the massive EEG abnormalities (and seizures) seen during intensive monitoring. The 96-h cassette–EEG was performed on the same medication, and she had paroxysmal EEG abnormalities before vigabatrin treatment.

What did I learn from this case?

I learned that an incessant search for an exact seizure and syndrome diagnosis is essential, especially if the clinical semiology is equivocal. This case reinforced the concept that aura-like phenomena are not infrequently seen in idiopathic generalized epilepsies.

I also learned that a prolonged EEG recording performed at the "wrong" time may not be informative in patients with idiopathic generalized epilepsies.

Finally, I learned that a prolonged EEG is not identical with intensive monitoring! I am now more careful to plan EEG monitoring when the chance of capturing clinical events is at its maximum.

FURTHER READING

Janz D. *Die Epilepsien. Spezielle Pathologie und Therapie.* Stuttgart: Thieme, 1969.

Lee AG, Delgado-Escueta AV, Maldonato HM, Swartz B, Walsh GO. Closed-circuit television videotaping and electroencephalographic biotelemetry (video/EEG) in primary generalized epilepsies. In: Gumnit RJ, ed. *Intensive neurodiagnostic monitoring. Advances in neurology,* vol 46. New York: Raven, 1987: 27–68.

Boylan LS, Labovitz DL, Jacksen SC, Starner K, Devinsky O. Auras are frequent in idiopathic generalized epilepsy. *Neurology* 2006;**67**:343–5.

Parker APJ, Agathonikou A, Robinson RO, Panaiyotopoulos CP. Inappropriate use of carbamazepine and vigabatrin in typical absence seizures. *Dev Med Child Neurol* 1998;**40**:517–19.

Absence Status Epilepticus in a 60-Year-Old Woman

Gerhard Bauer

HISTORY

In 1974, a 60-year-old woman was admitted to the hospital in a peculiar state. She was partially responsive and able to follow simple commands but unable to follow a conversation. She frequently smiled inappropriately and complained about dizziness. Eyelid fluttering was observed.

No neurologist had seen her before and her medical practitioner did not know of any history of paroxysmal events in the past. She was taking antihypertensive and cardiac medications.

EXAMINATION AND INVESTIGATIONS

The EEG showed continuously repeated runs of generalized 3-Hz spike-and-waves lasting up to 10–20 s. The short periods of interspersed activity revealed no gross abnormalities. Absence status was diagnosed and intravenous diazepam was administered, with prompt resolution of the status epilepticus.

The neurological examination after the episode resolved showed some mental slowing, exaggerated tendon reflexes, and a Babinski sign on the right side.

Pneumoencephalography revealed mild brain atrophy (ascribed to vascular encephalopathy) but was otherwise normal. Cerebrospinal fluid was also normal.

DIAGNOSIS

Absence status epilepticus occurring *de novo* in later life.*

*After the first edition of *110 Puzzling Cases of Epilepsy* several similar cases have been observed. These case reports are published under: Bauer G, Bauer R, Dobesberger J, Benke Th, Walser G, Trinka E. Absence status in the elderly as a late complication of idiopathic generalized epilepsies. *Epileptic Disord* 2007;9: 39–42.

TREATMENT AND OUTCOME

p0070　The patient was put on a combination of ethosuximide and phenobarbital, which at the time was the recommended therapy for epilepsies with absence seizures.

p0080　Two years later, I saw her in the outpatient clinic and she reported having had her first generalized tonic–clonic seizure at the age of 36 years, which was 24 years before her presentation with absence status epilepticus. Since that time, sporadic tonic–clonic seizures had occurred every year, but she never reported them to her family or to her doctors. Seizures occurred without exception in the morning hours, when she was alone at home.

p0090　She reported that no further seizures had occurred since the start of antiepileptic medications. The EEG at this time showed generalized spikes and slight diffuse slowing.

p0100　During the visit the patient was in an elated mood. She was accompanied by a school friend and the two women joked in the waiting room. I tried to find out why she had never reported her seizures and found myself dragged into a pleasant chat. To gain more information, I invited her school friend to take part. During the conversation, the patient's friend stated that the patient had always been a *Blinzelgeiß* (blinking goat). With this term the conversation turned serious, and it became clear that during her school years the patient had suffered daily absence seizures until they resolved spontaneously at the age of 14 years. No prolonged absence status epilepticus had occurred until the episode that had led to hospital admission in 1974. I also learned that a sister of the patient had experienced absences and generalized tonic–clonic seizures.

p0110　In light of this new information, I diagnosed generalized idiopathic epilepsy, childhood absence epilepsy followed by generalized tonic–clonic seizures on awakening, and absence status epilepticus. In addition, a diagnosis of vascular encephalopathy, hypertonia, and coronary heart disease was made.

p0120　On a subsequent visit, the patient noted mood changes and reported that she had been diagnosed with depressive mood disorder associated with menopause ("involutional depression") by a psychiatrist. Antidepressant medication was prescribed, but she was noncompliant with both the psychotropic and the antiepileptic medications. She continued to have generalized tonic–clonic seizures, scattered absence seizures, and prolonged periods of "dizziness." Because these episodes of "dizziness" had been treated successfully by her medical practitioner with intravenous diazepam, the diagnosis of repeated absence status epilepticus seemed to be justified.

p0130　In 1982, she was admitted to the hospital with cervical radiculopathy. Brain computed tomography showed slight brain atrophy. A trial of valproate led to an increase in absence seizures, and the former combination of ethosuximide and phenobarbital was re-established. After this admission the patient became compliant and free of seizures. The mood changes stabilized without antidepressant medication, and the patient lived a decent life until she died from a cerebrovascular accident at the age of 75 years.

COMMENTARY

p0140　Since the reappraisal of absence status by Andermann and Robb,[1] many forms of prolonged states of altered mental functions accompanied by ongoing spike activities in the EEG have been differentiated. Non-convulsive status epilepticus is now understood to include generalized absence status epilepticus and focal complex partial status epilepticus. Furthermore, it has become clear that generalized non-convulsive status epilepticus (absence status epilepticus) includes status epilepticus that occurs in association with known absence epilepsies, in Lennox–Gastaut syndrome, and *de novo* in later life.[2,3] Complex partial status epilepticus may be difficult to differentiate from absence status epilepticus during the episode, but the distinction usually becomes clear after clinical investigations have been performed.

When this patient first presented, absence status epilepticus occurring *de novo* in later life was diagnosed – this was a diagnosis that had been established in the literature 3 years earlier.[3] The EEG exhibited generalized 3-Hz spike-and-waves without any focal elements and against normal background activity. Although a focal component could not be excluded, the EEG and the prompt recovery led to the diagnosis of absence status epilepticus. Signs of a vascular encephalopathy were considered a comorbidity.

After learning of the patient's history of childhood absence epilepsy and generalized tonic–clonic seizures, the correct diagnosis was changed. The generalized character of the non-convulsive episode was confirmed, but it became clear that absence status epilepticus was not the presenting symptom but rather a manifestation of an idiopathic generalized seizure disorder.

Why absence status occurs as the late complication of an otherwise mild seizure disorder, which in this case was kept a secret by the patient (even from her family), remains an enigma. Some authors[4,5] consider that the condition is usually situational. Psychotropic drugs and withdrawal from benzodiazepines seem to be the most frequently observed precipitating factors.[2,6,7] Another entity – non-convulsive status epilepticus in a critically ill elderly patient – is unrelated to this discussion.[8]

This patient also suffered from cerebrovascular disease and a mood disorder. In the search of factors that may have triggered absence status, psychotropic agents could be ruled out, but the role of cerebrovascular insufficiency remains a speculation. Although the pathogenesis of absence status as a late complication of generalized idiopathic epilepsy is unknown, it is nonetheless a well-documented fact and might be syndrome related.[9] In rare cases, absence status epilepticus represents the very first symptom of a generalized idiopathic epilepsy with late onset.[10]

What did I learn from this case?

I learned a number of lessons from this case. First, I learned that the diagnostically relevant information was gained during an informal chat with the patient and her school friend. Besides a strictly medical interview, a personal conversation in a relaxed atmosphere represents an important part of taking a thorough history.

Second, her childhood absence seizures stopped spontaneously, without any medication. Her first generalized tonic–clonic seizure occurred many years later, at the age of 36. Thus, offering a good prognosis in cases of absence epilepsy, as is frequently done by pediatricians, may neglect the late complications, as in this case.

Third, if some patients with daily absence seizures do not come to medical diagnosis, as in this case, then the "true" incidence, prevalence and natural history of the epilepsy is open to question. Since this case is not a single observation, the figures given in the published literature might be too low.

Fourth, these uncertainties may also concern genetic studies. My patient's positive family history for seizures was only reported after repeated examinations. The degree to which a patient is affected may also be disguised in patients with a self-limited course that does not come to medical attention.

Fifth, elderly people often suffer from multiple diseases. A seizure disorder occurring in an elderly patient cannot be uncritically assumed to be symptomatic of an acute or remote brain insult. Likewise, labeling a mild brain condition as a triggering factor remains speculative. With late seizures, the possibility of an idiopathic seizure disorder in earlier life cannot be ruled out categorically. The second age peak can be due to an exaggeration of a pre-existing idiopathic generalized epilepsy (as in this case), or it can really be de novo.[10]

How did this case alter my approach to the care and treatment of my patients with epilepsy?

I do not draw final conclusions after the first visit even if my conclusion fits nicely with recently published papers. If a patient wants to have a personal conversation besides the formal interview, I indulge the patient and take my time. Decisive information is sometimes reported only in a relaxed atmosphere.

I realize now that patients with generalized idiopathic epilepsies are prone to seizures throughout their lives. Therefore, before I consider withdrawing antiepileptic drugs, I take a careful history, with special attention to "minor seizures." If appropriate, I also obtain long-term EEG monitoring to look for generalized paroxysmal EEG abnormalities. I recognize that an EEG is crucial in evaluating patients with altered states of consciousness during the episode.

Finally, even though multiple comorbidities are common in elderly patients, the causal relationship of these conditions to seizures should be judged critically.

REFERENCES

1. Andermann F, Robb JP. Absence status. A reappraisal following review of thirty-eight patients. Epilepsia 1972;13:177–87.
2. Bourrat Ch, Garde P, Boucher M, Fournet A. États d'absence prolongée chez des patients agés sans passé épileptique. Rev Neurol 1986;142:696–702.
3. Schwartz MS, Scott DF. Isolated petit mal status presenting de novo in middle age. Lancet 1971;ii:1399–401.
4. Thomas P, Beaumanoir A, Genton P, et al. "De novo" absence status of late onset: report of 11 cases. Neurology 1992;42:104–10.
5. Thomas P, Andermann F. Late-onset absence status epilepticus is most often situation-related. In: Malafosse A, Genton P, Hirsch E, et al., eds. Idiopathic generalized epilepsies: clinical, experimental and genetic aspects. London: John Libbey and Company, 1994: 95–109.
6. Brodtkorb E, Sand T, Kristiansen A, Torbergsen T. Non-convulsive status epilepticus in the adult mentally retarded. Seizure 1993;2:115–23.
7. Rumpl E, Hinterhuber H. Unusual "spike-wave stupor" in a patient with manic-depressive psychosis treated with amitryptiline. J Neurol 1981;226:131–5.
8. Litt B, Wityk RJ, Hertz S, et al. Nonconvulsive status epilepticus in the critically ill elderly. Epilepsia 1998;39:1194–202.
9. Agathonikou A, Panayiotopoulos CP, Giannakodimos S, Koutroumanidis M. Typical absence status in adults: diagnostic and syndromic considerations. Epilepsia 1998;39:1265–76.
10. Luef G, Schauer R, Bauer G. Idiopathic generalized epilepsy of late onset: a new epileptic syndrome? Epilepsia 1996;37(suppl 4):4.

Hemiplegia in a 76-Year-Old Woman with Status Epilepticus

Susanne Aull-Watschinger, Paolo Gallmetzer and Christoph Baumgartner

HISTORY

A 76-year-old woman was admitted to the emergency department because of focal motor status epilepticus consisting of clonic activity of the left face, arm, and leg. On admission the patient was stuporous. The patient was treated intravenously with clonazepam and phenytoin, which stopped the focal motor activity. However, the patient developed a left-sided hemiplegia and remained stuporous.

The patient experienced her first seizure half a year before this admission. This first seizure consisted of a focal motor seizure that evolved into a generalized tonic-clonic status epilepticus necessitating intubation and artificial ventilation. At that time a computed tomography (CT) scan showed a right posterior borderzone infarction and multiple lacunar vascular lesions that had not previously caused any transient or permanent neurological deficits. The patient recovered completely from status epilepticus and remained seizure-free on phenytoin. A follow-up CT scan performed 2 months before this admission showed a right parietal subdural hygroma (maximum width 15 mm). Because the hygroma did not exhibit a significant mass effect and the patient was completely asymptomatic and had no focal neurological signs, a conservative approach was undertaken.

EXAMINATIONS AND INVESTIGATIONS

On transfer to our ward (on day 2 after admission to the emergency department), the patient was stuporous (Glasgow coma scale 8) and showed a left-sided hemiplegia. A CT scan on admission was unchanged compared with the previous scan performed 2 months ago. Control CT scans performed on the following days also showed no significant changes. A magnetic resonance imaging scan essentially confirmed the CT scan findings. Cerebrospinal fluid showed a mild pleocytosis (14 cells/mm^3) consisting of granulocytes and lymphocytes as well as a total protein of 82 mg/dl, which f0010 FIGURE 31.1   EEG recording obtained during ictal hemiplegia showing PLEDs over the right hemisphere with maximum activity in the right central region.

was considered to be consistent with a non-specific meningeal irritation. An EEG showed periodic lateralized epileptiform discharges (PLEDs) over the right hemisphere (Figure 31.1). A repeat single-photon emission CT (SPECT) study showed marked hyperperfusion of the entire right hemisphere.

s0030 ## DIAGNOSIS

p0040 Non-convulsive focal status epilepticus with ictal hemiplegia.

s0040 ## TREATMENT AND OUTCOME

p0050 After the diagnosis of focal status epilepticus the patient was treated with high-dose benzodiazepines and intravenous phenytoin. However, while the state of vigilance slightly improved after this treatment, the hemiplegia remained unchanged. On day 5, therefore, it was decided to evacuate the hygroma via a burr-hole using a Jackson-Pratt drainage. The hygroma completely resolved after this intervention. On EEG, the PLEDs disappeared and the patient gradually woke up and she completely recovered from her hemiplegia over the next 2 weeks. A repeat single-photon emission CT (SPECT) study performed after her recovery showed – besides hypoperfusion in the right posterior border zone – a normal perfusion pattern and, specifically, no evidence of a hyperperfusion within the right hemisphere.

COMMENTARY

Why did we choose this case?

We chose this case for several reasons. First, this case shows that convulsive status epilepticus can evolve into non-convulsive status epilepticus after what seems like successful treatment. Thus, in one study,[1] 48% of 164 patients showed persistent EEG seizure activity after clinical control of convulsive status epilepticus and 14% of patients developed non-convulsive status epilepticus. Persistent EEG seizure activity was associated with a significantly higher mortality and a poorer outcome in this study, which underlines the importance of EEG monitoring after treatment of convulsive status epilepticus.

Secondly, the differential diagnosis of hemiparesis or hemiplegia in patients with seizures should include structural lesions such as tumors, vascular events and encephalitis as well as functional abnormalities such as postictal Todd's paresis and ictal hemiparesis. While some authors proposed a highly variable duration of Todd's paresis lasting from several minutes to 36 h,[2] in our own series Todd's paresis lasted 3 min on average, with a maximum duration of 22 min.[3] Therefore, the duration of several days for the hemiparesis in our patient would be a strong argument against a postictal phenomenon.

Thirdly, the true incidence of ictal paresis is unclear from the literature, owing to differences in definition. Some authors[4] have found a short ictal hemiparesis in up to 5% of patients with temporal lobe seizures, which most probably represents a motor neglect rather than a true hemiparesis. On the contrary, a real, prolonged paralysis caused by inhibitory motor seizures is an uncommon seizure symptom and most often occurs in patients with frontoparietal foci.[5,6]

Fourthly, this case may help to clarify the controversy about whether PLEDs represent a non-epileptiform or an epileptiform EEG abnormality and specifically whether PLEDs should be considered to be an interictal or an ictal phenomenon. PLEDs occur in a variety of disorders, most often in acute unilateral lesions such as ischemia, tumors or encephalitis. PLEDs are usually transient, and clinical seizures occur in approximately 70% of patients with PLEDs.[7] The findings of a hyperperfusion of the entire right hemisphere on SPECT scanning during hemiplegia as well as the appearance of a normal perfusion pattern after the resolution of the PLEDs and the resolution of hemiparesis, represent strong evidence that, at least in this specific patient, PLEDs were an ictal phenomenon. Our findings are in agreement with a positron emission tomographic study[8] that showed markedly increased mesiotemporal lobe glucose metabolism in a case with PLEDs and a SPECT study[9] where patients with focal neurological deficits and PLEDs showed a corresponding hyperperfusion on SPECT.

What did we learn from this case?

Apart from what we have outlined above, we were impressed by the existence of a long-lasting hemiplegia representing an ictal event. This case drew our attention towards non-convulsive status epilepticus as an important differential diagnosis in patients with unexplained mental obtundation, coma or focal neurological signs. We believe that EEG should be used more often in these patients. Finally, we think that

SPECT can be used to distinguish between the interictal and the ictal state in patients with EEG patterns of unclear significance.

REFERENCES

1. DeLorenzo RJ, Waterhouse E, Towne AR, *et al*. Persistent nonconvulsive status epilepticus after control of convulsive status epilepticus. *Epilepsia* 1998;**39**:833–40.
2. Rolak LA, Rutecki P, Ashizawa T, Harati Y. Clinical features of Todd's post-epileptic paralysis. *J Neurol Neurosurg Psychiatr* 1992;**55**:63–4.
3. Gallmetzer P, Leutmezer F, Serles W, *et al*. Postictal paresis in focal epilepsies – incidence, duration, and causes: a video-EEG monitoring study. *Neurology* 2004;**62**:2160–4.
4. Oestreich LJ, Berg MJ, Bachmann DL, Burchfiel J, Erba G. Ictal contralateral paresis in complex partial seizures. *Epilepsia* 1995;**36**:671–5.
5. Smith RF, Devinsky O, Luciano D. Inhibitory motor status: two new cases and a review of the literature. *J Epilepsy* 1997;**10**:15–21.
6. Villani F, D'Amico D, Pincherle A, *et al*. Prolonged focal negative motor seizures: a video-EEG study. *Epilepsia* 2006;**47**:1949–52.
7. Brenner RP, Schaul N. Periodic EEG patterns: classification, clinical correlation, and pathophysiology. *J Clin Neurophysiol* 1990;**7**:249–67.
8. Handforth A, Cheng JT, Mandelkern MA, Treiman DM. Markedly increased mesiotemporal lobe metabolism in a case with PLEDs: further evidence that PLEDs are a manifestation of partial status epilepticus. *Epilepsia* 1994;**35**:876–81.
9. Assal F, Papazyan JP, Slosman DO, Jallon P, Goerres GW. SPECT in periodic lateralized epileptiform discharges (PLEDs): a form of partial status epilepticus? *Seizure* 2001;**10**:260–5.

Persistence Pays Off

Mark D Bej

HISTORY

The first patient was 17 years of age when she was first seen after having had several blackout spells. She also complained of severe fatigue and abdominal pains that had started after the death of her grandmother. The pains had no relationship to meals and were described as "a weird sensation" and "reminding me of something," although she denied *déjà vu* when specifically asked. Two blackouts occurred on the same day while she was visiting friends. Another event occurred later while she was on the phone: she suddenly stopped talking and appeared to be in a trance. There were no automatisms or convulsions. She had previously been seen for chronic fatigue.

The second patient was seen when she was aged 35 years. She had had three episodes of loss of consciousness followed by some body jerking. A brain computed tomography (CT) scan was normal and she was placed on phenytoin. Another episode resulted in an emergency department evaluation, but the patient was discharged home. A third episode occurred in sleep. She was also having other episodes every couple of months, near the time of her menses. These episodes produced complaints of an unusual sensation without loss of consciousness. The only other significant history was that of being thrown out of the back of a truck at the age of 15 and suffering a wrist fracture (but no loss of consciousness). When she was evaluated, she had been, at different times, on phenytoin, carbamazepine, gabapentin, and phenobarbital, all of which had been stopped for various reasons. She had three EEGs; two were normal and one was read as demonstrating spike–wave activity. Despite the medications and consultations with several neurologists, the spells were not controlled.

The third patient was aged 13 years when she first presented with focal seizures. She was placed on carbamazepine, and over subsequent years the dosage of this medication needed to be slowly increased. When she was aged 16 or 17, it became clear that the dose increases were proportionally greater than her normal peripubertal weight gain. Eventually the side effects of carbamazepine became intolerable and she was switched to another antiepileptic drug.

s0020   # EXAMINATIONS AND INVESTIGATIONS

p0040   In the first patient, examination was normal, as were a CT scan, routine EEG and a subsequent 72-h ambulatory EEG during which seven of her episodes of abdominal pain were captured. A syncope clinic consultation with tilt table testing was sought; this revealed reduction of red cell mass and a marked hyperkinetic circulatory state in the supine position. She tolerated tilt for only 11 min, complaining of darkening vision. The test was terminated, owing to hypotension.

p0050   In the second patient, a 48-h EEG ordered at a local academic center demonstrated an electrographic seizure arising from the right temporal lobe. An epilepsy-protocol magnetic resonance imaging (MRI) scan was subsequently ordered and demonstrated a high-signal mass in the right hippocampus on fluid attenuation inversion recovery (FLAIR) and T2 weighting.

p0060   For the third patient, a thin-cut MRI scan was ordered. The scan demonstrated an area of focal cortical dysplasia in the right frontal lobe.

s0030   # DIAGNOSIS

p0070   Symptomatic partial epilepsy due to a low-grade glioma (Patient 1), and due to a hippocampal tumor (Patient 2), and cortical dysplasia (Patient 3).

s0040   # TREATMENTS AND OUTCOMES

p0080   The first patient was lost to follow-up until 2 years later when she presented to a local emergency department with a tonic–clonic seizure. Routine EEG was again normal but MRI scanning revealed a lesion in the right amygdalar area. The mass was excised and was felt to be a low-grade glioma with focal cortical dysplasia. Since surgery, the abdominal pains have resolved.

p0090   The second patient had appropriate ancillary testing of memory function, and her mass was then excised. The patient has been free of seizures since the surgery.

p0100   The third patient's seizures failed to respond to trials of three antiepileptic drugs over 2 years. After appropriate ancillary testing, she underwent an evaluation with subdural grid electrodes and ultimate excision of the dysplastic area of cortex, resulting in complete freedom from seizures.

s0050   # COMMENTARY

p0110   These three cases share a single common element: each patient was incompletely diagnosed during the early phases of their treatment. Definitive diagnosis was made only after a careful review of each patient's course; in two patients, the review occurred after referral or transfer to another neurologist.

p0120   It must be stated here that the simple fact that a diagnosis is not known with certainty is not of itself undesirable. This is true for more patients with epilepsy than any of us would like to admit. For medical, financial, or social reasons, it is not always practical to do a thorough diagnostic evaluation on initial presentation.

However, these three cases demonstrate the need for vigilance with each follow-up visit. Significant changes in the patient's seizure history should prompt the neurologist to investigate further. The first patient had a change in the type of event – events that had not, up to that time, even been definitively diagnosed as seizures. The second patient's significant change (which had admittedly occurred previously) was intractability to several medications. The third patient's change was considerably subtler – increasing intractability to her first medication in the form of breakthrough seizures.

What did I learn from the cases?

The most valuable lesson for me is the need for continued vigilance and the utility of maintaining a seizure calendar. Only by reviewing the prior history well – in the case of the third patient, more than once – did it become obvious that the new or continuing seizures were evidence of something more than "run-of-the-mill" epilepsy. Running a clinical practice often places significant pressures on one's time, and it is all too easy simply to increase dosages or add medications. One must watch for the "red flags" and, when they appear, review the case again.

How did these cases alter my approach to the care and treatment of my epilepsy patients?

I try to review every case when a patient requires dosage increases or a new anti-epileptic drug because of continuing seizures. If the epilepsy type has not been well defined, I order ambulatory EEG or inpatient video–EEG monitoring. If an epilepsy-protocol (thin-cut) MRI scan has not been done, then this is ordered. Ordering such studies has very often resulted in defining an etiology, defining the epilepsy syndrome and determining the best medications to use for the patient, even in cases where multiple routine EEGs were previously normal.

c00033

Drugs Did Not Work in a Little Girl with Absence Seizures

David B Bettis

HISTORY

s0010

p0010 J was a little girl with an angelic face and curly blonde hair. She was aged 2 years 8 months when her mother brought her to my office with a 6-month history of staring spells. These attacks occurred one to four times a day and consisted of a blank stare, eyelid fluttering, some jerking of the eyebrows, and rolling the eyes upward. They lasted 5–20 s. During this time she was motionless and unresponsive. The spells could not be interrupted. There was no associated urinary incontinence, although some urinary urgency occurred after the attacks. They were exacerbated by fatigue. Rarely, she had slight jerking movements of her arms. These spells had never caused her to fall or lose consciousness.

p0020 Her past medical history included being the product of an uncomplicated, full-term pregnancy. Birth weight was 3.5 kg. Her development had been normal to date. Her only medication was sulfasoxazole for prophylaxis of recurrent otitis media. Her family medical history was negative for epilepsy, seizures or other neurological disorders of significance. She had three healthy sisters.

EXAMINATION AND INVESTIGATIONS

s0020

p0030 Physical examination revealed a head circumference of 49.7 cm. General and neurological physical examinations were entirely normal and age-appropriate. Hyperventilation failed to elicit any events. Her EEG revealed multiple instances of 3-Hz spike-and-slow wave generalized epileptiform discharges, sometimes with a bifrontal predominance, which were slightly exacerbated by drowsiness. Photic stimulation was unremarkable.

DIAGNOSIS

Absence epilepsy.

TREATMENT AND OUTCOME

I counseled her mother on the typical benign prognosis of absence epilepsy, and started the patient on valproate. Her spells improved for a few weeks, but then relapsed. She was having 3–12 events a day. Ethosuximide was added; she again improved for a few weeks but then regressed again. She developed a sleep disturbance with restlessness, squirming, and hallucinations. Ethosuximide was discontinued and her symptoms improved. A few months later, she was having dozens of seizures a day. A repeat trial of ethosuximide improved her symptoms, but was associated with stomach upset and vomiting. She developed behavioral problems with uncharacteristically whiny and sometimes aggressive behavior. This improved when valproate was stopped and clonazepam was added. However, clonazepam was associated with behavioral side effects including crying and mood swings, and it was discontinued after a brief trial. She was having up to 20 absence spells a day.

A trial of amantadine improved her symptoms for 1 week, followed by yet another relapse. All medications were discontinued, and she improved, although she continued to have 20 seizures a day lasting 10–30 s. A repeat EEG revealed ongoing 3-Hz spike-and-wave generalized epileptiform discharges, but also some less frequent independent right and left parietal spike–wave discharges. A trial of phenytoin was not beneficial. This was followed by a trial of carbamazepine, which did not help. She was having up to 50 events per day, and was starting school.

Felbamate was initiated in September 1993, at a time when she was having 50 seizures a day. It did not help, and she was referred to a pediatric epileptologist at a major university. Review of several EEGs in the past confirmed typical changes for absence epilepsy. A trial of methsuximide was initiated and decreased the seizures frequency from 30 a day to 10 a day. This was the best seizure control that had been achieved in some time. Her family moved to a small town and she adjusted to her new school setting. Her seizures increased to 100 a day, and methsuximide was discontinued. She began having trouble in school. A trial of lamotrigine was discussed, but her mother was understandably hesitant to try a ninth medication. J continued to worsen and was having hundreds of events a day, associated with regression in school and occasional urinary incontinence.

In desperation, her mother asked about the ketogenic diet, a therapy that had recently been resurrected following some attention in the national media. After some discussion, and shortly after the ketogenic diet became available at our center, J was hospitalized and underwent fasting. She was placed on the ketogenic diet at a 4:1 ratio of fat to carbohydrate and protein calories. Her seizures immediately decreased to only a few per day; she had a slight exacerbation associated with an episode of otitis media and fever. She then became seizure-free for the first time in years. As weeks went by, her cognitive abilities improved. Her mother observed that the changes were "like taking a veil off of her brain." She exhibited improved abilities in reading and mathematics in school.

The diet was not without side effects. J was observed to be hungry, tired, and moody. She suffered a bout of renal stones after being on the diet for a little over 1 year.

However, she continued to make vast progress in school, and became a straight A student. She won the "most improved reader award."

p0100 After being seizure-free for 20 months, the ratio of her ketogenic diet was gradually decreased and a weaning process was started. After being seizure-free for 2 years, the diet was discontinued. A follow-up EEG was normal. She has remained seizure-free since that time.

p0110 J and her family were deservedly given the "winning kid with epilepsy award" from our local Epilepsy Foundation affiliate. Her mother shared this compelling story with a large audience. She has started on a college education.

s0050 ## COMMENTARY

p0120 Absence epilepsy of childhood is typically a benign condition that responds well to medication in more than 90% of cases. When a truly refractory case of absence epilepsy is encountered, effective treatment options are limited. Since this experience, I have become aware of at least one case of refractory absence epilepsy that responded well to a vagus nerve stimulator.

p0130 Although it is not possible to prove that the ketogenic diet was clearly responsible for curing this case of epilepsy, I cannot be convinced that her drastic improvement was mere coincidence after treating this child for more than 4 years with eight different anticonvulsant medications.

s0060 ### What did I learn from this case?

p0140 I once again learned a lesson that I had been taught in medical school and by my prior practice experience: the importance of remaining open minded to unconventional therapies when standard therapy is clearly unsuccessful. Because the vast majority of cases of absence epilepsy are responsive to medication, I persisted with medication trials for a prolonged period, even though the patient had nothing but a succession of side effects to show for undergoing those treatments.

s0070 ### How did this case alter my approach to the care and treatment of my epilepsy patients?

p0150 I am happier now about thinking of non-medication options when a reasonable trial of at least a few appropriate medications has failed. Those options include epilepsy surgery, the ketogenic diet, and the vagus nerve stimulator. I am haunted by the thought of how much sooner J would have improved had the ketogenic diet been tried earlier, and even more so by thoughts of other patients who have not been reached by non-medication therapies that could prove to be highly beneficial for their epilepsy.

"Alternative" Therapy for Partial Epilepsy – with a Twist

Nadir E Bharucha and Thomas Kuruvilla

HISTORY

A 20-year-old man presented with a 10-year history of partial seizures that had become generalized. A computed tomography scan of the brain, performed at the onset of the seizures, had shown a lesion, probably a tuberculous granuloma, in the right frontal cortex. He was started on antiepileptic drugs (carbamazepine and phenobarbital) and given a full course of antituberculous drugs. The seizures were well controlled and after about 5 years, anticonvulsants were discontinued.

About 1 year later, the seizures reappeared. Antiepileptic drugs were restarted but the seizures continued in spite of regular medication. This prompted the patient's relatives to consider alternative modes of therapy. The name of one doctor stood out prominently in this regard because he was widely advertised, even in leading newspapers, as a "specialist in the treatment of epilepsy, having treated more than 25,000 patients over the last 15 years." These claims were reinforced with highly favorable references from many prominent personalities. This was promising enough for a young man with uncontrolled epilepsy and he approached this doctor with hope of a cure. The antiepileptic drugs were discontinued and he was started on some tablets, which were to be taken daily. However, in spite of regular treatment, the seizures continued with a frequency of about one every month.

EXAMINATION AND INVESTIGATIONS

After several months, the patient came to Bombay Hospital for further advice. Clinical examination was normal. A magnetic resonance imaging scan of the brain showed a small cystic area in the right frontal cortex, probably representing the treated tuberculoma. His routine blood tests were normal. His blood was also sent for measurement of levels of the commonly used antiepileptic drugs. To our surprise, his serum phenytoin

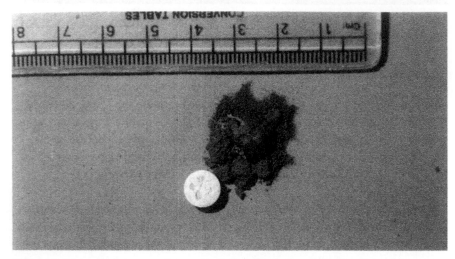

f0010 FIGURE 34.1   The "alternative" drugs that were given to the patient. The crushed, brown tablet contained a combination of phenytoin sodium and phenobarbital.

level was 13.1 μg/ml (which was in the therapeutic range) and his serum phenobarbital level was 14.8 μg/ml (slightly below the therapeutic level), even though he was supposedly not on either of these drugs! His medicines were then sent to an independent laboratory for analysis and one of the tablets was found to contain a combination of phenytoin sodium and phenobarbital (Figure 34.1).

s0030 ## DIAGNOSIS

p0040 Right frontal lobe epilepsy, probably due to a tuberculous granuloma.

s0040 ## TREATMENT AND OUTCOME

p0050 The "traditional" medicines were discontinued and replaced with conventional antiepileptic drugs. With adjustment of doses and regular serum assays, optimal seizure control was achieved.

s0050 ## COMMENTARY

s0060 ### Why did I choose this case?

p0060 Many patients have great faith in alternative systems of medicine. This is especially true in situations where modern medicine is considered to be either ineffectual or when the side effects of therapy are unacceptably severe. The merits of the alternative systems cannot be ignored, but it should be noted that the side effects of alternative drugs and drug interactions are often not clearly defined. Patients and even physicians tend to consider these medicines safe although there may be insufficient evidence to sub-stantiate this claim. Similarly, most physicians do not consider prescription of non-allopathic drugs at the same time as "conventional" drugs to be potentially harmful, and patients are rarely asked to discontinue "alternative" drugs when conventional drugs are prescribed. In addition, as with conventional drugs, quality control may at times be suboptimal.

I chose this case because it illustrates the dangers of simultaneous prescription of allopathic and non-allopathic drugs, especially when the quality of drugs is not ade-quately monitored. With this patient, if conventional antiepileptic drugs had been started without discontinuing the "alternative" ones, dangerous and even fatal toxic effects could have resulted.

What did I learn from this case?

The important lessons are:

- proper standardization and quality control are essential for all drugs, be they allopathic or non-allopathic;
- side effects and drug interactions of all drugs should be objectively studied and clearly defined;
- patients need to inform their physicians about other medications they may be taking; and
- physicians should inform their patients that drug interactions may occur even between allopathic and non-allopathic medicines, and care needs to be exercised when such drugs are used in combination.

ACKNOWLEDGEMENT

This case has been reproduced with the kind permission of the publishers of the *Journal of the Royal College of Physicians of London*, in which it was first published as a scientific letter. (Bharucha NE, Kuruvilla T. Co-prescription of conventional and "alternative medicines." *J Roy Coll Phys Lon* 1999;**33**:285.)

FURTHER READING

Angell M, Kassirer JP. Alternative medicine, the risks of untested and unregulated remedies. *N Engl J Med* 1998;**339**:839–41.

Jonas WB. Alternative medicine: learning from the past, examining the present, advancing to the future. *JAMA* 1998;**280**:1616–8.

Psychology Treats Epilepsy (advertisement). *Times of India*. Mumbai, 14 June 1998: 3.

c00035

A 19-Year-Old Man with Epilepsy, Aphasia, and Hemangioma of the Cranial Vault

Paulo Rogério M de Bittencourt

HISTORY

p0010

I first met the patient in 1996 when he was 19 years old. He was having daily seizures, could not speak, and was either hyperkinetic or autistic depending on the information that the mother chose to believe. He never slept well, never swallowed pills, and always had trouble swallowing food. He received excellent attention from his parents and two sisters.

p0020

His mother's pregnancy had been normal and his birth had been by forceps. Cyanosis was noted. A laryngeal cyst was diagnosed. Despite esophageal dilatation procedures, he aspirated frequently. At the age of 2 months, the cyst was resected. Five hours after surgery he went into cardiac arrest and was resuscitated, requiring a tracheotomy.

p0030

He held up his head at age 3 months, sat at 4 months, made sounds at 8 months, walked at 2 years, and controlled his sphincters at 4 years.

p0040

At 6 months of age, his sleep worsened. He did not sleep more than a few minutes at a time and was hyperkinetic during the day. When he was 4 years old, his physicians stopped treating him with sedatives because they made him more agitated.

p0050

At 5 years of age he developed absences, and Lennox–Gastaut syndrome was diagnosed. Soon after this, he developed drop attacks. At the age of 8 years, he began having tonic-clonic seizures. An eight-channel EEG showed bursts of generalized spike-waves, which were taken to be consistent with Lennox–Gastaut syndrome. An anesthetic accident that occurred during an attempted head computed tomography (CT) scan required resuscitation. Until he was 10 years of age, his buccal hygiene was poor because he would not allow contact with that area. He accepted only liquids and liquefied

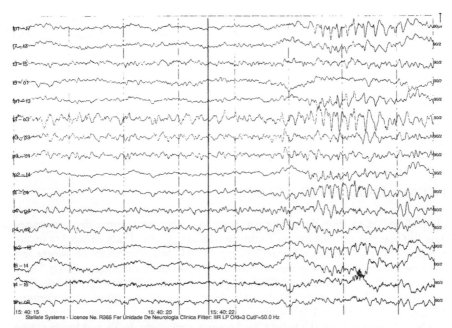

FIGURE 35.1   EEG showing continuous slowing in the left frontocentral region, which frequently spread widely through the left hemisphere.

foods, and then only at the end of every second day. This situation remained until 1996, when he was 19.

EXAMINATION AND INVESTIGATIONS

On presentation in 1996 the patient had an expressive aphasia, making grunts, and communicating by pointing out things with his eyes and hands. He understood most of what happened around him in spite of having brief absence seizures with eye blinking that occurred almost every minute. I estimated that his IQ, except for the aphasia, was in the 60s. He weighed 85 kg and was ataxic. There were no other physical or neurological abnormalities.

An EEG showed continuous slowing in the left frontocentral region, which frequently spread widely through the left hemisphere (Figure 35.1) and eventually evolved to frequent absence seizures with blinking and generalized irregular spike–wave discharges. The seizures lasted 4–20 s and occurred every 10–30 s.

The mother refused to allow further investigations because of the anesthetic accidents in childhood. Follow-up EEGs showed progressively less frequent abnormalities. Eventually, in late 1996, a waking background rhythm of 5–6 Hz was observed.

A very old CT scan was reportedly normal. In mid-1999, a 99-technetium ECD cerebral single photon emission CT scan showed decreased perfusion in the left perisylvian region. A 2.0 T magnetic resonance imaging (MRI) study showed a very large cranial vault hemangioma in the left parietal region. Five months later, a contrast

MRI scan followed by a bone-density CT scan showed that the hemangioma was unchanged, had no intracranial extension, and did not involve the meninges or cortex.

s0030   ## DIAGNOSIS

p0100   A diagnosis of epilepsy with aphasia was made, which was felt to characterize the patient's neurological condition more accurately than either autism or hyperkinetic behavior.

s0040   ## TREATMENT AND OUTCOME

p0110   On presentation in 1996 the patient was receiving valproate 2250 mg/day, carbamazepine 1800 mg/day, and clonazepam 10 mg/day. His therapy was slowly changed to oxcarbazepine 1600 mg/day and valproate 2000 mg/day. He lost 10 kg of excess weight and developed insomnia. He went into absence status epilepticus, vomiting profusely. Doses were changed to oxcarbazepine 1800 mg/day and valproate 1500 mg/day. In late 1997 he was having absences every few days. His drug regimen was changed to lamotrigine 150 mg/day and valproate 1000 mg/day.

p0120   Over the past 4 years, the patient has become a relatively docile and happy young man. He likes traveling by plane, riding cars, and playing, but he does not sleep continuously for more than 4 h. He enjoys his family and understands most of what happens. Some of his noises have become objective. His swallowing problem ended in late 1998, allowing him to take tablets regularly and to eat everything. His seizures stopped in early 1999. His only word is *Mae*, which is the word for Mum in Portuguese.

p0130   A thorough search of the literature and consultation with two expert neurosurgeons, including an uncle of the patient, as well as Dr. Fred Andermann of Montreal, did not reveal any relationship between the bone malformation and the patient's epilepsy or aphasia. After the follow-up MRI scan showed that the lesion had not changed, everybody decided to leave it alone.

s0050   ## COMMENTARY

p0140   This was a difficult case all around – the difficulties in successfully treating the seizures, the combination of seizures and aphasia, and the complex decision-making presented by the rare cranial vault hemangioma.

s0060   ### What did I learn from this case?

p0150   This case has reinforced my belief that benzodiazepines are as bad – or worse – than barbiturates. (One of my first publications dealt with this subject.) In my view, prescribing a benzodiazepine or a barbiturate to people with a chronic, long-standing disorder should only be a temporary maneuver. I also learned that Murphy's law applies to complex cases. Such patients may be victims of consecutive tragedies, rarities, and mysterious undiagnosable conditions. One can only be humble and take things as they come, just as the families of these patients do.

FURTHER READING

Bittencourt PRM, Richens A. Anticonvulsant-induced status epilepticus in Lennox–Gastaut syndrome: a case report. *Epilepsia* 1981;**22**:129–34.

Bittencourt PRM, Antoniuk AS, Bigarella MM, *et al.* Carbamazepine and phenytoin in epilepsies refractory to barbiturates: efficacy, toxicity and mental function. *Epilepsy Res* 1993;**16**:147–55.

Paillas JE, Grisoli F, Vincentelli F, Hassoun J. Hemangiomas of the cranial vault. Atypical forms: lacunar, pseudomeningiomatous, hyperostotic. *Neurochirurgie* 1977;**23**:475–90.

c00036

Severe Psychiatric Disorder in an 8-Year-Old Boy with Myoclonic–Astatic Seizures

Césare Maria Cornaggia, Alessandra Mascarini and Giuseppe Gobbi

s0010

HISTORY

p0010

An 8-year-old boy with epilepsy was initially diagnosed as autistic. Atypical absences had passed unobserved for a long time – consequently, epilepsy was not considered until he was 6 years old, when brief myoclonic–astatic seizures were recognized. The frequency of the seizures progressively increased until they were occurring more than once a day.

p0020

The initial EEG was performed when the patient was aged 6 years 3 months. It showed background slowing and frequent diffuse spike–wave discharges. Frequent atypical absences were also recorded. Valproate alone and in combination with lamotrigine led to good control of the drop attacks but was associated with a rash and persistent myoclonic head drops. Complete seizure control was obtained for a short period of time with the combination of valproate and clobazam, but at the cost of worsening of the psychiatric and behavioral disturbances.

p0030

His behavior problems were multiple. He jostled himself, avoided his parents, and developed marked phobias against strong male figures. He also reported seeing monsters and hearing sudden noises. In addition, regression and disorganization of his language, with a loss of communicative content, and an almost continuous use of the third person, were noted. His interests narrowed, and he scarcely involved himself in group activities and showed aggression toward his contemporaries, with little respect for group hierarchies and rules. Manual stereotypies were observed. At school, he subsequently developed marked learning difficulties in reading, writing, and arithmetic. In addition, marked attention and concentration deficits were described, to the extent that his scholastic performance was minimal and possibly nonexistent.

p0040

His behavior soon changed to almost continuous closure characterized by complete polarization of attention toward certain cartoon characters (Ninja turtles), which totally absorbed his interest, and the persistence of repetitive and stereotyped attitudes.

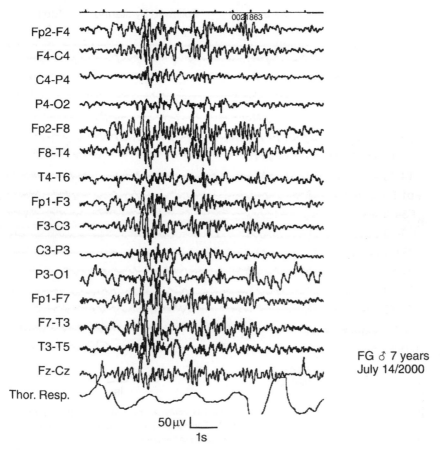

FIGURE 36.1   Burst of diffuse spike-and-wave discharges, maximal in the anterior regions.

EXAMINATION AND INVESTIGATIONS

When he presented in November 1999, the patient's behavior was characterized by impulsiveness with sudden changes in mood, little tolerance of frustration and thoughts that were concentrated on selective interests and motor hyperkinesia.

The neuropsychological assessment revealed markedly labile attention, deficits in concentration and learning (with no scholastic learning), and language atypias such as lexical impoverishment, a lack of relation to context, and the use of the third person.

The results of neurological and neuroimaging assessments were normal. EEG examination showed slowing of background activity and frequent diffuse spike–wave discharges, which were more frequent during sleep (Figures 36.1 and 36.2).

A few months later, he had a new MRI evaluation with thinner slices (instead of the 5 mm slices of the previous one): it was possible to identify a focal frontal dysplasia. He decided to continue the treatment in another medical center where he had surgery. We know that after the surgical removal he obtained a complete seizure control, but no improvements in behavior and cognitive functions were observed.

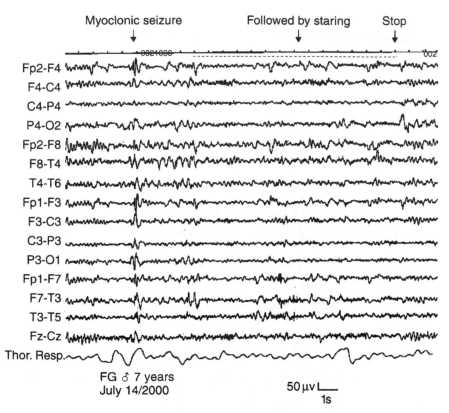

FIGURE 36.2   The seizure starts with a myoclonic jerk concomitant with a generalized spike-and-wave discharge and is followed by staring lasting 14s. During this phase, monomorphic theta activity interrupted by rapid rhythm appears bilaterally over the central regions.

DIAGNOSIS

Psychogenic disorder (DSM-IV 299.80) and "mental retardation" (DSM-IV 319); epilepsy with myoclonic–astatic seizures. Actually, after the last MRI the diagnosis of epileptic disease may be reviewed. Before we considered this patient as affected by a generalized epilepsy with myoclonic–astatic seizures. Now we believe that this patient has a focal frontal lobe epilepsy with severe evolution into a kind of epileptic encephalopathy with bilateral synchrony and myoclonic–astatic seizures. We also think that this diagnosis is better connected with the neuropsychological picture of "deficits in concentration and learning (with no scholastic learning) and language atypias such as lexical impoverishment."

TREATMENT AND OUTCOME

Treatment with felbamate (45 mg/kg/day) and valproate (34.6 mg/kg/day) before surgery controlled the drop attacks and markedly decreased the other seizures (such as myoclonic head drops) without causing any severe unwanted psychiatric effects. The improvement in epilepsy was actually accompanied by modest behavioral improvement, although the cognitive difficulties persisted.

COMMENTARY

Why did we choose this case?

We chose this case because it shows the interactions between epilepsy and psychiatric, cognitive, and behavioral disturbances. Psychiatric, cognitive, and behavioral disturbances can sometimes prevail over epileptic symptoms to the extent that the diagnosis of epilepsy is missed altogether for a number of years. Furthermore, in this case, the behavioral, relational, and communicative disturbances were associated with a cognitive deficit.

A number of severe epileptic conditions, such as some frontal lobe epilepsies with subcontinuous specific EEG activity (including rapid activity lasting for 1–1.5 s) are associated with severe behavioral disturbances (sometimes with psychotic symptoms) or schizophrenia-like or autism-like syndromes. The literature also includes cases of selective cognitive disturbances associated with EEG anomalies, such as the Landau–Kleffner syndrome.[1] There are also other cases in which an early disturbance of language function has led to a disturbance in communication and social interaction, such as the cases reported by Echenne et al.,[2] which others have included among the regressive autistic syndromes with epileptiform anomalies.[3] There are also extreme conditions involving severe and complex impairment of mental functions, such as the continuous spike-wave during sleep syndrome, in which cognitive deterioration (with deficits in attention, memory, problem solving, abstraction, and learning) is associated with a behavioral and psychiatric disturbance characterized by hyperkinesia, impulsiveness, perseveration, personality alteration with autistic regression, and disintegrative psychosis. Roulet-Perez et al.[4] and Patry et al.[5] have proposed the hypothesis of an acquired epileptic frontal syndrome in these cases.

Clearly, our case is not as severe as that of the continuous spike-wave during sleep syndrome, and no EEG picture typical of the continuous spike-wave during sleep syndrome has ever been recorded. But is our case less serious because there are fewer EEG findings? And are interictal EEG abnormalities really just that, or could they be the expression of subtle seizures? The extent to which subtle seizures or epileptiform EEG activity affect learning and behavior remains controversial. One wonders if some children who are diagnosed as having attention deficit disorders or autism may actually have undiagnosed manifestations of epilepsy.[6,7]

What did we learn from this case?

We believe that it is important to report cases such as this one because they are potential sources of serious diagnostic errors: the initial diagnosis of primary autism in this patient, also with the beginning of a psychotherapeutic treatment, was a mistake, because the psychiatric disturbance was secondary to the unrecognized epilepsy or secondary to epileptiform EEG discharges (not investigated) even in the absence of clinical seizures.

Secondly, cases such as this underline the need to clarify the causative role of epilepsy and non-convulsive EEG epileptiform discharges in childhood behavioral problems. We believe that the use of EEG in children with behavioral or learning disturbances should be strongly considered:[6] to have more clinical data to complete the diagnosis it would be useful to have an EEG evaluation not only during waking, but also during nocturnal sleeping.

A thorough neuropsychological evaluation could suggest involvement of specific cerebral areas to better orient the neuroimaging investigations. In this case the frontal dysplasia was observed after repeating the MRI for persistent seizures: in this way it was possible to correlate the neuropsychological findings with the location of the lesion.

We similarly believe that it is worthwhile to consider interventions to improve interictal EEG discharges, although we recognize that this requires particular prudence and has to be individually evaluated because antiepileptic drugs may, at least partly, disrupt cognitive processing.

In conclusion, we would like to underline that the use of an MRI capable of 2-mm slices instead of 5-mm slices had been essential in this case to make the right diagnosis.

The prognosis of a cognitive and behavioral disturbance of this type greatly depends on its duration, and so precious time may had been lost in this case as a result of the undiagnosed epilepsy.[8]

REFERENCES

1. Stephani U. The natural history of myoclonic astatic epilepsy (Doose syndrome) and Lennox-Gastaut syndrome. *Epilepsia* 2006;**47(Suppl. 2)**:53–5.
2. Echenne B, Cheminal R, Rivier F, *et al.* Epileptic electroencephalographic abnormalities and developmental dysphasias: a study of 32 patients. *Brain Dev* 1992;**14**:216–25.
3. Touchman R, Rapin I. Regression in pervasive developmental disorders: seizures and EEG correlates. *Pediatrics* 1997;**99**:560–6.
4. Roulet-Perez E, Davidiff V, Despland PA, Deonna T. Mental and behavioural deterioration of children with epilepsy and CWCS: acquired epileptic frontal syndrome. *Dev Med Child Neurol* 1993;**35**:661–74.
5. Patry G, Lyagoubi S, Tassinari CA. Subclinical 'electrical status epilepticus' induced by sleep in children. *Arch Neurol* 1971;**24**:242–52.
6. Cornaggia CM, Gobbi G. Learning disability in epilepsy: definitions and classification. *Epilepsia* 2001;**42(suppl 1)**:2–5.
7. Hughes JR, DeLeo AJ, Melyn MA. The electroencephalogram in attention deficit disorder: emphasis on epileptiform discharges. *Epilepsy Behav* 2000;**1**:271–7.
8. Besag FMC. Epilepsy, learning, and behaviour in childhood. *Epilepsia* 1995;**36(suppl 1)**:58–63.

A Girl with Two Epilepsy Syndromes

Marie-José Penniello, Isabelle Jambaqué, Christine Bulteau, Perrine
Plouin, Olivier Delalande and Olivier Dulac

HISTORY

The patient is a right-handed girl who was born at full term after normal pregnancy
and delivery. She had two healthy siblings and no familial antecedents of epilepsy.
Psychomotor development was initially normal. At the age of 41 months, she had her
first febrile convulsion, which consisted of loss of consciousness, trismus, and limb
hypertonia with massive jerks, mydriasis and cyanosis around the mouth. The convulsion lasted over 30 min, but because the onset was not noticed, the precise duration
could not be determined. It was followed by right hemiparesis that lasted for several
hours. Carbamazepine treatment was started.

At the age of 47 months, a second long-lasting but non-febrile seizure was also
followed by transient weakness of the right arm and leg. After recovery from the transient postictal paresis, neurological examination failed to demonstrate any motor defect
or pyramidal signs, but there was lack of speech, including very poor comprehension
and no expression. The child seemed to react to a few familiar noises, including those
produced by some animals, and to very high-pitched sounds, but she did not react
to speech. Indeed, during the child's third year of life, the parents had noticed the
insidious regression of speech abilities with aggressive behavior and poor interpersonal
communication resulting in schooling difficulties. However, they did not seek medical
advice for these troubles until the occurrence of the convulsions.

After the second seizure, an EEG showed paroxysmal focal spike–wave activity predominating in the left temporal area, becoming diffuse and continuous in sleep (Figure 37.1).

Transmission deafness could be excluded, and brainstem evoked potentials were
normal. Brain magnetic resonance imaging (MRI) disclosed no abnormality (Figure
37.2). Landau–Kleffner syndrome was diagnosed and carbamazepine was replaced
with the combination of valproate and diazepam. Within 3 months, the EEG tracings
returned to normal and the child showed major improvement in speech (both perception and expression). She started to read at the age of 7.5 years. Sodium valproate was
gradually tapered at the age of 7.75 years, and diazepam was stopped 8 months later.

Puzzling Cases of Epilepsy

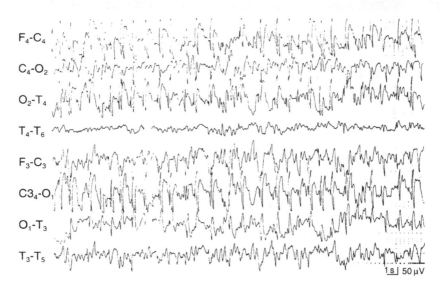

FIGURE 37.1   Sleep EEG recording at the age of 4 years, showing interictal paroxysmal spike-wave activity that is continuous and diffuse, although it predominates in the left temporal area.

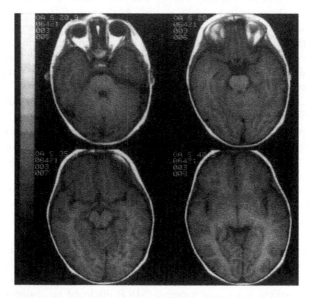

FIGURE 37.2   Normal MRI scan at the age of 4 years after the second episode of long-lasting unilateral convulsive seizure. There is no evidence of mesial temporal abnormality.

After cessation of treatment, the child remained seizure-free for the next 2.5 years, but at the age of 10.25 years, a new type of seizure occurred. It consisted of an arrest of activity and speech with fixed gaze, bilateral mydriasis, and head shaking that seemed to be automatic. When the child resumed normal activity, she complained of

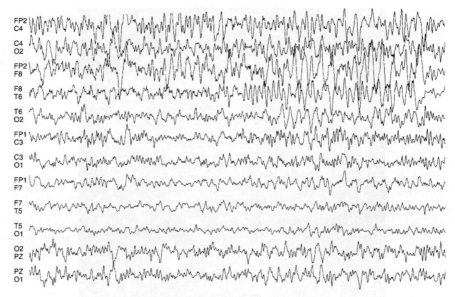

FIGURE 37.3   Ictal EEG recording at the age of 12 years, showing a right temporal focal seizure discharge. There was no concomitant clinical manifestation.

epigastric heaviness, and there was complete amnesia of the ictal event. These seizures lasted 30–60 s and occurred twice a week.

Pre-surgical evaluation was performed since these seizures suggested mesio-temporal epilepsy.

INVESTIGATIONS

On neuropsychological investigation, the child proved to have good attention. The Wechsler Intelligence Scale for Children (version III) disclosed clear dissociation between verbal abilities (a score of 56) and non-verbal abilities (a score of 90). There were phonological defects and articulation troubles. The Chevrie–Muller test revealed major difficulties in repetition of simple words as well as dyssyntaxia. Naming remained difficult, with phonemic paraphasias. In addition, memory for both verbal and non-verbal items was affected. While these neuropsychological findings are consistent with the Landau–Kleffner syndrome, the patient's persistent speech abnormalities meant that it was not possible to determine whether she was affected by additional cognitive dysfunction consistent with mesial temporal sclerosis.

Ictal EEG recording showed that most discharges affected the left temporal area, although a single seizure affected the right temporal area (Figure 37.3). An MRI scan showed left mesial temporal atrophy (Figure 37.4).

Long-lasting video–EEG with bilateral foramen ovale electrodes was obtained at the age of 12 years; 11 electro-clinical seizures were registered with onset in left mesio-temporal or fronto-temporal lobe. Discharges from right mesial temporal structures were always a reflection of the left-sided discharges and were asymptomatic. We

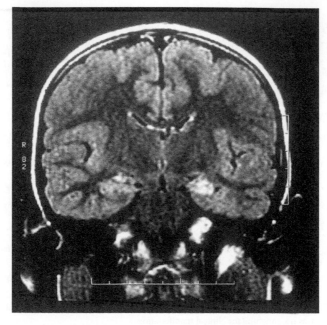

FIGURE 37.4   FLAIR MRI sequence at the age of 12 years, showing bilateral mesial temporal atrophy, predominating on the left, with hyperintensity signal on this side.

performed intracranial exploration with grids and depth electrodes placed in the left fronto-temporal region, which confirmed the left mesio-temporal onset of seizures.

TREATMENT AND OUTCOME

Treatment with valproate, gabapentin, and vigabatrin failed to control the seizures. A left internal and polar temporal resection was done at the age of 13 years. Histological analysis found hippocampal sclerosis and nodular heterotopias. After surgery, she became free of seizures and of antiepileptic drugs but developed severe depression. At the age of 17 years, she was doing well, pursuing professional training and had recovered normal affect.

DIAGNOSIS

Landau–Kleffner syndrome and mesial temporal lobe epilepsy with mesial temporal sclerosis.

COMMENTARY

Because epilepsy in childhood demonstrates such great variability, the use of epilepsy syndromes to categorize patients considerably helps the clinician to approach diagnosis in a pragmatic fashion[1,2] and to select optimal treatment.[3] However, the situation may be complicated when a patient seems to combine two epilepsy syndromes, as in this case.

To our knowledge, this is the first reported case combining Landau–Kleffner syndrome with mesial temporal epilepsy, at two different times in the same child. Although both types of epilepsy affect the temporal lobe, they are clearly distinct from each other. One exhibits no evidence of a brain lesion and mainly affects the neocortex during the course of development of speech, while the other results from focal atrophy and affects the mesial temporal lobe after speech is fully acquired. In this patient, both types of epilepsy were separated by a silent period of over 2 years.

The first signs of epilepsy in this case very probably consisted of speech deterioration, although it is only when the child experienced convulsive seizures that the parents considered this concern as a possible neurological disorder. Thus, features of Landau–Kleffner syndrome were the first to appear. EEG abnormalities and speech troubles were controlled when carbamazepine was stopped and replaced by valproate and a benzodiazepine. Corticosteroids are usually advocated to control continuous spike–wave activity in patients with Landau–Kleffner syndrome,[4] but this was not necessary in the present case. Carbamazepine is known to increase spike–wave activity and to eventually trigger the development of continuous spike-waves in slow sleep and its psychomotor correlates.[5] Stopping this drug is therefore a prerequisite for the treatment of this condition.

The other major and very unusual event in the history of this child was the occurrence of two long-lasting, focal motor seizures followed by transient motor deficit. When she presented with mesial temporal epilepsy, the MRI scan showed atrophy that predominated on the side contralateral to the transient postictal motor deficit. This finding was not present on the first MRI scan, which was performed when Landau–Kleffner syndrome was diagnosed.

As in this case, long-lasting seizures followed by motor deficits are known to precede mesial temporal atrophy by several years in a number of patients.[6] The fact that her MRI scan was normal just after the initial episode of status epilepticus suggests that atrophy did not precede this event but rather that it may have been a consequence of it.

In this case, complex partial seizures occurred over a period of 4 years after the disappearance of the continuous spike-waves in slow sleep. Ictal recording showed that these new seizures originated from the left temporal lobe, the site of the hippocampal sclerosis that was disclosed on MRI.

What did we learn from this case?

The relationship between Landau–Kleffner syndrome and mesial temporal sclerosis is difficult to establish. Mesial temporal sclerosis is not a usual finding in patients with Landau–Kleffner syndrome, in which the MRI scan is most often normal,[7] as was the case in this child when the syndrome was identified. In an attempt to improve speech in patients with Landau–Kleffner syndrome, temporal lobectomies have been performed, but without success.[8] The most striking characteristic of Landau–Kleffner syndrome is, in fact, the scarcity of ictal discharges. The animal model of continuous spike–wave activity developed by Barbarosie and Avoli[9] demonstrated the difficulty in eliciting tonic discharges, which are the hallmark of convulsive status epilepticus, as if continuous spike–wave activity could prevent tonic discharges.

p0190   Therefore, any cause-and-effect relationship between Landau–Kleffner syndrome and mesial temporal sclerosis in this case is most unlikely. However, both the epilepsy syndromes exhibited by this patient could in fact have resulted from a common predisposition to epilepsy that produced both status epilepticus and major spike–wave activity. Pre-existing anatomical anomalies that were not disclosed on either MRI scan, such as microdysgenesis, cannot be ruled out.

p0200   There is growing evidence that cognitive functions are affected differently in different epilepsy syndromes.[10] In this patient, the cognitive troubles were those of Landau–Kleffner syndrome, but memory disturbances related to mesial temporal sclerosis could not be identified because of the limited language function.[11] Therefore, this case taught us that the impact of continuous spike–wave activity on developing speech during childhood is so striking that it masks the later effects of hippocampal sclerosis and mesial temporal epilepsy.

p0210   Finally post-operative depression was quite surprising since mood disorders are usually improved after successful temporal lobe epilepsy. We could hypothesize that the implication of bilateral temporal lobe involvement in her medical history has made cognitive functions and emotional process recovery more difficult.[12,13]

REFERENCES

1. Roger J, Bureau M, Dravet C, Dreifuss F, Perret A, Wolf P. *Epileptic syndromes in infancy, childhood and adolescence.* London: John Libbey, 1991.
2. Commission on Classification and Terminology of the International League against Epilepsy. Proposal for revised classification of epilepsies and epileptic syndromes. *Epilepsia* 1989;**30**:389–99.
3. Dulac O, Leppik I. Initiating and discontinuing treatment. In: Engel J, Pedley J, eds. *Epilepsy: a comprehensive textbook.* New York: Lippincott–Raven, 1998: 1237–46.
4. Lerman P, Lerman-Sagie T, Kivity S. Effects of early corticosteroid therapy for Landau–Kleffner syndrome. *Dev Med Child Neurol* 1991;**33**:257–60.
5. Perucca E, Gram L, Avanzini G, Dulac O. Antiepileptic drugs as a cause of worsening seizures. *Epilepsia* 1998;**39**:5–17.
6. Cendes F, Andermann F, Dubeau F, et al. Early childhood prolonged febrile convulsions, atrophy and sclerosis of mesial structures, and temporal lobe epilepsy: an MRI volumetric study. *Neurology* 1993;**43**:1083–7.
7. O'Regan ME, Brown JK, Goodwin GM, Clarke M. Epileptic aphasia: a consequence of regional hypometabolic encephalopathy? *Dev Med Child Neurol* 1998;**40**:508–16.
8. Cole AJ, Andermann F, Taylor L, et al. The Landau–Kleffner syndrome of acquired epileptic aphasia: unusual clinical outcome, surgical experience, and absence of encephalitis. *Neurology* 1988;**38**:31–8.
9. Barbarosie M, Avoli M. CA3-driven hippocampal–entorhinal loop controls rather than sustains in vitro limbic seizures. *J Neurosci* 1997;**17**:9308–14.
10. Dulac O. Mechanisms, classification and management of seizures and epilepsies. In: Jambaqué I, Dulac O, Lassonde M, eds. *Neuropsychology of childhood epilepsy.* New York: Kluwer Academic/Plenum Press, 2001: 1–12.
11. Jambaqué I, Dellatolas G, Dulac O, Ponsot G, Signoret JL. Verbal and visual memory impairment in children with epilepsy. *Neuropsychologia* 1993;**31**:1321–37.
12. Devinsky O, Barr WB, Vickrey A, et al. Changes in depression and anxiety after resective surgery for epilepsy. *Neurology* 2005;**65**:1744–9.
13. Gilliam FG, Maton BM, Martin RC, et al. Hippocampal 1H-MRSI correlates with severity of depression symptoms in temporal lobe epilepsy. *Neurology* 2007;**68**:364–8.

38

The Obvious Cause of Seizures May Not Be the Underlying Cause

Keith R Edwards

HISTORY

The patient is a 48-year-old man with a previous history of alcohol and drug abuse. He presented to the emergency department following a generalized tonic–clonic seizure. He had no history of seizures and no history of head trauma, but he did have a recent history of alcohol abuse with decreasing amounts over the last several days, although he had not totally stopped drinking.

EXAMINATION AND INVESTIGATIONS

In the emergency department, the patient was initially postictal but without focal findings. A cranial computed tomography (CT) scan without contrast was unremarkable, and the patient quickly regained orientation. He was not started on any anticonvulsant therapy. Outpatient follow-up with EEG was scheduled in 1–2 weeks.

However, 48 h later, the patient returned in status epilepticus. He responded to lorazepam 2 mg intravenously. He was then given phenytoin 1 g intravenously without further seizures, but he had a prolonged postictal state that required careful observation. He aspirated and was treated for pneumonia. Repeat cranial CT with and without contrast was unremarkable. The patient could not cooperate for a magnetic resonance imaging (MRI) scan. EEG showed generalized slowing but no seizure activity.

INITIAL DIAGNOSIS

Seizures related to alcohol abuse and past history of head trauma (the patient had had numerous falls).

s0040

TREATMENT AND OUTCOME

p0050

Following the episode of status epilepticus, it was determined that long-term phenytoin was necessary. He was therefore discharged on phenytoin 300 mg daily and did well for the next 3 months. He attended Alcoholics Anonymous and remained free of further seizure activity. On two office visits 6 weeks apart, the patient had a normal examination, including a normal cognitive status.

p0060

The patient then began having right arm tremor associated with an altered state of consciousness and loss of speech lasting 5–10 min. He was seen in the emergency department and found to have undetectable phenytoin levels. He was given 500 mg phenytoin intravenously. He was felt to be non-compliant.

p0070

However, over the next 2 weeks, the patient continued to have intermittent complex partial seizures with a therapeutic phenytoin level.

p0080

The EEG was repeated, showing focal slowing in the left frontal region. Cranial MRI showed a neoplasm in the left frontal lobe. Craniotomy revealed high-grade malignancy consistent with glioblastoma multiforme.

s0050

COMMENTARY

p0090

The patient had an all-too-familiar seizure presentation associated with alcohol. However, when the seizure pattern changed to multiple complex partial seizures, further imaging was done with MRI scanning. The underlying neoplasm was found in a reasonably timely fashion but there was still considered to be some delay, owing to the multifactorial aspect of the patient's seizure etiology.

s0060

What did I learn from this case?

p0100

In this case, timely follow-up with the patient and listening to his complaints and those of his family saved the patient from a more delayed diagnosis, from which there may have been more disastrous results. I learned that patients may have multiple etiologies for seizures and to reconsider the underlying cause if the seizure type or frequency changes.

s0070

How did this case alter my approach to the care and treatment of my epilepsy patients?

p0110

Although alcohol abuse is a common cause of seizures, I am more alert to patients' breakthrough seizures, particularly with any focal type of symptomatology. The presentation of status epilepticus just 2 days after a first seizure, even with alcohol, should have prompted me to follow up with an MRI scan sooner than was done in this case, once the patient was stable and able to cooperate. The fact that he had continued seizures long after he was alcohol-free should have altered my thinking away from the patient's alcohol as a precipitating factor of his seizure to other etiologies.

Absence Seizures in an Adult

Edward Faught

HISTORY

The patient is a 53-year-old woman with a history of seizures beginning at the age of 5 years. The seizures occurred several times daily when she was a young child. Witnesses described a sudden blank stare, sometimes accompanied by humming or picking at her clothes. Occasionally she walked around during the episodes but she never fell down. Urinary incontinence occurred with some of the seizures up until the age of 12. Although she never had a warning or an aura, she usually knew when she had a seizure because she recalled a sensation "as if daydreaming." She specifically described this as not merely a loss of time but as a definite feeling. She has had only four generalized tonic–clonic seizures in her life, each proceeded by an odd feeling of "going down a tunnel."

Precipitating factors included the premenstrual state and "stress." As a car passenger, she noted that sunlight flickering through the trees made her feel as if she were going to have a seizure.

Previous treatments had included phenobarbital, ethosuximide, phenytoin, primidone, and acetazolamide. She had a previous EEG that was abnormal, but she reported that her doctors could not decide whether she had "petit mal" or "frontal" seizures. When I first saw her, she was 42 years old and was taking carbamazepine 1400 mg/day. She was having up to 20 seizures each day, and she stated that she had never gone more than 3 days in her life without seizures. Despite this, she had 13 years of education, was married, had children, and had a supervisory job.

EXAMINATION AND INVESTIGATIONS

General and neurological examinations were normal. The patient appeared to be of above-average intelligence. An EEG demonstrated hyperventilation-induced three-per-second spike–wave discharges with a generalized distribution and a bifrontal voltage maximum. One of these discharges lasted 14 s and was accompanied by staring, lip smacking and patting the thigh with the right hand. No photosensitivity was detected. A magnetic resonance imaging scan was normal.

DIAGNOSIS

Childhood-onset absence epilepsy persisting into adult life.

TREATMENT AND OUTCOME

Valproate was begun and gradually increased to 30 mg/kg/day, and carbamazepine was stopped. The patient improved immediately, but she still had one or two seizures each day. Over the next 5 years, addition of ethosuximide or felbamate to valproate was of little help. At the age of 47, a lamotrigine–ethosuximide combination rendered her seizure-free. After 3 years without seizures, at her request, and after a normal 24-h ambulatory EEG, first ethosuximide then lamotrigine was tapered and stopped, during a 6-month driving restriction. She has remained free of seizures, off all medications, for 3 years. A recent 24-h ambulatory EEG recording was normal.

COMMENTARY

This patient was treated with carbamazepine because she was thought to have complex partial seizures. This error could have been avoided by recognizing that

- automatisms occur in 38–63% of absence seizures;[1,2]
- in adults, generalized spike–wave discharges usually have a frontal voltage predominance, and may be asymmetrical[3]; and
- that patients with generalized epilepsies may have prodromal sensations and unusual perceptions.[4]

Nevertheless, differentiation of absence from frontal lobe complex partial seizures can be quite difficult. Bancaud et al.[3] demonstrated experimentally that stimulation of mesial frontal structures can produce symmetrical spike–wave discharges, and it is clear that this happens clinically. This EEG phenomenon is called "secondary bilateral synchrony." The assumption that adults with staring spells have complex partial seizures should be examined in each case.

Carbamazepine often worsens absence seizures,[5] so that this distinction is important. Eventual complete control of seizures in this patient required a prolonged, determined quest culminating in an exotic combination of medications – ethosuximide and lamotrigine.

Because 92% of patients with late persistent absences have generalized tonic–clonic seizures as well,[6] ethosuximide alone should not be relied on for therapy; it should be combined with valproate or a sodium channel blocking agent. Of the sodium channel blockers, lamotrigine may also have some antiabsence action, and phenytoin may be less likely to exacerbate absence than carbamazepine or oxcarbazepine. If valproate is unsatisfactory as monotherapy, another broad-spectrum drug such as lamotrigine, topiramate, zonisamide, or eventually felbamate may be considered.

Perhaps the most surprising feature of this case was the occurrence of a terminal remission of seizures after 49 years, including 42 years of therapeutic futility. Gastaut et al.[6] studied the course of primary generalized epilepsy with absences persisting after the age of 30 up to the age of 61 and found that remission was rare, although the frequency of seizures tended to diminish with time. Although it is not wise to raise false hopes, it is comforting to know that remissions may occur even after half a century of troubles.

What did I learn from this case?

A diagnosis of seizure type requires careful consideration of age of onset, seizure semiology, patient report, EEG pattern, and response to therapy — and is not always simple. Patients with generalized epilepsies may report experiential phenomena that are easy to interpret as aurae of partial-onset seizures.

Not all absence epilepsies are easily treated, but one should never give up. I found an odd but surprisingly effective medication combination, so an empirical trial of an unreported polytherapy may be worthwhile.

How did this case alter my approach to the care and treatment of my epilepsy patients?

I am less smug when informing patients with a new diagnosis of absence epilepsy that they have an easily treatable syndrome. I look more carefully at my patients with diagnoses of frontal lobe complex partial seizures to consider whether they might have a primary generalized disorder. I do not dismiss out of hand a patient's request to try a medication taper after years of absence seizures, but I do carefully negotiate the conditions of the discontinuation, including restrictions on driving. I also routinely obtain a 24–48 h EEG recording before beginning the process and again before removing activity restrictions at the end.

REFERENCES

1. Penry JK, Porter RJ, Dreifuss FE. Simultaneous recording of absence seizures with videotape and EEG. *Brain* 1975;**98**:427–40.
2. Stefan H, Burr W, Hildenbrand K, Penin H. Computer-supported documentation in the video analysis of absences; preictal–ictal phenomena: polygraphic findings. In: Dam M, Gram L, Penry JK, eds. *Advances in epileptology: the XIIIth Epilepsy International Symposium*. New York: Raven Press, 1981.
3. Bancaud J, Talairach J, Morel P, et al. "Generalized" epileptic seizures elicited by electrical stimulation of the frontal lobe in man. *Electroencephalogr Clin Neurophysiol* 1974;**37**:275–82.
4. Faught E, Falgout J, Nidiffer FD, Dreifuss FE. Self-induced photosensitive absence seizures with ictal pleasure. *Arch Neurol* 1986;**43**:408–10.
5. Snead OC, Hosey LC. Exacerbation of seizures in children by carbamazepine. *N Engl J Med* 1985;**313**:916–21.
6. Gastaut H, Zifkin BG, Mariana E, Pulg JS. The long-term course of primary generalized epilepsy with persisting absences. *Neurology* 1986;**36**:1021–8.

c00040

A Case Solved by Seizures During Sleep

Jacqueline A French

s0010

HISTORY

p0010

The patient was an 18-year-old right-handed woman who had seizures dating back to the age of 2 years. These initially consisted of staring, picking at clothes, automatisms, and pacing the room. She was treated through her childhood with phenobarbital, carbamazepine, phenytoin, and primidone. By her adolescence, the patient's seizures had changed in character. They were now described as thrashing, rocking back and forth, at times striking out in a seemingly purposeful way, and injuring herself, with resultant ecchymoses of the elbow and forehead. Seizures also increased in frequency, so that she was having multiple seizures each day, preventing her from attending school. Medication included primidone, valproate, and phenytoin.

p0020

The patient had a significant family history. Her maternal great-grandfather and first cousin had generalized tonic–clonic convulsions and her brother may have had a partial seizure. Her mother was institutionalized with schizophrenia.

s0020

EXAMINATION AND INVESTIGATIONS

p0030

Physical and neurologic examinations were normal, as were magnetic resonance imaging scan and EEG.

p0040

The patient was admitted for video–EEG monitoring. Standard and sphenoidal electrodes were placed. Background EEG was entirely normal. Eight typical events were recorded, consisting of clenching her teeth, clenching her fist, and shaking in a rhythmical fashion. She would frequently utter sentences or fragments of sentences that might include obscenities. There was no apparent alteration of consciousness, and the patient was able to respond to commands to move extremities during the event. She seemed anxious and upset during these events, and she had full recollection of them afterward. During the events there was no discernible electrographic discharge. Because of this, a diagnosis of psychogenic seizures was made.

p0050

The patient continued to have frequent events and was therefore transferred to a psychiatric unit. After discharge, daytime events decreased markedly in frequency for several months. However, the patient presented again after about 6 months. Her father reported that he had witnessed no daytime events but that episodes were occurring nightly during sleep.

The patient was readmitted for video–EEG monitoring. Multiple nocturnal events were recorded. These events had identical clinical characteristics as had been seen during the first monitoring session and, again, no ictal or interictal EEG changes were noted. However, some events occurred directly out of stage 2 sleep, and the patient returned directly to sleep afterward. This prompted subsequent intracranial EEG monitoring, which confirmed that both the diurnal and the nocturnal events were frontal lobe complex partial seizures.

DIAGNOSIS

Frontal lobe complex partial seizures.

TREATMENT AND OUTCOME

A right mesial frontal resection was performed. Pathology revealed microdysgenesis and gliosis.

COMMENTARY

This patient had many characteristics that led to a diagnosis of psychogenic seizures

- a family history of psychiatric disease;
- a change in seizure semiology from her childhood seizures;
- events with no loss of awareness, purposeful movements, and full recall; and
- normal ictal and interictal EEGs.

In fact, she was having frontal lobe complex partial seizures. Several characteristics of her seizures might have raised suspicion of this diagnosis, including the fact that the events were brief and stereotyped, with rapid return to normal function. Another clue was the occurrence of stereotyped events in sleep, without awakening. These characteristics have been identified in several articles on frontal lobe epilepsy.[1,3] These articles also report characteristic seizure manifestations in patients with frontal lobe complex partial seizures, including:

- bilateral movements and complex automatisms, which are often bizarre;
- vocalizations; and
- a high seizure frequency.

The absence of an ictal or interictal correlate, although rare, may be seen in patients with frontal lobe foci.[1,2]

It is important to distinguish patients with frontal lobe complex partial seizures from those with non-epileptic seizures. Usually, diagnosis requires admission to a video–EEG monitoring unit and withdrawal of any antiepileptic drugs. Such withdrawal may increase seizure spread, causing identifiable EEG ictal changes. Inpatient monitoring may allow recognition of seizures beginning directly out of stage 2 sleep, as in this case. Such findings are rarely or never seen in patients with psychogenic events.[3]

If a diagnosis of frontal lobe complex partial seizures is confirmed and the patient has been demonstrated to be refractory to antiepileptic drug therapy, referral for surgical management should be considered. Up to 67% of patients with an identified frontal focus may become seizure-free after surgical resection.[1]

What did I learn from this case?

I learned that there is a great deal of overlap between the characteristics of pseudo-seizures and those of frontal lobe complex partial seizures. Both may cause events that are bizarre in appearance. The presence or absence of an ictal discharge does not absolutely distinguish between the two. Patients may be responsive throughout a bizarre ictal event that is physiological in nature.

How did this case alter my approach to the care and treatment of my epilepsy patients?

I am always very aware of the characteristics that may indicate frontal lobe complex partial seizures. I am careful to ask family members about nocturnal events that mimic events seen during the day. I will not rush to a diagnosis of psychogenic seizures based on one or two brief events seen in the monitoring unit if these events have any characteristics of frontal lobe complex partial seizures. In these patients, I will withdraw antiepileptic drugs while continuing monitoring. Also, I feel that some patients who have received a diagnosis of psychogenic seizures deserve a second evaluation if seizures do not remit.

REFERENCES

1. Laskowitz DT, Sperling MR, French JA, O'Connor MJ. The syndrome of frontal lobe epilepsy: characteristics and surgical management. *Neurology* 1995;**45**:780–7.
2. Williamson PD, Spencer DD, Spencer SS, Novelly RA, Mattson RH. Complex partial seizures of frontal lobe origin. *Ann Neurol* 1985;**18**:497–504.
3. Saygi S, Katz A, Marks DA, Spencer SS. Frontal lobe partial seizures and psychogenic seizures: comparison of clinical and ictal characteristics. *Neurology* 1992;**42**:1274–7.

Alternative Psychosis in an Adolescent Girl?

Andres M Kanner

HISTORY

The patient is a 17-year-old adolescent girl with a history of partial epilepsy of unknown etiology. Her seizures began at 17 months of age and have consisted primarily of complex partial seizures and less frequently of secondarily generalized tonic–clonic seizures. The semiology of her seizures and her ictal recordings are suggestive of frontal lobe epilepsy.

EXAMINATION AND INVESTIGATIONS

Prolonged video–EEG monitoring studies with scalp and intracranial electrodes failed to identify the exact location of the ictal onset. No abnormalities were identified with high-resolution brain magnetic resonance imaging scans. Testing revealed an IQ in the mild mentally retarded range.

DIAGNOSIS

Probable frontal lobe onset seizures.

TREATMENT AND OUTCOME

The patient's seizures had failed to respond to multiple trials of antiepileptic drugs and to vagus nerve stimulation. At the age of 15, after being started on clonazepam (in combination with carbamazepine) and reaching a dose of 1.5 mg/day, her seizures stopped completely.

After being seizure-free for a period of 6 weeks, her parents noted a change in her behavior – she became irritable and refused to use the toilet to urinate. The patient claimed that "she was a baby" and she therefore insisted on wearing diapers. She refused to go to the bathroom when she had the urge to urinate and would often hold the urine until she would become incontinent. Treatment with sertraline (selective serotonin reuptake inhibitor) and behavioral strategies were unsuccessful.

p0060   After several weeks, her behavior became increasingly more erratic. She seemed to be responding to auditory hallucinations and a thought disorder became apparent. Sertraline was discontinued and she was started on haloperidol. Failure to respond to neuroleptic medication led me to taper clonazepam off at a rate of 0.25 mg/week. Her psychiatric symptoms disappeared 2 days after she experienced a generalized tonic–clonic seizure that occurred upon reaching a daily dose of clonazepam of 0.25 mg/day.

p0070   In the past 2 years, this patient has had two additional prolonged seizure-free periods. The first period, while she was on a combination of valproate and lamotrigine, lasted for 4 months; the second period (while she was on levetiracetam, valproate, and lamotrigine) has so far lasted 9 months. In the course of these seizure-free periods, the patient has not had a recurrence of psychotic symptoms, despite the fact that she had been restarted on clonazepam after the seizures recurred while on valproate and lamotrigine. She does experience frequent episodes of increased irritability and poor frustration tolerance that have occasionally been associated with short bouts of aggressive behavior. This cluster of symptoms has been controlled to a certain degree with two selective serotonin reuptake inhibitors (sertraline and paroxetine).

p0080   During a recent attempt to taper off valproate, the patient developed insomnia, pressured speech, and increased energy. Sertraline was discontinued but these symptoms disappeared only after she was placed back on higher doses of valproate.

COMMENTARY

s0050

p0090   I chose this case because it exemplifies the complex relationship between epilepsy and psychiatric disorders. The psychotic episode that followed a complete cessation of seizure activity could be an example of the phenomenon of "alternative psychosis."[1] At first I could not exclude the possibility that clonazepam may have been the culprit for this patient's psychiatric symptoms. Yet a significant reduction of its dose failed to yield any improvement in her psychiatric symptoms, which remitted only after she experienced a generalized tonic–clonic seizure. Furthermore, a subsequent reintroduction of clonazepam was not associated with recurrence of these symptoms.

p0100   The concept of alternative psychosis was developed from observations by Landolt in 1953 of an inverse relationship between control of seizures and occurrence of psychotic symptoms.[2] In fact, Landolt described a "normalization" of EEG recordings with the appearance of psychiatric symptoms and coined the term "forced normalization." Wolf and Trimble suggested the term "paradoxical normalization" while Tellenbach proposed the term of "alternative psychosis."[1]

p0110   This phenomenon is rare. Landolt reported 47 cases between 1951 and 1958. Single case studies were reported by others,[3] and in 1988, Schmitz estimated the prevalence of alternative psychosis to be 1% among 697 patients followed at a university epilepsy center.[4]

p0120   Forced normalization has been reported in patients with temporal lobe epilepsy and generalized epilepsy. The psychotic manifestations were identified after a relatively long duration of the seizure disorder. Wolf reported a 15-year history of epilepsy in 23 patients.[5] Both Landolt and Wolf reported a pleomorphic clinical presentation, with a paranoid psychosis without clouding of consciousness being the most frequent manifestation. As with other types of psychosis in epilepsy, a richness of affective symptoms is a characteristic finding.

As stated above, although the psychotic episodes in this patient could be construed as an expression of an "alternative psychosis" phenomenon, subsequent prolonged seizure-free periods have not resulted in a recurrence of psychotic symptoms or bizarre behavior. In fact, after 9 months of being seizure-free on levetiracetam, valproate, and lamotrigine and a low dose (5 mg/day) of paroxetine, the patient is attending school on a daily basis. With the exception of occasional outbursts of anger and irritability, she is functioning well. This may, in fact, be one of the unusual features of this case: namely, that it exemplifies that the phenomenon of "alternative psychosis" need not be a chronic process but can occur as an isolated event. On the other hand, I cannot exclude the possibility that the mood-stabilizing properties of valproate and lamotrigine[6] are "protecting" this patient from subsequent psychotic episodes.

What did I learn from this case? How did this case alter my approach to the care and treatment of my epilepsy patients?

This case highlights the multiple variables that can operate in the psychiatric comorbidity of patients with epilepsy. I am now more careful to perform a thorough assessment of the role of negative and positive psychotropic properties of antiepileptic drugs, the patient's risk factors for psychopathology (i.e. past personal and familial psychiatric history), and the actual impact of seizure occurrence versus seizure control as determinants of psychopathology.

REFERENCES

1. Tellenbach H. Epilepsie als Anfallseiden und als Psychosen. Über alternative psychosen paranoider Pragung bei "forcierter Normalisierung" (Landoldt) des Elektroencephalogramms Epileptischer. *Nervenarzt* 1965;**36**:190.
2. Landoldt H. Some clinical electroencephalographical correlations in epileptic psychosis (twilight states)[abstract]. *Electroencephalogr Clin Neurophysiol* 1953;**5**:121.
3. Ried S, Mothersill IW. Forced normalization: the clinical neurologist's view. In: Trimble MR, Schmitz B, eds. *Forced normalization and alternative psychoses of epilepsy*. Petersfield: Wrightson Biomedical Publishing, 1998: 77–94.
4. Schmitz B. Psychosen bei Epilepsie. Eine epidemiologische Untersuchung. PhD Thesis, West Berlin.
5. Wolf P. The prevention of alternative psychosis in outpatients. In: Janz D, ed. *Epileptology*. Stuttgart: Thieme, 1976: 75–9.
6. Kanner AM, Palac S. Depression in epilepsy: a common but often unrecognized comorbid malady. *Epilepsy Behav* 2000;**1**:37–51.

c00042

Exacerbation of Seizures in a Young Woman

Pavel Klein

s0010

HISTORY

p0010

A 31-year-old woman suffered head trauma with transient coma at the age of 3 years and developed seizures at the age of 16 years. The seizures consisted of feeling strange and vertiginous, with a feeling of impending doom, word-finding difficulties, speech perseveration, and inability to focus her thoughts. They lasted 4–5 min and were followed by drowsiness. They occurred once or twice a month, mostly 2–3 days after the onset of menstruation or at the time of ovulation. Rarely (five or six times during 15 years), the patient had secondary generalization. Over the past 2–3 years, her seizures became more frequent – three or four times a month – and the perimenstrual worsening became less apparent, although the patient still felt that the seizures and her menses were related.

p0020

She was treated with phenytoin 300 mg at bedtime. Past treatments had included carbamazepine, phenobarbital, and valproate.

p0030

Past medical history was positive for recent gingivectomy. Family history was significant for hypothyroidism and anxiety but negative for epilepsy. The patient's menarche had occurred at the age of 13 years, with initially regular menses that had become irregular, every 5–10 weeks, 3 years earlier. She had developed hirsutism during the past 3 years.

s0020

EXAMINATION AND INVESTIGATIONS

p0040

The patient was mildly overweight and mildly hirsute (on the face, arms, and legs). The rest of the general and neurological examinations were normal.

p0050

Evaluations included an EEG, which showed occasional left anterior spike discharges and theta slowing, and a normal magnetic resonance imaging scan.

p0060

Reproductive endocrine evaluations showed mild hyperandrogenism (free testosterone level 0.3 ng/dl, normal <0.2 ng/dl), elevated ratio of luteinizing hormone to follicular stimulating hormone (menstrual cycle day 3 luteinizing hormone 12.4 IU, follicular stimulating hormone 4.7 IU; normal LH/FSH ratio <2.5), and the presence of anovulatory menstrual cycles with impaired luteal ovarian progesterone secretion (menstrual cycle day 22 estradiol level 182 pg/ml, normal 50–270 pg/ml; progester-one 1.2 ng/ml (normal >6 ng/ml)). These findings were consistent with the diagnosis of polycystic ovarian syndrome with mild hyperandrogenism. An ovarian ultrasound showed a couple of ovarian cysts bilaterally.

Trough phenytoin level was 21.4 μg/ml on menstrual cycle day 22 and 16.1 μg/ml on menstrual cycle day 1. Triphasil, an estrogen-containing oral contraceptive prepa-ration, was started by the patient's gynecologist for the treatment of the polycystic ovarian syndrome. Seizures worsened so that they were occurring five or six times a month, and the patient had three secondarily generalized seizures in 2 months. Repeated estradiol level on Triphasil was 661 pg/ml.

DIAGNOSES

Polycystic ovarian syndrome and anovulatory menstrual cycles. Seizure exacerbation related to polycystic ovarian syndrome and to estrogen-containing therapy.

TREATMENT AND OUTCOME

An increase of phenytoin dose to 400 mg at bedtime produced mild somnolence and diplopia with a level of 24.0 μg/ml. The dose was reduced back to 300 mg at bedtime. Oral progesterone was added at 600 mg/day in three divided doses on days 1–12 of each calendar month, with taper over days 13–15. After three menstrual cycles, the menses became more regular – every 30–35 days – and the progesterone administra-tion was changed to days 15–28 of each menstrual cycle. Seizure frequency decreased to one seizure every 2 months, often at the time of progesterone withdrawal, which was improved further by a slow taper over 4 days. On menstrual cycle day 22, the estradiol level was 89 pg/ml and the progesterone level was 28 ng/ml. The patient experienced mild breast discomfort and feeling of fullness and a 3-kg weight gain. The mastalgia improved with progesterone dose reduction to 500 mg/day in three divided doses (200, 100, and 200 mg).

COMMENTARY

This patient had partial complex seizures with perimenstrual and periovulatory exac-erbation of seizures (catamenial epilepsy types 1 and 2).[1] Twelve years after the onset of seizures, she developed a reproductive endocrine disorder (polycystic ovarian syn-drome), with concomitant exacerbation of her seizures. The customary gynecological treatment of this condition further exacerbated her seizures. Treatment with natural progesterone improved both the seizures and the polycystic ovarian syndrome.

Temporal lobe epilepsy is associated with increased risk of reproductive endocrine disorders.[2] Left-sided temporal lobe epilepsy is associated with an increased inci-dence of polycystic ovarian syndrome, while right-sided temporal lobe epilepsy may be associated with hypothalamic hypogonadism.[2,3] In either case, the reproductive endocrine consequence is the development of anovulatory cycles.[4] During anovula-tory cycles, the ovary continues to secrete estrogen, but secretion of progesterone is minimal. Estrogens have proconvulsant properties, whereas progesterone has potent anticonvulsant properties.[4,5] Thus, the development of reproductive endocrine disorders such as polycystic ovarian syndrome or hypothalamic hypogonadism in women with temporal lobe epilepsy may lead to exacerbation of seizures, as occurred in this case. Progesterone is a potent inhibitor of neuronal excitation because of its potentiating effect on gamma-aminobutyric acid A receptors. This effect is exerted indirectly, via allopregnanolone, a metabolite of progesterone, but it is very potent, equal to the most potent of benzodiazepines.[4,6,7] Progesterone may thus be used as an adjunct anticonvulsant and has been shown to be effective in several open label studies in women with temporal lobe epilepsy, refractory seizures, and reproductive endocrine disorders.[8] An NIH-funded double-blind, randomized, placebo-controlled multi-center study is currently evaluating its efficacy as adjunctive treatment in women with refractory localization-related epilepsy.

p0120   In women with perimenstrual seizure exacerbation, reduced serum levels of phenytoin and possibly of other antiepileptic drugs that induce hepatic enzymes may also be associated with perimenstrual seizure exacerbation, as may have occurred in the present case.[9,10] When menses are predictable, increase in the dose of the antiepileptic drug 7–10 days before expected menstruation may be an effective treatment. Because this patient's menses were irregular, it was not feasible to adjust the phenytoin dose perimenstrually. Adjunctive treatment with natural progesterone may be beneficial in such cases, as it was here.

s0060   ## What did I learn from this case?

p0130   I learned that chronic temporal lobe epilepsy can lead to the development of a reproductive endocrine disorder, and that the development of such a reproductive endocrine disorder may be associated with worsening of previously stable seizures. I also learned how important it is to pay attention to the hormonal treatment of a reproductive endocrine disorder – one treatment (an estrogen-containing oral contraceptive) exacerbated the patient's seizures,[11] whereas another treatment (progesterone) improved both the reproductive endocrine disorder and the seizures.

s0070   ## How did this case alter my approach to the care and treatment of my epilepsy patients?

p0140   I pay attention to reproductive history in women with epilepsy. I include a history of hormonal factors in my evaluation of possible exacerbating factors of a seizure disorder. In my female patients with temporal lobe epilepsy, I look for clinical evidence of anovulatory cycles, such as menstrual cycles that are too short (under 23 days) or too long (over 35 days), and also for other evidence of reproductive endocrine dysfunction, such as hirsutism. I work closely with my gynecological colleagues to decide on the most appropriate hormonal treatment for patients with epilepsy and reproductive endocrine dysfunction. I also keep in my mind the possibility of hormonal therapy as adjunct treatment for seizures in women with refractory epilepsy and reproductive endocrine dysfunction.

REFERENCES

1. Herzog AG, Klein P, Ransil BJ. Three patterns of catamenial epilepsy. *Epilepsia* 1997;**38**:1082–8.
2. Herzog AG, Seibel MM, Schomer DL, *et al*. Reproductive endocrine disorders in women with partial seizures of temporal lobe origin. *Arch Neurol* 1986;**43**:341–6.
3. Drislane FW, Coleman AE, Schomer DL, *et al*. Altered pulsatile secretion of luteinizing hormone in women with epilepsy. *Neurology* 1994;**44**:306–10.
4. Klein P, Herzog AG. Hormonal effects on epilepsy in women. *Epilepsia* 1998;**39(suppl 8)**:S9–S16.
5. Scharfman HE, MacLusky NJ. The influence of gonadal hormones on neuronal excitability, seizures, and epilepsy in the female. *Epilepsia* 2006;**47**:1423–40.
6. Paul SM, Purdy RH. Neuroactive steroids. *FASEB J* 1992;**6**:2311–22.
7. Hosie AM, Wilkins ME, da Silva HM, Smart TG. Endogenous neurosteroids regulate GABAA receptors through two discrete transmembrane sites. *Nature* 2006;**23(444)**:486–9.
8. Herzog AG. Progesterone therapy in women with complex partial and secondary generalized seizures. *Neurology* 1995;**45**:1660–2.
9. Roscizewska D, Buntner B, Guz I, *et al*. Ovarian hormones, anticonvulsant drugs and seizures during the menstrual cycle in women with epilepsy. *J Neurol Neurosurg Psychiatry* 1986;**49**:47–51.
10. Foldvary-Schaefer N, Falcone T. Catamenial epilepsy: pathophysiology, diagnosis and management. *Neurology* 2003;**61**:S2–S15.
11. Cantero J, Klein P. Effect of estrogen-containing contraceptives on seizure frequency in women with epilepsy. *Epilepsia* 2002;**43(suppl 7)**:242.

c00043

Genetic Counseling in a Woman with a Family History of Refractory Myoclonic Epilepsy*

Dick Lindhout

s0010

HISTORY

p0010
A woman with therapy-resistant epilepsy was referred for genetic counseling. Her first male child had moderate mental retardation. The patient wanted to know the cause of her epilepsy, while hoping that this would lead to a better treatment resulting in seizure freedom. Her husband was more concerned about the risk of epilepsy and mental retardation to subsequent offspring.

p0020
At the age of 10 years, the patient had her first generalized tonic–clonic seizure while watching television. Subsequently, myoclonic seizures developed, initially during the morning shortly after awakening but gradually more evenly distributed over the day. The seizures predominantly affected the trunk and the proximal extremities. Generalized tonic–clonic seizures continued infrequently.

p0030
The patient's past medication history consisted of an extensive list of different antiepileptic drugs used singly and in combinations, including 6 years of phenytoin. However, the myoclonic seizures had persisted. During the past treatment with phenytoin, her mental performance had deteriorated progressively and signs of ataxia had developed. Her son with mental retardation had been exposed to phenytoin throughout the pregnancy.

p0040
At the time of referral, the patient was on valproate 2000 mg/day and clonazepam.

p0050
The patient had a mildly affected sister who was treated with valproate and ethosuximide. This sister had finished high school. The patient also had an affected brother who had a severe and progressive course of disease and who had been on long-term

*This case history has been modified for privacy reasons and educational purposes and should not be included in any kind of meta-analysis without prior consultation of the author.

phenytoin medication. He had died of aspiration pneumonia during a period of phenobarbital intoxication. The patient's parents were healthy, non-consanguinous, and native Dutch.

EXAMINATION AND INVESTIGATIONS

Physical examination of the patient confirmed the myoclonus of the trunk and proximal extremities, and signs of ataxia. She was mentally subnormal. The EEG showed generalized polyspike-waves and photosensitivity.

The patient's son was confirmed to be mentally retarded, and he showed hypertelorism, a depressed nasal bridge, and distal phalangeal hypoplasia.

Mutation analysis of the cystatin B gene in the mother showed only an expanded dodecamer repeat and no normal-sized allele. Subsequently, the same DNA result was obtained in her affected sister. The parents were not available for DNA analysis.

DIAGNOSIS

Progressive myoclonus epilepsy of Unverricht–Lundborg in the mother. Fetal hydantoin syndrome in her son.

TREATMENT AND OUTCOME

The patient's medication was adjusted by dividing the total daily dose of valproate of 2000 mg in four equal dosages of 500 mg each. Clonazepam was discontinued and low-dose folic acid supplementation (0.5 mg/day) was started.

The patient was informed about the following risks to future offspring above standard population risks:

- risk of recurrence of epilepsy: less than 1%;
- risk of recurrence of the fetal hydantoin syndrome: zero, provided that phenytoin is not used; and
- risk of teratogenesis from valproate use: 5% risk of congenital abnormalities, including a 1–2% risk of neural tube defects.

The patient was offered prenatal diagnosis of congenital abnormalities in the fetus by means of amniotic fluid analysis (alpha-1-fetoprotein level) and structural ultrasound examination.

COMMENTARY

To the patient and her husband, the risk of recurrence of epilepsy in their children was unexpectedly low. This can be explained by the autosomal-recessive mode of inheritance of progressive myoclonus epilepsy of Unverricht–Lundborg.

p0170   Each child of a patient will inherit one of the two abnormal genes from the patient. However, the disease may only occur if the other parent is a carrier (heterozygous) for the same disease. This chance is low when the other parent has no family history of epilepsy and is not related to the patient. In addition, one may offer carrier detection to the healthy partner for currently known mutations in the cystatin B gene. A normal result (the most likely outcome) would further decrease the risk to the offspring, whereas the finding of a mutation (the less likely outcome) would increase the risk toward 50%.

p0180   Adjustment of the dosage scheme for valproate was made in order to reduce peak levels that are possibly related to the risk of teratogenesis. Clonazepam was discontinued in view of reports that suggest potentiation of teratogenic risks with the combination of valproate and clonazepam.

p0190   Low-dose folic acid supplementation was prescribed according to the guidelines of the Dutch Health Council. High-dose folic acid supplementation is reserved for women with a previous child with an open neural tube defect. Effectiveness as well as safety of the high-dose folic acid is proven only in women at increased risk because of a previous child with a neural tube defect, but not in women at increased risk because of other risk factors such as maternal use of antiepileptic drugs.

p0200   This case was chosen in order to outline the complex issues that may be encountered when dealing with maternal epilepsy and maternal use of antiepileptic drugs. Genetic counseling in epilepsy should always explore and address three main questions:

u0040   • What is the etiology and recurrence risk of epilepsy?
u0050   • Can seizures during pregnancy damage the mother or the unborn child?
u0060   • What is known about the effects of maternal antiepileptic drugs on the developing embryo and fetus?

s0060   ## What did I learn from this case?

p0240   Until this case, progressive myoclonus epilepsy of Unverricht–Lundborg existed for me only in the textbooks. The discovery of the cystatin B gene currently provides an efficient and specific diagnostic tool. Some reports suggest that the course of the disease is less severe and the prognosis is favorable when valproate is used and phenytoin and carbamazepine are avoided.

p0250   Since this case, I have diagnosed seven other cases in a short period of time. Many of these patients were initially diagnosed as juvenile myoclonus epilepsy. The clinical presentation of progressive myoclonus epilepsy of Unverricht–Lundborg may show considerable overlap with juvenile myoclonus epilepsy, especially at onset. Atypical occurrence of myoclonias, therapy-resistant myoclonias, progression of the disease, development of ataxia or mental regression, parental consanguinity or parental origin from the Baltic, the Mediterranean or the Middle East should suggest the diagnosis and lead to DNA analysis of the cystatin B gene.

p0260   This case underscores the importance of early diagnosis for better prognosis and optimal genetic counseling, and it illustrates one of the many new benefits of genetic research.

FURTHER READING

Berkovic SF, Cochius J, Andermann E, Andermann F. Progressive myoclonus epilepsies: clinical and genetic aspects. *Epilepsia* 1993;**34(suppl 3)**:S19–S30.

Eldridge R, Iivanainen M, Stern R, Koerber T, Wilder BJ. "Baltic" myoclonus epilepsy: hereditary disorder of childhood made worse by phenytoin. *Lancet* 1983;**2**:838–42.

Laegreid L, Kyllerman M, Hedner T, Hagberg B, Viggedahl G. Benzodiazepine amplification of valproate teratogenic effects in children of mothers with absence epilepsy. *Neuropediatrics* 1993;**24**:88–92.

Lehesjoki AE, Koskiniemi M. Progressive myoclonus epilepsy of Unverricht–Lundborg type. *Epilepsia* 1999;**40(suppl 3)**:23–8.

Lindhout D, Omtzigt JGC. Latest report on teratogenic effects of antiepileptic drugs: implications for the management of epilepsy in women of childbearing age. *Epilepsia* 1994;**35(suppl 4)**:19–28.

Samrén EB, van Duijn CM, Christiaens GC, Hofman A, Lindhout D. Antiepileptic drug regimens and major congenital abnormalities in the offspring. *Ann Neurol* 1999;**46**:739–46.

c00044

"Funny Jerks" Run in the Family

Heinz-Joachim Meencke

HISTORY

p0010 A 21-year-old right-handed woman was seen in the outpatient department of an epilepsy center, 1 week after a generalized tonic–clonic seizure.

p0020 The report from the emergency room described tongue biting, and I got an unequivocal description of a generalized tonic–clonic seizure from the patient's mother. The seizure happened 1 h after awakening. She had not slept adequately for several days because she was studying for an examination.

p0030 I asked them about a previous history of other seizures and epilepsy, which both she and her mother denied strongly. Then I discussed specific signs and symptoms of seizures. When I demonstrated jerks with my arms and shoulders, the patient told me that this was very familiar to her and that she often had similar jerks in the morning, dating back to when she was aged 12 or 13.

p0040 However, these jerks, in her mind, had nothing to do with her seizure. To her, they were just a personal mode of behavior. Her mother admitted to having the same problem beginning in her school years, which she described as "funny jerks." She strongly denied having any "blackouts." Doctors, she noted, had explained the jerks as just tics. She had been satisfied with this explanation because her aunt was also reported to have these "funny jerks." It seemed that in this family, to some extent, jerks were acceptable behavior in the women.

s0020

EXAMINATION AND INVESTIGATIONS

p0050 Physical and neurological examinations were normal. A magnetic resonance imaging scan showed slight frontoparietal parasaggital atrophy. The routine EEG showed increased generalized intermittant rhythmic slowing that was excessive for her age. With sleep deprivation, bilateral polyspike-and-wave complexes were seen, which were intermittently accompanied by bilateral myoclonic jerks of the upper extremities.

p0060 An EEG of the mother was obtained, which showed increased generalized intermittent rhythmic slowing but no epileptiform potentials, even after sleep deprivation.

DIAGNOSIS

Juvenile myoclonic epilepsy (impulsive petit mal, Janz syndrome, generalized idiopathic epilepsy).

TREATMENT AND OUTCOME

It was very difficult to explain to the patient and her family that the myoclonic jerks were, in fact, a feature of generalized epilepsy. We counseled her about seizure-provoking factors, especially sleep deprivation, and started monotherapy with valproate 1500 mg/day. At 1-year follow-up, the myoclonic jerks had stopped and she had had no more tonic–clonic seizures. She did not return for a further appointment.

COMMENTARY

What did I learn from this case?

First, I learned that what initially appears to be a first seizure is very often not, in fact, the first seizure. This case taught me that it is absolutely necessary to ask carefully for other signs and symptoms of seizures and that it is mandatory to demonstrate signs and symptoms of different seizure types. Very subtle ictal behavioral change might be misinterpreted as "personal" or idiosyncratic behavior. In this case, earlier initiation of appropriate antiepileptic drug therapy together with adequate lifestyle counseling may have avoided the development of generalized tonic–clonic seizures.

Second, this case shows that the phenotypic expression of idiopathic generalized epilepsies may be very mild over many generations and may be manifested only as myoclonic jerks that may never be identified as epilepsy. The psychological and social consequences of epilepsies are strongly influenced by the type of epilepsy syndrome.

Third, this case highlights the problem of underdiagnosing juvenile myoclonic epilepsy, a syndrome that responds very favorably to appropriate treatment.

Bearing these lessons in mind will positively influence my strategy for choosing an appropriate therapy after a so-called first seizure.

c00045

Side Effects That Imitate Seizures

George Lee Morris III

George Lee Morris III

s0010

HISTORY

p0010

The patient is a 41-year-old woman who developed seizures in her early teens. Her seizures consisted of premonitory sensations for a day before the events and an aura of language difficulties – she understood that speech was occurring but could not determine what was being said to her. Episodes of loss of consciousness with or without preceding auras occurred several times a month. Auras without subsequent loss of consciousness occurred rarely.

p0020

Her past medical history included minor surgeries, two uneventful pregnancies with normal children, and the occasional treatment of depression with tricyclic antidepressants. There was no history of head trauma, febrile seizures, or previous hospitalization. Prior medications included divalproex, phenytoin, felbamate, gabapentin, and lamotrigine. Each was unsuccessful in stopping her seizures and several had significant cognitive effects.

p0030

She used low-estrogen oral contraceptives and daily multivitamins. She was married with two children of elementary-school age, and she had worked as a nurse before her second child. She did not drink alcohol or smoke tobacco. Her health was currently good and she reported a positive mood. Her current medication for seizures was carbamazepine 1400 mg/day in three divided doses.

s0020

EXAMINATION AND INVESTIGATIONS

p0040

The patient's general appearance, physical examination, and neurological examination were normal.

p0050

She had a routine EEG that showed left mid-temporal spike and slow-wave discharges and intermittent slowing in the left temporal lobe. Cranial magnetic resonance imaging scanning was normal and showed symmetric hippocampal structures.

s0030

DIAGNOSES

p0060

Complex partial seizures, with and without preceding simple partial seizures. Intractable, cryptogenic left temporal lobe localization-related epilepsy.

TREATMENT AND OUTCOME

The patient was presented with the options of further medication trials, vagus nerve stimulation, or hospitalization for seizure confirmation via video–EEG monitoring for a potential surgical epilepsy treatment. The patient elected to try an additional medication. She reviewed the benefits and risks of each of the available medications, including commercially available and investigational drugs, and she chose tiagabine. A gradual titration over 6 weeks to 32 mg/day in three divided doses was begun.

Three weeks later the patient called to report that her auras were occurring early in the morning, after her children went to school, but she was without further complex partial seizures and no side effects had appeared. In several additional phone calls over the following weeks, the patient expressed concern over lengthy morning auras that were stronger. No loss of consciousness occurred but she was having more trouble speaking.

She then had a complex partial seizure. Because she was currently taking tiagabine 32 mg/day, her carbamazepine dose was lowered in the hope of raising the tiagabine level. However, the patient was now reporting daily auras for 30 min or more. She requested video–EEG monitoring.

The patient was hospitalized and her medications were tapered over 3 days. EEGs over 7 days showed occasional left mid-temporal epileptiform discharges but no seizures. Sleep-deprivation, hourly hyperventilation, and light stimulation were performed, and the patient requested discharge so that she could return to caring for her children. Both medications were started again at their prehospital doses. The patient's discharge was planned for the following morning.

The following morning the patient motioned to the technician to come in her room. She was unable to speak and could not read. She appeared sedated and motioned that she felt dizzy. The patient's EEG was reviewed and found to be unchanged during the episode.

COMMENTARY

The paroxysmal nature of epilepsy vexes a physician's diagnosis in several ways. The variable presentation of medication side effects is a particularly difficult area.

Whereas a transient side effect from an antiepileptic drug can be readily attributed to rapidly escalating or high plasma concentrations, ictal symptoms are generally differentiated by their longer duration. Indeed, antiepileptic drugs produce a variety of clinical symptoms that may be similar to a seizure phenomenon. The unusual or "indescribable" feeling of limbic seizures begins as undefinable by the patient, making it difficult for a patient to separate these sensations from a drug-induced sensation. Dizziness, paresthesias, vision alteration, and various cognitive difficulties may all overlap and be paroxysmally related to peak concentration of these medications.

On further questioning, this patient related that these "seizures" occurred only on school days and that her breakfast was limited to tea because she was busy getting her children ready for school. The rapid absorption of tiagabine produced by administration on an empty stomach led to these transient symptoms that were similar to her habitual auras.

s0060   **What did I learn from this case?**

p0150   An issue that I raise constantly with patients is the need to confirm that events they experience are seizures. Direct confirmation by video–EEG recordings is invaluable in patient management. The correct diagnosis may be suspected before monitoring but the outcome that was seen in this case is always a possibility.

s0070   **How did this case alter my approach to the care and treatment of my epilepsy patients?**

p0160   In my daily practice I use such illustrative cases with my patients. Describing to them the various potential outcomes from monitoring educates them as to the many benefits of disease confirmation and makes the process of managing patients who have been unresponsive to medications much easier. This patient's outcome is one that I use frequently when describing how patients may benefit from hospitalization for video–EEG monitoring.

46

Epilepsy, Migraine, and Cerebral Calcifications

Willy O Renier

HISTORY

When the patient was 5 years old, he suffered two events while at school that were characterized by nausea, sweating, and confusion. Examination at that time was normal, as was blood and urine screening, except for a mild anemia. The EEG was described as normal for age but with some sharp theta-wave activity over the left temporo-occipital region. An EEG after sleep deprivation did not contribute further to the diagnosis. The events were interpreted as non-specific vegetative reactions, and iron supplementation was prescribed.

Six months later, another event occurred during the holidays. After a flight of 22 h, the boy awoke in his hotel room in a confused state, complained of visual hallucinations ("moving walls"), and had verbal dyspraxia. One hour later, left-sided hemiclonic jerks occurred for 2 min. After two similar seizures within 1 h, the boy was transferred to a hospital.

General examination was again normal. EEG showed irregular sharp theta waves over both posterior regions. A computed tomography (CT) scan (Figure 46.1) showed bilateral parieto-occipital calcifications with a garland pattern. Laboratory investigations revealed a microcytic anemia. The boy was administered diazepam 5 mg and the parents were advised to contact a neurologist.

Two uneventful weeks later, the neurological examination was normal. It was concluded that the seizures had been provoked by fatigue. Over the following months, the patient suffered two additional episodes of nausea – one at the end of a 4-day sport meeting and the other during an episode of flu. He was referred to my department for a second opinion.

When the history was explored in greater detail with the patient's mother, she expressed her feeling that her son was having migraines. Migraine was well known in her family because she herself, her sister, her brother, and the younger brother of the patient regularly suffered from migraine headaches. When the general medical history was taken, she reported that her son had mild chronic intestinal problems and had regularly taken ferrous salts for anemia since the age of 3.

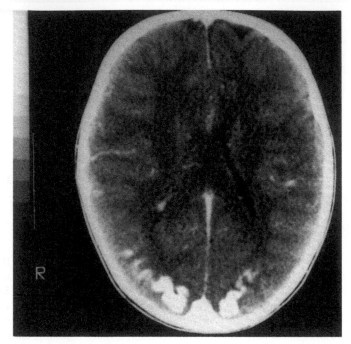

t0010 FIGURE 46.1   Cerebral CT scan with typical calcifications in the parieto-occipital lobes.

EXAMINATION

The patient was a hyperactive but otherwise normal child.

DIAGNOSIS AND FURTHER INVESTIGATIONS

Celiac disease with epilepsy. Further laboratory investigations confirmed the diagnosis of celiac disease (Table 46.1).

TREATMENT AND OUTCOME

The boy was treated with a gluten-free diet and carbamazepine 100 mg at bedtime. Three months later, the mother described her son as "a completely new child." He was more alert, more pleasant, and had better school performance. The EEG was normal. After having been seizure-free for 1 year, carbamazepine was stopped. Four years later, the boy is still doing well without seizure recurrence on a gluten-free diet.

COMMENTARY

Migraine-like seizures have been described in occipital lobe epilepsy[1] and in this case could have been related to the occipital calcifications. The association of migraine-like t0010

TABLE 46.1   Laboratory Investigations Confirming the Diagnosis of Celiac Disease
(Glutenteropathy). In Addition, Duodenal Biopsy Showed Villous Atrophy

Test	Result before therapy	Result 8 months after therapy	Normal values
Hb (mmol/l)	6.4	6.8	6–9
Iron (μmol/l)	7	17	10–25
Iron-binding capacity (μmol/l)	68	54	45–75
Folic acid (nmol/l)	3.3	21	5.5–40
Anti-gliadine IgG (U/ml)	49	Negative	<12
Anti-gliadine IgA (U/ml)	5	Negative	<4
Anti-reticuline IgA (U/ml)	+++	±	
Anti-endomysium IgA (U/ml)	++	+	

TABLE 46.2   The Syndrome of Parieto-Occipital Calcifications with Celiac Disease and
Epilepsy

t0020

Clinical characteristics

Epilepsy

- In most cases, partial seizures with the characteristics of occipital paroxysms (migraine-like headache, nausea, visual complaints); cognitive disturbances and deterioration (with great individual variability)   u0010

Celiac disease

- First signs and symptoms in infancy, toddler age, or childhood (dysphoric episodes, dystrophic habitus, loss of appetite, growth retardation, puffed belly)   u0020
- Frequent association with HLA-B8 and HLA-DW3   u0030

Neuropathology

- Calcifications at the corticomedullary junction   u0040
- Patchy glial angiomatosis ("Sturge-Weber" without cutaneous angiomas)   u0050

Possible mechanisms of pathogenesis:

- Chronic iron and folic acid deficiency   u0060
- HLA related auto-immune pathology   u0070

Evoluation

- Can lead to severe encephalopathy in cases without treatment   u0080

Treatment

- Start as early as possible with a gluten-free diet and iron and folic acid; continue the gluten-free diet   u0090
- Antiepileptic drugs when seizures recur   u0100

seizures, parieto-occipital calcifications and intestinal complaints with chronic anemia are pathognomonic for celiac disease with epilepsy (Table 46.2).[2,3]

The case illustrates the pitfalls in the diagnosis of epilepsy. The final diagnosis was based on the description of the seizure pattern, a detailed history of all body systems and the typical appearance of the cerebral calcifications.

Visual auras followed by hemisensory or hemiconvulsive attacks (or both) have been described in benign epilepsy of childhood with occipital paroxysms. The varied manifestations of occipital lobe epilepsy resulting from multiple spread patterns to the temporal, frontal, supplementary motor, or parietal regions are a source of diagnostic error. Interictal surface EEG is helpful in localizing the seizure focus in only approximately 20% of cases.

Another confounding factor is the family history of migraine. The mother was familiar with signs and symptoms of migraine and, therefore, was not aware of the possibility of epileptic events. In families of children with benign epilepsy of childhood with occipital paroxysms, a history of epilepsy is present in 30% and a history of migraine is present in 15%.

Paroxysmal neurovegetative events, a normal neurological examination and non-specific EEGs do not necessarily exclude the diagnosis of epilepsy or signify a non-lesional epilepsy. In parietal and occipital lobe epilepsy, there is frequently a poor correlation between clinical and EEG features.

Chronic gastrointestinal complaints and anemia are common complaints in children, particularly in hyperactive children, but they can also be the expression of celiac disease. The typical garland configuration of parieto-occipital calcifications should alert the physician to this diagnosis.

What did I learn from this case?

The case illustrates that the diagnosis of epilepsy is primarily a clinical one and that clinical epileptology is based on experience, knowledge of the literature, and good visual memory. Once you have seen the typical calcifications on CT scans in cases of celiac disease, you remember the picture.

Taking a history from patients with seizures and their family members should be as complete as possible and not restricted to the description of the seizure pattern, though the information has to be interpreted with caution. The brain is not an isolated organ. Therefore, attention should be paid to complaints other than neurological ones. Developing knowledge about metabolic disorders should be part of the training of neurologists. In symptomatic epilepsy, treating the underlying cause at an early stage can prevent further deterioration and, in some cases, avoid antiepileptic drug treatment.

REFERENCES

1. Gastaut H. Benign epilepsy of childhood with occipital paroxysms. In: Roger J, Bureau M, Dravet Ch, Dreifuss FE, Perret A, Wolf P, eds. *Epileptic syndromes in infancy, childhood and adolescence*, 2nd ed. London: John Libbey, 1992: 201–17.
2. Gobbi G, Sorrenti G, Santucci M, *et al*. Epilepsy with bilateral occipital calcifications: a benign onset with progressive severity. *Neurology* 1988;**38**:913–20.
3. Gobbi G, Bouquet F, Greco I, *et al*. Coeliac disease, epilepsy, and cerebral calcifications. *Lancet* 1992;**340**:439–43.

An Unusual Application of Epilepsy Surgery

Edward H Bertram and Jaideep Kapur

HISTORY

The patient is a 57-year-old, right-handed woman who had two kinds of seizures. The first type occurred primarily during the day and consisted of *déjà vu* followed by staring, confusion, orofacial automatisms, and dystonic posturing of the left hand. The second type consisted of distressing nocturnal episodes of abrupt arousal from sleep followed by severe pain in the left hand and arm accompanied by screams of pain, a frightened look on the face and brief confusion.

Seizures started at the age of 43 without a clear epilepsy risk factor. Her seizures were not reliably triggered by any particular events, but she did note that seizures recurred periodically two or three times each month in clusters. Her anticonvulsant was topiramate 400 mg/day in two divided doses. Carbamazepine, valproate, phenytoin, and gabapentin administered in various combinations had not controlled her seizures. Lamotrigine was discontinued because of a rash. Other medications were estrogen–progesterone for prevention of osteoporosis and propranolol for poorly documented "palpitations."

She had no significant past medical history. There was no history of epilepsy in the family. Her mother died from carcinoma of the stomach and father from lung carcinoma. She is married and has four healthy children. She stopped working as a receptionist as a result of her epilepsy.

EXAMINATION AND INVESTIGATIONS

Physical and neurological examinations were unremarkable. The patient was admitted for video–EEG monitoring to determine the nature of the two events and, if appropriate, localize the site of seizure onset.

The seizures with staring and lip smacking were associated with electrographic seizures over the right mid-temporal region. EEG activity during the episodes of nocturnal left arm pain was partially obscured by artifact, but there were rhythmic changes over the right hemisphere.

A magnetic resonance imaging (MRI) scan of the brain disclosed dual pathology of right hippocampal atrophy and a subtle right parietal cortical malformation.

Neuropsychological testing revealed mild generalized cognitive dysfunction and no clear lateralization of deficits as well as a significant level of depression and anxiety.

p0070 To localize the site of origin of the two seizure types, in part to determine if they originated from one or multiple foci, intracranial monitoring was performed using subdural strip electrodes and bilateral intrahippocampal–depth electrodes. Intracranial EEG disclosed two distinct seizure foci – a right temporal focus corresponding to the complex partial seizures and a right parietal focus corresponding to the nocturnal ictal pain.

s0030 ## DIAGNOSIS

p0080 Symptomatic localization-related epilepsy with independent right mesial temporal and right parietal epileptic foci.

s0040 ## TREATMENT AND OUTCOME

p0090 The right parietal focus was resected following cortical mapping with a subsequently implanted subdural grid. Microscopic evaluation of the samples taken from the right parietal lobe revealed focal cortical dysplasia with gliosis.

p0100 Since surgery, the frequency and intensity of nocturnal ictal pain declined, and now occur only several times a year and cause tingling but no severe pain or screaming. Because the seizures are only minimally disturbing, the patient is comfortable with traveling. Before successful surgery she did not want to stay at hotels, as she was afraid that her nocturnal screaming would be disturbing to others and possibly be misinterpreted by other hotel guests.

p0110 The seizures of ictal pain were her biggest concern, but once they resolved, the limitations placed by her other complex partial seizures became more bothersome, so, approximately 2 years following the first surgery, she underwent a second surgery, an anterior temporal lobectomy, to control these other seizures. Following this surgery she had no further complex partial seizures, although the occasional episode of left-hand paresthesias continued every several months. She has resumed driving following the second surgery.

s0050 ## COMMENTARY

p0120 This case demonstrates that two types of seizures in a patient can arise from two different seizure foci and that seizures arising from two different regions of the brain are differentially susceptible to circadian modulation. In addition, this case demonstrates that the two separate foci can be treated with two surgeries.

p0130 Patients with partial epilepsy sometimes have two or more types of seizures arising from a single focus. A common example of this phenomenon is the patient who has simple partial, complex partial, and secondarily generalized tonic–clonic seizures, all arising from a single mesial temporal focus. In addition, some patients have two distinct types of events, one epileptic and the other nonepileptic.[1]

p0140 Several clinical features, however, suggested that this patient had two distinct seizure foci causing two different seizure types. The clinical features of the daytime seizures – *déjà vu*, orofacial automatisms, and arm dystonia – suggested a temporal lobe origin.

None of these features were present in the nocturnal spells, which were characterized by distressing pain. The brain MRI scan and the scalp and intracranial EEG monitoring further supported the association of two seizure types with two distinct seizure foci. The fact that resection of the dysplastic area in the parietal cortex reduced the intensity and frequency of the nocturnal spells further suggests that these seizures originated in the parietal lobe and that the daytime seizures were arising from the temporal lobe.

The present case also illustrates that the endogenous circadian clock modulates seizure recurrence depending on the location of seizure foci. Seizures that involve the limbic system may be especially sensitive to circadian modulation as mediated by the hypothalamus, since the limbic system and the hypothalamus share anatomic and functional interconnections.[2,3] Cortically based seizures that spare the limbic system may be more susceptible to mediators of cortical excitation, such as the rhythm of the sleep–wake cycle. Furthermore, the sleep–wake cycle may contribute to both limbic and non-limbic seizure patterns, with limbic seizures facilitated by wakefulness (or resistant to effects of sleep) and extralimbic seizures promoted by sleep (or inhibited by the waking state). Transition states are particularly seizure-provoking for a variety of epileptic syndromes and may be a strong factor independent of syndrome.

What did we learn from this case?

We learned that two distinct seizure types can result from two separate seizure foci in a single patient. We also learned that seizures disable patients for different reasons. The nocturnal episodes of ictal pain robbed the patient of a comfort in traveling. The temporal lobe seizures limited her in her activities of daily living. Ultimately the patient decided to have both seizure types treated surgically in order to have a normal life.

How did this case alter our approach to the care and treatment of our epilepsy patients?

When patients have two types of seizures with distinct signs and symptoms, we carefully evaluate them for evidence of two seizure foci. We also learned that we could safely treat two distinct and separate seizure foci with two surgeries.

REFERENCES

1. Henry TR, Drury I. Non-epileptic seizures in temporal lobectomy candidates with medically refractory seizures. *Neurology* 1997;**48**:1374–82.
2. Quigg M, Clayburn H, Straurne M, Menaker M, Bertram EH. Hypothalamic neuronal loss and altered circadian rhythm of temperature in a rat model of mesial temporal lobe epilepsy. *Epilepsia* 1999;**40**:1688–96.
3. Quigg M, Clayburn H, Straurne M, Menaker M, Bertram EH. Effects of circadian regulation and rest-activity state on spontaneous seizures in a rat model of limbic epilepsy. *Epilepsia* 2000;**41**:502–9.
4. Cotter DR, Honavar M, Everall I. Focal cortical dysplasia: a neuropathological and development perspective. *Epilepsy Res* 1999;**36**:155–64.

c00048

All is Not What it Seems

William E Rosenfeld and Susan M Lippmann

s0010 HISTORY

p0010 The patient is a 35-year-old white man referred for evaluation of an increased number of seizures. He is the manager of a pediatric practice.

p0020 Eleven years before referral, in May 1989, the patient was moving furniture and hit his head in the right temporal region on a steel beam and a dresser. He fell, with loss of consciousness that lasted several minutes. A few days later he had jerking of the left lower extremity and was told he had post-traumatic seizures. He was placed on divalproex sodium.

p0030 In June 1996, the patient reported sustaining a right hemispheric stroke, resulting in a visual field cut, left hemiparesis, and left hemianesthesia. The stroke was felt to be cardioembolic-aortic valvular in etiology and was non-hemorrhagic on brain computed tomography (CT) scanning.

p0040 Six months later, the patient was seen for increased expressive aphasia and left-sided weakness. A stroke was suspected and a CT scan was negative. Shortly after this, he was admitted again with increased left upper extremity weakness and numbness as well as slurred speech. Again there was the impression that the patient had had a right cerebral infarction of possible embolic etiology. The possibility of a conversion reaction was also suspected.

p0050 In July 1997, the patient was admitted with severe anemia, which was thought to be secondary to low-grade hemolysis caused by his artificial heart valve. At this time, he had his "first major motor seizure" and was treated with phenytoin. He remembers having an "aura" of a sensation of smelling a grapefruit and then losing consciousness.

p0060 One year later, the patient suddenly fell. In the emergency department, his phenytoin level was undetectable. He left the hospital against medical advice. Subsequently, he had three traffic violations, possibly related to seizures.

p0070 In the month before coming to our office, the patient recorded up to one seizure a day. He reported his aura as consisting of a "citrus smell, weird feelings, and then I don't remember." He noted that his roommates heard him "flopping around." He reported biting his tongue, occasionally chipping his teeth, and occasionally being incontinent of urine.

p0080 When we first saw the patient, he reported being under treatment for a brain tumor. He stated that his brain magnetic resonance imaging (MRI) scan showed a tumor the size of a walnut and that a biopsy approximately 2 weeks earlier had revealed a grade IV astrocytoma. He reported participating in a "phase I chemotherapy trial" and receiving intramuscular chemotherapy. He stated that another "phase I procedure"

Puzzling Cases of Epilepsy

was tried. He said that a craniotomy was performed and that "the tumor was zapped twice with a laser," resulting in 95% tumor eradication. He could not give us the names of the neurologist, neurosurgeon, or oncologist who had treated him. He stated that he did not want us to look at previous records because he was afraid that this would interfere with his work.

The patient's past medical history was notable for a diagnosis of presumptive connective tissue disorder, which had eventually led to aortic valve replacement in October 1994. He also has a history of supraventricular tachycardia.

EXAMINATION AND INVESTIGATIONS

The patient appeared in our office with 10 bottles of "study drugs." These included phenytoin, clonazepam, phenobarbital, primidone, alprazolam, amitriptyline, temazepam, omeprazole, atenolol, and warfarin.

On examination, the patient had a scalp incision with staples in the right posterior parietal region. His motor examination was inconsistent. Strength in the left upper and lower extremities was at least 4/5. On gait examination the patient occasionally dragged his left lower extremity but did not circumduct it. His heart examination revealed a holosystolic murmur that was greater over the aorta. In his extremities there was mild pitting edema.

Previous studies included a brain MRI scan from August 1998 that was normal. A brain CT scan from September 1998 was similarly negative, as was a follow-up MRI.

On the day that the patient was to be hospitalized in the epilepsy monitoring unit (in September 1998), he appeared in the emergency department after falling. His prothrombin time was 81.3 s and his international normalized ratio was 8.5.

On admission to the epilepsy monitoring unit, he underwent Minnesota Multiphasic Personality Inventory testing, which showed increased scales for hysteria, depression, and histrionics. Phenytoin, primidone, phenobarbital, and clonazepam were withheld. EEGs over the next 5 days showed no evidence of interictal or ictal abnormalities. He then had a generalized tonic–clonic seizure that was documented on video–EEG, and he was reloaded with phenytoin.

DIAGNOSES

Four diagnoses were made:

- Munchausen's syndrome with regard to the history of tumor (pseudoglioblastoma multiforme);
- generalized tonic–clonic seizure documented by a physiological seizure in the epilepsy monitoring unit;
- a history of supraventricular tachycardia with ablation and subsequent aortic valve replacement; and
- warfarin toxicity from an overdose.

COMMENTARY

The patient has an obvious psychiatric disturbance that manifested as Munchausen's disorder with regard to "the tumor" and, possibly, the history of "strokes." His presentation may also have included conversion reactions and non-epileptic episodes. Nonetheless, his testing confirmed that he also did have truly epileptic generalized tonic–clonic seizures.

s0050   **What did we learn from the case?**

p0210   We learned that psychological disorders can manifest in many different ways, including self-mutilation (incision and surgical staples). Secondly, this case demonstrated that patients with Munchausen's syndrome, conversion disorder, and non-epileptic episodes could still have physiological seizures. Therefore, such patients must be carefully monitored so that appropriate therapies can be instituted.

s0060   **How did this case alter our approach to the care and treatment of our epilepsy patients?**

p0220   We are careful to evaluate a patient's episodes thoroughly before jumping to conclusions. Too often, patients receive a diagnosis of non-epileptic episodes without undergoing thorough video–EEG monitoring.

FURTHER READING

Wyllie E, Glazer JP, Benbadis S, Kotagal P, Wolgamuth B. Psychiatric features of children and adolescents with pseudoseizures. *Arch Pediatr Adolesc Med* 1999;**153**:244–8.

Kalogjera-Sackellares D, Sackellares JC. Intellectual and neuropsychological features of patients with psychogenic pseudoseizures. *Psychiatry Res* 1999;**86**:73–84.

Torta R, Keller R. Behavioral, psychotic, and anxiety disorders in epilepsy: etiology, clinical features, and therapeutic implications. *Epilepsia* 1999;**40(suppl 10)**:S2–S20.

Barry E, Krumholz A, Bergey GK, Chatha H, Alemayehu S, Grattan L. Nonepileptic posttraumatic seizures. *Epilepsia* 1998;**39**:427–31.

Sigurdardottir KR, Olafsson E. Incidence of psychogenic seizures in adults: a population-based study in Iceland. *Epilepsia* 1998;**39**:749–52.

Devinsky O. Nonepileptic psychogenic seizures: quagmires of pathophysiology, diagnosis and treatment. *Epilepsia* 1998;**39**:458–62.

Scheepers B, Clough P, Pickles C. The misdiagnosis of epilepsy: findings of a population study. *Seizure* 1998;**7**:403–6.

Bowman ES. Pseudoseizures. *Psychiatr Clin North Am* 1998;**21**:649–57.

Westbrook LE, Devinsky O, Geocadin R. Nonepileptic seizures after head injury. *Epilepsia* 1998;**39**:978–82.

Davard G, Andermann F, Teitelbaum J. Epileptic Munchausen's syndrome: a form of pseudoseizures distinct from hysteria and malingering. *Neurology* 1998;**38**:1628–9.

A Patient Whose Epilepsy Diagnosis Changed Three Times Over 20 Years

Masakazu Seino and Yushi Inoue

HISTORY

A 42-year-old, right-handed housewife had a cerebral contusion from a fall at the age of 4 years. At the age of 18 years, she experienced her first seizure, with loss of consciousness followed by a convulsion. Subsequently, she repeatedly had seizures consisting of right-sided hemifacial spasms and slight turning of the head and eyes toward the right; these seizures occurred several times a day. Seizures with impairment of consciousness lasting 20–30 min preceded by an indiscernible aura and accompanied by automatisms were also observed.

During a follow-up of more than 20 years, absence-like seizures characterized by momentary loss of consciousness were often observed, in addition to the focal motor seizures and long-lasting impairment of consciousness with automatisms mentioned above, each occurring independently. At 38 years of age, she had an episode of convulsive status epilepticus as a result of taking her antiepileptic drugs irregularly.

EXAMINATION AND INVESTIGATIONS

Because her seizures were resistant to drug treatment, the patient was hospitalized at our center four times over a period of 20 years and investigations were carried out.

At 19 years of age, short bursts of bisynchronous spike-and-wave or polyspike-and-wave activity slightly slower than 3 Hz were observed (Figure 49.1). Coincident with the generalized and diffuse spike-and-wave discharges was a brief arrest of motion, which was documented by video–EEG monitoring. The bursts of bisynchronous and diffuse discharges persisted into the patient's 20s and 30s although spike-and-wave formation became less discrete, transforming to high-voltage slow wave rhythms (Figure 49.2). Immediately after the cessation of discharges, she could sometimes

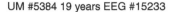

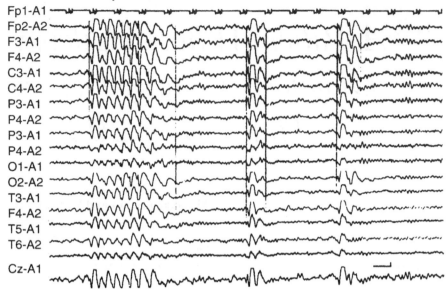

f0010 FIGURE 49.1   Awake EEG at 19 years of age.

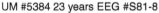

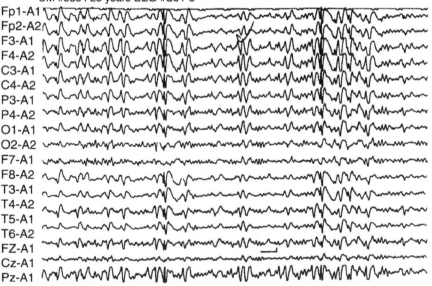

f0020 FIGURE 49.2   Awake EEG at 23 years of age.

recognize an interruption of awareness or difficulty speaking. Ictal EEGs that were associated with a slight deviation of head and eyes showed flattening of background activities followed by a gradual build-up of spike–wave rhythms without focal findings. In other words, these two seizure events were electro-clinically independent.

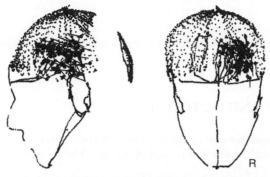

FIGURE 49.3   Magnetoencephalography (BTi, Magnes, 74 channel).   f0030

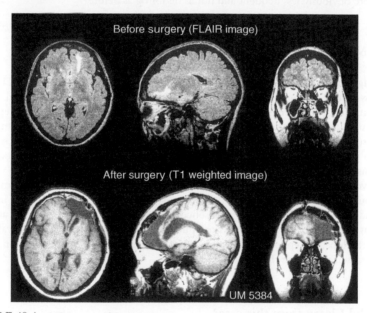

FIGURE 49.4   MRI; pre- and post-surgery.   f0040

Magnetoencephalography demonstrated that the localization of estimated dipoles of the spike component of the spike-waves clustered diffusely in the left frontal lobe (Figure 49.3). Magnetic resonance imaging of the brain revealed a wedge-shaped, T2-weighted, high-signal lesion in the left frontal lobe (Figure 49.4). An ictal technetium-99 ECD (ethyl cysteinate dimer) revealed an area of hyperperfusion in the mesial basal part in the left frontal lobe.

The patient's IQs as measured by the Wechsler Adult Intelligence Scale (Revised) were within a subnormal range, with a comparatively lower IQ in the verbal domain. On the Wisconsin Card Sorting Test, categories achieved were six. A Wada test showed that speech and memory dominance were on the left.

s0030   ## DIAGNOSIS

p0070   Frontal lobe epilepsy with focal motor seizures, occasionally secondarily generalized, and absence-like seizures.

s0040   ## TREATMENT AND OUTCOME

p0080   Phenytoin, carbamazepine, and valproate, often in combination, were administered at maximal dosage with insufficient control of seizures. The seizures occurred on a daily to weekly basis.

p0090   The patient underwent a left frontal resection at the age of 41. Scar tissue was found at surgery in the antero-inferior portion of the left frontal lobe. Seizures subsided for 6 months, but then simple and complex focal seizures recurred, although they were obviously less frequent and not as disabling as before.

s0050   ## COMMENTARY

p0100   The diagnosis of this patient during more than 20 years of follow-up has changed twice, with three different diagnoses – idiopathic generalized epilepsy with absences, symptomatic generalized epilepsy with atypical absences, and frontal lobe epilepsy with simple and complex focal seizures. Once subtle but definite focal motor and dysphasic seizure manifestations became evident, there was no doubt that her seizures were of frontal lobe origin. Furthermore, the outcome of her surgery supports this diagnosis.

p0110   However, at least in her 20s, episodes of brief and abrupt loss or impairment of consciousness accompanied by bisynchronous spike-and-wave rhythms, both interictally and ictally, were interpreted as absence seizures, even though they were atypical in terms of EEG expression. Since the epileptogenic zone was proven to localize in the frontal lobe, the episode of impairment of consciousness was, by definition, complex focal seizures rather than absence.

s0060   ### What did I learn from this case?

p0120   A time-honored term, secondary bilateral synchrony, was first described by Jasper *et al.*, nearly half a century ago, as bursts of high-amplitude synchronous slow spike-and-wave complexes that are more or less symmetrical over both hemispheres and are caused by a unilateral epileptogenic lesion of the mesial surface of the frontal or temporal lobe. The term originally referred to an interictal EEG expression and not to an ictal manifestation. For the past two decades, it has been reported that patients having focal seizures with secondary bilateral synchrony may have non-convulsive seizures that mimic absences, especially when an epileptogenic focus is localized in the frontal lobe.

p0130   Differentiation between idiopathic generalized epilepsy and frontal lobe epilepsy, or between symptomatic generalized epilepsy of the Lennox–Gastaut type and symptomatic partial epilepsy with secondary bilateral synchrony, has been a subject of controversy. It can be difficult to differentiate absence seizures from complex focal seizures of frontal origin. The choice of drug treatment, the evaluation for surgical interventions, and the prognosis of the disorder considerably differ between these two conditions.

This patient showed that secondary bilateral synchrony might be associated with ictal phenomena that mimic absences. This case also teaches us that long-term follow-up may be necessary to define an epileptic syndrome, whether focal or generalized.

FURTHER READING

Blume W. Lennox-Gastaut syndrome and secondary bilateral synchrony: a comparison. In: Wolf P, ed. *Epileptic seizures and syndromes.* London: John Libby, 1994: 285–97.

Holthausen H. Lennox-Gastaut syndrom vs. sekundäre bilaterale Synchronie. In: Fröscher W, Kramer G, Ried S, Vassella F, eds. *Das Lennox-Gastaut syndrom.* Berlin: Blackwell, 1998: pp. 65–102.

Gastaut H, Zifkin B, Maggauda A, *et al.* Symptomatic partial epilepsies with secondary bilateral synchrony: differentiation from symptomatic generalized epilepsies of the Lennox-Gastaut type. In: Wieser HG, Elger CE, eds. *Presurgical evaluation of epileptics.* Berlin: Springer, 1987: 308–17.

Kudo T, Sato K, Yagi K, *et al.* Can absence status epilepticus be of frontal lobe origin? *Acta Neurol Scand* 1995;**92**:472–7.

Lombroso CT. Consistent EEG focalities detected in subjects with primary generalized epilepsies monitored for two decades. *Epilepsia* 1997;**38**:797–812.

Roger J, Bureau M. Distinctive characteristics of frontal lobe epilepsy versus idiopathic generalized epilepsy. In: Chauvel P, Delgado-Escueta AV, eds. *Advances in neurology,* vol 57. New York: Raven, 1992: 399–410.

Yagi K. Evolution of Lennox-Gastaut syndrome: a long-term longitudinal study. *Epilepsia* 1996;**37(suppl 3)**:48–51.

c00050

If You Don't Succeed, Investigate

Michael R Sperling

s0010

HISTORY

p0010

A woman first came to the epilepsy center at the age of 28 for management of uncontrolled seizures. Her seizures had begun at the age of 7, immediately after a bout of measles with high fever. She had previously been in good health and had no antecedent risk factors for epilepsy. The seizures were characterized by staring and unresponsiveness that started without warning and lasted for less than 1 min. At the age of 12 she began to experience tonic–clonic seizures, which began with a feeling of restlessness and the urge to defecate. Next, she lost her ability to speak, blinked her eyes and paced back and forth for half a minute, and her head would then turn to the left. This was followed by generalized tonic–clonic activity. She was confused for several hours after each seizure and was sleepy for the remainder of the day.

p0020

Until the age of 28, she had one seizure at the start of each menstrual period approximately 10 times per year. At the age of 28, the seizures became more frequent. She reported between 5 and 10 seizures separated by 15–60 min in a single day at the onset of menses. She had been treated with phenytoin, phenobarbital, carbamazepine, mephenytoin, trimethadione, primidone, acetazolamide, and chlorazepate in the past without benefit.

p0030

At the time of her initial evaluation, she was taking phenytoin, carbamazepine, and chlorazepate. A maternal second cousin and paternal aunt had a history of seizures, but the patient could not provide any details about their condition. She was married and had two healthy children. She had formerly worked as a keypunch operator but had lost her job on account of the seizures. She also complained of poor memory.

s0020

EXAMINATION AND INVESTIGATIONS

p0040

The general physical examination was normal. She weighed 72 kg and had normal vital signs. Her neurological examination was remarkable for moderately impaired long-term memory and nystagmus on horizontal gaze in either direction. The remainder of the examination was normal. A magnetic resonance imaging scan showed two small, high-signal intensity lesions in the left centrum semiovale. Her first EEG showed intermittent left temporal theta activity and the second EEG showed left mid-temporal sharp waves in sleep. Neuropsychological testing revealed a full-scale IQ of 84, mild to moderate impairment of verbal and visuospatial memory, and markedly impaired naming, phonemic verbal fluency, and repetition.

She was given a provisional diagnosis of catamenial partial epilepsy, with monthly bouts of status epilepticus. She expressed a decided lack of interest in having an inpatient evaluation, and elected to continue to try medical therapy. Her drug regimen was changed to carbamazepine and acetazolamide without benefit. A combination of phenytoin and carbamazepine was then used, but she continued to experience monthly episodes of tonic–clonic status epilepticus. Another further interictal EEG again showed left temporal sharp waves.

She was admitted to the hospital during a bout of status epilepticus and had video–EEG monitoring. The EEG showed generalized, frontally predominant spike–wave discharges during her "interictal" confusional period and generalized spikes followed by muscle artifact during the tonic–clonic activity. When the cluster of seizures ended, the EEG showed diffuse background theta and delta waves for several days without interictal spikes. Her serum carbamazepine level was subtherapeutic, and she was discharged on increasing doses of carbamazepine and phenytoin.

Her monthly clusters of status epilepticus continued. She was instructed to discontinue carbamazepine, and valproate was prescribed at doses sufficient to produce a therapeutic level. The seizures persisted on a combination of phenytoin and valproate, although they diminished in frequency to one a month. Eight months later, phenytoin was discontinued and the seizures stopped.

DIAGNOSIS

Based on the observed ictal behavior, EEG findings of a generalized spike–wave pattern, the remarkable response to valproate and the strong family history of epilepsy, the patient was given a diagnosis of generalized epilepsy. The etiology remains uncertain, with weak evidence for an underlying static encephalopathy, although an idiopathic generalized epilepsy is possible in light of her response to valproate. A unilateral neocortical focus with secondary bilateral synchrony in the EEG is also possible but unproven.

TREATMENT AND OUTCOME

She had no seizures for the subsequent 12 years while taking valproate 1250 mg/day. Her serum levels have ranged between 55 and 70 mg/l. Her weight increased to 107 kg in the first 6 months after beginning valproate, and she then stabilized at 113 kg. She experienced a single recurrent seizure in late 1999, and has remained free of seizures since then on a dose of valproate 1500 mg/day. Although somewhat dissatisfied with her weight gain, the patient finds it preferable to recurrent bouts of status epilepticus.

COMMENTARY

This patient had uncontrolled tonic–clonic seizures that were refractory to a variety of antiepileptic drugs. Her condition worsened over time despite therapy, so that she experienced monthly bouts of status epilepticus with its attendant risks before her condition was controlled. This happened in part because of an incorrect diagnosis and, as a result, treatment for presumed partial epilepsy without knowledge and, later, attention to the generalized spike–wave findings on EEG.

p0110   Several features in the history and EEG were misleading. The seizures began after a bout of measles, which is often associated with encephalitis and consequent focal brain injury. The childhood seizures, which were probably absence attacks, lasted longer than usual and complex partial seizures were suspected. Moreover, the tonic–clonic seizures began with what resembled an aura, and the late head turning also suggested the possibility of a focal process. Her early interictal EEGs suggested a focal disturbance, with left temporal sharp waves noted on two occasions.

p0120   Only after ictal recording was performed did the generalized nature of her epilepsy begin to reveal itself. Her condition began to improve only when she was treated with valproate for generalized epilepsy. Combining phenytoin and valproate did not completely stop the seizures, and it was necessary to use valproate in monotherapy to abolish her seizures. The favorable response to valproate helped to establish the diagnosis and confirm the clinical impression.

p0130   This case history demonstrates the importance of accurately diagnosing the seizure type and epilepsy syndrome. Accurate diagnosis leads to appropriate therapy, which offers the best chance of a successful result. Although other antiepileptic drugs are sometimes effective in idiopathic generalized epilepsy, many patients with generalized spike–wave discharges respond only to valproate.[1,2] Older antiepileptic drugs such as phenobarbital, phenytoin and carbamazepine are often less effective than valproate or produce only a partial response. Rarely, antiepileptic drugs other than valproate exacerbate some types of generalized seizures. For example, carbamazepine may exacerbate absence seizures.[3] Several of the newer antiepileptic drugs such as topiramate and lamotrigine are also beneficial in treating generalized epilepsy; others such as zonisamide and levetiracetam are promising for these conditions as well.[4,5] There are no published studies comparing the efficacy of different antiepileptic drugs in the generalized epilepsies, and such trials are desirable. At present, valproate remains the first–line choice for most patients after due consideration of its potential side effects.

p0140   These side effects should also be mentioned, however briefly. Valproate is associated with many potential adverse reactions. These include fatigue, tremor, hair loss, teratogenic effects, polycystic ovarian disease, idiosyncratic liver and hematopoetic reactions, and weight gain.[6] The patient in this case experienced serious weight gain. Her weight quickly ballooned by more than 30 kg and has not diminished over the succeeding decade. Nonetheless, her sensible opinion is that the benefits of seizure control far outweigh the detriment of obesity. Usually this decision must be made by the patient, who ultimately bears the burden both of the illness and the treatment.

s0060   ## What did I learn from this case?

p0150   I learned that it is important to question the diagnosis early when the treatment is not working. In retrospect, I used ineffective therapy for too long and should have insisted on obtaining an ictal EEG recording sooner. In addition, therapy for generalized epilepsy should have been instituted earlier rather than continuing to use carbamazepine. This case history also reinforces the importance of using valproate as monotherapy in generalized epilepsy and in patients whose EEG shows generalized spike–wave discharges when the etiology is uncertain. Valproate is often most effective when used alone. This case history demonstrates the value of using valproate in monotherapy despite the lack of seizure control at the same serum levels when used in conjunction with another agent.

How did this case alter my approach to the care and treatment of my epilepsy patients?

I question my original diagnosis more readily if seizures do not respond to therapy, and I advise video–EEG or ambulatory EEG monitoring early if seizures remain uncontrolled. I spend more time verifying the seizure history and family history during follow-up office visits, and have somewhat less faith in the interictal EEG as a guide for therapy.

REFERENCES

1. Davis R, Peters DH, McTavish D. Valproic acid: a reappraisal of its pharmacological properties and clinical efficacy in epilepsy. *Drugs* 1994;**47**:332–72.
2. Simon D, Penry JK. Sodium di-*n*-propylacetate (DPA) in the treatment of epilepsy: a review. *Epilepsia* 1975;**22**:1701–8.
3. Liporace JL, Sperling MR, Dichter MA. Absence seizures and carbamazepine in adults. *Epilepsia* 1994;**35**:1026–8.
4. Matsuo F. Lamotrigine. *Epilepsia* 1999;**40(suppl 5)**:S30–S36.
5. Glauser TA. Topiramate. *Epilepsia* 1999;**40(suppl 5)**:S71–S80.
6. Dreifuss FE, Langer DH. Side effects of valproate. *Am J Med* 1988;**84**:34–41.

Should He or Shouldnt't He? Is It Reasonable to Prescribe Carbamazepine after Lamotrigine-induced Stevens–Johnson Syndrome?

Fahmida Chowdhury and L Nashef

s0010

HISTORY

A 23-year-old right-handed man first presented at age 21 years with generalized tonic–clonic seizures lasting for about 4–5 min. These occurred without warning, and resulted in minor injury on several occasions. There were no other seizure types. There was no previous history of febrile seizures, meningitis, encephalitis, or severe head injury. There was no family history of epilepsy. He had worked as a maintenance worker but had been unable to do so for about a year due to uncontrolled seizures. He previously consumed about 8 pints of beer a week, cutting down to 2. He did not take recreational drugs and was otherwise well. Despite sodium valproate, he continued to have seizures at least once a month. Lamotrigine was added, starting at 25 mg/day increased to 50 mg/day after 2 weeks, a higher starting dose than recommended in the data sheet as add-on treatment to valproate. Unfortunately, this led to Stevens–Johnson syndrome requiring hospitalization. The patient later recalled being warned about the possibility of a rash but not of mouth ulcers, this resulting in some delay in presentation. Lamotrigine was stopped with full recovery. He was then prescribed levetiracetam which was associated with an apparent increase in seizure frequency. At the time he was referred to our service, he was taking sodium valproate and levetiracetam and was experiencing seizures once a week.

s0020

INVESTIGATIONS

p0030

MRI brain scan was normal. EEG showed focal epileptiform activity with frequent sharp waves and sharpened slow waves over the right temporal electrodes in the awake

Puzzling Cases of Epilepsy

EEG and runs of focal polyspikes lasting 1–3 s in a right frontotemporal distribution during sleep. These fast discharges raised the possibility of underlying cortical dysplasia. On subsequent telemetry, his interictal EEG again showed the same relatively frequent focal epileptiform discharges. One partial seizure with secondary generalization was recorded which showed right-sided onset and early bilateral spread. MEG showed a right temporo-sylvian focus with consistent spiking during the awake stage with sparing of the mesial temporal structures.

DIAGNOSIS

MRI negative refractory partial epilepsy with rapid secondary generalization.
Stevens–Johnson syndrome secondary to lamotrigine.

TREATMENT AND OUTCOME

Levetiracetam was gradually withdrawn. Other treatment options were discussed with the patient. Carbamazepine is a first choice effective medication in partial epilepsy. The patient previously had been led to understand that it was contraindicated given his history of Stevens–Johnson syndrome. Despite structural similarity, our Medicine Information Service confirmed that there was no good evidence for specific cross-reactivity between lamotrigine and carbamazepine. T-cell reactivity to antiepileptic medications was tested *in vitro*.[a] This was negative for all drugs tested including carbamazepine and lamotrigine. He was started on carbamazepine as add-on to valproate. This was introduced slowly at 100 mg/day of the slow release preparation increased every 2 weeks to 200 mg twice/day; further increases were guided by clinical response. There was no evidence of allergic reaction. On slow release carbamazepine 400 mg twice/day, seizure frequency improved from once a week to one nocturnal seizure in the last 6 months with no further daytime seizures. He has been able to take up employment again. Assessment for possible epilepsy surgery has been put on hold.

COMMENTARY

The epilepsy history in this case is suggestive of an underlying cortical dysplasia with unprovoked relatively frequent seizures presenting at the age of 21. There was frequent focal epileptiform activity on EEG. MRI was normal as is the case in about 30% of patients with cortical dysplasia.[1]

We chose this case in view of the concern for potential cross-reactivity when starting another AED in a patient with previous hypersensitivity reaction. In this case the patient had suffered Stevens–Johnson syndrome, a rare but potentially life-threatening reaction, secondary to lamotrigine. The patient and his family were understandably anxious about the possibility of further reactions.

Dermatological hypersensitivity reactions to antiepileptic drugs range from a mild maculopapular rash to severe reactions such as Stevens–Johnson syndrome and toxic epidermal necrolysis. Minor skin rash has been reported in up to 10% of people

[a]1 We are grateful to Professor Munir Pirmohamed, Department of Pharmacology and Therapeutics, University of Liverpool , UK, for arranging for the test to be performed in his laboratory.

started on lamotrigine.[2] The rash is usually maculopapular in appearance, generally appears within 8 weeks of starting treatment and resolves on withdrawal of lamotrigine. The incidence of Stevens–Johnson syndrome in clinical trials is approximately 1 in 1000.[3] The risk is higher in younger children and in patients on co-medication with valproate and with rapid dose escalation.[4] For carbamazepine, the incidence of minor skin rash has been reported as between 5% and 10%[5] and Stevens–Johnson syndrome reportedly occurs in approximately 1 in 10,000.[6]

p0100   It is thought that the mechanism of hypersensitivity in Stevens–Johnson syndrome/toxic epidermal necrolysis (Lyell Syndrome) with aromatic amines such as carbamazepine, phenytoin, and phenobarbitone is through induction of cytochrome P450 enzymes leading to production of reactive oxidative intermediates.[7,8] MHC-dependent clonal proliferation of T-cell lymphocytes is also thought to be involved. A study in Han Chinese patients found that carbamazepine-induced Stevens–Johnson syndrome correlated strongly with the HLA-B 1502 allele,[9] present in all 44 patients with this reaction, compared with 3 of 101 patients without and 8 of 93 healthy controls. This may explain the higher incidence of Stevens–Johnson syndrome in Chinese patients and argues for genetic testing in this population before starting carbamazepine. Two European studies have also studied this allele. One study found no correlation between carbamazepine-induced hypersensitivity and HLA-B 1502 in a group of Caucasian patients.[10] The other found that 4 out of 12 patients with carbamazepine-induced Stevens–Johnson syndrome/toxic epidermal necrolysis were heterogenous for HLA-B 1502 and remarkably all four had oriental ancestry.[11]

p0110   The mechanism of lamotrigine-induced hypersensitivity is less well understood but is thought to be similar due to shared structures. Valproic acid inhibits glucuronidation, the major elimination pathway for lamotrigine[7] and prolongs the half-life of lamotrigine significantly up to 60 h.[5] Studies indicate that valproic acid can increase the risk of hypersensitivity with lamotrigine and it has been suggested that diversion from glucuronidation to an oxidative elimination pathway results in the production of a reactive epoxide intermediate.

p0120   In view of the structural similarities between carbamazepine and lamotrigine, there was concern that the patient was at an increased risk of Stevens–Johnson syndrome with carbamazepine. Cross-reactivity can occur between the aromatic antiepileptic drugs. There is evidence in the literature of both in vitro and in vivo cross-reactivity of carbamazepine with other aromatic compounds including phenytoin, phenobarbitone, and oxcarbazepine but not specifically with lamotrigine.[12–14] A recent study which looked at 1890 patients on antiepileptic mediations reported that the rate of an antiepileptic drug rash is approximately five times greater in patients with another antiepileptic drug rash than those without.[15] The reported cases of hypersensitivity to more than one antiepileptic have generally involved the aromatic antiepileptics. However, there has been a single case report of a patient who had developed Stevens–Johnson syndrome with phenytoin and carbamazepine, who then developed a skin rash attributed to gabapentin, usually considered safe in this situation.[16]

p0130   Hypersensitivity reactions can be reduced by introducing drugs at a low dose and slowly increasing the dose.[4] The outcome can be improved with rapid recognition of the syndrome and immediate discontinuation of the offending drug. On the evidence available, it was felt reasonable to introduce carbamazepine at a low dose and increase this slowly. Some reassurance was provided by T-cell testing. T-cells are thought to be actively involved in hypersensitivity reactions as cytoxic effector cells.[17] This T-cell response test measures the proliferation of T-cells to a drug in vitro. If T-cells react to a particular drug then, theoretically, a reaction is more likely. However, sensitivity is limited (approximately 60%) and the clinical value of such testing is currently unproven.

What did we learn from this case?

This case highlights the importance of hypersensitivity reactions to antiepileptic medication, the potential of cross-reactivity between drugs and possible genetic predisposition to such reactions. In time, it may be possible to test for such a predisposition before a particular medication is prescribed. For now, in all but emergency situations, it is advisable to introduce medications at a slow rate, as this may reduce the incidence of hypersensitivity reactions. Furthermore, reliable data on comparative incidence of severe hypersensitivity reactions with different AEDs are needed, as this should influence choice of AED. It is also important to warn patients of potential serious side effects so that medication is withdrawn early.

REFERENCES

1. Tassi L, Colombo N, Garbelli R, et al. Focal cortical dysplasia: neuropathological subtypes, EEG, neuroimaging and surgical outcome. Brain 2002;**125**:1719–32.
2. Guberman AH, Besag FM, Brodie MJ, et al. Lamotrigine associated rash: risk/benefit consideration in adults and children. Epilepsia 1999;**18**:281–96.
3. Walia SW, Khan EA, Ko DH, et al. Side effects of antiepileptics – a review. Pain Pract 2004;**4(3)**:194–203.
4. Lawrence JH, Weintraub DB, Buchsbaum R, et al. Predictors of lamotrigine associated rash. Epilepsia 2006;**47(2)**:318–22.
5. Shorvon S. Handbook of epilepsy treatment, 2nd ed. Blackwell Publishing, 2005.
6. Novartis Pharmaceuticals UK Ltd. Summary of product characteristics for Tegretol Retard tablets, www.emc.medicines.org.uk, downloaded on May 14, 2007.
7. Krauss G. Current understanding of delayed anticonvulsant hypersensitivity reactions. Epilepsy Currents 2006;**6(2)**:33–7.
8. Friedmann PS, Strickland I, Pirmohamed M, Park BK. Investigation of mechanisms in toxic epidermal necrolysis induced by carbamazepine. Arch Dermatol 1994;**130**:598–604.
9. Chung WH, Chung WH, Hong HS, et al. Medical genetics: a marker for Stevens–Johnson syndrome. Nature 2004;**428(6982)**:486–586.
10. Alfirevic A, Jorgensen AL, Williamson PR, et al. HLA–B locus in Caucasian patients with carbamazepine hypersensitivity. Pharmacogenomics 2006;**7(6)**:813–8.
11. Lonjou C, Thomas L, Borot N, et al. A marker for Stevens–Johnson syndrome…: ethnicity matters,. Pharmacogenomic J 2006;**6**:265–8.
12. Misra UK, Kalita J, Rathore C. Phenytoin and carbamazepine cross-reactivity: report of a case and review of literature. Postgrad Med J 2003;**79**:703–4.
13. Sierra NM, Garcia B, Marco J, et al. Cross-hypersensitivity syndrome between phenytoin and carbamazepine. Pharm World Sci 2005;**27**:170–4.
14. Knowles SR, Shapiro LE, Shear NH. Anticonvulsant hypersensitivity syndrome: incidence, prevention and management. Drug Saf 1999;**6**:489–501.
15. Arif H, Buchsbaum R, Weintraub D, Koyfman S, Salas-Humara C, Bazil CW, Resor SR, Hirsch LJ. Comparison and predictors of rash associated with 15 antiepileptic drugs. Neurology 2007;**68(20)**:1701–9.
16. DeToledo JC, Minagar A, Lowe MR, Ramsay RE. Skin eruption with gabapentin in a patient with repeated AED-induced Stevens–Johnson's syndrome. Ther Drug Monit 1999;**21(1)**:137–8.
17. Pichler WJ, Tilch J. Review article: the lymphocyte transformation test in the diagnosis of drug hypersensitivity. Allergy 2004;**59**:809–20.

The Value of Repeating Video–EEG Monitoring and the Importance of Concomitant ECG Tracings in the Evaluation of Changes in Seizure Semiology

c00

Meriem K Bensalem-Owen and Toufic A Fakhoury

HISTORY

s0010

The patient is a 60-year-old right-handed woman with a history of seizures since the age of 21. Her seizures were characterized by aphasia, staring, and at times manual automatisms lasting 30 s to 1 min. She has no significant past medical history. She does not have any epilepsy risk factors.

p0010

EXAMINATION AND INVESTIGATIONS

s0020

Her general and neurologic examinations were normal. MRI of the brain was normal and showed no pathology in the temporal lobes. She had inpatient video EEG monitoring. Several typical seizures were recorded and the study localized the epileptogenic focus to the left temporal lobe.

p0020

p0030

Within a few months of discharge from the hospital, her seizure semiology changed. The patient and her husband reported more severe events. The onset was similar to her typical seizures but some were associated with loss of consciousness leading to falls every 3 weeks or so. Her medications included carbamazepine and valproic acid.

A second admission for prolonged EEG-closed circuit television (EEG-CCTV) study was undertaken in order to better characterize the nature of her new events. Four typical complex partial seizures were recorded. Clinically they were characterized by behavioral arrest, staring, language disturbance, and manual automatisms. In addition, two of these events were associated with eye closure (the patient was lying in bed and her head was resting on the pillow when these episodes occurred).

Electrographically, all four seizures had a left temporal onset. Concomitant ECG recording with the two episodes associated with eye closure revealed asystole lasting as long as 16 s (Figure 52.1).

DIAGNOSIS

Partial epilepsy of left temporal lobe origin causing asystole.

TREATMENT AND OUTCOME

The patient had a demand cardiac pacemaker implanted. She later underwent resective epilepsy surgery and has been seizure-free since then.

COMMENTARY

We present a case in which repeating video–EEG monitoring for changes in seizure semiology was crucial not only for a correct diagnosis, but for potentially life-saving intervention.

The patient presented illustrates a case where a diagnosis of partial onset epilepsy was already confirmed. However, the patient's seizures evolved to more severe episodes of falls associated with loss of consciousness without any jerking activity or tonic posturing. One consideration in this patient would be late-onset drop attacks associated with temporal lobe epilepsy also known as temporal lobe syncope[1] versus syncope of different etiology. In such cases, EEG/ECG co-registration may be the only method of differentiating between an epileptic seizure and neurogenic or vasovagal syncope. In our patient ECG recordings revealed asystole.

Our patient was referred for cardiologic consultation. Since inpatient monitoring typically only captures a few seizures, and since ictal asystole or bradycardia may not occur with every seizure, a thorough cardiologic evaluation and insertion of a loop recorder may be warranted to capture these events. Cardiac arrhythmias are frequently observed during seizures, but the specific relation between cerebral ictal activity and cardiac rhythm is not completely understood. Nearly 40% of patients with medically intractable focal epilepsy display cardiac rhythm or repolarization abnormalities during or immediately after seizures.[2] Epileptic activity can produce a spectrum of cardiac abnormalities: supraventricular and sinus tachycardia, sinus bradycardia, sinus arrest, atrioventricular block, and asystole. Of those, ictal and peri-ictal tachycardia are the most frequent ECG abnormalities. They have been found in 86–99% of temporal

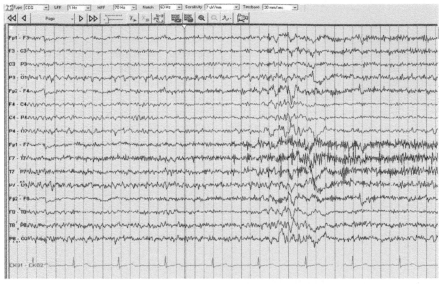

(A)

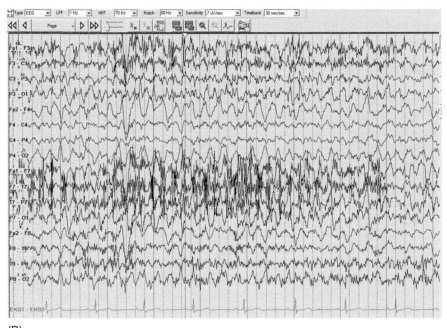

(B)

FIGURE 52.1   (A–D) Four consecutive pages of continuous EEG with concomitant ECG illustrating a seizure of left temporal onset associated with bradycardia then asystole in the patient presented.

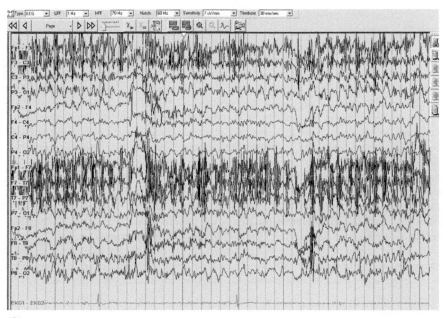

(C)

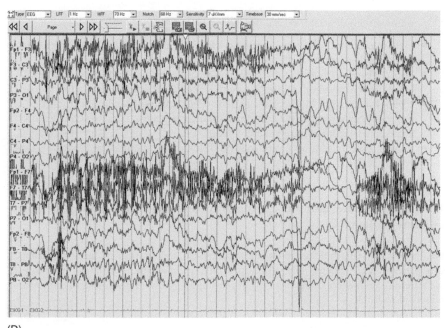

(D)

FIGURE 52.1   (*Continued*).

lobe seizures, often preceding scalp EEG changes.[3-6] Almost a century ago, Russell clinically observed the cessation of the pulse during a seizure in a young woman.[7] Since then, several anecdotal cases have been reported in which ictal episodes were accompanied by slowing of the heart rate or asystole. Ictal asystole is a rare feature of patients with focal epilepsy as reported in a recent paper from Schuele et al.,[8] occurring in 0.27% of the 6825 patients in their database who had undergone video-EEG monitoring. However, Rugg-Gunn et al. noted that 16% of the 20 patients with epilepsy investigated by an implantable ECG loop recorder had one or more episodes of ictal asystole.[9] Rocamora et al. noted that seizure-induced asystole appeared only in focal epilepsy and lateralized to the left hemisphere.[10] Altenmüller et al. reported that electrical stimulation of the temporal limbic structures, frontal lobe, and the insula in patients with implanted electrodes can cause changes in heart rate and blood pressure to the point of asystole.[11]

Documenting ictal or peri-ictal arrhythmias associated with epileptic seizures is relevant in a patient's management for two main reasons, namely to avoid undesirable cardiac side effects of AEDs and to prevent potentially life-threatening events such as sudden unexpected death in epileptic patients. Cardiac arrhythmias together with central apnea and neurogenic pulmonary edema have been hypothesized to be relevant to the pathogenesis of sudden unexplained (or unexpected) death in epilepsy (SUDEP).[12]

What did we learn from this case?

The case presented illustrates several interesting points.

- First, one should have a low threshold for repeating video–EEG monitoring in patients who develop a change in seizure semiology.
- Second, careful attention should be paid to concomitant ECG recording since heart rate changes may sometimes be the only clinical sign of a seizure.
- Third, it is prudent for the management of patients with symptomatic and prolonged ictal bradycardia and/or asystole to implant a cardiac pacemaker, in addition to optimizing antiepileptic drugs.
- Fourth, assessment of ictal cardiac arrhythmias may be crucial in monitoring the risk of SUDEP.

How did this case alter our approach to the care and treatment of our epilepsy patients?

We have a low threshold in repeating video–EEG monitoring in the evaluation of our patients with epilepsy who develop a change in seizure semiology. In addition, we carefully review concomitant ECG recordings in view of possible arrhythmogenic effects of seizures.

REFERENCES

1. Gambardella A, Reutens DC, Andermann F, et al. Late-onset drop attacks in temporal lobe epilepsy: a reevaluation of the concept of temporal lobe epilepsy. Neurology 1994;44(6):1074–8.

2. Nei M, Ho RT, Sperling MR. EKG abnormalities during partial seizures in refractory epilepsy. *Epilepsia* 2000;**41**:542–8.
3. Leutmezer F, Schernthaner C, Lurger S, *et al.* Electrographic changes at the onset of epileptic seizures. *Epilepsia* 2003;**44(3)**:348–54.
4. Mayer H, Benninger F, Urak L, *et al.* EKG abnormalities in children and adolescents with symptomatic temporal lobe epilepsy. *Neurology* 2004;**63(2)**:324–8.
5. Opherk C, Coromilas J, Hirsh LJ. Heart rate and EKG changes in 102 seizures: analysis of influencing factors. *Epilepsy Res* 2002;**52(2)**:117–27.
6. Di Gennero G, Quarato PP, Sebastiano F, *et al.* Ictal heart rate increase precedes EEG discharge in drug-resistant mesial temporal lobe seizures. *Clin Neurophysiol* 2004;**115(5)**:1169–77.
7. Russel AE. Cessation of the pulse during the onset of epileptic fits. *Lancet* 1906;**2**:152–4.
8. Schuele SU, Bermeo AC, Locatelli ER, Burgess RC, Dinner DS, Foldvary-Schaefer N. Video-electrographic and clinical features in patients with ictal asystole. *Neurology* 2007;**69**:434–41.
9. Rugg-Gunn FJ, Simister R, Squirell M, Holdright DR, Duncan JS. Cardiac arrhythmias in focal epilepsy: a prospective long-term study. *Lancet* 2004;**364**:2212–9.
10. Rocamora R, Kurthen M, Lickfett L, von Oertzen J, Elger CE. Cardiac asystole in epilepsy: clinical and neurophysiologic features. *Epilepsia* 2003;**44(2)**:179–85.
11. Altenmüller D-M, Zehender M, Schulze-Bonhage A. High-grade atrioventricular block triggered by spontaneous and stimulation-induced epileptic activity in the left temporal lobe. *Epilepsia* 2004;**45**:1640–4.
12. Nashef L, Hindocha N, Makoff A. Risk factors in sudden death in epilepsy (SUDEP): the quest for mechanisms. *Epilepsia* 2007;**48(5)**:859–71.

Unforeseen Complications and Problems

A 35-Year-Old Man with Poor Surgical Outcome after Temporal Lobe Surgery

Gus A Baker

HISTORY

The patient is a 35-year-old man with a long-standing history of temporal lobe epilepsy.

Despite intractable seizures, he had managed to attend mainstream schooling and obtain his school certificates in six subjects. He left school at the age of 16 years and worked for 4 years as a television salesman. Unfortunately his seizures became more frequent and as a consequence he was forced to give up work in 1983. He tried a combination of antiepileptic drugs but was unable to obtain satisfactory control.

He lived at home with his parents and had never been in a romantic relationship. His family was reluctant to explore the possibility of surgery for the control of his seizures because they were fearful that he might be left disabled by the operation. However, after his father died suddenly from a cardiovascular disorder, the patient decided to reconsider the surgical option. He underwent a number of investigations and was considered a good candidate for surgery.

EXAMINATION AND INVESTIGATIONS

Results from the surgical assessment (EEG, brain magnetic imaging, intracarotid sodium amytal test [ICSA], neuropsychology) confirmed that right mesial temporal sclerosis was responsible for his seizures.

DIAGNOSIS

Right mesial temporal sclerosis with nocturnal seizures and occasional daytime seizures.

s0040

TREATMENT AND OUTCOME

p0060
A right anterior temporal lobectomy was carried out in 1997. The operation was complicated by a right third nerve palsy and mild expressive dysphasia. No significant changes in neuropsychological functioning from the pre-operative baseline were noted.

p0070
Initially there was a reduction in the frequency and severity of his nocturnal seizures. However, at a 12-month assessment, his seizures had returned to their pre-operative status.

s0050

COMMENTARY

p0080
I chose this case for several reasons. First, despite the impressive results obtained from epilepsy surgery programs in the USA and Europe, not all patients fare well. In this case, a young man who underwent a right temporal lobectomy did not have a good surgical outcome. While there was an initial reduction in the frequency of seizures, within 6 months his seizures returned to the level that existed before his surgery.

p0090
Second, the patient had a number of expectations of the surgery, the most important being that he would become more independent as a result of being rendered seizure-free. At the time of the operation he was heavily reliant on his mother, who was in her late 70s and not in good health. He had two siblings who lived away from the family home. His family was naturally concerned about his future, particularly if his mother's health deteriorated further.

p0100
Third, he showed great courage in going for the surgery, particularly as both he and his family were concerned about the risk of something awful going wrong during the surgery and of him being left severely disabled.

p0110
Fourth, despite the failure of the surgery to meet his expectations, the patient did not suffer any significant psychosocial consequences. This may have been because he felt that had he not gone for the surgical option, he would always have regretted not knowing whether or not it would have worked.

s0060

What did I learn from this case?

p0120
It is important to recognize that, for many patients and their families, the idea of brain surgery may create a number of anxieties. It is important for the epilepsy surgery team to be sure that the patient and the patient's family have a clear conception about what surgery will entail. Furthermore, there should be discussion about the relative risks and benefits associated with the procedure. In my practice, it is not uncommon to put prospective candidates in touch with others who have been through the surgery program.

p0130
This case highlights the importance of spending time with patients and their families to discuss their expectation of surgery. Patients will undoubtedly have varying expectations of the surgery. The way they react to the outcome of such a radical intervention is influenced by a number of factors, including whether they are rendered seizure-free or not, their own and their family's expectations of surgery, whether there are any emotional changes associated with the surgery, their premorbid psychological and neuropsychological functioning, and the level of social support they have both before and after surgery.

Clinical experience from my own surgical series suggests that even when surgery is successful it is not always accompanied by an improved quality of life. Equally, as in this case, the failure to render a patient seizure-free does not necessarily lead to a reduction in quality of life. This patient was grateful for the opportunity at least to see if surgery could help with the management of his seizures.

FURTHER READING

Engel J (ed.). *Surgical treatment of the epilepsies*, 2nd ed. NY: Raven, 1993.

Hermann BP, Seidenberg M, Wendt G, Bell B. Neuropsychology and epilepsy surgery: optimizing the timing of surgery, minimizing cognitive morbidity and maximizing functional status. In: Schmidt D, Schachter S, eds. *Epilepsy: problem solving in clinical practice*. London: Martin Dunitz, 2000: 279–90.

Wilson S, Saling MM, Kincade P, Bladin PF. Patient expectations of temporal lobe surgery. *Epilepsia* 1998;**39**:167–74.

c0054

When More is Less

Carl W Bazil

s0010 ## HISTORY

p0010   A 42-year-old woman was admitted because of exacerbation of her chronic seizure disorder. Her pertinent history began at the age of 13 years, when she began to experience frequent seizures consisting of head dropping, eye blinking, and eye deviation, sometimes with loss of awareness. She occasionally sustained injury during the head drops as a result of suddenly falling to the floor. She also had very rare secondarily generalized seizures.

p0020   The patient was found to have aqueductal stenosis and hydrocephalus. A ventricular shunt was placed; however, her course was complicated by multiple shunt revisions and infections. She had been treated with virtually all antiepileptic drugs, often in combination, including bromides and mephenytoin. She was placed on vigabatrin 5 years ago, which resulted in excellent seizure control. However, she developed visual symptoms over the following 2 years and was found to have vigabatrin-related visual field loss. Topiramate treatment resulted in severe word-finding difficulty, and the initial dose had to be decreased.

p0030   Two years before admission, she developed a new seizure type, which consisted of sudden unresponsiveness with eyes closed and all limbs limp. She was evaluated with video–EEG monitoring, and these episodes were found to be non-epileptic. They resolved with psychotherapy, including training in self-hypnosis. Tiagabine was also started at this time, resulting in improved seizure control. Over the 2 weeks before admission, however, she began to have prolonged episodes of confusion, which were sometimes associated with violent behavior. These episodes were described by her family as being unlike all previous seizure episodes – longer (lasting several hours) and usually associated with some purposeful behavior. Oral diazepam led to resolution of some of these episodes within seconds or minutes. However, owing to the increasing frequency of seizures, she was admitted for monitoring and further treatment.

p0040   Medications on admission were:

u0010   • extended-release carbamazepine 800 mg three times a day;
u0020   • topiramate 25 mg three times a day;
u0030   • tiagabine 20 mg in the morning and 16 mg twice a day;
u0040   • zolpidem 5 mg at bedtime as needed;
u0050   • folic acid 1 mg once daily.

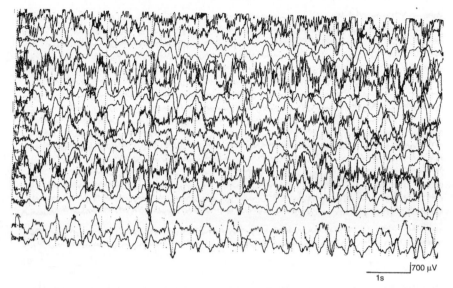

f0010

FIGURE 54.1   EEG from the patient during an episode of confusion and irregular movements. A diffuse, irregular spike–wave discharge was seen most prominently in the anterior region.

EXAMINATION AND INVESTIGATIONS

The general and neurological examinations were normal. The patient was admitted to the epilepsy monitoring unit for video–EEG monitoring. On the day after admission she had a 3-h episode of prolonged confusion with staring and irregular movements. The EEG during this time showed an irregular, generalized spike–wave discharge that was more pronounced on the right at times (Figure 54.1). Diazepam was administered, initially rectally then (after 30 min) intravenously. She began to improve 10 min after the intravenous administration, although nearly 2 h passed before there was complete resolution of the clinical symptoms and the EEG changes. Figure 54.2 shows her EEG 10 h later.

DIAGNOSIS

The diagnosis was non-convulsive status epilepticus.

TREATMENT AND OUTCOME

Non-convulsive status epilepticus has been described as an unusual complication of tiagabine. However, this patient had responded well to tiagabine for control of her other seizures. Tiagabine was, therefore, decreased to a total of 28 mg/day. She had another, briefer episode of confusion associated with irregular spike–wave discharges during the taper. She has remained now on this dose of tiagabine for 18 months, with no recurrence of non-convulsive status epilepticus.

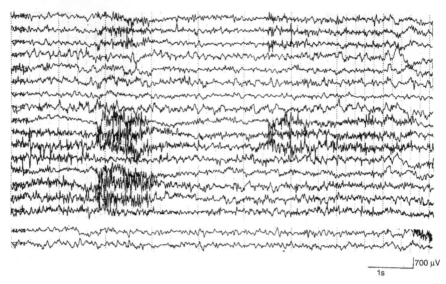

700 µV

1s

f0020

FIGURE 54.2   EEG from the same patient 10h later, after resolution of the symptoms. There is mild diffuse slowing, probably caused by benzodiazepines.

s0050

COMMENTARY

p0130

It is well known that epileptic and non-epileptic seizures frequently coexist. For this reason, both diagnoses must be considered in any patient with epilepsy who develops a new seizure type. As clinicians, we always operate at a disadvantage since we are usually unable to observe the symptom (the seizure) directly. The history is necessarily biased, and any caregiver (no matter how experienced and knowledgeable about epilepsy) can inadvertently give misleading information.

p0140

My initial thought in this patient was that she was experiencing a new type of non-epileptic event. From the history, the episodes had a number of characteristics that would be unusual for epileptic seizures. First, they were variable in quality and duration. Second, she was reported to be unresponsive and yet able to perform purposeful tasks during the episodes. Third, although the episodes resolved with benzodiazepines, this was described as occurring within seconds to minutes of an oral dose – not enough time for absorption of oral diazepam and therefore suggestive of a placebo effect. Finally, most of the episodes lasted several hours whereas typical complex partial seizures last no more than 2 min.

p0150

However, I have been humbled a number of times when attempting to make such a diagnosis by history alone. Furthermore, this patient was already known to suffer both epileptic and non-epileptic seizures. It was fortunately my standard to admit such complicated patients for definitive diagnosis using video–EEG monitoring. It was also fortunate that her seizures were frequent enough for this to be feasible.

s0060

What did I learn from this case?

p0160

This case illustrates the possibility of new seizure types induced by medication changes. Most commonly, partial seizures change somewhat in quality; for example, a psychic aura may appear when none was present before, or nonsensical speech may occur as a result of a change in the pattern of spread. Rarely (as in this case) a totally new seizure type can emerge. The most common example is myoclonus induced by phenytoin, carbamazepine or gabapentin, which can occur in patients with no history of myoclonus. These patients probably have an underlying susceptibility to such seizures and most would have a typical spike–wave or polyspike–wave discharge on EEG. Tiagabine has been described as inducing non-convulsive status epilepticus in a few patients.

How did this case alter my approach to the care and treatment of my epilepsy patients?

I now recognize the need for healthy skepticism with patients who have complicated epilepsy. Whenever the treatment does not work as expected or the described event does not make neurological sense in the context of the patient's known disease, I consider alternative explanations. Although, in a few cases, it might be appropriate to treat empirically first (e.g. with an increase in medication dosage), I now realize that most such patients will require video–EEG monitoring.

c0055

Change of Antiepileptic Drug Treatment for Fear of Side Effects in a 45-Year-Old Seizure-Free Patient

Elinor Ben-Menachem

s0010

HISTORY

p0010
The patient, born in 1956, was healthy until the age of 2 years, when he began to have seizures. First he had some jerks accompanied by short periods of unconsciousness and then had a few generalized tonic–clonic seizures. The diagnosis of juvenile myoclonic epilepsy was made.

p0020
The seizures slowly increased in frequency; by the time he was 16, he was in and out of hospital with repeated episodes of status epilepticus. He was treated with combinations of carbamazepine, phenobarbital, phenytoin, and valproate, but he had daily seizures in spite of adequate serum concentrations.

s0020

EXAMINATION AND INVESTIGATIONS

p0030
The patient had a normal neurological and psychiatric examination. Video–EEG monitoring showed evidence of bifrontal epilepsy.

s0030

DIAGNOSIS

p0040
Partial seizures of bifrontal lobe onset, with occasional secondary generalization and status epilepticus.

TREATMENT AND OUTCOME

In 1987, at the age of 31, the patient weighed 120 kg, mainly because of previous valproate therapy that caused a large weight increase. He was prescribed vigabatrin 50 mg/kg per day (6 g/day) and instantly became seizure-free. Phenobarbital was titrated down and stopped in 1989 and he remained on carbamazepine and vigabatrin. After becoming seizure-free, the patient began full-time work, learned to drive, and established a family with a wife and two children. He has lived, in other words, a normal life.

During the last few years, there has been a lively discussion of the appropriateness of vigabatrin therapy in the light of its association with irreversible visual field defects in up to 40% of patients, even though most patients are asymptomatic. However, 60–80% of patients on vigabatrin do not experience this side effect. When our patient heard of the possibility of visual field defects, although he had normal visual field testing, he was reluctant to continue on vigabatrin. Moreover, he was found to have anemia, which can be caused by vigabatrin, so the decision was made to slowly downtitrate the drug and replace it with topiramate.

Over 4 months, vigabatrin was titrated down to 1 g/day and topiramate up to 400 mg/day. His dose of carbamazepine stayed the same. At a vigabatrin dose of 4 g/day the patient began to have myoclonic jerks and occasional generalized tonic–clonic seizures again. He had to stop driving and often stayed home from work. His children were in a state of shock to see their father have seizures because they had not witnessed them before. The patient's anemia resolved with iron replacement therapy and was thought to be due to a low iron content in his diet – an extensive investigation found no other cause.

The patient lost weight on topiramate, became extremely irritable, and had trouble expressing himself. Finally the situation deteriorated with such frequent generalized tonic–clonic seizures that he was hospitalized in March 2000. Topiramate was stopped and vigabatrin was reinstated at a dose of 5 g/day. He immediately became seizure-free again and regained his usual personality. His hemoglobin count and visual fields are being regularly monitored.

COMMENTARY

This case illustrates the dilemma that patients and doctors find themselves in concerning vigabatrin. It is still a very effective antiepileptic drug and not all patients experience side effects. This drug has changed the lives of many patients with refractory epilepsy for the better, and changes in this medication should be made with the greatest caution.

What did I learn from this case?

Overly enthusiastic elimination of vigabatrin from a patient's therapy may ruin his or her life, as happened with my patient until vigabatrin was started again. Both the pros and cons of discontinuing any treatment must be discussed with the patient in detail before it is stopped.

c0056

Personality and Mood Changes in a Teenager

Ahmad Beydoun, Ekrem Kutluay and Erasmo Passaro

s0010

HISTORY

p0010

The patient is a 17-year-old woman whose present medical illness started in February 2000 when she was diagnosed with a left frontal abscess complicating a pansinusitis. She underwent a left frontal craniotomy with an evacuation of the left frontal brain abscess and her sinuses. Perioperatively, she was treated with antibiotics and put on phenytoin prophylaxis for 3 weeks. She remained seizure-free and was discharged home with no apparent neurological sequelae.

p0020

She remained asymptomatic until early July 2000, when she experienced two generalized tonic–clonic seizures and multiple complex partial seizures that were characterized by staring and unresponsiveness. She was treated with intravenous lorazepam and loaded with phenytoin.

p0030

Over the next few days, she had two brief staring spells and developed personality changes, which were characterized by an unusual amount of energy, racing thoughts, inappropriate laughter, irritability, and a reduced attention span. However, she remained fully alert, oriented, and conversant. The phenytoin level was 19 mg/l.

s0020

EXAMINATION AND INVESTIGATIONS

p0040

She was admitted to the hospital for an evaluation. During the 3 days of monitoring, her awake EEG revealed well-modulated posterior 8–9 Hz activity, a left frontal breach rhythm, continuous slowing over the left frontal region, and intermittent bifrontal spike-wave activity, which occurred occasionally in bursts of up to 5 s; in addition, a total of five electrographic partial seizures without clinical accompaniment were recorded. The seizures consisted of rhythmic 5–7 Hz sharp wave activity lasting for 15–45 s over the left frontal and frontopolar regions with a maximal field at the F7 electrode site (Figure 56.1).

s0030

DIAGNOSIS

p0050

Non-convulsive status epilepticus of frontal lobe origin.

Puzzling Cases of Epilepsy

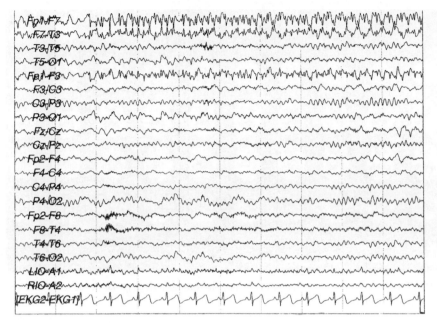

FIGURE 56.1   Ictal EEG during one of the patient's typical electrographic seizures, showing rhythmic 6–7 Hz sharp wave activity over the left frontal electrode sites.

f0010

TREATMENT AND OUTCOME

The patient was discharged home on carbamazepine and then converted to levetiracetam monotherapy because of a rash. Approximately 2 weeks later, during a 30-min outpatient EEG, she had more than 20 electrographic seizures of left frontal origin and was diagnosed with non-convulsive status epilepticus.

She was readmitted for video–EEG monitoring. She was alert and oriented but had persistent personality changes. Her short-term and long-term memory were intact, she could spell appropriately, she could calculate, and she could follow three-step commands without difficulty. Her general neurological examination was normal. During the 24 h of monitoring, 32 subclinical electrographic seizures originating from the left frontal region were recorded. During these electrographic seizures, her examination and cognitive abilities did not differ from baseline: she was able to carry on a conversation, was fully alert and oriented, and was totally unaware of the seizures when they occurred. The only detectable clinical correlate was subtle hesitancy while performing complex calculations.

On the insistence of the patient and her mother, she was discharged home the next day on levetiracetam 1500 mg/day and divalproex 1250 mg/day. A brain magnetic resonance imaging scan showed an area of encephalomalacia in the left frontal lobe at the site of her known previous abscess. Several weeks later, nine electrographic seizures originating from the left frontal region lasting 10–144 s were recorded over a period of 82 min. The doses of levetiracetam and divalproex sodium were gradually increased. In spite of this, she remained in electrographic partial status epilepticus and a subtraction ictal single photon emission computed tomography showed increased perfusion in the left orbitofrontal region, adjacent to the area of encephalomalacia (Figure 56.2).

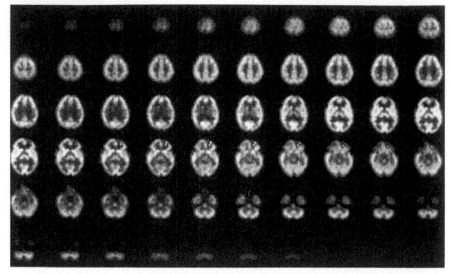

f0020

FIGURE 56.2   Subtraction ictal SPECT study showing increased uptake in the left frontal and frontopolar regions.

p0090

On the combination of levetiracetam 3000 mg/day and divalproex 1500 mg/day she was seizure-free on prolonged EEG monitoring and her personality returned to baseline.

s0050

COMMENTARY

p0100

The interesting feature of this case was the dissociation between the electrographic findings and the clinical manifestations. Status epilepticus is a medical emergency that requires immediate and aggressive treatment in order to prevent mortality or significant morbidity. Non-convulsive status epilepticus is usually suspected when there is a sudden and persistent change in mental status or behavior and confirmed by EEG.

p0110

Based on the ictal EEG findings, non-convulsive status epilepticus is divided into two categories:

u0010
u0020

- generalized non-convulsive status epilepticus and
- partial non-convulsive status epilepticus.

p0140

Although the majority of cases of partial non-convulsive status epilepticus originate from the temporal lobes, extratemporal non-convulsive status epilepticus is usually of frontal lobe origin, as in this case.

p0150

The fascinating feature of this case is how subtle the clinical manifestations were. Even during her electrographic seizures, she was fully aware of her environment and cognitively unimpaired except for minimal hesitancy during calculations. The behavioral abnormalities were perceived by her mother but were unimpressive to her examiners except for occasional inappropriate comments and irritability that could normally be observed in any teenager.

As illustrated by this patient, non-convulsive status epilepticus of frontal lobe origin frequently occurs without alteration in the level of awareness, in contrast to non-convulsive status epilepticus of temporal lobe origin. When this is the case, as in our patient, a diagnosis of simple partial non-convulsive status epilepticus should be made. Since mood disturbances are a frequent clinical manifestation, it is not uncommon for patients with non-convulsive status epilepticus of frontal lobe origin to be initially diagnosed with hypomania or hysteria. This indicates that non-convulsive status epilepticus should be considered if a patient has an unexplained subacute change in behavior.

What did we learn from this case?

Although the patient was functioning well, we were concerned about the potential cognitive morbidity that could be caused by prolonged partial non-convulsive status epilepticus. At various times, we considered aggressive medical treatment, including drug-induced coma or surgical intervention. Both the patient and her mother were understandably concerned about our recommendations for aggressive interventions since she was otherwise performing well. After numerous discussions with the family, we decided to maximize dual therapy with levetiracetam and divalproex, titrated to tolerability. If this had failed to abort the non-convulsive status epilepticus, she would have had surgical resection of the encephalomalacia with electrocorticography to guide the margins of the resection.

Her long-term prognosis remains uncertain. Data from the largest series to date on non-convulsive status epilepticus of frontal lobe origin suggest that recurrence of status epilepticus is uncommon in this patient population. Despite being in non-convulsive status epilepticus for more than 1 month, this patient did not have detectable cognitive sequelae, although formal neuropsychological testing was not done.

How did this case alter our approach to the care and treatment of our epilepsy patients?

We now approach the treatment of simple partial non-convulsive status epilepticus of frontal lobe origin conservatively before more aggressive interventions are considered. Our case illustrates that non-convulsive status epilepticus of frontal lobe origin may present with behavioral changes not associated with impairment of awareness. In fact, had our patient not had video–EEG monitoring, the diagnosis would have been unrecognized. Our case underscores the pleomorphic clinical features of non-convulsive status epilepticus for which a high index of suspicion is necessary for prompt diagnosis and management.

FURTHER READING

Thomas P, Zifkin B, Migneco O, Lebrun C, Darcourt J, Andermann F. Nonconvulsive status epilepticus of frontal origin. *Neurology* 1999;**52**:1174–83.

Thomas P. Status epilepticus with confusional symptomatology. *Neurophysiol Clin* 2000;**30**:147–54.

Kaplan PW. Assessing the outcomes in patients with nonconvulsive status epilepticus: nonconvulsive status epilepticus is underdiagnosed, potentially overtreated, and confounded by comorbidity. *J Clin Neurophysiol* 1999;**16**:341–52.

Krumholz A, Sung Y, Fisher RS, Barry E, Bergey GK. Complex partial status epilepticus accompanied by serious morbidity and mortality. *Neurology* 1995;**45**:1499–504.

Monitoring Patients May Be More Important Than Their Laboratory Tests

c0057

Jane Boggs

HISTORY

s0010

The patient is a 56-year-old white woman with a 3-year history of seizures, presumably due to known cerebrovascular disease. Her moderately demented husband brought her to the emergency department for evaluation because she had remained lethargic on the kitchen floor (for 3 days) after a single witnessed seizure. Although she was treated with phenytoin, her compliance was suspected because her home situation was somewhat unsupervised.

p0010

A neurologist had never previously seen her. Her first known seizure occurred 8–12 months after having a stroke that caused right-sided weakness and difficult-to-understand speech. A computed tomography (CT) scan reportedly showed a "stroke" but was unavailable for review. The patient's husband could not remember the name of the hospital where it was performed.

p0020

The patient's family described the initial seizure as "grand mal", and phenytoin 300 mg at bedtime was the only antiepileptic drug ever prescribed. Refills had been generated by rotating clinic physicians and by episodic visits to local emergency departments for "occasional" seizures. No EEG, repeat neuroimaging, or laboratory investigations had been done as far as the patient's husband could remember.

p0030

The patient's past medical history was significant for diabetes mellitus, mild congestive heart failure following three-vessel coronary artery bypass graft surgery 4 years previously, chronic obstructive pulmonary disease, depression, rheumatoid arthritis, and colostomy for resected colon cancer. Medications included phenytoin as above, insulin (Humulin 70/30) 20 units subcutaneously in the morning and 10 units in the evening, clopidogrel 75 mg/day, amitriptyline 25 mg/day at bedtime and sertraline 100 mg/day in two divided doses. Her only known allergy was to penicillin. She had a previous history of smoking, no history of alcohol or drug abuse and a strong family history of diabetes and coronary artery disease in middle age.

p0040

EXAMINATION AND INVESTIGATIONS

p0050   Vital signs on presentation were blood pressure 110/68 mmHg, pulse 96 beats/per minute, regular respirations 16 per minute and unlabored, and rectal temperature 37.3°C. Her general examination was remarkable for the following: mild diabetic retinal changes; dependent decubitus stage IV ulcers over her left hip, sacrum, arm, and lower face with mildly purulent oozing; dry oral mucosa; and a clean colostomy with heme-negative contents in the colostomy bag.

p0060   Her neurological examination revealed normal cranial nerve function, but assessment of cranial nerves I, XI, and XII was not possible. She had increased tone on passive movement of the right arm and leg, with a mild flexion contracture of the right elbow. There were no spontaneous movements and withdrawal to pain was better on the left side than on the right. Reflexes were minimally brisker on the right side than on the left, and ankle jerks were absent. Plantar responses were bilaterally extensor. She moaned with uncomfortable parts of the examination, but was otherwise unresponsive and followed no commands. She was intubated because of failure to protect her airway adequately.

p0070   A CT scan of the head revealed multiple old lacunae bilaterally. A lumbar puncture documented mildly elevated cerebrospinal fluid protein of 75 mg/dl, but otherwise normal studies and no growth on cultures. Phenytoin level was 9.8 μg/ml with a normal level serum albumin of 3.0 g/dl and a creatinine level of 1.6 mg/dl. Serum ammonia was 98 μmol/1. Blood chemistry, liver function tests, and blood counts were otherwise surprisingly normal, but urinalysis and culture indicated a pseudomonal urinary tract infection. Wound cultures also grew *Pseudomonas* spp. Troponin levels and electrocardiography suggested a subacute subendocardial myocardial infarction.

p0080   The neurology team was consulted after the patient's mental status remained unimproved after 24 h of antibiotics and gentle hydration. An EEG revealed diffuse slowing with superimposed 2–3 Hz, rhythmic, sharply contoured biphasic and triphasic waveforms maximally expressed in the left frontotemporal region. This activity did not change with painful, auditory or visual stimulation, but was replaced within 2 min by irregular, reactive theta activity after a total of 10 mg of intravenous diazepam. The patient was treated with intravenous fosphenytoin, which raised her phenytoin level to 16 μg/ml.

p0090   Her mental status and EEG still did not improve, and occasional myoclonic jerks of the right arm were noted, with concomitant spiking seen at electrode F7; this spiking persisted after administering clinically effective paralytics. This activity persisted despite a total of 20 mg of intravenous diazepam, which resulted in a 20 mmHg drop in mean arterial pressure. The activity was stopped by valproate 500 mg intravenously, and the patient was placed immediately on maintenance intravenous fosphenytoin and valproate. The EEG improved to generalized theta waves, left slower than right (but non-rhythmic and reactive to stimulation). Within 24 h she had spontaneous limb movements and opened her eyes to auditory stimulation. Within 1 week she was extubated and was able to answer yes–no questions appropriately.

p0100   For an unclear reason, her serum ammonia was repeated at this point and was found to be 150 μmol/l. The medical team abruptly discontinued the valproate. Three days later she answered questions more hesitantly and inappropriately. The EEG revealed recurrence of her previous left hemispheric ictal pattern. Raising her phenytoin dose to achieve a free level of 3.0 μg/ml failed to resolve the recurrent complex partial status epilepticus. Phenobarbital, gabapentin, and topiramate were also tried without success.

    After much discussion, the medical team agreed to resume valproate, and the EEG   p0110
ictal pattern resolved. Within 24 h she again showed clinical improvement, but required

2 weeks to regain her previous verbal skills. Serial serum ammonia levels remained between 200 and 300 μmol/1.

DIAGNOSIS

s0030

Recurrent left complex partial status epilepticus responsive to valproate. Asymptomatic hyperammonemia secondary to valproate.

p0120

TREATMENT AND OUTCOME

s0040

Six months later, the patient was brought to the emergency department again for altered mental status. The nursing home physician had discontinued oral generic valproate about 3 months previously because of gastrointestinal distress, and so she was receiving only oral phenytoin. Once again, the EEG showed ictal left hemispheric patterns, which were responsive to intravenous valproate. She was discharged on phenytoin and divalproex after 3 weeks. Because she maintained a clinically improving picture, measurement of serum ammonia levels was not repeated.

p0130

COMMENTARY

s0050

This patient had the typical clinical presentation of complex partial status epilepticus, which in her case came from the left frontotemporal region. Although no specific cerebrovascular lesion was identified as the culprit, remote stroke or new-onset cortical stroke were the most likely inciting events. Because she had been left on the kitchen floor for 3 days, the documentation of a new, small cerebral lesion would have required more detailed neuroimaging (e.g. magnetic resonance imaging scans with Fluid Attenuated Inversion Recovery [FLAIR] images), which was unfortunately difficult to perform in such an unstable patient.

p0140

Her initial outpatient management with phenytoin, although a reasonable choice, appeared to have been incompletely successful and upward adjustment of the dose or consideration of another antiepileptic drug should have been considered before the subsequent acute events. Other factors that probably contributed to lowering the seizure threshold in this patient were infection, non-antiepileptic medications (particularly antibiotics) and possible chronic hypoxia.

p0150

Clearly, however, phenytoin appeared insufficient to abort non-convulsive status epilepticus in this patient. Increasing the serum level was an appropriate first attempt at treatment, although this patient's slightly decreased creatinine clearance and the concomitant use of other competitive protein-bound drugs probably raised the free fraction of phenytoin anyway.

p0160

Even so, the most common error in the early treatment of status epilepticus is administering too little of the initial antiepileptic drug. Adding a second agent is necessary when higher doses of the first drug are ineffective. All parenteral antiepileptic drugs other than valproate have some potential for causing cardiovascular instability. The relatively inert cardiovascular profile of valproate makes it an appropriate choice in any patient who has cardiac disease or who has had documented hypotensive responses to other antiepileptic drugs. In the unstable patient who requires urgent treatment,

p0170

even rapid intravenous infusions of valproate have not caused significant hypotension.[1] Although valproate is not licensed in the USA for the treatment of status epilepticus, recent studies have documented success in this indication.[2,3]

Hyperammonemia is a well-known metabolic cause of altered mental status. Valproate formulations are among the drugs that may result in elevated serum ammonia levels, especially in patients with defects in the urea cycle.[4] Asymptomatic hyperammonemia should not routinely prompt discontinuation of an effective medication.[5] This patient's clinical improvement despite the higher level of ammonia after addition of valproate is supportive of an incidental laboratory finding with no evidence of clinical toxicity. It is, however, prudent to monitor steadily increasing ammonia levels in any patient with altered mental status. The risk of precipitating recurrent status epilepticus should be balanced against the risks of continuing all components of the medication regimen that aborted the seizures. Perhaps a more logical medication to consider discontinuing in this case was phenytoin, since it had failed to control both individual seizures and status epilepticus without the addition of another agent.

What did I learn from this case?

I learned that elevations in serum ammonia concentrations could occur with short-term use of valproate. The elevation may be as high as those that usually cause altered mental status. In an asymptomatic and indeed improving patient, discontinuation of valproate may risk recurrent seizures. Ongoing neurologic consultation is often helpful to non-neurologists in such complex patients, even after seizures are controlled.

How did this case alter my approach to the care and treatment of my epilepsy patients?

I am now more insistent that the neurology service remains involved in the care of inpatients after the neurological crisis has seemingly ended. Although this can create a large list of "inactive" patients, it is far easier to remedy a problem acutely than after the fact. I also make sure that I mention in my consult notes that ammonia levels need not necessarily be measured in the absence of related clinical symptoms.

REFERENCES

1. Venkataraman V, Wheeless JW. Safety of rapid intravenous infusion of valproate loading doses in epilepsy patients. *Epilepsy Res* 1999;**35**:147–53.
2. Kaplan PW. Intravenous valproate treatment of generalized nonconvulsive status epilepticus. *Clin Electroencephalogr* 1999;**30**:1–4.
3. Chez MG, Hammer MS, Loeffel M, Nowinski C, Bagan BT. Clinical experience of three pediatric and one adult case of spike-and-wave status epilepticus treated with injectable valproic acid. *J Child Neurol* 1999;**14**:239–42.
4. Murphy JV, Marquardt K. Asymptomatic hyperammonemia in patients receiving valproic acid. *Arch Neurol* 1982;**39**:591–2.
5. Wyllie E, Wyllie R, Rothner AD, Erenberg G, Cruse RP. Valproate-induced hyperammonemia in asymptomatic children. *Cleveland Clin Q* 1983;**50**:275–7.

Depression in a Student with Juvenile Myoclonic Epilepsy

c0058

Enrique J Carrazana

HISTORY

The patient is a 19-year-old man who had his first convulsion at the age of 18 during a week of intense studying for his college final examinations. The event occurred during his chemistry examination, and witnesses' accounts were suggestive of a generalized tonic–clonic seizure. The patient was seen at a local hospital, loaded with 1 g of fosphenytoin and then started on phenytoin 300 mg at bedtime. A brain computed tomography scan was unremarkable.

His second convulsion occurred 6 months later at his fraternity house, the day after a night of heavy drinking with friends. Urinary incontinence and a violent postictal phase were noted in the paramedics' report. His phenytoin level was therapeutic at 17 mg/l. The seizure was attributed to alcohol withdrawal; nevertheless, a neurological evaluation was requested.

In review of the patient's history, it was noted that he had frequent "morning jerks" and that these were more frequent during anxiety-provoking situations, at times of sleep deprivation and on the morning after heavy alcohol consumption.

EXAMINATION AND INVESTIGATIONS

The patient's physical and neurological examinations were unremarkable.

An EEG revealed frequent brief generalized bursts of 3–4 Hz polyspike–wave complexes that lasted less than 1–2 s. These complexes were superimposed over a normal background. Hyperventilation induced the occurrence of the discharges accompanied by bilateral arrhythmic myoclonic jerks of the arm and facial musculature.

DIAGNOSIS

Juvenile myoclonic epilepsy.

s0040   ## TREATMENT AND OUTCOME

p0070   The antiepileptic drug regimen was changed to valproate. At a follow-up visit 2 months later, the patient reported being seizure-free and was no longer experiencing myoclonic jerks. The valproate level was 105 mg/l and his EEG had normalized.

p0080   Two months later, a psychologist at the patient's college contacted me with concerns about the patient. Following his second seizure, he had become more withdrawn and isolated. He moved out of the fraternity house to a small studio apartment somewhat distant from the campus. His grades were less than optimal, which he blamed on poor concentration. He dropped out of intramural softball, which he had not only enjoyed in the past but was also quite good at. He expressed feelings of hopelessness, frustration, and inferiority. He had a fear of having another seizure in front of his classmates and verbalized concerns about becoming the subject of cruel jokes and gossip.

p0090   Depression was diagnosed, and treatment was initiated with citalopram 20 mg/day together with weekly psychotherapy sessions. The patient had a positive response to the psychiatric intervention with gradual lifting of his depression.

p0100   He has remained seizure-free on valproate monotherapy and has commented that excellent seizure control was important to him in establishing his self-confidence and calming his fears. He is currently completing a doctorate program and is in a committed serious relationship.

s0050   ## COMMENTARY

p0110   Depression is an important concomitant of epilepsy. Community-based studies have reported depression in 20–30% of patients with epilepsy. The importance of diagnosing depression is highlighted when the frequency of suicide in the epileptic population is considered, especially in patients with temporal lobe epilepsy.

p0120   While the definition of depression may be quite obvious, the condition is often underdiagnosed in epileptic patients. Thus, it is important to review the presentation and diagnosis of depression.

p0130   Patients with depression will often present with:

u0010   • feelings of worthlessness, guilt, discouragement, hopelessness, or sadness;
u0020   • significant loss of interest in pleasurable activities;
u0030   • feelings of being overwhelmed by ordinary, everyday situations;
u0040   • insomnia or hypersomnia;
u0050   • anxiety, panic attacks (pseudoseizures), obsessive–compulsive traits, or irritability;
u0060   • abnormal appetite and weight change;
u0070   • sexual dysfunction, and
u0080   • suicidal ideation.

p0220   According to the DSM-IV diagnostic criteria, at least five symptoms (including depressed mood or anhedonia) that significantly interfere with the patient's life need to be present for over 2 weeks in order to establish a diagnosis of major depression.

p0230   Because the etiology of depression is often multifaceted, the treatment approach towards the depressed patient with epilepsy should encompass several factors. Initially, a clinical assessment of the severity of the depression should be made because of the increased risk of suicide. In addition, seizure frequency and type, antiepileptic drug regimen, and psychosocial variables need to be examined. Other medical causes for a depression should be considered, such as structural brain lesions, hypothyroidism, vitamin B12 deficiency, and substance abuse.

Antidepressants should be chosen carefully. Safety, tolerability, efficacy, cost, and simplicity of dosing need to be considered. While tricyclic antidepressants such as amitryptiline and desipramine are relatively inexpensive, side effects such as sedation, memory impairment, constipation, and weight gain are common. Cardiac arrhythmias are of concern at higher doses. Monoamine oxidase inhibitors are problematic in patients with epilepsy. Of the atypical antidepressants, bupropion should be used with caution because of the increased risk of seizures.   p0240

Selective serotonin reuptake inhibitors are generally well tolerated and safe in this setting, as was the case with my patient. Common side effects of the selective serotonin reuptake inhibitors include nausea, sleep disturbance, and sexual dysfunction, although these tend to occur in a small minority of patients.   p0250

Seizure control needs to be optimized. Although loss of seizure control may certainly lead to a depressed state, the reverse is possible as well. A change in sleep patterns or the loss of compliance with the antiepileptic drug regimen may lead to an increase in seizure frequency.   p0260

Psychotherapy is of paramount importance in the management of depressed patients with epilepsy. Psychologists and social workers can be particularly beneficial for helping the patient establish a support system. A reactive depression as a result of discrimination, loss of driving privileges, loss of employment, and unfounded fears can often be managed by psychotherapy alone or by psychotherapy together with patient education.   p0270

What did I learn from this case?   s0060

I was reminded that depression commonly occurs in patients with epilepsy and that it is frequently unrecognized and undertreated. As physicians, we need to encourage our patients to discuss their feelings and troubles openly and we need to respond by diagnosing and treating depression and other mood disorders appropriately.   p0280

How did this case alter my approach to the care and treatment of my epilepsy patients?   s0070

I am careful to inquire about symptoms that could be suggestive of an underlying depression and refer patients for psychiatric consultation and treatment when indicated.   p0290

FURTHER READING

Barraclough B. Suicide and epilepsy. In: Reynolds ER, Trimble MR, eds. *Epilepsy and psychiatry.* Edinburgh: Churchill Livingstone, 1981: 72–6.

Diagnostic and statistical manual of mental disorders, 4th ed., text revision (DSM-IV-TR). Washington DC: American Psychiatric Association, 2000.

Kanner AM, Palac S. Depression in epilepsy: a common but often unrecognized comorbid malady. *Epilepsy Behav* 2000;**1**:37–51.

Mendez MF, Cummings JL, Benson F. Depression in epilepsy: significance and phenomenology. *Arch Neurol* 1986;**43**:766–70.

Robertson MM, Trimble MR. The treatment of depression in patients with epilepsy: a double-blind trial. *J Affect Disord* 1985;**9**:127–36.

Osteomalacia in a Patient Treated with Multiple Anticonvulsants

c0059

Joost PH Drenth, Gerlach FFM Pieters and Ad RMM Hermus

HISTORY

s0010

A 67-year-old farmer was admitted because of suspicion of osteomalacia. His medical history revealed epilepsy caused by cerebral trauma in 1947, an implanted dynamic hip screw for a right femur neck fracture in 1991 and a fracture of the left humerus in 1996.

p0010

He complained of progressive difficulty in walking because of generalized weakness, but he denied bone pain. He had a limited walking span that prevented him from going out but he enjoyed adequate sun exposure. Three weeks before admission he fractured his left femur neck after a fall, necessitating a total hip prosthesis. Further, he had noticed diarrhea after fatty meals but denied any other abdominal symptoms.

p0020

Despite an impressive daily regimen of carbamazepine (600 mg), valproate (2100 mg), phenytoin (250 mg), vigabatrin (100 mg), and acetazolamide (250 mg), the patient experienced repetitive absence seizures.

p0030

EXAMINATION AND INVESTIGATIONS

s0020

When we first saw him in February 1998 the patient had a waddling gait. On admission in March 1998, both hips showed signs of the surgical procedures but muscle atrophy was absent. There was no apparent muscular dysfunction, and neurological testing was normal.

p0040

Laboratory testing revealed reduced serum calcium (1.86 mmol/l) and phosphate (0.77 mmol/l), high alkaline phosphatase (378 U/l), high parathyroid hormone (45 pmol/l, normal below 6.5 pmol/l), and low levels of 25-hydroxy vitamin D_3 (5 nmol/l, normal 25–72.5 nmol/l) and 1,25-dihydroxy vitamin D_3 (37 pmol/l, normal 80–200 pmol/l).

p0050

Lumbar bone mineral density was 3.2 standard deviations below the mean value of a reference group of 30-year-old males (T-score). A bone biopsy specimen demonstrated osteomalacia and signs of secondary hyperparathyroidism. These findings led to a presumptive diagnosis of osteomalacia and secondary hyperparathyroidism due to hypovitaminosis D.

Because dietary intake of vitamin D and calcium in our patient was normal, malabsorption of vitamin D remained as a possibility. We therefore embarked on a search for a cause of malabsorption of vitamin D. Liver disease was absent and a small bowel enema yielded normal results. A biopsy specimen of the proximal jejunum showed only minor atrophy of villi. Antiendomysium and antigliadin antibodies were absent, ruling out a gluten-sensitive enteropathy. A 24-h stool specimen contained 34 g fat (normal below 7.2 g). Skeletal X-rays showed chalky depositions in the pancreas, suggesting that the steatorrhoea could be caused by chronic pancreatitis. This was surprising because our patient had never had significant abdominal symptoms. A specific cause for the chronic pancreatitis was not found.

DIAGNOSES

Osteomalacia due to anticonvulsant therapy and vitamin D deficiency; malabsorption due to chronic pancreatitis with exocrine dysfunction.

TREATMENT AND OUTCOME

The patient was treated with high dosages of vitamin D, calcium and pancreatic enzymes. After 1 year this treatment resulted in complete disappearance of clinical symptoms, increased weight (by 13.5 kg), increased lumbar bone density (T-score of −1.4), and normalization of biochemical parameters (Figure 59.1).

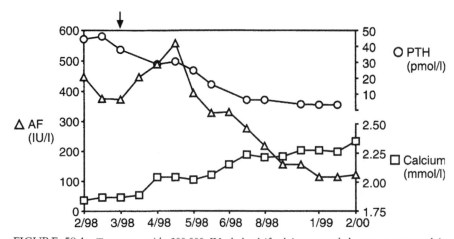

FIGURE 59.1 Treatment with 300,000 IU cholecalciferol intramuscularly was commenced in March 1998 (arrow) and repeated every 6 months. Effects on serum alkaline phosphatase (AF, left axis), serum calcium (right lower axis), and parathyroid hormone concentrations (right upper axis) are shown.

COMMENTARY

s0050

Vitamin D is made available to the body by photogenesis in the skin and by absorption from the intestine. It is hydroxylated in the liver to 25-hydroxy vitamin D_3 and further in the kidney to 1,25-dihydroxy vitamin D_3. Anticonvulsants impair bone metabolism by induction of hepatic microsomal enzymes, resulting in increased catabolism of 25-hydroxy vitamin D_3 and perhaps through inhibition of intestinal transport of calcium. Although clinical and biochemical findings in our patient could be explained by the long-term use of anticonvulsants, osteomalacia is rare in these patients when they are well nourished and normally active. Almost invariably, other factors must be present before the complete clinical picture develops.
p0100

Anticonvulsant-related osteomalacia is an insidious disorder that may lead to considerable morbidity if not detected at an early stage. Our case shows the need for monitoring vitamin D levels in patients using anticonvulsants.
p0110

Supplementation of vitamin D in our patient led to an impressive improvement of clinical symptoms. It reminds us that vitamin D therapy should be considered in patients who are taking multiple antiepileptic drugs and who are at the greatest risk of developing osteomalacia, such as those with malabsorption, as in this case, or reduced sun exposure or poor dietary intake.
p0120

What did we learn from this case?

s0060

We knew that antiepileptic drugs could cause hypovitaminosis D. This case taught us that additional factors such as malabsorption or inadequate sun exposure need to be present for osteomalacia to develop. Because our patient was normally active and his dietary intake of calcium and vitamin D was normal, we suspected an additional factor and searched for other causes. We learnt that a systematic analysis of the metabolic pathway of vitamin D in these cases will be needed in order to yield the eventual diagnosis.
p0130

ACKNOWLEDGEMENT

s0070

Published in and copyright by *The Lancet* 2000;**355**:1882. Adapted and reprinted here with permission.
p0140

FURTHER READING

Hahn TJ. Drug-induced disorders of vitamin D and mineral metabolism. *Clin Endocrinol Metab* 1980;**9**:107–29.

Hahn TJ, Birge SJ, Scharp CR, Avioli LV. Phenobarbital-induced alteration in vitamin D metabolism. *J Clin Invest* 1972;**51**:741–8.

Shafer RB, Buttall FQ. Calcium and folic acid absorption in patients taking anticonvulsant drugs. *J Clin Endocrinol Metab* 1975;**41**:1125–9.

Francis RM, Selby PL. Osteomalacia. *Baillieres Clin Endocrinol Metab* 1997;**11**:145–63.

c0060

Parkinsonism and Cognitive Decline in a 64-Year-Old Woman with Epilepsy

Manuel Eglau, Peter Hopp and Hermann Stefan

s0010

HISTORY

p0010

A 64-year-old woman with symptomatic epilepsy caused by perinatal brain damage was admitted to the hospital because of progressive deterioration of her general health over the preceding 2 weeks, intermittent clouding of consciousness, dizziness, and nausea. Parkinsonism had been diagnosed recently on the basis of tremor and motor slowing. Current complaints were constant whole body tremor and a mostly frontal headache.

p0020

Her seizures, which were complex partial and secondary generalized tonic–clonic, had been well controlled over the years with valproate 3000 mg/day and lamotrigine 200 mg/day, a regimen that the patient had tolerated well until 2 weeks before admission. No apparent cause for her deterioration, such as infection or dehydration, was found.

s0020

EXAMINATION AND INVESTIGATIONS

p0030

On neurological examination, the patient was awake but disoriented. Her psychomotor performance was impaired. A remarkable resting tremor of the whole body was found, as well as increased muscle tone and impaired motor coordination with bilateral bradykinesia and severe limb ataxia. Standing or walking was impossible. The other neurological and general physical findings were normal.

p0040

The initial EEG revealed background slowing in the theta range with bilaterally synchronous high-voltage slow wave activity. No epileptiform activity was recorded.

p0050

Laboratory studies showed elevated levels of blood urea nitrogen (35 mg/dl, normal range 8–20 mg/dl) and ammonia (123 μg/dl, normal range 19–82 μg/dl). The serum concentration of valproate was 134.6 mg/l (normal range 50–100 mg/l), and of lamotrigine was 19.9 mg/l. No other abnormalities were found, including on liver function tests. An abdominal ultrasound was normal except for liver steatosis.

DIAGNOSIS

Valproate-induced encephalopathy.

TREATMENT AND OUTCOME

As the valproate dose was reduced, her physical and cognitive condition improved significantly. Valproate was then completely withdrawn, resulting in complete remission of both the cognitive impairment and the parkinsonian syndrome. Subsequently, the EEG showed normalization of the background activity and resolution of the generalized epileptiform activity.

COMMENTARY

What did we learn from this case?

First, we learned that although valproate may be well tolerated over many years, changes in alertness, disorientation, a worsened general health condition, and impairment of motor coordination can occur without any obvious underlying cause as manifestations of valproate-induced encephalopathy.

In addition, this case shows that treatment with valproate may cause a syndrome that imitates Parkinson's disease. The insidious onset of valproate-associated movement disorder – after months or years of otherwise well-tolerated treatment with valproate – increases the probability that these symptoms may be mistaken for a neurodegenerative disease.[1,2,4]

In this case, clinical symptoms, hyperammonemia and EEG findings led to the diagnosis of valproate-induced encephalopathy. It should be noted that the serum valproate concentration was only moderately elevated above the therapeutic range. This observation is consistent with several reports that valproate-induced parkinsonism is independent of valproate serum concentrations.[3]

Different pathophysiological mechanisms underlying valproate encephalopathy have been proposed.[4] A crucial factor seems to be hyperammonemia, which interferes with excitatory and inhibitory neurotransmission and causes deficits in cerebral energy metabolism. Consequently, ammonia concentrations should be measured in cases of suspected valproate encephalopathy.

REFERENCES

1. Armon C, Shin C, Miller P, et al. Reversible Parkinsonism and cognitive impairment with chronic valproate use. Neurology 1996;**47**:626–35.
2. Nouzeilles M, Garcia M, Rabinovicz A, Merello M. Prospective evaluation of Parkinsonism and tremor in patients treated with valproate. Parkinsonism Rel Disord 1999;**5**:67–8.
3. Butterworth RF. Effects of hyperammonaemia on brain function. J Inherit Metab Dis 1998;**21(suppl 1)**:6–20.
4. Göbel R, Görtzen A, Bräunig P. Enzephalopathien durch Valproat. Fortschr Neurol Psychiatr 1999;**67**:7–11.

FURTHER READING

Onofrj M, Thomas A, Paci C. Reversible Parkinsonism induced by prolonged treatment with valproate. *J Neurol* 1998;**245**:794–6.

Problems in Managing Epilepsy during and after Pregnancy

Cynthia L Harden

HISTORY

A 30-year-old woman had a history of epilepsy since the age of 13. Her epilepsy began with myoclonic jerks of the hands and arms, occasionally associated with falling down. She also developed brief staring spells associated with thought interruptions, and she had extremely rare convulsions.

She underwent trials of valproate, carbamazepine, ethosuximide, and phenytoin, but had difficulty with side effects from each medicine.

At the age of 17, she was diagnosed with pseudoseizures after seeking a second opinion. Consequently, she was taken off antiseizure medicines and continued to have myoclonus, with menstrual exacerbations. After having an escalation of myoclonus associated with falls at the age of 23, just before her marriage, she was restarted on valproate on the assumption that her seizures were epileptic, and she tolerated the sprinkle formulation. She then had complete resolution of all seizures types after a slow increase of the dose to 875 mg/day.

Past medical history was negative. There was no history of febrile seizures, head trauma, or brain infection, and there was no family history of epilepsy.

EXAMINATION AND INVESTIGATIONS

The patient's general and neurological examinations were unremarkable. A brain magnetic resonance imaging scan was normal and an EEG on medication was normal. Her valproate level was 62 mg/l. A muscle biopsy was negative for ragged red fibers.

DIAGNOSIS

Juvenile myoclonic epilepsy.

TREATMENT AND OUTCOME

p0070   The patient wanted very much to get pregnant, but had a history of prolonged menstrual cycles of 39–40 days since the onset of menarche at the age of 12. She noted no change in her menses when she began taking valproate regularly, but she was told by her gynecologist that she was likely having anovulatory cycles. She was currently taking folate 4 mg/day. There was no family history of birth defects, including spina bifida.

p0080   The patient became pregnant while taking valproate at 875 mg/day and folate. At 16 weeks' gestation, fetal ultrasound showed evidence of spina bifida, cleft palate, and hydrocephalus. The pregnancy was terminated. Consultation with a geneticist about the outcome of the pregnancy was obtained, with the opinion that perhaps not all of the fetal malformations could be attributed to valproate. Both parents were Hispanic of Jewish heritage.

p0090   The patient wanted to become pregnant again but insisted on not taking any medicine to prevent seizures this time. She continued a high-folate diet and also took a prenatal vitamin preparation plus an additional 3 mg/day of folate (with her prenatal vitamin preparation she would be getting 4 mg), since it was thought that a genetic component was present in the outcome of the first pregnancy. However, she noted that now that she was off valproate, taking the extra folate seemed to produce myoclonic jerks and she gradually tapered off the folate with resolution of the myoclonus. She gradually developed increasing myoclonus as the pregnancy advanced, but she did not take antiepileptic drugs. A normal girl was delivered at term.

p0100   Postnatally, she was restarted on valproate, but she had continued myoclonus with doses up to 1750 mg/day and she had two generalized convulsions associated with exhaustion. She is currently stable with the addition of topiramate 200 mg/day and clonazepam 0.25 mg/day. Valproate has been reduced to 750 mg/day.

COMMENTARY

p0110   This case illustrates many of the difficulties in managing women of reproductive potential with epilepsy. The American Academy of Neurology guidelines for the management of women with epilepsy state that women should be maintained on the antiepileptic drug that best controls seizures,[1] given the low risk of fetal malformations with exposure to antiepileptic drugs and the lack of clear-cut safety or superiority of any single antiepileptic drug in this setting, combined with the risk of seizures to the fetus during pregnancy. The fetus in this case developed abnormally in the presence of valproate, although the patient was taking a low dose, which decreases the risk of fetal malformations.[1,2] The case was further compounded by the question raised of an independent genetic component producing the abnormal fetal outcome.

p0120   This patient was taking a higher dose of folate than is generally advocated by epileptologists, yet this did not prevent spina bifida. Paradoxically, when she was not taking valproate, the high-dose folate seemed to exacerbate her myoclonic seizures. There is some evidence in animals and in a few clinical studies that high doses of folate may be epileptogenic. Intracerebral injections of folate have produced myoclonus in chronically implanted, nonepileptic rats.[3] A study of eight patients with epilepsy and low initial folate levels found that injection of very high doses of folate (7–20 mg) produced seizures and EEG activation in six of the patients.[4] In another study of 15 schizophrenic patients with comorbid epilepsy, folate administration improved mood and decreased aggressiveness, but was associated with an increase in seizures in three of the patients and increased EEG epileptiform activity in six of the patients.[5] As suggested in one case report, an altered blood–brain barrier may be a factor in increasing the risk of seizures in a patient with epilepsy taking supplemental folate.[6]

Finally, after the pregnancy, the formerly effective treatment regimen was no longer nearly as effective, and this may be at least in part due to situational factors, such as sleep deprivation and increased stress.

What did I learn from this case?

It was reinforced to me that even low doses of valproate can be associated with birth defects. I did not expect it in this case because of the low dose of valproate used together with the high dose of folate.

Furthermore, I realized that resuming medication after a medication-free pregnancy (during which many seizures occurred) may not produce the same stellar results it had before the pregnancy, for reasons that are probably complex but that must include situational factors.

Finally, I learned that my patient's reliable reports of increased seizures with high-dose folate may be supported by existing literature.

How did this case alter my approach to the care and treatment of my epilepsy patients?

I am more careful now to assess seizure frequency when using more than 1 mg/day of folate, and I realize that the "right" dose for women with epilepsy is unclear at this time. I also feel more cautious about reassuring patients that resuming medications after a prolonged medication-free period, particularly if seizures have occurred during the medication hiatus, can once again produce seizure control. Although situational factors were probably present in this case, I am nagged by the possibility that this patient's seizures during pregnancy may have been epileptogenic in origin.

REFERENCES

1. Report of the Quality Standards Subcommittee of the American Academy of Neurology. Practice parameter: management issues for women with epilepsy (summary statement). *Neurology* 1998;**51**:944–8.
2. Omtzigt JG, Nau H, Los FJ, Lindhout D. The disposition of valproate and its metabolites in the late first trimester and early second trimester of pregnancy in maternal serum, urine, and amniotic fluid: effect of dose, co-medication, and the presence of spina bifida. *Eur J Clin Pharmacol* 1992;**43**:381–8.
3. Tremblay E, Berger M, Nitecka L, Cavalheiro E, Ben-Ari Y. A multidisciplinary study of folic acid neurotoxicity: interactions with kainate binding sites and relevance to the aetiology of epilepsy. *Neuroscience* 1984;**12**:569–89.

4. Ch'ien LT, Krumdieck CL, Scott CW Jr, Butterworth CE Jr. Harmful effect of megadoses of vitamins: electroencephalogram abnormalities and seizures induced by intravenous folate in drug-treated epileptics. *Am J Clin Nutr* 1975;**28**:51–8.
5. Ueda S, Shirakawa T, Nakazawa Y, Inanaga K. Epilepsy and folic acid. *Folia Psychiatr Neurol Jpn* 1977;**31**:327–37.
6. Eros E, Geher P, Gomor B, Czeizel AE. Epileptogenic activity of folic acid after drug induced SLE. *Eur J Ostet Gynecol Reprod Biol* 1998;**80**:75–8.

Status Epilepticus in a Heavy Snorer

Peter Höllinger, Christian W Hess and Claudio Bassetti

HISTORY

A 50-year-old railwayman suffered from idiopathic absence seizures until the age of 16 years and had been seizure-free without antiepileptic treatment since then. Hypothyroidism and arterial hypertension were adequately treated. He was a heavy, habitual snorer. His wife witnessed nocturnal apneas and he reported excessive daytime sleepiness (e.g. falling asleep when watching television or when traveling in the train, or in the car as a passenger). One day after lunch he was tired and nervous and shortly thereafter had three generalized tonic–clonic seizures in succession, corresponding to tonic–clonic status epilepticus. The patient was treated with intravenous benzodiazepines, phenytoin, and muscle relaxation, followed by intubation. He was transferred to our department.

EXAMINATION AND INVESTIGATIONS

On admission the patient was intubated and unconscious as a result of the sedatives and relaxants. His body mass index was 42.5, indicating that he was massively overweight. There were no focal neurological deficits, and a computed tomography scan of the brain was normal.

The patient became seizure-free after intubation and muscle relaxation and he was able to be extubated the next day. An EEG performed 1 day after the status epilepticus showed a mild slowing of the background activity (around 8 Hz) but was otherwise normal. An EEG performed 2 days after the status epilepticus was completely normal. A magnetic resonance imaging scan of the brain and a lumbar puncture also revealed normal results.

The Epworth Sleepiness Score estimated for the 3 months before the status epilepticus was abnormal, with 19 points (a normal score being less than 10); this was consistent with the history of excessive daytime sleepiness.

Polysomnography performed 9 days after admission showed severe obstructive sleep apnea with an apnea–hypopnea index of 74 (a normal index being less than 10) and 53 oxygen desaturations per hour (normal being less than 3) (Figure 62.1).

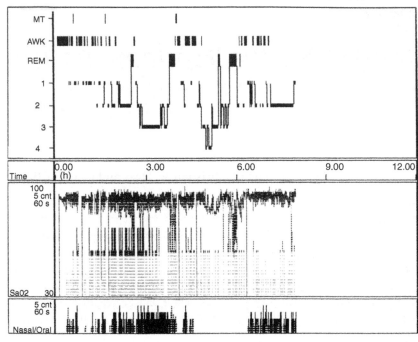

f0010
FIGURE 62.1   Tests performed 9 days after admission. The patient's hypnogram (top) (MT, movement time; AWK, awake). Oxygen saturation (middle). The occurrence of apneas and hypopneas (bottom).

The mean oxygen level during desaturations was 83, and the minimal oxygen desaturation level was 68%. Sleep latency was 21 min, total sleep time was 357 min, rapid eye movement (REM) latency was 123 min, stage transitions numbered 144 and sleep efficiency was 74%. Stage 1 sleep accounted for 18% of the sleep period, stage 2 for 24%, REM sleep for 8%, and slow wave sleep for 18%.

s0030

DIAGNOSIS

p0060
Generalized idiopathic epilepsy with status epilepticus and obstructive sleep apnea.

s0040

TREATMENT AND OUTCOME

p0070
Treatment with nocturnal continuous positive airway pressure (CPAP) was initiated, with good compliance. Owing to the history of absence seizures in childhood, the phenytoin was replaced with valproate, which, however, had to be discontinued because of severe generalized exanthema. Carbamazepine was not tolerated either (again because of generalized exanthema). Finally, phenylbarbital (phenobarbital) was tried and found to be well tolerated.

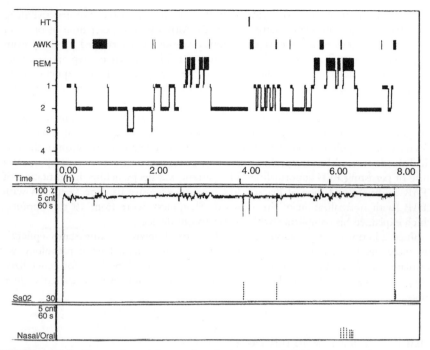

FIGURE 62.2   Tests performed 1 year after the initiation of CPAP treatment. The hypnogram (top) is much less fragmented than the earlier test and there is more REM sleep. There are no episodes of oxygen desaturation (middle). There are no episodes of apnea or hypopnea.

f0020

In the absence of clinical seizures, EEGs 4 and 9 months later showed frequent generalized epileptiform activity in the form of spike–wave bursts without clinical correlates, occurring approximately every 6 min.

A control polysomnography performed 1 year after the initiation of CPAP treatment showed normal findings with an apnea–hypopnea index of less than 1, and 0.3 oxygen desaturations an hour (Figure 62.2). Sleep latency was 6 min, total sleep time was 384 min, REM latency was 155 min, stage transitions numbered 78, and sleep efficiency was 85%. Stage 1 sleep accounted for 20% of the sleep period, stage 2 for 52%, REM sleep for 14%, and slow wave sleep for 2%.

The Epworth Sleepiness Score had normalized to five points and the multiple sleep latency test was also normal, with a mean sleep latency of 12.5 min (normal being less than 10 min).

Two years after the status epilepticus, the patient remains seizure-free on 300 mg phenylbarbital (phenobarbital), works to full capacity, and is highly satisfied with his CPAP treatment.

COMMENTARY

Why did we choose this case?

This patient's history highlights one possible pathogenic interaction between obstructive sleep apnea and epilepsy. We hypothesize that this patient's childhood epilepsy remained asymptomatic for many years until the detrimental effect of obstructive sleep apnea triggered an episode of status epilepticus. Although the exact time of onset of signs and symptoms of obstructive sleep apnea cannot be determined precisely from the patient's history, he clearly exhibited symptoms of obstructive sleep apnea (snoring, apneas, and sleepiness) for a few months before the episode of status epilepticus. In addition he was massively overweight, which is a well-known risk factor for obstructive sleep apnea.

Furthermore, the patient remained clinically seizure-free after treatment with antiepileptic drugs and CPAP, despite the persistence on EEG of generalized spike–wave activity. Control polysomnography demonstrated a complete normalization of the initial sleep disordered breathing, thus excluding persistent obstructive sleep apnea as a cause of persisting EEG abnormalities. The patient was sleepy before the initiation of CPAP treatment and showed marked lessening of excessive daytime sleepiness with CPAP (with normalization of the Epworth Sleepiness Score from 19 to 5 points), which explained his compliance with the treatment device.

Since additional investigations excluded factors known to cause status epilepticus, including for example fever or inflammatory or structural brain pathology, we postulate that status epilepticus arose from an idiopathic predisposition for generalized epilepsy (as manifested by childhood absence seizures) and severe obstructive sleep apnea.

What did we learn from this case?

In patients with a hitherto well-controlled seizure disorder and recently increasing seizure frequency, new onset of epileptic seizures, or status epilepticus, it is obviously important to exclude such causes as degenerative, structural or inflammatory brain disease, or poor compliance to drug treatment. In the absence of such factors, one should also ask about symptoms of obstructive sleep apnea such as snoring, observed apneas, and excessive daytime sleepiness. Fatigue or sleepiness in patients under antiepileptic drug treatment should not automatically be attributed to the drug, since a treatable sleep disorder, including obstructive sleep apnea, might underlie this specific complaint.[1] In the presence of obstructive sleep apnea, CPAP treatment should be considered, although at best 80% of patients in larger series may be compliant with this treatment.[2] Poor compliance is especially likely in patients who do not report excessive subjective daytime sleepiness.

Our group has shown that the frequency of epilepsy and obstructive sleep apnea is higher than what could be estimated by pure coincidence, suggesting a specific pathogenic link. Obstructive sleep apnea induces sleep fragmentation caused by recurrent arousals and thus leads to sleep deprivation, which is well known to precipitate epileptic seizures.

Obviously, obstructive sleep apnea represents only one of several potential pathogenic mechanisms in the etiology of seizures. Hence, despite optimal treatment with CPAP, seizures may persist. The effect of CPAP treatment on seizure frequency in a single patient may be difficult to estimate considering the fact that most patients already receive antiepileptic drug treatment and that CPAP is prescribed only as an adjunctive treatment. Prospective studies with larger samples of patients with obstructive sleep apnea and epilepsy are needed.

REFERENCES

1. Malow BA, Fromes GA, Aldrich MS. Usefulness of polysomnography in epilepsy patients. *Neurology* 1997;**48**:1389–94.
2. Strollo PJ, Rogers RM. Obstructive sleep apnea. *N Engl J Med* 1996;**334**:99–104.

FURTHER READING

Höllinger P, Bassetti C, Gugger M, Hess CW. Epilepsy and obstructive sleep apnea. *Neurology* 2000;**54(suppl 3)**:A27.

c0063

A Boy with Epilepsy and Allergic Rhinitis

Kazuie Iinuma and Hiroyuki Yokoyama

s0010

HISTORY

p0010
A five-year-old boy with partial epilepsy and allergic rhinitis was hospitalized for optimal seizure control. Eventually, combined antiepileptic treatment with valproate 400 mg/day, zonisamide 80 mg/day, and clonazepam 0.8 mg/day resulted in complete seizure control.

p0020
About 6 months later, he was given ketotifen 1.0 mg/day for treatment of allergic rhinitis. A few days later, he started having partial seizures, with or without loss of consciousness, two or three times a day. According to his mother, his seizures had previously been aggravated by ketotifen when it has been prescribed by a local doctor during the spring and autumn.

p0030
Thereafter, ketotifen was replaced with terfenadine 60 mg/day. After the switch from ketotifen to terfenadine, the patient regained excellent seizure control. There was no obvious change in the serum concentrations of his anticonvulsant medications when the allergy medication was changed.

s0020

EXAMINATION AND INVESTIGATIONS

p0040
We examined the effect of intravenous D-chlorpheniramine, a centrally acting histamine H_1 antagonist, on the patient's EEG after signed informed consent was obtained from his parents. The occurrence of spikes was calculated before and after administration of D-chlorpheniramine to evaluate its effect on seizure susceptibility.

p0050
The administration of D-chlorpheniramine significantly increased the number of spikes compared with those observed before treatment (Figure 63.1). Figure 63.2 shows an increase of spikes on the EEG after D-chlorpheniramine administration.

s0030

DIAGNOSIS

p0060
Partial epilepsy with seizure exacerbation by ketotifen, an antihistaminic agent.

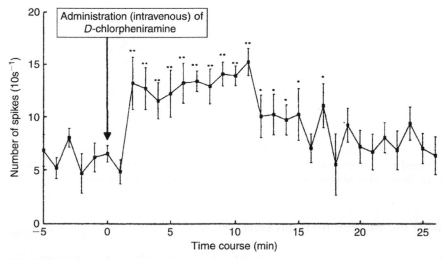

FIGURE 63.1   EEG activation by *D*-chlorpheniramine. Spikes were measured over a 10-sec period, and averaged during 1 min before and after the administration of intravenous *D*-chlorpheniramine. Administration of *D*-chlorpheniramine significantly increased the number of spikes, compared to pre-treatment. Significant differences: $^*p < 0.05$, $^{**}p < 0.01$ versus the number of spikes before the administration, as determined by ANOVA followed by Duncan's test.

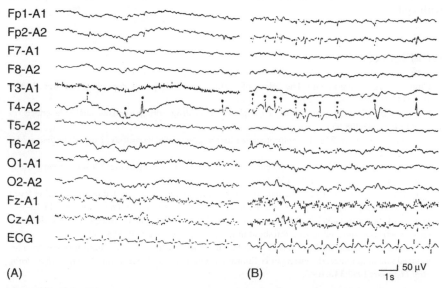

FIGURE 63.2   Sample EEG before (A) and after (B) the administration of *D*-chlorpheniramine.

TREATMENT AND OUTCOME

After switching from ketotifen to terfenadine, the patient was seizure-free for 8 years. His antiepileptic drugs were then gradually reduced and discontinued.

COMMENTARY

p0080   According to the literature, histamine H_1 antagonists occasionally produce convulsions in healthy children, especially pre-school age children.[1-4] The antihistamines are commonly used in patients with allergic disorders, including patients with epilepsy.

p0090   Our patient lost optimal seizure control during treatment with ketotifen; epileptic discharges markedly increased after loading with D-chlorpheniramine, a histamine H_1 antagonist; however, terfenadine, one of the new generation antihistamines with little penetration into brain, did not exacerbate seizures in this patient. These observations strongly support the contention that his seizure exacerbation was due to ketotifen and was probably the result of the blockade of central histamine H_1 receptors. Experiments have shown an inhibitory effect of histamine in a variety of seizure models.[5-7]

s0060   **What did we learn from this case?**

p0100   First, we learned that histamine H_1 receptor antagonists might aggravate seizures.

p0110   Secondly, we observed that terfenadine did not exacerbate the patient's seizures, possibly because of minimal brain penetration.

p0120   Thirdly, we discovered that EEG monitoring during D-chlorpheniramine administration could be used to examine the susceptibility of particular patients with epilepsy to antihistamines. We now believe that this class of drugs should be avoided in patients with epilepsy.

REFERENCES

1. Churchill JA, Gammon GD. The effect of antihistaminic drugs on convulsive seizures. *JAMA* 1949;**141**:18–21.
2. Mueller MD. Phenylpropanolamine, a nonprescription drug with potentially fatal side effects. *N Engl J Med* 1983;**308**:653.
3. Bernstein E, Diskant BM. Phenylpropanolamine: a potentially hazardous drug. *Ann Emerg Med* 1982;**11**:311–5.
4. Schwartz JF, Patterson JH. Toxic encephalopathy related to antihistamine–barbiturate antiemetic medication. *Am J Dis Child* 1978;**132**:37–9.
5. Onodera K, Tuomisto L, Tacke U, Airaksinen M. Strain differences in regional brain histamine levels between genetically epilepsy-prone and resistant rats. *Meth Find Exp Clin Pharmacol* 1992;**14**:13–6.
6. Freeman P, Sturman G, Wilde P. Elevation of histamine levels but not H2-receptor blockade influences electrically-induced seizure threshold in mice. *J Psychopharmacol* 1990;**4**:313.
7. Yokoyama H, Onodera K, Maeyama K, *et al.* Histamne levels and clonic convulsions of electrically-induced seizures in mice: the effects of α-fluoromethylhistidine and metoprine. *Naunyn-Schmiedeberg Arch Pharmacol* 1992;**346**:40–5.

Seizures and Behavior Disturbance in a Boy

Sookyong Koh

HISTORY

The patient is a 12–year-old, right-handed, sixth-grade boy with complex partial seizures, oppositional defiant disorder, attention deficit hyperactivity disorder, depression, psychosis, and a non-enhancing lesion in the left medial temporal lobe.

He initially presented at 4 years of age with 6 h of unresponsiveness and decreased respiratory effort that required intubation. The head computed tomography (CT) scan was normal. Two years later, he returned because of monthly episodes of forceful swallowing, staring, and fidgeting with his hands followed by a period of disorientation. With these spells, which lasted "a couple of minutes," he would talk rapidly and incoherently with slurred and garbled speech about things that did not apply to the current situation such as "the cat is in the refrigerator." At times, he would not recognize his mother and would respond to his mother, placing her hand on his back, by saying, "that's a policeman's hand." His sister once asked him "Are you all right?" and he responded, "I will be if you wake me up."

He also described visual changes associated with the spells. For example, while looking at a chair it might become a table, a table might become a television, and so on. He described apparent auras consisting of a feeling of "weirdness" or "fuzziness in my head." Besides reporting "sometimes I find myself in a different place than when I started", he had been found lying next to his bicycle, his bed and his school desk, apparently after falls.

In addition to his typical complex partial seizures with rare generalization, he experienced multiple daily episodes of "floaty feelings," during which he felt "fuzzy" and "floaty" as if in a cloud. He also complained of "dead feelings," when he became limp and unable to move his limbs. He described "room seizures," when he did not know where he was, thought he was in a room where he had previously been and felt he was going back in time.

He also experienced severe headaches that were "caused by balls permeating from my head rolling down my face." During these headaches, he clutched his head, screamed with pain, and became completely limp and unresponsive for a brief period. After these headaches he would vomit. Once, after four successive episodes, he described vivid visual hallucinations, such as seeing his dead aunt or seeing evil and good fighting on the wall.

p0060   He related a story about his imaginary friends Shelly, who is good, and Philip, who is bad. Philip has been with him almost constantly and interfered with his everyday activities since he was 5 years old. Philip tells him to punch himself at times, and it was Philip who also told him to swallow broken glass (which he had done). It was Philip, too, who caused "floaty feelings" and "dead feelings." Gabapentin made Philip more visible whereas methylphenidate "fights off Philip and makes Philip calm." He referred to valproate as a "shield" against Philip and carbamazepine as a "sword."

p0070   The patient was maintained on high therapeutic doses of both carbamazepine and valproate. He had been on carbamazepine monotherapy for the first 2 years after diagnosis. Gabapentin was tried for 3 months before being discontinued because of worsening "dead feelings." He has had a fluctuating response to his antiepileptic drugs – at best, one or two seizures a month, at worst, three seizures a week with multiple daily episodes of "floaty feelings."

p0080   Over the years, he has had escalating behavioral dyscontrol, leading to many crises at school and home, fist fights, confrontation with teachers and threats of expulsion. He had tried to hurt himself by swallowing shards of glass and overdosing on his anticonvulsants. He has reported feeling very, very sad and helpless. He has been treated by a psychiatrist with methylphenidate and haloperidol.

s0020   ## EXAMINATION AND INVESTIGATIONS

p0090   The patient was admitted to the hospital for presurgical evaluation with video–EEG monitoring. On the admission examination, he presented with "I am a dickweed" written across his abdomen. He was talkative and inattentive. He had difficulty reciting a short story from memory and wrote, with poor penmanship, "this season seems like an endless conclusion compared to our winter it seems an illusion". There was posturing of the right hand on stressed gait and clumsy rapid alternating movements. While his antiepileptic drugs were withheld over the ensuing few days, he became increasingly agitated, ripped his telemetry wires off his head, jumped over the bed and ran out of the room. The outburst escalated and finally necessitated four-point leather restraints, as well as the administration of diazepam, chloral hydrate, and lorazepam.

p0100   The interictal EEG showed focal sharp waves and continuous slowing over the left mid to anterior temporal lobe. His "floaty feelings" were without concomitant EEG correlate.

p0110   A head magnetic resonance imaging (MRI) scan showed a non-enhancing T2-weighted hyperintense lesion that involved the entire anterior tip and undersurface of the left temporal lobe and extended posteriorly to involve the medial portion. The lesion measured approximately 4 cm by 2.5 cm by 3 cm and had not changed in appearance or size on yearly head MRIs over a 6-year period.

p0120   Neuropsychological testing showed a large discrepancy between verbal IQ (120) and performance IQ (79).

s0030   ## DIAGNOSIS, TREATMENT, AND OUTCOME

p0130   The patient underwent left temporal lobe lesionectomy under the guidance of intraoperative electrocorticography at the age of 12½ years after the initial presentation of partial seizures. Pathology revealed a hamartoma.

After the operation, the patient suffered no neurological deficit, but rather could recall remote childhood memories. He is not only free of seizures, but also free of psychosis. The patient continues on valproate, carbamazepine, and methylphenidate for continued aggression and "mood swings," and he attends a residential school for behavioral modification. He remains seizure-free on last follow-up, nearly 3 years after the surgery.

COMMENTARY

Neuropsychiatric consequences of poorly controlled temporal lobe epilepsy can be truly devastating. This is particularly evident for seizures that begin in childhood. In one study, nearly one-quarter of the 100 children with temporal lobe seizures followed to adulthood had IQs of less than 70; only 15 of all these children were recorded as showing no form of personality difficulty at any time; 26 suffered from the hyperkinetic syndrome; 36 exhibited catastrophic rage, and 9 developed schizophreniform psychosis.[1]

This case illustrates the central focus of many patients with epilepsy and of their families – behavioral difficulties. Behavioral problems, once the seizure disorder has become less psychologically dramatic to people in the child's environment, are often considered by the parents and teachers as more difficult to cope with than the epilepsy itself.[2] In addition, a study on long-term prognosis of seizures with onset in childhood[3] reports the startling finding of significantly increased risk of death in patients with epilepsy, especially in those whose seizures were not in remission. Patients with epilepsy since childhood were also more likely to remain unmarried, unemployed, and childless.

What did I learn from this case?

I often wondered, together with the patient's family, what would have happened if the surgery was performed earlier. Could we have prevented this child's school failure, psychosis, depression, suicidal attempts, and behavioral deterioration, as well as his seizures, if the surgery had been performed at the time of his initial presentation? What if, at age 4, a head MRI had been done instead of a CT scan and the hamartoma had been detected and then removed? Early surgery in my patient may not only have stopped the seizures but may also have prevented further brain injury from the seizures and the side effects of the antiepileptic drugs. Removal of the abnormal tissue might have spared the patient and his family 6 years of ordeal and allowed the remainder of his developing brain to be free of the undesirable influences of the abnormal epileptic tissue.[4]

How did this case alter my approach to the care and treatment of my epilepsy patients?

Surgery for intractable, catastrophic seizures in young children has become more established in recent years. This case impressed me that treatment of seizures, especially for the developing brain, should be "decisive and prompt."[5] I now consider early surgery under the appropriate circumstances.

REFERENCES

1. Lindsay J, Ounsted C, Richards P. Long-term outcome in children with temporal lobe seizures: 3. Psychiatric aspects in childhood and adult life. *Dev Med Child Neurol* 1979;**21**:630–6.
2. Gillberg C. Psychiatric and behavioral problems in epilepsy, hydrocephalus and cerebral palsy. In: Aicardi J, ed. *Diseases of the nervous system in childhood (Clinics in Developmental Medicine No 115–118)*. London: Mac Keith Press, 1992.
3. Sillanpää M, Jalava M, Kaleva O, Shinnar S. Long-term prognosis of seizures with onset in childhood. *N Engl J Med* 1998;**338**:1715–22.
4. Holmes GL. Surgery for intractable seizures in infancy and early childhood. *Neurology* 1993;**43(suppl 5)**:S28–S37.
5. Moshe SL. Intractable seizures in infancy and early childhood. *Neurology* 1993;**43(suppl 5)**:S2.

Abulia in a Seizure-Free Patient with Frontal Lobe Epilepsy

Ennapadam S Krishnamoorthy and Michael R Trimble

HISTORY

A 32-year-old medically retired civil servant was referred to our clinic by his general practitioner. He had a history of epilepsy from the age of 16 years, and 3 years earlier, on referral to a university hospital, he had been correctly diagnosed with frontal lobe epilepsy. Neuroimaging studies had shown right frontal pathology. Therapy with topiramate had been instituted, which led to complete cessation of seizures. However, over the 18-month period between then and his consultation with us, he had developed a very prominent lack of motivation, though he remained seizure-free. This was diagnosed as depression and treated with fluoxetine for 18 months with little effect. In addition there was a complaint of erectile dysfunction and impaired ejaculation that appeared to predate these complaints.

While waiting to be seen in our clinic his clinical condition worsened significantly. He became profoundly withdrawn, stopped taking care of himself, did not eat for days on end, had not opened his mail, and had not washed for a considerable time. While he was somewhat depressed, the most prominent feature was his profound lack of will to engage in goal-directed behavior (abulia). Unlike people with depression that is severe enough to result in significant self-neglect, he did not have mood-congruent delusions or hallucinations, nor did he entertain nihilistic or suicidal ideas.

His general practitioner replaced fluoxetine with reboxetine, and his family intervened and took care of him. He was also seen by a local psychiatrist, who documented these developments, and by the uroneurologist in our hospital, who recommended sildenafil for the erectile dysfunction.

With the institution of reboxetine, and perhaps the use of sildenafil (on one occasion), his seizure control was destabilized and he developed a flurry of seizures. Nonetheless, his motivation improved, he began to engage in purposeful goal-directed behavior, his appetite became better, and he began to gain weight. Although there was no change in his mood and he remained somewhat miserable, his clinical state improved markedly and his abulia ceased.

s0020

EXAMINATION

p0050

When examined in the clinic, the patient was somewhat anxious and he reported long-standing low self-esteem. He attributed his low self-esteem, as well as his sexual dysfunction, to epilepsy. There were no psychotic features or major depressive ideation. He did, however, give a good account of the very prominent syndrome characterized by lack of motivation that he had suffered from, in the absence of seizures, while on treatment with topiramate, and which had remitted when his seizures returned.

s0030

DIAGNOSIS

p0060

Alternative psychosis in a patient with frontal lobe epilepsy presenting as a frontal lobe syndrome characterized by abulia.

s0040

TREATMENT AND OUTCOME

p0070

Because the patient's symptoms had remitted with the reemergence of seizures, it was recommended that the dose of anticonvulsant drugs should be titrated to allow the occasional breakthrough seizure. The patient was referred to a sexual dysfunction clinic. When last reviewed in our clinic, his improvement with regard to abulia was maintained and he continued to have the occasional seizure.

s0050

COMMENTARY

p0080

This case clearly illustrates the complex relationships between epilepsy and psychiatric disorders, ranging from the more common and better-accepted agonistic relationship, to the less common and often hotly debated antagonistic relationship – the forced normalization of Landolt[1] and the alternative psychoses of Tellenbach.[2]

p0090

This case also shows that distinct, possibly localization-related, neuropsychiatric syndromes do exist in epilepsy and are often mistaken for common psychiatric disorders such as depression.

p0100

Furthermore, this case aptly demonstrates the significance of the disability that sometimes results from anticonvulsant-induced neuropsychiatric disorders, which may arise, paradoxically, as a consequence of seizure control.

s0060

What did we learn from this case?

p0110

This case taught us several important lessons.

p0120

First, it is automatically assumed that good seizure control is the panacea for all the patient's ills. While this is certainly true for the vast majority of patients, there is a distinct subset of patients in whom we see an antagonistic relationship between seizure control and mental health. We learned from this case that it may be better for some patients to have the occasional seizure, rather than aggressively pursuing the ideal of complete seizure control. As Landolt somewhat crudely put it: "It appears that there are some patients with epilepsy who need to have seizures in order to be mentally sane."[3]

Secondly, a number of people fail to recognize the distinct behavioral syndromes that accompany neurological and neuropsychiatric disorders. Abulia, the inability to engage in goal-directed behavior, is one such syndrome, commonly seen with lesions of the basal ganglia and frontal lobes.[4] According to experts that we have surveyed, the syndrome does have some very distinct characteristics, such as difficulty in initiating and sustaining purposeful actions, reduced social interactions and reduced interest in usual pastimes, reduced emotional responsiveness and spontaneity, and reduced spontaneous speech and movement.[5] Abulia is often mistaken for depression and treated as such. In this case, treatment with antidepressant drugs was beneficial in that it destabilized the patient's seizure control, leading to remission of the abulia.

Thirdly, even those clinicians who acknowledge the existence of the antagonistic relationship between epilepsy and psychiatric disorders often believe that the only presentation of the psychiatric disorders is with psychotic symptoms. This could not be further from the truth. The alternative psychoses, often accompanied by forced normalization of the EEG, are a spectrum of disorders that range from traditional psychosis to affective disorder, anxiety disorder and even non-organic complaints.[6] In our experience, alternative psychoses can also present as discrete neuropsychiatric syndromes such as abulia and even the syndrome of episodic dyscontrol. Putative mechanisms include kindling in subcortical structures, secondary epileptogenesis and alternating states of GABAergic and glutaminergic preponderance, influenced by complex interactions with dopamine.[7] Anticonvulsant drugs, particularly those such as topiramate that increase γ-aminobutyric acid levels, are well known to lead to alternative psychosis with or without forced normalization of the EEG.[8]

Furthermore, although the alternative psychoses are usually acute, they often develop insidiously. We have proposed criteria for the diagnosis of this condition that we hope will encourage epileptologists to establish prospective studies.[9]

Fourthly, most anticonvulsant drugs (both new and old) do produce neuropsychiatric symptoms or syndromes in some patients that are often ignored or remain undiagnosed. These syndromes can cause a significant level of disability, as this case highlights, and need to be identified and managed properly.

Finally, this case serves to remind us that psychotropic drugs, especially antidepressants, are proconvulsant and may precipitate seizures. On this occasion the offending agent was reboxetine, a newer antidepressant. The seizure, however, ironically proved helpful in the patient's diagnosis and remission.

REFERENCES

1. Landolt H. Serial EEG investigations during psychotic episodes in epileptic patients and during schizophrenic attacks. In: Lorentz De Haas AM, ed. *Lectures on epilepsy*. Amsterdam: Elsevier, 1958: 91–133.
2. Tellenbach H. Epilepsie als Anfallsleiden und als Psychose. *Nervenar* 1965;**36**:190–202.
3. Schmitz B. Forced normalization: history of a concept. In: Trimble MR, Schmitz B, eds. *Forced normalization and alternative psychoses of epilepsy*. Petersfield: Wrightson, 1998: 7–24.
4. Bhatia KP, Marsden CD. The behavioural and motor consequences of focal lesions of the basal ganglia in man. *Brain* 1994;**117**:859–76.
5. Vijayaraghavan L, Krishnamoorthy ES, Brown RB, Trimble MR. Abulia: a survey of British neurologists and psychiatrists. *Mov Disord* 2002;**17(5)**:1052–7.

6. Wolf P. Acute behavioural symptomatology at disappearance of epileptiform EEG abnormality: paradoxical or forced normalization. In: Smith D, Treiman D, Trimble MR, eds. *Neurobehavioural problems in epilepsy*. NY: Raven Press, 1991: 127–42.

7. Krishnamoorthy ES, Trimble MR. Mechanisms of forced normalization. In: Trimble MR, Schmitz B, eds. *Forced normalization and alternative psychoses of epilepsy*. Petersfield: Wrightson, 1998: 193–207.

8. Trimble MR. Forced normalization and the role of anticonvulsants. In: Trimble MR, Schmitz B, eds. *Forced normalization and alternative psychoses of epilepsy*. Petersfield: Wrightson, 1998: 169–78.

9. Krishnamoorthy ES, Trimble MR. Forced normalization: clinical and therapeutic relevance in mood disturbances, psychoses and epilepsy. *Epilepsia* 1999;**40(suppl 10)**:S57–S64.

The Continuing Place of Phenobarbital

Fumisuke Matsuo

HISTORY

This male patient experienced his first seizure in 1978 at the age of 15. It was a generalized convulsion that occurred early in the morning during sleep and lasted approximately 5 min, as have all of his subsequent seizures. EEG was abnormal and his family doctor initiated phenobarbital 120 mg/day. The phenobarbital dose was raised to 180 mg/day after his second seizure 9 months later.

A subsequent EEG in 1981 was normal. The phenobarbital was reduced by 60 mg every other day. Soon after this, the patient suffered another seizure, and phenobarbital was increased back to 180 mg/day. In October 1982, he left for an 18-month church mission, which radically altered his eating and sleeping habits. Two seizures occurred over the next 6 months and his phenobarbital was increased to 240 mg/day. The dose was further increased to 360 mg/day in January 1984 after another seizure that was unrelated to non-compliance. After being seizure-free for 2 years, the patient decreased phenobarbital to 300 mg/day.

Over the next 12 years, in consultation with a neurologist, he attempted further phenobarbital dosage reductions down to 200 mg daily, but breakthrough seizures occurred and the dose was continued at 300 mg/day.

INVESTIGATIONS

The patient's sister, 7 years younger, suffered refractory generalized epilepsy from the age of 2, with a frequency of four or five seizures a month. She died a sudden and unexplained death at the age of 24. The family doctor arranged for all six siblings to undergo EEGs when our patient experienced his first seizure. Two of the siblings had abnormal EEGs, but neuroimaging was normal in both of these siblings.

s0030

TREATMENT AND OUTCOME

p0050

At his wife's urging, the patient saw another neurologist when he was aged 36. The neurologist felt that the patient's quality of life would be better with a different medication, and initiated carbamazepine. When the carbamazepine dose reached 800 mg/day, the phenobarbital dose was reduced by 50 mg every 3 weeks. During the transition, the patient had two seizures; by October 1999 the phenobarbital dose was 50 mg/day and the carbamazepine dose was 1200 mg/day. The next month, he had a mild seizure, noted involuntary muscle jerking and began experiencing severe double vision.

p0060

Phenobarbital was discontinued and he had several additional seizures over the next few months. Lamotrigine was added and titrated over 2 months to 400 mg/day in two divided doses, and carbamazepine was reduced to 800 mg/day in two divided doses.

p0070

The patient continued to have seizures and therefore restarted phenobarbital. On a regimen of phenobarbital 100 mg/day, carbamazepine 200 mg/day and lamotrigine 400 mg/day in two divided doses, he suffered from tiredness but his seizures were completely controlled.

s0040

DIAGNOSIS

p0080

Syndrome of familial epilepsy with nocturnal recurrences.[1]

s0050

COMMENTARY

p0090

Phenobarbital was able to control this patient's seizures, although the patient and his wife were concerned about adverse neurobehavioral symptoms at high doses. Carbamazepine not only failed to control the seizures at maximally tolerated doses, but it may also have precipitated non-convulsive generalized seizures.[2] Lamotrigine may prove satisfactory in this patient, but ultimate control may require the use of valproate as monotherapy or in combination.[3]

s0060

What did I learn from this case?

p0100

I learned that it might take decades in some patients with very infrequent seizures to assess the results of different treatment regimens. This patient suffered an average of one seizure a year, including some precipitated by minor changes in antiepileptic drug regimens. This patient's history also highlights the difficulty involved in evaluating possible discontinuation of prophylaxis with antiepileptic drugs even after prolonged periods of freedom from seizures.[4] This case illustrated to me that the efficacy of antiepileptic drugs is notoriously difficult to assess in certain provoked epilepsy syndromes, and that such assessments may result in negative notions about the role of antiepileptic drugs in such patients.[5]

s0070

How did this case alter my approach to the care and treatment of my epilepsy patients?

p0110

I am more sensitive now to the fact that the lives of patients with very infrequent seizures could be disrupted by the occurrence of a seizure, even when they are exclusively nocturnal as in this patient. I am also more cautious about discontinuing phenobarbital.[6]

REFERENCES

1. Berkovic SF, Scheller IE. Genetics of the epilepsies. *Curr Opin Neurol* 1999;**12**:177–82.
2. Snead OC, Hosey LC. Exacerbation of seizures in children by carbamazepine. *N Engl J Med* 1985;**313**:916–21.
3. Brodie MJ, Yuen AW. Lamotrigine substitution study: evidence for synergism with sodium valproate. *Epilepsy Res* 1997;**26**:423–32.
4. American Academy of Neurology. Practice parameter: a guideline for discontinuing antiepileptic drugs in seizure-free patients: summary statement. *Neurology* 1996;**47**:600–2.
5. Friis ML, Lund M. Stress convulsions. *Arch Neurol* 1974;**31**:155–9.
6. Buchthal F, Svenmark O, Simonsen H. Relation of EEG and seizures to phenobarbital in serum. *Arch Neurol* 1968;**19**:567–72.

c0067

A Patient with Epilepsy Slips Down Some Attic Stairs

Rajesh C Sachdeo

s0010

HISTORY

p0010

A 63-year-old white man was admitted to a community hospital with status epilepticus and then transferred to my facility the next day for further evaluation and management.

p0020

The patient had a history of seizures since the age of 16 (etiology and type unknown) and had been well controlled on phenobarbital and phenytoin since then. His seizures consisted of arm and leg shaking with loss of consciousness and occasional incontinence. Six months before admission, he slipped down some stairs and sustained head trauma with loss of consciousness for 10 min. At that time, he did not seek medical attention because he felt well. Over the ensuing 6 weeks, the patient developed increasing lethargy, memory impairment, decreased sensation on the right side of his body, headache, and visual impairment.

p0030

A subdural hematoma was diagnosed and evacuated. He initially did well, but after several weeks he developed increasing lethargy progressing to loss of consciousness. He had a second burr hole (3 months before the present admission) and again he did well but required a third evacuation about 3 weeks before admission.

p0040

Beginning about that time, his seizures increased to a frequency of about five a day. They were typically nocturnal and characterized by focal shaking of the right arm or leg with secondary generalization. He had recently been prescribed sustained-release oral theophylline for asthma control in addition to prednisone, and his seizure exacerbation was attributed to the theophylline.

p0050

At the time of admission, the patient was on:

u0010
- carbamazepine 800 mg/day in four divided doses;

u0020
- phenobarbital 180 mg/day in three divided doses;

u0030
- phenytoin 400 mg/day in four divided doses;

u0040
- sustained-release theophylline 800 mg/day in two divided doses; and

u0050
- prednisone 15 mg/day.

EXAMINATION AND INVESTIGATIONS

On examination, the patient had a decreased attention span, poor performance of serial sevens, dysdiadochokinesia and mild tremor. An EEG done on admission revealed bilateral mild slowing. A computed tomography (CT) scan of the brain showed postsurgical changes of the left calvarium and a left parietal subdural fluid collection. The carbamazepine level was low.

DIAGNOSIS

Seizures since childhood, assumed to be partial onset, and recent head trauma.

TREATMENT AND OUTCOME

Based on the absence of seizures on EEG, phenobarbital and phenytoin were discontinued. The carbamazepine dose was increased over 3 days to 1600 mg/day. The patient was seizure-free for 2 days and then had a generalized tonic–clonic seizure, which was initially thought to be secondary to phenobarbital withdrawal. However, when the EEG showed epileptiform discharges in the right frontotemporal area and generalized spike–wave activity, valproate 750 mg/day in three divided doses was started.

The next day, the patient developed complex partial status epilepticus, terminated with intravenous diazepam. The carbamazepine dose was then increased to 1800 mg/day. In addition, theophylline was discontinued and replaced by albuterol with consultation of the pulmonary service. After 1 week on valproate, the patient developed intolerable vertigo and nystagmus, which necessitated discontinuation of the drug. He was then discharged from the hospital 2 days later.

Three days after discharge, the patient was readmitted because of two generalized seizures, and he had two more seizures on the day after admission. He had sustained a laceration of his left eyebrow. A CT scan showed no new changes, but an EEG showed focal epileptiform discharges as well as generalized spike–wave discharges. He was successfully treated with phenytoin 200 mg intravenously and then with oral phenytoin; he was started again on valproate 1000 mg/day and carbamazepine reduced to 1400 mg/day.

An EEG 18 months later showed mild generalized slow wave activity together with sharp and slow wave complexes in the right anterior temporal region. Four years after the initial presentation, the patient had a normal EEG and was eventually weaned off the carbamazepine.

COMMENTARY

This patient had an antecedent history of seizures since the age of 16, which were not well characterized but were assumed to be partial onset. At the age of 63 he sustained a fall, which required three surgical evacuations of a subdural hematoma. The head trauma clearly was a risk factor for partial seizures. An EEG demonstrated right fronto-temporal epileptiform discharges that generalized, thereby confirming partial epilepsy.

p0180   On the assumption that the patient had partial seizures and that polytherapy may not have been necessary, his drug regimen was simplified to carbamazepine monother-apy. At that point, generalized tonic–clonic seizures emerged, suggesting the possibility that the patient's lifelong seizure disorder was due to a generalized epilepsy syndrome. Valproate was therefore added.

p0190   It is well known that carbamazepine can exacerbate generalized epilepsies such as childhood absence epilepsy, juvenile myoclonic epilepsy, generalized tonic–clonic sei-zures, and atonic or myoclonic seizures. A subsequent EEG in this patient confirmed two types of epileptiform abnormalities – focal discharges with secondary generaliza-tion and generalized epileptiform patterns consistent with primary generalized epilepsy.

s0060   ## What did I learn from this case?

p0200   Ockham's razor does not always prevail! William of Ockham was a Franciscan logi-cian who lived in England in the 13th century. Ockham is credited with the saying "entities should not be multiplied unnecessarily." Thus, the principle of parsimony has been called Ockham's razor. The practice of clinical neurology is predicated upon this rule of parsimony – we strive to localize a single lesion that explains all the symptoms under one diagnosis. In this case, Ockham's razor failed us, since the patient had two different types of seizure disorders at once – complex partial seizures with secondary generalization and primary generalized tonic–clonic seizures.

p0210   Furthermore, this case points out the importance of obtaining a complete history of any antecedent seizures. This patient's seizure at the age of 16 was considered to be of uncertain etiology. Perhaps, if the patient's chart or an earlier EEG had been avail-able, his epilepsy would have been more accurately characterized. At times, a family history of epilepsy can also be helpful.

s0070   ## How did this case alter my approach to the care and treatment of my epilepsy patients?

p0220   This case taught me that different seizure types, as identified by the international clas-sification system, are not mutually exclusive. Now I do not rule out the possibility of the co-occurrence of a primary generalized epilepsy and an acquired symptom-atic complex partial seizure disorder in appropriate patients. I am mindful of choosing antiepileptic drug regimens for such patients that are likely to be beneficial and not potentially detrimental.

s0080   ## What would I do different today?

p0230   Firstly I would have put him on oxcarbazepine instead of carbamazepine. Oxcarbazepine is much less of an enzyme-inducer compared with carbamazepine. It has fewer drug–drug interactions and very similar efficacy for partial seizures.

Therefore the dose of valproate that would be required to control this patient's generalized seizures could be reduced to half. Also oxcarbazepine seems less prone to precipitate myoclonic and absence seizures.

FURTHER READING

Snead OC, Hosey LC. Exacerbation of seizures in children by carbamazepine. *N Engl J Med* 1985;**313**:916–21.

c0068

Bilateral Hip Fractures in
a 43-Year-Old Woman
with Epilepsy

Dieter Schmidt

s0010

HISTORY

p0010
A 43-year-old heavy smoker had a history of idiopathic generalized epilepsy with absences since childhood and generalized tonic–clonic seizures, often on awakening.

p0020
She stopped taking primidone on the recommendation of her neurologist in July 1998 after being completely seizure-free for several years. In October of the same year she was hospitalized for an ischemic middle cerebral artery stroke with transient left-sided hemiplegia and received low-dose heparin while she was bedridden. At 0730 hrs in the morning of October 10 she had a generalized tonic–clonic seizure that lasted 1–2 min according to the nurse's report. Afterwards the patient complained about moderate pain in both upper legs and difficulty moving her legs in bed. She received an intravenous infusion of 4 mg clonazepam over several hours and oral carbamazepine treatment was started. At 1400 hrs she had her second tonic–clonic seizure.

s0020

DIAGNOSIS

p0030
Bilateral hip fracture in a patient with idiopathic generalized epilepsy following a relapse of tonic–clonic seizures.

s0030

INVESTIGATIONS

p0040
Two hours later, an X-ray revealed bilateral hip fractures (Figure 68.1), which were successfully operated on the next day. The surgeon told the neurologist who had cared for her in the hospital that he was surprised how brittle her bones had been.

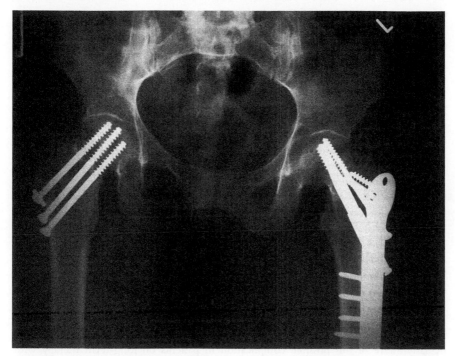

FIGURE 68.1   Bilateral hip fracture in a 43-year-old woman with epilepsy following a single tonic–clonic seizure. A second one occurred several hours later. The X-ray shown here was taken following surgery the next day. A medial femoral neck fracture is seen on the right side and a pertrochanteric fracture on the left side.

OUTCOME

A lawyer acting on behalf of the woman later charged that better treatment after the first seizure would have prevented the second one and the fractures, and for good measure suggested that bodily violence against the patient by hospital staff might have caused the fractures. I learnt about the case when I was asked to give an expert opinion in the ensuing legal controversy.

COMMENTARY

Why did I choose this case?

I chose this case for two reasons. First, I was interested in why a middle-aged patient would suffer from bilateral hip fractures while having a tonic–clonic seizure in bed, and second, I had never heard about bilateral leg pain following a seizure, which is different from the well-known postictal back pain or general muscle ache.

What did I learn from this case?

When I first heard about this case, I had known from experience that tonic–clonic seizures in bed – without falls – may cause compression fractures of the lower thoracic or upper lumbar spine, resulting in back pain for a few weeks. Enzyme-inducing antiepileptic drugs may uncommonly cause osteomalacia in otherwise healthy people, putting them at risk for fractures. Patients with poor nutrition or gastrointestinal disease may be at even higher risk. The relative risk for fractures is increased twofold in patients with epilepsy (CI 1.5–2.5).[1] Bilateral fractures have been reported in individual patients[2] and one report singled out bilateral hip fractures in institutionalized patients with epilepsy.[3,4] In a further report, muscular contractions were identified as the cause of bilateral hip fractures during a tonic–clonic seizure, as occurred in our patient.[5] In total, about 0.3% of patients with epilepsy suffer fractures after seizures, not including those after falls. In summary then, the patient suffered from seizure-related bilateral hip fractures, a rare but nevertheless well-described complication of a tonic–clonic seizure.

How did this case alter my approach to the care and treatment of my epilepsy patients?

If a patient complains about pain immediately following a seizure, I look for bone fractures even when the patient did not fall as a consequence of the seizure. I am particularly aware of this possible complication in patients on long-term therapy with enzyme-inducing antiepileptic drugs, because of their increased risk for latent or overt osteomalacia and seizure-associated bone fractures. Further, I try to use non-enzyme-inducing antiepileptic drugs, if possible, to minimize the risk of anticonvulsant-induced osteomalacia.

Finally, I am more cautious when withdrawing antiepileptic drugs in adult patients who have had a remission of their seizures for at least 2 years because of the morbidity associated with recurrent seizures.

REFERENCES

1. Vestergaard P, Tigaran S, Rejnmark L, Tigaran C, Dam M. Fracture risk is increased in epilepsy. *Acta Neurol Scand* 1999;**99(5)**:269–75.
2. Lohiya GS, Tan-Figueroa L. Eighteen fractures in a man with profound mental retardation. *Ment Retard* 1999;**37(1)**:47–51.
3. Ribacoba-Montero R, Puig Salas J. Simultaneous bilateral fractures of the hip following a grand mal seizure. An unusual complication. *Seizure* 1997;**6(5)**:403–4.
4. Desai KB, Ribbans WJ, Taylor GJ. Incidence of five common fracture types in an institutional epileptic population. *Injury* 1996;**27(2)**:97–100.
5. Van Heest A, Vorlicky L, Thompson RC. Bilateral central acetabular fracture dislocations secondary to sustained myoclonus. *Clin Orthop* 1996;**324**:210–13.

Picking a Wrong
Antiepileptic Drug for a
9-Year-Old Girl

Peter Uldall

HISTORY

This patient was diagnosed with childhood absence epilepsy at the age of 4 by the local pediatric department. She was treated with valproate with a good result. She developed normally and was seizure-free for 3 years. When she was 7 years old, her mother tapered off the medicine by herself. The next year passed apparently without seizures – at least nobody noticed any. By the time she was 9 years, however, it became obvious that she was having frequent absences, and valproate treatment was re-instituted by the local pediatric department. Now, however, she complained of adverse effects, including vomiting, abdominal discomfort, and weight gain. She was re-admitted three times and a new EEG was performed. At this time, some focal traits were seen in the EEG (Figures 69.1 and 69.2).

On suspicion of complex partial seizures, a trial of vigabatrin was undertaken. The seizures increased; she was re-admitted and treatment was changed to valproate syrup. The adverse events continued, however, and she refused to take any medicine orally. Then she was put on valproate suppositories. This resulted in unstable plasma levels, diarrhea, and continuing absences. Furthermore, she was wetting the bed and she had learning disabilities, no friends and no self-confidence. She had never had generalized tonic–clonic seizures.

EXAMINATION AND INVESTIGATIONS

The patient, together with her mother, was admitted to a tertiary epilepsy hospital for 4 weeks. Her mother was a single, insecure woman who had two other children and was only just able to manage to keep her job. Video–EEG showed typical absences. During admission she was observed in the school at the hospital. The girl and her mother were intensively informed and educated about epilepsy. A neuropsychological

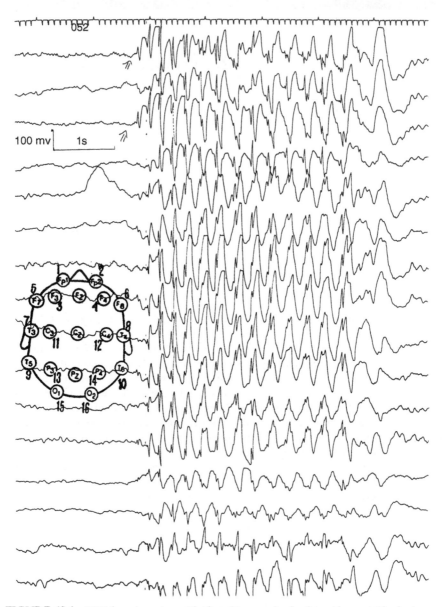

f0010 FIGURE 69.1   EEG from the patient with idiopathic generalized epilepsy (absences). The focal onset (left prefrontal and left frontal regions) of the generalized spike–wave discharge can be seen (arrows).

examination showed that the patient had normal intelligence and only subtle cognitive problems. The neurological examination was normal.

s0030 ## DIAGNOSIS

p0040 Childhood absence epilepsy.

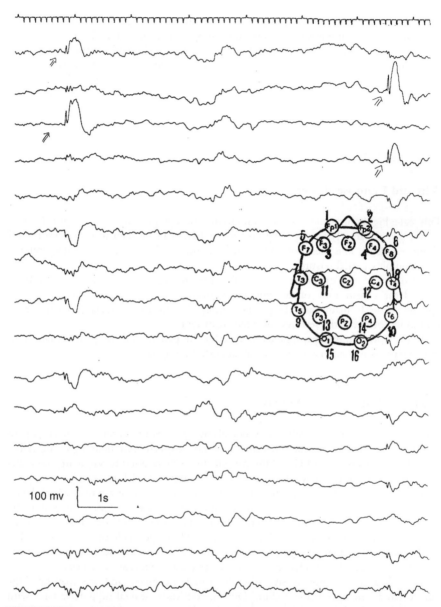

FIGURE 69.2   (Light sleep), two independent frontal spike–wave discharges are seen (arrows).   f0020

TREATMENT AND OUTCOME

When the mother and the girl were shown the video–EEG, they realized what the problem was and finally became motivated to try a new drug. The girl was started on ethosuximide syrup without any adverse events. The absences disappeared and the child slowly regained her self-confidence. It was possible to get leave for the mother from her job for 2 months so that she could support the child. The daughter was able to regain her confidence about her school performance. The bed-wetting disappeared after the valproate was tapered off (it had previously been unsuccessfully treated with a reward of 5 Danish kroner for each dry night and a penalty of 2 Danish kroner for each wet night). At discharge the patient could return to her school without problems, and the EEG was normal.

COMMENTARY

Why did I choose this case?

This case highlights issues that are important for the pediatric neurologist. First, it shows that apparently focal paroxysms on the EEG can be seen in otherwise typical absence epilepsy. This must not lead to the conclusion of a localization-related epilepsy with complex partial seizures.

Second, the case underlines the fact that the management of epilepsy extends far beyond the classification of the epilepsy syndrome and the prescription of an anti-epileptic drug. In many cases the psychological, educational and social problems are at least as important as the seizures and their treatment.

Information on epilepsy and acceptance by the patient and the patient's family of the epilepsy is mandatory in order to obtain good compliance.

What did I learn from this case?

The diagnosis of absence epilepsy is not always easy. Some absences can last up to 20–30s with elements of automatisms. If a non-experienced neurologist describes some focal traits on the EEG and the patient does not respond to valproate, the clinician may erroneously believe that it is a case of complex partial seizures.

Because of the failure of treatment resulting from the use of a wrong antiepileptic drug (vigabatrin in this case) and an unsuitable route of administration, as well as the adverse events that resulted, the confidence of the patient and her mother in treatment and in the doctors was lost. The mother could not persuade the child to take her medicine and because of ongoing seizures and adverse events (such as bed-wetting) the child lost her self-confidence at school. In this way, a vicious cycle began.

In such a case, comprehensive re-evaluation is necessary, and this may be difficult to handle in an outpatient clinic. During admission, several supportive talks with other girls with epilepsy, the nurses, schoolteachers, and psychologists made it possible to change the situation. A video–EEG is a very powerful tool, not only for diagnostic purposes, but also for education of patients and relatives. In this case the girl and her mother could see for themselves what was going on, and they both realized the importance of treatment. Even a video without EEG could be used in this situation. The neuropsychological examination was necessary to convince the girl herself and her teachers that she had sufficient abilities to continue in her mainstream school. Adverse events must always be taken seriously, even minor ones. Bed-wetting is often overlooked. In this case, the treatment may actually have been worse than the disease.

In conclusion, this case illustrates that information and correct syndrome diagnosis are crucial not only in the severe intractable cases of childhood epilepsy, but also in the benign syndromes, when we should be able to give our patients a normal life.

An important message from this case and from several audit studies, not least in teenagers, is that the treatment process should include management of global health and daily function of the child from the social, educational and psychological points of view – then it will be possible to change the lives of children with epilepsy.

c0070

With Epilepsy
You Never Know

Walter van Emde Boas

s0010

HISTORY

p0010
AQ1
While living in the tropics, Mrs. F had her first generalized convulsion at the age of 3.5 years in association with a fever, which was possibly malarial. She was born after a normal pregnancy of healthy Caucasian parents and had normal psychomotor development.

p0020
Seven years later she had a second generalized convulsion, which was provoked by sleep deprivation. At that time a neurologist examined her. Physical examination was normal. The EEG showed right posterior focal slowing but no epileptiform discharges. A computed tomography (CT) scan showed a small, contrast-enhancing lesion in the right frontal lobe. After a negative angiography study, the tentative diagnosis of angioma was changed to cerebral cysticercosis, although cerebrospinal fluid titers remained negative.

p0030
Anticonvulsant treatment with phenytoin and carbamazepine was started but did not prevent occasional generalized seizures, which were consistently provoked by sleep deprivation and jet lag after long flights. Brief absence-like episodes, sometimes with mild automatisms, started at the age of 14 years and continued despite treatment up to maximum tolerated doses with carbamazepine and phenytoin. When she was 16 years old, phenytoin was replaced by valproate because of progressive gingival hyperplasia but this had no effect on the seizures. The possible option of epilepsy surgery was suggested but rejected by the patient and her parents until they could return permanently to The Netherlands.

s0020

EXAMINATION AND INVESTIGATIONS

p0040
The first time I saw Mrs. F she had just turned 18. Generalized seizures had not occurred for more than 20 months but she reported between one and three brief

"absence" spells a day and complained about drowsiness and impaired concentration caused by her medication (valproate 1000 mg/day in two divided doses and carbamazepine 800 mg/day in two divided doses).

Physical examination was normal, as before, but the interictal EEG now showed irregular slow waves and occasional spike–wave discharges over the right anterior region without consistent focal characteristics. A magnetic resonance imaging scan of the brain showed a small (approximately 2.5 cm), well-demarcated round lesion in the anteriomedian part of the right frontal lobe, probably a cavernoma, without signs of progression in comparison to the previous CT scans.

During EEG with video monitoring, the "absences" turned out to be brief complex partial seizures with arrest reaction, loss of contact, and partial amnesia but without additional clinical signs. An ictal EEG showed some attenuation of ongoing activity, followed by an increase of irregular theta and delta activity over both anterior regions, with slight preponderance to the right but otherwise without convincing lateralizing or localizing features.

DIAGNOSIS

Symptomatic frontal lobe epilepsy characterized by complex partial seizures with anterior frontal or frontopolar clinical characteristics.[1]

TREATMENT AND OUTCOME

Epilepsy surgery was discussed again. At that time (1989) it was believed that intracranial EEG and video monitoring were mandatory in all cases without unequivocal scalp EEG localization, even in the presence of a lesion. Mrs. F and her parents did not consider her sufficiently socially or medically impaired to warrant such studies. Furthermore she wanted to finish high school during that summer and it was decided to postpone further procedures.

She switched to controlled-release carbamazepine, which improved her diurnal alertness, and she successfully took her final examinations. She immediately applied for and obtained a scholarship for a 3-year college education in the USA, starting within 3 months. Presurgical evaluation was thus further postponed.

Over the next 3 years her complex partial seizures gradually became more severe, and secondary generalized seizures recurred occasionally. The dose of controlled-release carbamazepine was increased to 1200 mg/day in two divided doses, and phenytoin was added but then withdrawn again when disfiguring hirsutism developed. Repeat EEG with video monitoring during a brief holiday in The Netherlands (in 1991) showed more elaborate complex partial seizures, including vocalizations, oro-alimentary automatisms, and some hypermotor automatisms of the arms.[2] The ictal EEG remained poorly localizing.

After graduation, Mrs. F returned to The Netherlands for further consultation. At this time her seizure pattern had become more disabling and included frequent urinary incontinence during complex partial seizures. A third video–EEG suggested clinical involvement of the anteriofrontal area as well as the anterior cingulate, insular-opercular, and mesial frontobasal areas,[1] suggesting a progressive type of frontal lobe epilepsy.[3] Ictal scalp EEG still remained equivocal but late ictal and postictal slowing predominated over the right frontal lobe. Our surgical approach of lesional epilepsy had changed, following the second Palm Desert Meeting on Epilepsy Surgery,[4] and surgery was offered without further invasive procedures.

p0130   A partial right frontal lobe resection was performed, including complete lesionectomy, and Mrs. F became seizure-free as of December 1992. She successfully completed health care–related studies and started a private practice in yet another faraway country. Treatment was gradually reduced to monotherapy with controlled-release carbamazepine 200 mg/day, and follow-up consultations became rare.

p0140   In 1998 she wrote to me saying that she was experiencing a problem with insurance because of her epilepsy, despite having been seizure-free for more than 5 years. I advised her to consider herself healed, and to stop her controlled-release carbamazepine gradually over the next 4 months and then to try again with the insurance company. I included a letter to the company, stating that in her case the epilepsy had been surgically cured and that seizure recurrence was extremely unlikely. Four months later I learned that she had relapsed. Since then she has been on controlled-release carbamazepine 800 mg/day in two divided doses, without significant side effects and thus far without further seizures.

s0050   ## COMMENTARY

s0060   ### What did I learn from this case?

p0150   First of all I learnt from her that epilepsy is a disorder that people can cope with. Despite significantly disabling seizures, this brave and motivated young woman, assisted by an understanding and supportive family, managed to pursue and achieve the goals of her own choosing, most often on her own terms.

p0160   Secondly, I learnt that epilepsy surgery is indeed an elective type of surgery – medical urgencies can be offset by social urgencies and the process of evaluation and surgery must be optimized accordingly.

p0170   From the case of Mrs. F I also learnt that epilepsy can be a progressive disorder, even in lesional epilepsy that is associated with a static, non-malignant structural lesion.[3]

p0180   From her, more than from others, I learnt that epilepsy surgery rarely relieves patients from their seizure disorder. In most patients who undergo surgery, we are able to change an intractable epilepsy into a treatable condition, yet with the need for lifelong drug treatment of a perennial lingering and threatening disorder.

p0190   Finally I learnt to realize my own limitations better. I had advised this young woman that she was cured of her epilepsy because I wanted to believe her to be cured, *not* because I knew that she was.

p0200   With epilepsy you never know.

REFERENCES

1. van Emde Boas W, Velis DN. Frontal lobe epilepsies. In: Meinardi H, vol ed. *The epilepsies, part II.* In: Vinken PJ, Bruyn GW, eds. *Handbook of clinical neurology (revised series)* vol 73(29). Amsterdam: Elsevier;2000:37–52.

2. Lüders H, Acharaya J, Baumgartner C, *et al.* Semiological seizure classification. *Epilepsia* 1998;**39**:1006–13.
3. van Emde Boas W. Longitudinal evolution of frontal lobe complex partial seizures: a progressive seizure syndrome? In: Wolf P, ed. *Epileptic seizures and syndromes.* London: John Libbey, 1994: 408–15.
4. Engel J (ed.). *Surgical treatment of the epilepsies,* 2nd ed. New York: Raven, 1993.

Unexpected Solutions

When Antiepileptic Drugs Fail in an Infant with Seizures, Consider Vitamin B6

Mary R Andriola

HISTORY

A 3½-year-old girl had a normal perinatal history, normal growth and development, and a negative family history.

She first presented at 8 months of age with partial seizures involving the left hand and arm. A routine EEG and a video–EEG, without an event, were normal, as was a magnetic resonance imaging (MRI) scan of the brain. She was treated with carbamazepine and was seizure-free for 2 months.

She then presented with partial motor seizures, which again began in the left hand but then generalized. Her carbamazepine regimen was adjusted. Two weeks later, at 11 months of age, she was hospitalized with recurrent multiple seizures. These still had a focal component with twitching of the left face but frequent generalization. In the pediatric intensive care unit she received intravenous fosphenytoin, phenobarbital, and lorazepam. There was only a partial clinical response at first and then the seizures became intractable with decreased interictal responsivity.

EXAMINATION AND INVESTIGATIONS

When the patient presented at 11 months of age with left facial twitching, she was noted to have spike–polyspike–wave activity from the right hemisphere. Video–EEG monitoring revealed seizures developing independently and multifocally from either the right or the left hemisphere. Following treatment with intravenous antiepileptic drugs in the pediatric intensive care unit, the EEG was diffusely slow. When the seizures became intractable, the EEG was markedly abnormal with polymorphic slow wave activity and frequent rhythmic 1-Hz slow-and-sharp wave activity. With the administration of intravenous pyridoxine (Vit B$_6$) 100 mg, the sharp wave activity was rapidly replaced by diffuse slowing, which persisted for a number of days.

s0030   ## DIAGNOSIS

p0050   Pyridoxine-dependent seizures.

s0040   ## TREATMENT AND OUTCOME

p0060   Carbamazepine and phenobarbital were quickly tapered and the patient was maintained on pyridoxine 100 mg/day. Her mental status gradually improved, as did her developmental skills. At 1 year of age, approximately 1 month after beginning pyridoxine therapy, she had a normal neurological examination, a normal EEG and a normal MRI scan.

p0070   She has continued to grow and develop normally, and is maintained on pyridoxine 100 mg/day. She experienced a single seizure at about 2 years of age when she had a febrile illness and had missed a dose of pyridoxine. This was a brief and self-limited seizure. Her parents were instructed to give her pyridoxine 200 mg whenever she has a febrile illness.

s0050   ## COMMENTARY

p0080   This girl first presented when she was 8 months old with partial seizures that initially responded to carbamazepine. When her seizures recurred, with partial onset but secondary generalization, they became intractable and EEGs suggested multifocal onset, eventually showing diffuse slowing and 1-Hz spike-and-slow wave activity.

p0090   The intravenous administration of pyridoxine was both diagnostically and therapeutically specific for pyridoxine-dependent seizures. This was an unusual presentation, out of the neonatal period, with partial seizures that initially appeared to respond to carbamazepine. Such unusual or atypical cases have been reported but there are less than 100 total cases of pyridoxine-dependent seizures in the literature. Cases have been reported with onset up to 3 years of age.

s0060   ### What did I learn from this case?

p0100   Pyridoxine-dependent seizures require a high index of suspicion. From this case, I learned that intractable seizures in an infant may be related to pyridoxine dependency even if the seizures do not have their onset in the neonatal period. The most important aspects of this infant's gradual clinical evolution were progressively abnormal EEGs and decreased responsivity of the patient in spite of multiple antiepileptic drugs that were being appropriately administered. This had to be distinguished from the sedating effects of medications.

How did this case alter my approach to the care and treatment of my epilepsy patients?

I consider administering intravenous pyridoxine to a child whose seizures become intractable and refractory to antiepileptic drugs when there is no known etiology. A markedly abnormal interictal EEG also suggests that a metabolic etiology should be pursued. Pyridoxine-dependent seizures is a rare disorder, and a high index of suspicion must be present if it is to be diagnosed properly; treatment of affected children can be almost miraculously effective.

FURTHER READING

Bankier A, Turner M, Hopkins IJ. Pyridoxine-dependent seizures: a wider clinical spectrum. *Arch Dis Child* 1983;**58**:415–8.

Goutieres F, Aicardi J. Atypical presentations of pyridoxine-dependent seizures: a treatable cause of intractable epilepsy in infants. *Ann Neurol* 1985;**17**:117–20.

Krishnamoorthy KS. Pyridoxine-dependency seizure: report of a rare presentation. *Ann Neurol* 1983;**13**:103–4.

Mikati MA, Trevathan E, Krishnamoorthy KS, Lombroso CT. Pyridoxine-dependent epilepsy: EEG investigations and long-term follow-up. *Electroencephalogr Clin Neurophysiol* 1991;**78**:215–21.

c0072

A 12-Year-Old Boy with Daily Clonic Seizures

Eloy Elices and Santiago Arroyo

s0010

HISTORY

p0010

A 12-year-old right-handed boy started to have seizures at the age of 5. At first the seizures consisted of clonic jerking of the left lower extremity, most prominent in the foot.

p0020

Within a few weeks, the seizures evolved into epilepsia partialis continua, which was eventually controlled, several months later, on a combination of carbamazepine and clobazam.

p0030

Soon after this, the patient started to have:

u0010 • daily clonic seizures of his left lower extremity (again most prominent in the foot);
u0020 • left-sided motor seizures occurring between six and eight times a month and beginning either in the foot or hand, followed by Todd's paralysis for several minutes; and
u0030 • several myoclonic jerks of the left leg each day.

p0070

At the age of 11, the patient reported three new types of episodes:

u0040 • left-hand paresthesias lasting up to 1 min;
u0050 • episodes of bilateral auditory or visual illusions; and
u0060 • right versive seizures with drooling, abnormal pharyngeal sensation, and preserved consciousness.

p0110

These events occurred on a weekly to monthly basis despite multiple trials of antiepileptic drugs (phenytoin, valproate, carbamazepine, primidone, phenobarbital, clonazepam, piracetam, clobazam, and prednisone) used at different doses and in different combinations. He also received three 5-day courses of immunoglobulins without significant success.

p0120

The patient's motor development was normal. After the age of 6, he became progressively slower when performing his usual tasks, which his parents and teachers attributed to difficulties with attention and concentration. Moreover, he was increasingly more hyperactive and impulsive. These behaviors did not improve with several changes in his antiepileptic drugs.

Beginning at the age of 12, the patient developed a slowly worsening left hemiparesis, more pronounced in the leg, which progressed in a step-wise fashion.

The patient's parents were not related to each other and there had been no problems with his delivery. His past medical history was unremarkable and he had normal developmental milestones. A maternal uncle, who had a few convulsive seizures during infancy that were easily controlled with medication, had been seizure-free for many years without medication.

EXAMINATION AND INVESTIGATIONS

Neurological examination when the patient was 9 had shown a left hemiparesis with hyperreflexia (before this his strength and reflexes had been normal). The hemiparesis was symmetrical, mild (4/5), and stable for several years, when it rapidly progressed over 2–3 months to complete functional loss of the hand, left motor neglect, and mild hypoesthesia of the left hand. No neurological deficits were found on the right side.

A brain magnetic resonance imaging (MRI) scan performed at age 7 was reported as normal but subsequent MRI scans showed radiological deterioration (Figure 72.1).

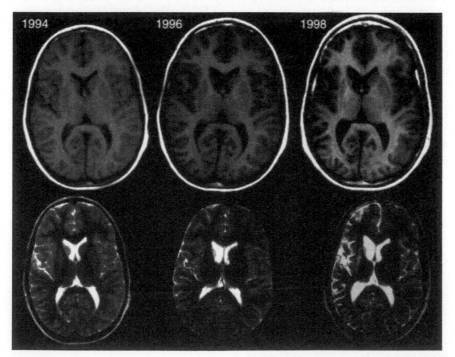

FIGURE 72.1 Progressive atrophy of the right hemisphere, first seen in the basal ganglia, leading eventually to the near-disappearance of the caudate and lenticular nuclei. In addition, hyperintensity of these nuclei was seen in the early stages. No radiographic abnormalities were seen in the left hemisphere.

p0170   Video–EEG monitoring at age 11 showed independent multifocal right hemisphere seizures – simple partial motor seizures (left leg clonic activity), secondarily generalized seizures (with motor component prominent over the left extremities), and simple partial auditory seizures.

p0180   Serial neuropsychological tests showed a continuous decline in his neuropsychological performance, including cognitive slowing.

p0190   A right temporal pole biopsy was performed in 1998 when he was 12 years old. This confirmed the diagnosis of Rasmussen's encephalitis. No viral inclusions were found in the tissue and cerebrospinal fluid studies for viral serologies and GluR3 antibodies were negative.

s0030 ## DIAGNOSIS

p0200 Rasmussen's encephalitis.

s0040 ## TREATMENT AND OUTCOME

p0210 When the patient lost function in his left hand at the age of 12, a functional hemispherotomy was carried out. Following the operation, his seizures greatly improved – he only had occasional right frontal onset EEG-confirmed simple partial seizures (bilateral blinking), and these were easily controlled with adjustments to his drug dosages. His intellectual performance improved significantly, as did his behavior. The left hemiparesis did not prevent him from walking within 2 weeks after surgery and he is undergoing intense rehabilitation for his left arm.

s0050 ## COMMENTARY

p0220 Although Rasmussen's encephalitis has been a fairly well-known disease for over 40 years, its incidence is very low. Our patient presented with several interesting and characteristic features:

u0070 - He had several types of seizures, which included motor signs, somatosensory symptoms, and auditory and visual semiology. The presence of multiple unilateral seizure types and epilepsia partialis continua is very suggestive of Rasmussen's encephalitis.

u0080 - The hemiparesis appeared 4 years after the onset of the seizures and was very mild until 3 years later, when it became rapidly progressive (in 2 months he was hemiplegic).

u0090 - Brain MRI scans showed striking and progressive hemispheric changes – hemiatrophy, hyperintense signals, and basal ganglia involvement.

s0060 ### What did we learn from this case?

p0260 Although there are no prospective studies of serial MRI scans in patients with Rasmussen's encephalitis, our patient's studies provide a good example of the radiological progression typical of this disease. We have looked with particular interest at these MRI abnormalities, because we are not aware of any other disease that shares similar characteristics. Since a certain diagnosis can only be achieved by brain biopsy, we have become aware of the need for diagnostic studies that would point to the diagnosis before brain atrophy occurs.

How did this case alter our approach to the care and treatment of our patients with epilepsy?

We waited until the child lost the functional use of his hand to do the biopsy and then perform the hemispherectomy, even though the diagnosis of chronic encephalitis had already been assumed. The optimal time to perform surgery is a controversial subject. Some clinicians propose waiting until the patient has hemiparesis and others advocate performing the hemispherectomy before the hemiparesis is complete in order to avoid the neuropsychological impairment, years of seizures, and social handicap that are associated with this otherwise relentless disease. The debate is still ongoing.

FURTHER READING

So NK, Andermann F. Rasmussen's encephalitis. In: Engel J, Pedley T, eds. *Epilepsy. A comprehensive textbook*. Philadelphia: Lippincott–Raven, 1997: 2379–88.

Tien RD, Ashdown BC, Lewis DV, *et al*. Rasmussen's encephalitis: neuroimaging findings in four patients. *Am J Roentgenol* 1992;**158**:1329–32.

Vining EP, Freeman JM, Brandt J, *et al*. Progressive unilateral encephalopathy of childhood (Rasmussen's syndrome): a reappraisal. *Epilepsia* 1993;**34**:639–50.

c0073

A Child with Attention-Deficit Disorder, Autistic Features and Frequent Epileptiform EEG Discharges

Frank MC Besag

s0010

HISTORY

p0010
This male patient first presented to our service at 6.5 years of age. Although there was no history suggestive of birth trauma, seizures commenced at 6 days of age with a prolonged period of unconsciousness that lasted 2 or 3 days, during which he had several convulsions. After this illness he was initially lethargic.

p0020
His milestones were delayed. He crawled at 12 months of age, walked at 20 months and was not able to utter more than three words until 20 months of age. At 23 months he fell off the bed when playing and struck his head. Although he was not knocked unconscious, he fell deeply asleep the following day and had a series of seizures in which he appeared blank for a few seconds and his pupils were dilated. Two months later he had a prolonged convulsion that had to be terminated with emergency treatment in the hospital.

p0030
He continued having prolonged convulsions at 2-week to 3-month intervals, usually stopped with 15 mg rectal diazepam. From about 5 years of age he also developed blank spells during which he stared and was unresponsive. These occurred three to six times a day for 4–7 days a week. From age 5 he also developed episodes in which his eyeballs flicked up to the left side while his mouth was pulled down to the left; his left hand came up and adopted a claw-like posture. These episodes lasted between 40 s and 1 min. They occurred three or four times weekly when he was first seen.

s0020

EXAMINATION AND INVESTIGATION

p0040
When the patient first presented to our service at 6.5 years of age, he was very overactive. It was difficult to obtain EEGs because of the overactivity, but they showed

copious spike–wave activity. At that time he was being treated with carbamazepine and phenytoin. In addition to very poor concentration span and a high degree of motor overactivity, he also had some striking autistic features. He appeared to be in a world of his own, could not carry out a conversation and gave poor, fleeting eye contact. However, he had developed a special skill of reciting nursery rhymes. If someone uttered the first few words of a nursery rhyme he would continue with the rhyme. At around 6 years of age his ability to recite nursery rhymes was far superior to that of any other child at his school or indeed any of the adults.

Dilated ventricles were noted on a computed tomography (CT) scan at 2.5 years of age. A repeat CT scan at 10 years of age showed marked atrophy of the right hemisphere. He had a very mild left hemiparesis, tending to drag his left leg when walking. However, he could run quite fast and play football.

DIAGNOSIS

Attention–deficit disorder, frequent epileptiform discharges, and autistic features.

TREATMENT AND OUTCOME

Following a review of the antiepileptic medication, the phenytoin was tailed off and valproate was added. He was also treated with acetazolamide for a period. The epileptiform discharges on the EEG resolved. He became calm, lost his motor overactivity, and was able to engage in rewarding two-way conversations. He began to enjoy social interaction greatly.

It was subsequently possible to discontinue both the acetazolamide and the valproate, leaving him on carbamazepine monotherapy. By the age of 19 years, he typically had no more than one seizure a year and the EEG showed only a nonspecific excess of slow-wave activity with occasional right-sided sharp-waves of dubious significance. Although he enjoyed social interaction and derived great pleasure from interacting with his parents and carers, he was markedly eccentric. The intonation and content of his speech was typical of an individual with Asperger syndrome. He had developed many skills of daily living but continued to require a moderate degree of supervision to enable him to live within society.

COMMENTARY

This case illustrates that epilepsy may present in ways that lead to evaluation and management by psychiatrists or pediatricians rather than pediatric neurologists. This patient's initial presentation at 6.5 years was striking both because of gross attention-deficit disorder and overactivity and because of the autistic features. It appears that both of these clinical disorders were the result of frequent epileptiform discharges that were fragmenting his concentration and affecting his ability to interact with the world around him. When these frequent epileptiform discharges responded successfully to treatment he was able to develop rewarding interactions with other people, and the gross overactivity and attention-deficit resolved. However, he then presented with a different clinical picture, reminiscent of Asperger syndrome.

I have now seen several young people who have presented with a similar clinical picture in the mid-to-late teenage years, having gone through a period in earlier child-hood when frequent epileptiform discharges occurred. It would appear that children who have frequent epileptiform discharges that largely prevent them from having the easy two-way interaction with the world that most children experience may subse-quently have difficulties with social interaction even after the epileptiform discharges have resolved. It appears that this is the reason why this patient presented with strong features of Asperger syndrome in his late teenage years even though the epileptiform discharges were well controlled at that time.

What did I learn from this case?

First, I learnt that children who present with attention-deficit disorder and overactiv-ity may be having frequent epileptiform discharges that are breaking up their ability to concentrate and to interact with others. Treatment of these discharges can result in the resolution of the attention-deficit disorder and overactivity and can enable them to have a meaningful, rewarding interaction with the world around them.

Second, if a child is prevented from having the usual two-way social interaction with the world around him or her during a critical phase of development because of frequent epileptiform discharges, he or she may continue to have social interaction problems, presenting with an Asperger-like picture, long after the discharges have been treated or have resolved.

Third, the implication of these cases is that early energetic treatment of epilepti-form discharges might both resolve the autistic features at that time and even prevent the development of permanent Asperger-like characteristics with the accompanying social interaction difficulties.

FURTHER READING

Asperger H. Die "Autistischen Psychopathien" im Kindesalter. *Archiv fur Psychiatric und Nervenkrankheiten* 1944;**117**:362–8.

Wing L. Asperger's syndrome: a clinical account. *Psychol Med* 1981;**11**:115–29.

Harris JC. *Developmental neuropsychiatry. Assessment, diagnosis, and treatment of developmental disorders*, vol. II. Oxford: Oxford University Press, 1995. (221–8).

Complete Seizure Control in a 14-Year-Old Boy after Temporal Lobectomy Failed

Martin J Brodie

HISTORY

A 14-year-old autistic, learning-disabled boy had been experiencing fortnightly clusters of 10–20 partial and secondary generalized seizures before his referral in July 1992.

He had been born by emergency caesarian section in response to fetal distress and had an Apgar score of 4 on delivery. Seizure activity developed following three prolonged febrile convulsions early in his first year of life and continued throughout childhood, despite removal of a damaged left temporal lobe at the age of 3 years. He was aggressive before the clusters of seizures, which were always followed by complex automatisms. His parents found his constant wandering particularly difficult to cope with. Treatment on referral was with phenytoin monotherapy. He had received carbamazepine, valproate, phenobarbital, and bromide in the past.

Adding vigabatrin to the phenytoin did not improve his seizure control and worsened his behavior. Lamotrigine produced a modest reduction in the number of seizures. The patient's family then moved from the area. When he was referred again in November 1996, his treatment consisted of phenytoin 300 mg/day (concentration 80 μmol/l) and lamotrigine 500 mg/day (concentration 21 μmol/l). Seizure frequency had worsened. The numbers of bimonthly clusters had not increased, but each cluster now consisted of 20 or more complex partial seizures with frequent secondary generalization over a period of 2–3 days.

EXAMINATION AND INVESTIGATIONS

Neurological examination was essentially normal. The patient had stereotypic behavior and marked gum hypertrophy. A surface EEG showed excess slow wave activity but no epileptiform discharges. Brain imaging was not undertaken.

DIAGNOSIS

Partial-onset seizures secondary to perinatal hypoxic brain damage in an autistic, learning-disabled young man.

TREATMENT AND OUTCOME

Phenytoin was withdrawn and the lamotrigine dose was increased to 800 mg/day in two divided doses. This regimen produced a modest reduction in the frequency and severity of seizures. The cautious addition of low-dose topiramate led to a marked improvement in alertness and behavior.

This young man has remained seizure-free since September 1998 on lamotrigine 800 mg/day in two divided doses (concentration 66 µmol/l) and topiramate 75 mg/day (25 mg in the morning and 50 mg at bedtime; concentration 6 µmol/l).

COMMENTARY

The combination of high-dose lamotrigine and low-dose topiramate resulted in complete seizure control with improvement in the patient's quality of life and that of his family. Temporal lobectomy and previous treatment with carbamazepine, valproate, phenobarbital, bromide, phenytoin, phenytoin–vigabatrin, and phenytoin–lamotrigine had been unsuccessful.

My recent studies suggest that in nearly 40% of patients, seizures will not come under control with a single antiepileptic drug. It is therefore essential to develop therapeutic strategies for combining antiepileptic drugs in patients with difficult-to-control epilepsy. Without a detailed knowledge of the pathophysiology underlying seizure generation and propagation, it seems reasonable to choose drugs with different and potentially complementary modes of action. Attention also needs to be paid to the range of efficacy, side-effect profile, and propensity for adverse interaction. This strategy is particularly relevant for patients with learning disabilities, who often present with multiple seizure types and always represent a major management challenge. The best evidence in support of this approach has been provided by results with lamotrigine and valproate, which is universally regarded as a "synergistic" combination.

When taking the history from a patient with refractory epilepsy, the clinician must review not just previous attempts at single-drug therapy, but also what combinations of antiepileptic drugs (and in what dosages) have been tried. A range of different strategies should be used until the best outcome is obtained. Some patients respond best to three-drug combinations, particularly valproate, lamotrigine, and topiramate. The older agents clobazam and acetazolamide should not be forgotten. The aim should be seizure freedom unless there is a good reason to be less ambitious. Sometimes the patient and doctor need to take a "time out" from manipulations of antiepileptic drugs. Nevertheless, if at first you don't succeed, try, try and try again!

What did I learn from this case?

There is now an increasingly wide range of new antiepileptic drugs to try in addition to the traditional agents. Using these drugs in rational combinations results in substantial

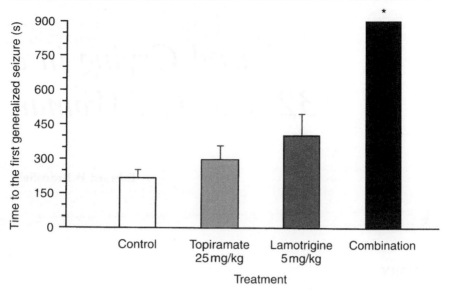

FIGURE 74.1   Effect of lamotrigine and topiramate singly and in combination in preventing pen-tylenetetrazol-induced seizures in adult Imperial Cancer Research mice.

improvement in seizure control in many more patients than ever before. I believe that both lamotrigine and topiramate contributed to the excellent outcome in this patient in a way that we do not yet fully understand. This sort of observation sets up a hypothesis that can be tested scientifically (Figure 74.1).

This patient represents one in a small series that has changed my clinical practice. We now have an ongoing research program exploring the use of adjunctive topiramate in patients with learning disability that involves a prospective baseline and predetermined end points. So far, 64 patients have been recruited to the study. The preliminary results look encouraging with 25% of patients being seizure-free.

FURTHER READING

Brodie MJ, French JA. Management of epilepsy in adolescents and adults. *Lancet* 2000;**356**:323–9.

Brodie MJ, Yuen AWC and the 105 Study Group. Lamotrigine substitution study: evidence for syner-gism with sodium valproate? *Epilepsy Res* 1997;**26**:423–32.

Dichter MA, Brodie MJ. New antiepileptic drugs. *N Engl J Med* 1996;**334**:1583–90.

Hannah JA, Brodie MJ. Epilepsy and learning disabilities: a challenge for the next millennium. *Seizure* 1998;**7**:3–13.

Kwan P, Brodie MJ. Early identification of refractory epilepsy. *N Engl J Med* 2000;**342**:314–9.

Stephen LJ, Sills GJ, Brodie MJ. Lamotrigine and topiramate may be a useful combination. *Lancet* 1998;**351**:958–9.

Stephen LJ, Sills GJ, Brodie MJ. Topiramate in refractory epilepsy: a prospective observational study. *Epilepsia* 2000;**41**:977–80.

c0075

Ictal Crying in a 32-Year-Old Woman

Edward B Bromfield

s0010

HISTORY

p0010

A 32-year-old woman, who had had a single febrile seizure at the age of 1, was well until a head-on motor vehicle collision at the age of 24, caused by another driver. She had 2-day retrograde amnesia and 5-day anterograde amnesia, subdural and subarachnoid hemorrhages, and bifrontal and left inferior temporal contusions.

p0020

She was treated prophylactically with antiepileptic drugs. She developed a rash from phenytoin and phenobarbital but not from carbamazepine. She later began having episodes of palpitations and a strange bodily sensation, followed by right upper and lower extremity paresthesias with nausea and inability to speak. These episodes lasted 1–2 min each. There was a sense of confusion, with variable preservation of comprehension and memory. Months later, when she had a prolonged confusional state that culminated in three convulsions, these episodes were recognized as seizures. Her dosage of carbamazepine was increased, but seizures persisted at a frequency of one or two a week. Lamotrigine was added but was then stopped when she had a second episode of status epilepticus. Gabapentin was added, possibly with some benefit, but later she was weaned off gabapentin in favor of valproate. Increasing doses of carbamazepine and valproate resulted in gastrointestinal distress, sedation, and dizziness without improvement in seizure control.

p0030

Despite residual naming and memory problems after rehabilitation, she was able to complete law school and pass the bar exam. She tried working for a law firm but had to resign, more because of seizures than cognitive limitations. She and her husband were highly motivated to have a child, although they were concerned about the potential risks of seizures and the patient's antiepileptic drug on the baby. The patient decided to attempt conversion to gabapentin monotherapy. This was accomplished over several months, with no change in seizure frequency or severity.

EXAMINATION AND INVESTIGATIONS

Examination was notable for mild dysnomia, right-sided clumsiness, and right hyper-reflexia. Neuropsychological testing demonstrated average global functioning, decreased naming, and memory deficits greater for verbal memory than for visuospatial memory.

A magnetic resonance imaging scan showed prominent central and cortical atrophy and two areas of encephalomalacia in the inferior left temporal lobe.

Inpatient video–EEG monitoring showed bilateral anterior–mid-temporal sharp waves and spikes occurring 20 times more frequently on the left than the right. After gabapentin was reduced, she had two complex partial seizures arising from the left anterior temporal lobe, the second of which generalized after 10 min. During the seizures, she held her left hand over her mouth, extended her right arm, and opened and closed the right hand; she appeared in profound distress and cried intermittently. Ictal single photon emission computed tomography showed marked hyperperfusion in the inferolateral left temporal region.

Subsequently, left temporal and frontoparietal subdural electrodes were implanted. Numerous interictal discharges and electrographic seizures were recorded from the left inferior temporal lobe. Because of the patient's reluctance to taper gabapentin aggressively, only one clinical seizure was recorded, showing a regional left inferior temporal onset. Language mapping showed interference with naming and reading when posterior temporal contacts were stimulated.

An intracarotid amobarbital test initially showed poor memory bilaterally. She recognized only two stimuli out of eight on left-sided injection and three out of eight on right-sided injection; however, she had profound shivering and anxiety during the left-sided injection. When this test was repeated during invasive monitoring, she recognized seven stimuli out of eight after left-sided injection.

DIAGNOSIS

Post-traumatic neocortical temporal lobe epilepsy.

TREATMENT AND OUTCOME

A tailored left temporal lobectomy was performed, using intraoperative language mapping and confirmatory electrocorticography. Pathological examination revealed neuronal loss and gliosis in the neocortex and hippocampus, together with focal neocortical hemosiderosis.

Three months after surgery, the patient's gabapentin was tapered and she had a secondarily generalized seizure. Gabapentin was increased, birth control was stopped, and she conceived within 1 month. She has since remained seizure-free except for a single aura during the second trimester of her pregnancy. One year after temporal lobectomy, she gave birth to a healthy baby boy. Repeat neuropsychological testing showed stable naming deficits and some memory improvement. She now works part-time for an advocacy organization.

s0050   COMMENTARY

p0120   This patient had post-traumatic left temporal lobe, neocortical epilepsy. Her seizures included prominent contralateral somatosensory manifestations, which probably reflected spread to the second sensory area in the frontal operculum. This area mediates sensation either contralaterally or bilaterally, often in the distal extremities.[1] She also had the unusual phenomenon of ictal crying.[2]

p0130   In the setting of phenytoin and possible phenobarbital allergies, partial response to gabapentin, and poor response to carbamazepine and valproate, the patient tolerated gradual conversion to gabapentin monotherapy without any increase in the frequency or severity of her seizures. Although gabapentin has shown efficacy as a sole agent,[3] it has not been systematically compared to other antiepileptic drugs, and meta-analyses have shown a lower response rate.[4]

p0140   Tailored left temporal lobectomy resulted in freedom from seizures, excluding an unsuccessful early postoperative attempt at medication reduction[5] that was done because of the patient's desire to minimize medications before conception.[6] Despite the multifocal nature of the insult, post-traumatic temporal lobe epilepsy can have a high surgical success rate.[7]

s0060   **What did I learn from this case?**

p0150   I learned that gabapentin monotherapy can be as effective as other drugs that are generally viewed as more potent. The case also reinforced the possibility of contralateral somatosensory symptoms and ictal crying as manifestations of temporal lobe (neocortical) epilepsy, and also the possibility of a good surgical outcome despite a known multifocal injury.

p0160   This patient also taught me how strongly a patient's desire to minimize risk during pregnancy can guide decision making, even with limited information. Finally, I realized how social supports and a realistic view of one's limitations and capacities can lead to excellent recovery from a potentially devastating injury.

s0070   **How did this case alter my approach to the care and treatment of my epilepsy patients?**

p0170   I am more likely now to view gabapentin monotherapy as a viable option in selected patients. I am also more positive about surgical and psychosocial prognosis after major head injury that leads to intractable epilepsy.

REFERENCES

1. Penfield W, Jasper H. *Epilepsy and the functional anatomy of the human brain.* Boston: Little, Brown, 1954.
2. Offen ML, Davidoff RA, Troost BT, Richley ET. Dacrystic epilepsy. *J Neurol Neurosurg Psychiatry* 1976;**39**:824–34.
3. Chadwick DW, Anhut H, Greiner MJ, *et al.* A double-blind trial of gabapentin monotherapy for newly diagnosed partial seizures. *Neurology* 1998;**51**:1282–8.

4. Chadwick DW, Marson T, Kadir Z. Clinical administration of new antiepileptic drugs: an overview of safety and efficacy. *Epilepsia* 1996;**37(suppl 6)**:S17–S22.
5. Schiller Y, Cascino GD, So EL, March WR. Discontinuation of antiepileptic drugs after successful epilepsy surgery. *Neurology* 2000;**54**:346–9.
6. Quality Standards Subcommittee, AAN. Practice parameter: management issues for women with epilepsy (summary statement). *Neurology* 1998;**51**:944–8.
7. Mathern GW, Babb TL, Vickrey B, Melendez M, Pretorius JK. Traumatic compared to non-traumatic clinical–pathologic associations in temporal lobe epilepsy. *Epilepsy Res* 1994;**4**:129–39.

Healing Begins with Communicating the Diagnosis

cOO

Orrin Devinsky

HISTORY

s001

The patient is a 48-year-old right-handed man with a history of atypical noctur-   p001
nal behaviors. There was a vague history that as a child he had episodes during sleep
that were similar to the recent episodes witnessed by his wife. The frequency and the
intensity of these events had increased over the past 5 years. He had been evaluated
by six neurologists, including two epileptologists, and had undergone two video–EEG
monitoring studies and three admissions to sleep disorder centers for polysomnography.
Various diagnoses were made, the most common of which was conversion disorder
with non-epileptic seizures.

During a 3-day inpatient video–EEG monitoring study that was conducted   p002
6 weeks before our initial evaluation, he had multiple nocturnal episodes. During a
typical episode, he awakened with return of posterior alpha-wave activity and then
suddenly grabbed his left knee, screaming in pain and calling for assistance as soon
as possible. Previous medical, rheumatological, and orthopedic evaluations of his left
knee were unremarkable. During some episodes, there was mild clonic activity in the
left upper extremity. The episodes were associated with intense emotional expression,
tachycardia, diaphoresis, facial flushing, and increased respiratory rate. The episodes
would occur over a period of 20–45 min. After the recent video–EEG monitoring
study he was sent home after a supportive discussion of non-epileptic conversion episodes and a recommendation for psychiatric counseling and possible psychopharmacology if an underlying mood disorder was identified. An anxiety disorder was also
considered.

The patient was seen in outpatient follow-up 2 weeks later, and both he and his   p003
wife were very resistant to the diagnosis of conversion disorder. During a prolonged
discussion he expressed his frustration with the medical system and what he perceived
as the lack of a clear answer despite very extensive testing. This reflected his failure to
accept the diagnosis of conversion non-epileptic events. He was admitted for another

video–EEG monitoring study to review his episodes and to look more carefully at his sleep activity to make certain that there was no evidence of an atypical parasomnia. However, before the admission he suffered an anterior wall myocardial infarction and underwent emergency angioplasty. He continued to have the nocturnal episodes, which were witnessed in the coronary care unit. A different group of neurologists was called in for consultation and thought that these episodes were psychiatric in origin. An additional neurologist suggested the diagnosis of an atypical Tourette's syndrome.

The patient was sent home. One week later he had another myocardial infarction in a different cardiac distribution and ruptured a papillary muscle, requiring emergency open heart surgery for mitral valve repair and three-vessel bypass. He continued to have the nocturnal episodes in the postoperative period, causing significant concerns that they would contribute to additional cardiac injury.

He was readmitted for video–EEG monitoring and again his atypical episodes were recorded. His alpha rhythm would return out of sleep and he would grab his left knee. He would then curse and scream. He would be belligerent toward the nursing staff who attended him, and was in a state of heightened sympathetic nervous system activity for a period of 20–45 min.

On discussion with the patient that there were no EEG correlates, he and his wife again became very upset and said, "We knew that already. What is the diagnosis? Don't tell us it is a conversion disorder."

A review of the literature revealed that some patients with panic disorder had their episodes exclusively limited to night-time, possibly accounting for up to 2.5% of all patients with panic disorder. This diagnosis was made and the biological nature of panic disorder was emphasized.

DIAGNOSIS

Panic disorder.

TREATMENT AND OUTCOME

The patient was started on clonazepam 0.5 mg at bedtime, which was increased to 1.0 mg at bedtime. He has been free of episodes since that time (12 weeks), with stable cardiovascular function.

COMMENTARY

This patient has episodes for which the ultimate diagnosis is still uncertain and controversial. This man, like many others, was very hesitant to accept the diagnosis of a conversion disorder, although it is likely that part of his disorder was attributable to that entity. However, the repeated presentation of this diagnosis to him and appropriate counseling did not lead to any improvement in his symptoms and unfortunately may have contributed to some of the stress that ultimately precipitated two myocardial infarctions and the need for angioplasty and open heart surgery.

What did I learn from this case?

s00!

The borderline between neurology and psychiatry is a shifting one. In this case, finding a biological explanation (panic disorder) that may not have been the best scientific
answer (or even a justifiable clinical explanation) was nonetheless clearly beneficial for
the patient's clinical condition and psychological well-being.

p01

How did this case alter my approach to the care and treatment of my epilepsy patients?

s006

I am now more willing to change my shift of attention and style of presentation to
patients and their families in a very individualized manner.

p01

An Unusual Case of Seizures and Violence

c0077

Robert S Fisher

HISTORY

s0010

The patient was a 24-year-old right-handed man with convulsions, postictal psychosis, and seizure-associated aggressive behavior. He had been well until the age of 11, when he developed viral encephalitis, which resulted in coma and acute seizures. No causative organism was isolated. He recovered, suffering only some residual short-term memory and attentional problems. Seizures recurred several months after the encephalitis. These were of a complex partial type, often with secondary generalization. The first warning of seizure onset was a sense of fear, followed by confusion, growling like a "caged bear," and hyperalertness. The patient would be unaware of conversation, and would not recall episodes that transpired during the seizures.

p0010

Seizure frequency increased over the next few years until he was having many seizures a week. By the age of 18, the patient was beginning to experience elements of postictal psychosis, with religious rumination and a sense that he was somehow "special" in the scheme of the world. Intrusive paranoid thoughts about people trying to harm him also were expressed during the postictal state. As time progressed, postictal psychosis became more frequent and more prolonged, and the patient did not return to a baseline normal psychiatric state between seizures.

p0020

By the age of 20, the patient would jump up during a seizure from a reclining or seated position and run across the room, sometimes slamming into objects and injuring himself. If he encountered people during his seizure, he might strike them or push them away. On one occasion, he physically lifted his father and hurled him into a wall. The most disturbing incident occurred when he had a seizure onset while sitting next to his mother, who was going through the day's mail. During the seizure, he picked a letter opener off the table, and stabbed his mother in the side. Fortunately, her physical injury was slight.

p0030

The patient was committed involuntarily to a hospital for the criminally insane, when no other facility would accept him. While in this hospital he attacked several of the other patients during seizures. During one seizure, he put his fist through a glass window and pulled back against a glass shard, cutting his hand severely. He then ran

p0040

around the room brandishing the shard. Following this behavior he was locked in a padded room in isolation.

EXAMINATION AND INVESTIGATIONS

The neurological examination fluctuated with proximity to a seizure. Within days of most seizures the patient showed an organic psychosis with religious preoccupation and failure to recognize place and time. At a time more than 1 week from a seizure, he was fully oriented, conversant, and without focal neurological signs, but depressed about his life circumstances. One seizure was observed in the clinic – he roared and then leapt up and out of the room. He ran straight down the clinic corridor toward an open door connecting with the clinical laboratory, screaming all the way. Laboratory phlebotomists heard and saw him coming and slammed the door shut. The patient ran forcibly into the closed door, slumped to the ground, and had a tonic–clonic convulsion.

Routine EEGs, video–EEG monitoring, and invasive recordings from eight electrodes (eight contacts on each) disclosed multifocal bilateral seizure onset in the temporal amygdalar and superior frontal regions, as well as diffuse interictal spiking. A magnetic resonance imaging scan showed no focal lesion and no specific mesial temporal sclerosis.

DIAGNOSIS

Multifocal partial epilepsy with postictal violence.

TREATMENT AND OUTCOME

Most of the usual seizure medications that were available at the time (before 1994) were tried, either without benefit or with intolerable side effects. Given the desperate and unusual nature of this case, a meeting was convened of the hospital ethics committee together with the parents (his legal guardians) to review all possible therapeutic options.

A decision was made to perform bilateral stereotaxic amygdalotomies, since both amygdalas appeared to be heavily involved in the origin of his seizures. The hippocampi were spared. This procedure was technically successful but completely ineffective against his epilepsy and provided no benefit for his postictal violence.

A decision then was made to perform stereotaxic radiofrequency lesions of the cingulate bundles bilaterally in the anterior superior medial frontal regions. The rationale for this procedure was two-fold:

- interruption of the spread of seizures via the circuit of Papez and the cingulum bundle and
- possible benefit of cingulotomy for intractable violence.

After the cingulotomies, the patient was lethargic and nearly mute for approximately 5 days. He then began to talk and became normally animated, appearing less depressed than before surgery. Memory and cognitive functions showed no decline from the preoperative (somewhat impaired) baseline.

After the cingulotomy, the patient's seizures and intermittent psychotic rumina- p0140
tions continued as before, but over 3 years of follow-up, none of the seizures led to
running or violent actions. He was released from hospital to home on conventional
antiepileptic and neuroleptic medications. One day, when sitting on the couch next to
his mother, he suddenly stood up, roared like a bear, then turned to her and said, "Just
kidding." She was not amused!

COMMENTARY s0050

People with epilepsy very rarely harm anyone but themselves during seizures.[1] A review p0150
of videotapes from 5400 people with epilepsy, including 19 with reported aggressive
behavior during seizures, showed violence during or after a seizure to be uncommon.[2]
The so-called epilepsy defense – claiming that a crime was due to epilepsy – is rarely
justified or effective,[3] although exceptions do occur.[4]

This was one of my most memorable cases as an exception to the rule of non- p0160
aggression during seizures. Even in this extreme instance, however, the aggression was
unfocused, non-directed, unplanned, and along the line of a striking out at anything in
the field of attention.

The association of aggression with postictal psychosis may not be coincidence, since p0170
at least one study[5] has found the risk for violent postictal behavior to be much higher
in those with postictal psychosis. Details of the seizures and EEG patterns may be less
important for assessing the risk of epilepsy-associated aggression than several variables
related to baseline psychopathology and cognitive ability.[6] These factors may also be of
key importance as well for interictal violence.[7]

The use of stereotaxic lesions to treat epilepsy in this context raises several con- p0180
troversial practical and ethical questions. Were we treating the patient's epilepsy, his
behavior or both? Was this a type of psychosurgery, a set of techniques with dubious
background?[8] Stereotaxic cingulotomy has been claimed to be effective for uncontrolled aggression, obsessive–compulsive disorder, and several other psychiatric conditions.[9] The ethics of such surgery were considered in this case, and the relevant ethical
issues have also been discussed in the medical literature.[10]

What did I learn from this case? s0060

Epilepsy is such a broad and varied family of disorders that blanket statements rarely p0190
hold true without exception. Most seizures do not precipitate violence, but some do.
Any violence is likely to be unplanned, undirected, and inadvertent. Unusual cases
call for "out-of-the-box" thinking about therapies. In such circumstances, help from
objective ethical review and human consent committees can help to make sure that
the actions that are taken are likely to be in the best interests of the patient.

How did this case alter my approach to the care and treatment of my epilepsy patients?

I advise families, friends, and health-care workers to be cautious in their delivery of
first aid to all delirious patients, including those in the midst of or in the wake of a

seizure. The best approach is usually one of gentle guidance, reorientation, and reassurance, rather than physical restraint.

REFERENCES

1. Fenwick P. The nature and management of aggression in epilepsy. *J Neuropsychiatry Clin Neurosci* 1989;**1**:418–25.
2. Delgado-Escueta AV, Mattson RH, King L, *et al.* Special report. The nature of aggression during epileptic seizures. *N Engl J Med* 1981;**305**:711–6.
3. Treiman DM. Violence and the epilepsy defense. *Neurol Clin* 1999;**17**:245–55.
4. Ramani V, Gumnit RJ. Intensive monitoring of epileptic patients with a history of episodic aggression. *Arch Neurol* 1981;**38**:570–1.
5. Kanemoto K, Kawasaki J, Mori E. Violence and epilepsy: a close relation between violence and postictal psychosis. *Epilepsia* 1999;**40**:107–9.
6. Mendez MF, Doss RC, Taylor JL. Interictal violence in epilepsy. Relationship to behavior and seizure variables. *J Nerv Ment Dis* 1993;**181**:566–9.
7. Devinsky O, Bear D. Varieties of aggressive behavior in temporal lobe epilepsy. *Am J Psychiatry* 1984;**141**:651–6.
8. Diering SL, Bell WO. Functional neurosurgery for psychiatric disorders: a historical perspective. *Stereotact Funct Neurosurg* 1991;**57**:175–94.
9. Ballantine HT Jr, Bouckoms AJ, Thomas EK, Giriunas IE. Treatment of psychiatric illness by stereotactic cingulotomy. *Biol Psychiatry* 1987;**22**:807–19.
10. Bouckoms AJ. Ethics of psychosurgery. *Acta Neurochir Suppl (Wien)* 1988;**44**:173–8.

c0078

Attacks of Generalized Shaking without Postictal Confusion

James S Grisolia

HISTORY

s0010

A 36-year-old woman was admitted for dilatation and curettage following a sponta- p0010
neous abortion. This was one of multiple miscarriages in her attempt to have a child
with her husband. After the procedure, she began to have multiple attacks of generalized shaking that lasted about 30s each. Although the patient appeared unconscious
during each attack, she often reported the sense of being able to hear health personnel
talking during the attacks, and she suffered no postictal change whatsoever.

The patient had already received diazepam 10mg intravenously followed by phenyt- p0020
oin 1g intravenously before neurological consultation. There was a previous history of
rare apparent faints with a few tonic movements, generally occurring perimenstrually,
and a history of multiple sclerosis, with minor residual coordination loss in the right leg.

EXAMINATION AND INVESTIGATIONS

s0020

The patient was somnolent owing to the effect of the intravenous medications, but she p0030
was easy to rouse. There was nystagmus in all directions of movement, which had not
been present during the examination on admission. The remainder of the neurological examination was remarkable only for reduced rapid alternating movements in the
right foot, which from the history was a residual effect of her multiple sclerosis.

The patient's EEG, blood pressure, and cardiac rhythm were monitored during the p0040
episodes. No changes were seen in any studies.

DIAGNOSIS

s0030

Psychogenic pseudoseizures. p0050

s0040

TREATMENT AND OUTCOME

p0060

The patient was gently confronted with the fact that these attacks were "stress-induced" attacks rather than "epileptic" attacks. She offered the observation that as she went into each attack, she had a feeling that she was "going away," just as she would "go away" when her mother beat her when she was a little girl.

p0070

Further inquiry established that she had a very difficult and stressful relationship with her mother, who subjected her to emotional and physical abuse. Sexual abuse by the mother or anyone else was denied. When offered the suggestion that her miscarriage undoubtedly was a significant acute stressor, she agreed, saying that she and her husband very much wanted children. I suggested that her maternal desire might include a desire to repair the relationship with her own mother by a healthy relationship with her own daughter, and that the frustration of this desire by the miscarriage might have triggered the "going away" response from her youth. The patient looked astonished for an instant, then readily agreed. I offered the hope that now that she understood the process and its origins, she was unlikely to have further pseudoseizures.

p0080

Under the vicissitudes of managed care, she was lost to follow up until 6 years later, when she was referred back to me for follow-up of her stable multiple sclerosis. In the interim, she and her husband had weathered five miscarriages to have a lovely daughter. On occasion, she has had rare attacks conforming to a clinical diagnosis of convulsive syncope, but has never had sustained shaking or repetitive attacks.

s0050

COMMENTARY

p0090

The association of psychogenic pseudoseizures with early life trauma is now well recognized. However, pseudoseizure cases that are commonly encountered in clinical practice demonstrate significant psychiatric morbidity, conforming to diagnoses of borderline personality organization, somatization disorder or other character pathology. Overall, the pathologies associated with early life trauma form a complex spectrum, with well-established neuroendocrine and cognitive pathologies still under study.

p0100

The profound character pathology associated with many pseudoseizure patients frustrates all clinicians. While much of this pathology arises from the original trauma and the reaction to it, prolonged ineffective treatment of pseudoseizures could contribute significantly to learned dependency, somatic preoccupations, depression, and distrust of health-care providers.

s0060

What did I learn from this case?

p0110

This patient was unique in presenting as a high-functioning person who responded to an acute psychodynamic intervention, with apparent cure over a very long follow-up. Her case follows a less complicated psychodynamic conversion paradigm, responding to a traditional "talking cure."

How did this case alter my approach in the care and treatment of my patients with epilepsy?

s0070

My experience with this patient has encouraged me to attempt to diagnose pseudo-seizures early, rather than at the end of a long, failed course of multiple medications. While direct intervention is usually unlikely to be as successful as it was in this case, I try to clarify the difference between "epileptic" and "stress-induced" seizures for the patient and the family, attempting to impart this opinion in a manner that is congenial with their medical beliefs and understanding. I avoid distinguishing between "real" and "fake" seizures. The revelation that anticonvulsants and emergency trips to the hospital are unavailing comes as good news to some and as a threat to others. When there is significant character pathology, maintaining supportive contact with the patient appears valuable, both to avoid a fresh round of misdiagnosis and to provide reassurance to psychotherapists and others involved in the patient's care.

p0120

FURTHER READING

Arnold LM, Privitera MD. Psychopathology and trauma in epileptic and psychogenic seizure patients. *Psychosomatics* 1996;**37**:438–43.

Krumholz A. Nonepileptic seizures: diagnosis and management. *Neurology* 1999;**53(suppl 2)**:576–83.

Lesser RP. Psychogenic seizures. *Neurology* 1996;**46**:1499–507.

Van der Kolk BA, Pelcovitz D, Roth S, *et al.* Dissociation, somatization and affect dysregulation: the complexity of adaptation to trauma. *Am J Psychiatry* 1996;**153**:83–93.

c0079

Lennox–Gastaut Syndrome with Good Outcome Associated with Perisylvian Polymicrogyria

Marilisa M Guerreiro

s0010
HISTORY

p0010
A 10-year-old right-handed boy had a history of dysarthria and seizures. He started having seizures at 3 years of age. They began with generalized tonic–clonic seizures. After a couple of weeks he started having drop-attacks and absence spells, which progressively increased in frequency, occurring up to 50–60 a day.

p0020
He was diagnosed with Lennox–Gastaut syndrome and underwent several unsuccessful trials of valproate, clobazam, phenobarbital, clonazepam, phenytoin, carbamazepine, and lamotrigine. Excellent control was finally achieved with topiramate 200 mg/day; for the past 4 years, he has averaged one generalized tonic–clonic seizure a year.

p0030
He was born after an uneventful pregnancy. Delivery was normal. Psychomotor development was borderline (walking at 18 months) but speech development was delayed. He has marked dysarthria and has a history of choking and feeding difficulties during infancy. He also has a history of learning disabilities but made progress in his studies and now attends a regular class, two grades behind the expected level for his age.

p0040
His younger brother is followed by a speech therapist and his mother has articulation problems under stress.

s0020
EXAMINATION AND INVESTIGATIONS

p0050
On examination, he presented with striking dysarthria, drooling, moderate restriction of tongue movements (he is unable to protrude his tongue completely), difficulty in

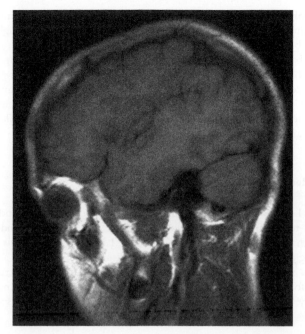

FIGURE   79.1   Sagittal T1-weighted   image   showing   diffuse   polymicrogyria   around   the   f0010
sylvian fissure.

whistling and blowing, and an abnormally brisk jaw jerk. Deep tendon reflexes were
hyperactive. The remainder of the neurological examination was normal.

Brain magnetic resonance imaging (MRI) revealed bilateral perisylvian polymicrogyria (Figure 79.1). His brother had asymmetrical perisylvian polymicrogyria on MRI
and his mother had similar, unilateral findings.

DIAGNOSIS

Lennox–Gastaut syndrome due to perisylvian polymicrogyria.

COMMENTARY

The main features of perisylvian syndrome are pseudobulbar palsy, cognitive deficits, and
epilepsy. The variability of the clinical picture is remarkable. Not all patients present with
all the main features. On the contrary, they may present with soft signs, as was the case in
this patient's mother. She had no complaints and had never been examined. Dysarthric
speech seems to be the main feature of this syndrome, and it occurs in approximately
75% of patients. Variable cognitive deficits and epilepsy occur in 50–75% of patients.

Imaging findings show a broad spectrum of abnormalities. Unilateral polymicrogyria correlates with milder or absent pseudobulbar signs, and bilateral, extensive

anatomic involvement correlates with worse pseudobulbar symptoms and signs. Bilateral asymmetric lesions may be present in affected people even though malformations may not be detectable with current MRI techniques.

A genetic basis in some patients with cortical dysplasia is becoming increasingly apparent. Band heterotopia or the double cortex syndrome and bilateral periventricular nodular heterotopia have been associated with X-linked transmission. Perisylvian syndrome may be familial. In this case it appears to be genetically heterogeneous. There are some families in which autosomal dominance is the most likely mode of inheritance; patterns in other families suggest X-linked transmission.

What did I learn from this case?

I learnt that Lennox–Gastaut syndrome may be medically treated and sometimes responds well to treatment with antiepileptic drugs. It is an age-dependent epilepsy syndrome with many different possible etiologies. I believe its prognosis depends on the underlying cause more than on the treatment itself.

In addition, we are learning that cortical dysgenesis comprises a spectrum of developmental malformations with different intrinsic epileptogenicity according to the specific pathology. Polymicrogyria probably stands on the benign side of this spectrum.

FURTHER READING

Guerreiro MM, Andermann E, Guerrini R, et al. Familial perisylvian polymicrogyria: a new familial syndrome of cortical maldevelopment. Ann Neurol 2000;48:39–48.

Kuzniecky R, Andermann F, Guerrini R, et al. Congenital bilateral perisylvian syndrome: study of 31 patients. Lancet 1993;341:608–12.

Palmini A, Gambardella A, Andermann F, et al. Intrinsic epileptogenicity of human dysplastic cortex as suggested by corticography and surgical results. Ann Neurol 1995;37:476–87.

Temporal Lobe Resection in a Patient with Severe Psychiatric Problems

c0080

Reetta Kälviäinen

HISTORY

s0010

A 40-year-old right-handed woman had suffered from asphyxia at birth and began to have frequent epileptic seizures from the first day of her life.

p0010

At first the seizures were generalized tonic–clonic seizures, but later the dominant seizure type was complex partial seizures with *déjà vu* and amnesia lasting for 1–2 min. While amnestic, the patient usually had orofacial automatisms and sometimes rhythmic movements with her right lower extremity.

p0020

During childhood the patient had suffered from difficult-to-control seizures and was overprotected by her parents. However, she became independent when her generalized seizures were controlled with dual therapy with carbamazepine and valproate. Because she still had one or two complex partial seizures a month, she was offered surgical evaluation, but she refused.

p0030

She married and had two children, and eventually she owned her own small firm. Suddenly, at the age of 30, she suffered a series of six generalized seizures, became psychotic, and was hospitalized. The psychotic episode relapsed after 1 year and the patient became severely depressed, requiring treatment with high-dose neuroleptics, antidepressants, and benzodiazepines.

p0040

The patient had to give up working. Her husband left her, taking their children. She had to move back in with her father, who had not coped well with her epilepsy when she was a child. Moreover, he abused alcohol.

p0050

When she was 37, she was put on olanzapine and the dosages of her other psychoactive drugs were reduced.

p0060

EXAMINATION AND INVESTIGATIONS

s0020

The patient underwent a surgical evaluation at the age of 38. Magnetic resonance imaging (MRI) clearly revealed left-sided hippocampal sclerosis. Additionally, the posterior

p0070

part of the left hemisphere was smaller than the right and there was white matter hyperintensity behind the trigonum consistent with the history of asphyxia at birth.

Multiple interictal scalp EEGs had been performed over the years, demonstrating left temporal abnormalities. During video–EEG monitoring, only one complex partial seizure was recorded. Although she stared motionlessly, there were no EEG changes. Subsequently left temporal sharp theta activity was recorded. Interictally, sharp theta activity was also recorded maximally from the region of the left sphenoidal electrode. Difficulties in memory tasks were predominantly verbal; no frontal deficits were seen.

DIAGNOSIS

Mesial temporal lobe epilepsy.

TREATMENT AND OUTCOME

The patient's psychiatrist felt that she needed full psychiatric support but was capable of going through epilepsy surgery. Her antiepileptic drug regimen was optimized before surgery with carbamazepine, topiramate, and clobazam. She remained on olanzapine and had frequent discussions with psychiatrists.

A left hippocampectomy and amygdalectomy were performed at the age of 39. Pathologic analysis of the resected tissue demonstrated severe focal neuronal loss in the hippocampus. In the first year after surgery, she had no seizures, moved to her own apartment, and started to work again.

COMMENTARY

This case shows that MRI is helpful in selecting optimal candidates for surgical treatment of temporal lobe epilepsy. Before high-resolution MRI was available, surgical candidates frequently required invasive EEG monitoring with depth or strip electrodes in the temporal lobe.

More recently, preoperative investigations have been limited to scalp EEG monitoring, MRI, neuropsychologic testing, and – at some centers – positron emission tomography or single photon emission computed tomography. This is a significant advance, particularly for patients like this woman who have MRI evidence of hippocampal pathology and who do not have to undergo invasive monitoring, which might have predisposed her to the possible psychiatric complications of long-term subdural or depth EEG monitoring.

What did I learn from this case?

The relative contraindications to epilepsy surgery include interictal psychosis, persistent interictal thought disturbance or depression, and severely dysfunctional family dynamics. My patient did suffer from all of these conditions, yet I still believed that many of these problems were related to her intractable mesial temporal lobe epilepsy. Fortunately, her temporal lobe epilepsy could be clearly and effectively localized, and she did in fact benefit from surgery. Consistent with my impression, her seizure control and also her behavioral situation and overall quality of life improved.

FURTHER READING

Engel J, Shewmon DA. Who should be considered a surgical candidate? In: Engel J, ed. *Surgical treatment of the epilepsies*. New York: Raven Press, 1993: 23–34.

Flor-Henry P. Ictal and interictal psychiatric manifestations in epilepsy: specific or nonspecific? A critical review of some of the evidence. *Epilepsia* 1972;**13**:767–72.

Thadani VM, Williamson PD, Berger R, *et al*. Successful epilepsy surgery without intracranial EEG recording: criteria for patient selection. *Epilepsia* 1995;**36**:7–15.

Trimble M. *The psychoses of epilepsy*. New York: Raven Press, 1991.

An Open Mind Can Benefit the Patient

c00*

Kaarkuzhali Babu Krishnamurthy

HISTORY

s001

A 35-year-old right-handed woman had a history of recurrent seizures since the age of 2. She was the product of a full term, uneventful pregnancy and delivery, and she achieved her developmental milestones at the appropriate ages. At first, her seizures were associated with high fever, but they later began occurring without fever. A typical seizure for her began with an aura of a bad taste, followed by nausea and a rising abdominal sensation. This would progress to loss of awareness, during which she would run or wander. She could converse relatively normally during the postictal period, but was quite aggressive and amnesic. Bystanders often mistook her postictal behavior for drunkenness and assumed she was mentally ill.

She completed high school, but could not begin college or hold down any type of employment. She was married briefly, and was the sole parent of a 6-year-old child. She had tried eight antiepileptic drugs in monotherapy and combinations without improvement in her seizure frequency. A magnetic resonance imaging (MRI) scan revealed a left frontal lobe heterotopia.

p002

She was referred to me for a presurgical evaluation. At the time of my initial evaluation, she was experiencing between 6 and 12 seizures a month.

p003

EXAMINATION AND INVESTIGATIONS

s0020

Surface video–EEG monitoring demonstrated independent, bitemporal interictal discharges. Clinical seizures were poorly localized. Neuropsychological testing suggested subtle left frontal dysfunction.

p004

Since there was lack of concordance between her clinical and EEG data, the patient underwent depth electrode monitoring. The onset of her clinical seizures localized to the right amygdala, but the ictal activity then spread rapidly to the left hippocampus. Electrical stimulation through the implanted depth electrode in the right amygdala

p005

reproduced her clinical symptoms without affecting her EEG, while stimulation through the left hippocampal electrode produced some EEG changes without reproducing her clinical symptoms.

DIAGNOSIS

Right temporal lobe epilepsy and left frontal heterotopia.

TREATMENT AND OUTCOME

The patient underwent a right temporal lobectomy. Pathological examination of the resected tissue was consistent with hippocampal sclerosis. During the year that elapsed after our initial meeting, her father was diagnosed with Alzheimer's disease, her mother developed breast cancer, and a close male friend was diagnosed with testicular cancer.

Since the lobectomy, she has been maintained on carbamazepine monotherapy. Approximately twice a year, she attempts to decrease her dose by 100–200 mg/day, which inevitably leads to breakthrough seizures. Otherwise, she has been seizure-free. Neuropsychological testing 18 months after surgery revealed only a mild decline in her nonverbal memory compared to presurgery performance, which was not an unexpected finding. After completing a vocational rehabilitation program, she went to work as an office manager and executive secretary. Most recently, she began a romantic relationship with a man whom she met at a self-help program and is contemplating marriage and, perhaps, pregnancy.

COMMENTARY

This patient's life was complicated by seizures as well as difficult social and family situations, which became exacerbated during the period leading up to her surgery. She did not have the support system in place to help her through the presurgical evaluation and recovery period. However, with the input of the epilepsy treatment team, we concluded that her social situation was likely to get significantly worse in the near future because of the nature of the illnesses of her parents and friend, and that her loved ones would be happier knowing that she was helping herself.

What did I learn from this case?

This case serves as a nice reminder that dual pathology can occur in epilepsy. Her clinical semiology was strongly suggestive of a temporal focus, but the presence of the left frontal heterotopia was what prompted her referral for a surgical evaluation. Fortunately, we pursued invasive monitoring to clarify the picture, because resection of the appropriate region resulted in a significant improvement in seizure control and overall quality of life. This is contrary to suggestions in the literature that resection of the lesion as well as the epileptic focus are important. In this woman's situation, however, resection of the visible lesion would probably have resulted in some loss of motor function. Thus, we must treat the patient as an individual, distinct from group statistics in the literature.

The second significant point for me is that, while psychosocial support is very important for patients considering epilepsy surgery, there is no absolute level of support quality or quantity that should determine whether to proceed to surgery. I initially considered this patient's unfortunate home situation to be a contraindication for surgery. I was convinced, however, by her epilepsy nurse specialist that the time of anticipated surgery was likely to be a "calmer" period in this patient's life than the next few months.

How did this case alter my approach to the care and treatment of my epilepsy patients?

I now keep a very open mind when working with patients who are considering epilepsy surgery. Before resorting to neuroimaging or EEG monitoring, I find it most helpful to localize seizure onset based on a description of the seizures by the patient or witnesses. Then, if the MRI data does not match the localization as predicted by the clinical features of the patient's seizures, I am reminded by this case that the presence of a single visible lesion does not preclude a second lesion, perhaps not apparent on the MRI, that may be responsible for the patient's epilepsy.

I value the multidisciplinary approach to epilepsy surgery that I am able to provide patients. Having epilepsy nurse specialists and social workers advise me about the pros and cons of the timing of epilepsy surgery was the key to this patient's successful outcome. If my original view had prevailed, her surgery would have been delayed and she might not have been able to rise above her grief.

FURTHER READING

Li LM, Cendes F, Andermann F, et al. Surgical outcome in patients with epilepsy and dual pathology. *Brain* 1999;**122**:799–805.

Clarke DB, Olivier A, Andermann F, Fish D. Surgical treatment of epilepsy: the problem of lesion/focus incongruence. *Surg Neurol* 1996;**46**:579–85.

An Unexpected Lesson

c0082

Paul M Levisohn

HISTORY

s0010

I first met G, an almost 3-year-old boy from southern Colorado, on July 5, 1995. He p0010
and his family were referred to me for treatment of his poorly controlled epilepsy.
G had experienced his first seizure 2 years earlier, just short of his first birthday. Like
most families, his parents sought an explanation for his seizures that had meaning to
them;[1] they believed at the time that his seizure had occurred because of a fall and
bump to the head.

Five months later, G experienced two further seizures, both with generalized motor p0020
activity. He was started on phenobarbital, which proved ineffective, as would many other
antiepileptic drugs. He experienced frequent seizures as well as several episodes of status epilepticus despite serial treatment with carbamazepine, valproate, and clonazepam.
Associated symptoms included insomnia, irritability, and severe language delay. He was
treated with melatonin and chloral hydrate for sleep and carnitine for potential valproate
toxicity. Episodes of status epilepticus were treated with rectally administered diazepam.

Seizures became more complex. He experienced events that began with behavioral p0030
arrest, followed by lateralized automatisms and tonic eye deviation to either side, perhaps more frequently to the left. Other less well-defined spells also occurred. Trials of
other antiepileptic drugs, including investigational medications, proved ineffective.

Developmental testing at the age of 2 years demonstrated severe language delays p0040
but otherwise normal developmental functioning. However, his language had deteriorated as his seizures became more frequent; over time, there were concerns regarding
more extensive developmental delays.

EXAMINATION AND INVESTIGATIONS

s0020

Multiple EEGs were all normal. Imaging studies revealed a benign congenital arachnoid p0050
cyst in the right temporal fossa. In October 1996, an evaluation for possible resective
epilepsy surgery was initiated. Video–EEG monitoring suggested lateralization to the
right hemisphere both in seizure semiology and EEG, although localization was unclear.
Ictal single photon emission computed tomography (SPECT) study demonstrated

multifocal areas of abnormal activity. A positron emission tomography (PET) scan revealed hypometabolism on the right, including the frontal cortex, the temporal cortex, and the parietal cortex.

s0030   ## DIAGNOSIS

p0060   Medically refractory seizures (right hemisphere onset) with developmental delay.

s0040   ## TREATMENT AND OUTCOME

p0070   Before initiating further workup for surgery, the family wanted to try the ketogenic diet. The diet resulted in a 3-week seizure-free interval. However, daily seizures then resumed; the seizures were now predominantly asymmetric tonic seizures, along with occasional seizures with a Jacksonian march. He also began to experience episodes of left Todd's paresis and dysphasia.

p0080   At about this time, his parents divorced, an event which surprised my staff and me since both parents had always attended clinic together with him on a regular (and frequent) basis and seemed to work extremely well together as they sought what was best for their son.

p0090   In June 1998 (4 years after he had experienced his first seizure), G underwent a craniotomy for placement of subdural grid electrodes. The study confirmed that many of his seizures were of right frontal origin although the site of onset of others was undefined. Recognizing that a "cure" was unlikely, his parents nevertheless agreed to proceed with a right frontal lobectomy. They reasoned that perhaps his most troublesome seizures, those leaving him with an increasing amount of left hemiparesis, would resolve.

p0100   Unfortunately, the surgery had little impact on G's epilepsy. His subsequent course was punctuated by status epilepticus with associated liver failure from which he gradually recovered; a fractured left arm from a fall related to ataxia (a residual effect of his almost fatal bout of status epilepticus and hepatic failure); poor weight gain, and significant neurobehavioral dysfunction that was suggestive of pervasive developmental disorder. A vagus nerve stimulator was placed in July 1998 but appeared to have little impact. His parents requested that the stimulator be removed. However, shortly after turning the stimulator off, his parents noted that his seizures and behavior worsened and stimulation was reinstituted at low current settings. Clobazam was introduced in May 1999 after all commercially available antiepileptic drugs had been tried without success.

p0110   Whether because of this unusual combination of vagus nerve stimulation and clobazam or because of the "natural history" of his disorder, G's epilepsy has recently improved. Most of his seizures now occur in sleep and there are no significant postictal residua. His behavior and learning, although still significantly impaired, have improved and he has developed limited language abilities. His mother has completed her bachelor's degree despite developing and apparently surviving ovarian cancer.

p0120   Both parents attend clinic together with G despite their divorce. They clearly have agreed to work together to do whatever is necessary for their son. I have suggested treatment with some of the newest antiepileptic drugs but they are not anxious to make any changes at this time. G is doing reasonably well and they have no desire to "upset the apple cart."

COMMENTARY s0050

Most of us, I believe, see G's story as a tragedy. A previously normal child develops epilepsy just before his first birthday and despite aggressive treatment with the new tools available for patients with intractable epilepsy, he experiences the full brunt of this disorder – progressive cognitive dysfunction, medication toxicity, injury, nearly fatal status epilepticus, and hepatic failure. His parents, too, have born the impact of his disorder, in addition to their divorce and the mother's illness. p0130

Even so, I always look forward to visits from G and his family. His parents are intelligent and warm people who are active participants in their son's care. They welcome my advice and heed my recommendations, but only when it appears appropriate within the context of their lives. They bear no obvious malice or anger for the troubles that their son has experienced. They do not see their son's life or their own lives as tragic. p0140

G has been my teacher. He has tested my skills and learning as I have struggled to deal with his seizures and their impact. In his few years, he has become a textbook of epilepsy treatment at the end of the 20th century – from phenobarbital, the oldest of the antiepileptic drugs, to clobazam, an unapproved drug in the USA, from the ketogenic diet to vagus nerve stimulation, from magnetic resonance imaging to functional imaging, he has run the gauntlet. Because of G, I have been forced to rethink what I thought I knew. PET and SPECT studies suggested that resective surgery might indeed result in seizure control, despite the lack of an identifiable lesion.[2–4] However, when intracranial monitoring failed to define a single zone of ictal onset, my goal for resective epilepsy surgery for G was modified from full control of seizures to improved control, a goal accepted by his parents. (Taylor et al.[5] provide a discussion about adjusting one's hoped-for outcomes from epilepsy surgery.) p0150

Although I am unconvinced about the role of the ketogenic diet in children with localization-related epilepsy, I was willing to try the diet and have done so subsequently with greater success. At the time of his vagus nerve stimulator implant, G was the youngest child who had been implanted at my hospital and he was the only one from whom I have removed the stimulator.[6] As we have tried to help G, his parents have actively participated in his care, asking appropriate questions, and carefully responding to my recommendations. p0160

What did I learn from this case? s0060

G's journey has been mine also, and I am a better physician because of him. The most important lesson I have learned from G and his family has nothing to do with pharmacology or neurophysiology. Rather, it is that as a physician, I have a limited ability to truly alter some patients' lives. If all goes well, I can significantly help children and families with the new tools that are available to me. But for too many children, this is not possible. p0170

And I wonder at the responses of so many families. The families who do best despite apparently tragic circumstances seem to grow in strength under their burden. They bring to life the words of Emily Pearl Kingsley, the mother of a child with Down's syndrome, who wrote a brief essay entitled "Welcome to Holland" in 1987 (reprinted with permission).

Welcome to Holland

p0190   I am often asked to describe the experience of raising a child with disability – to try to help people who have not shared that unique experience to understand it, to imagine how it would feel. It's like this…

p0200   When you're going to have a baby, it's like planning a fabulous vacation trip – to Italy. You buy a bunch of guidebooks and make your wonderful plans. The Coliseum. The Michelangelo. David. The gondolas in Venice. You may learn some handy phrases in Italian. It's all very exciting.

p0210   After months of eager anticipation, the day finally arrives. You pack your bags and off you go. Several hours later, the plane lands. The stewardess comes in and says, "Welcome to Holland."

p0220   "Holland?!?" you say. "What do you mean Holland?? I signed up for Italy. I'm supposed to be in Italy. All my life I've dreamed of going to Italy."

p0230   But there's been a change in the flight plan. They've landed in Holland and there you must stay.

p0240   The important thing is that they haven't taken you to a horrible, disgusting, filthy place, full of pestilence, famine, and disease. It's just a different place.

p0250   So you must go out and buy new guidebooks. And you must learn a whole new language. And you will meet a whole new group of people you would never have met.

p0260   It's just a different place. It's a slower pace than Italy, less flashy than Italy. But after you've been there a while and you catch your breath, you look around… and you begin to notice that Holland has windmills… and Holland has tulips. Holland even has Rembrandts.

p0270   But everyone you know is busy coming and going from Italy… and they are all bragging about what a wonderful time they had there. And for the rest of your life, you will say, "Yes, that's where I was supposed to go. That's what I had planned."

p0280   And the pain of that will never, ever, ever go away… because the loss of that dream is a very, very significant loss.

p0290   But… if you spend your life mourning the fact that you didn't get to Italy, you may never be free to enjoy the very special, the very lovely things… about Holland.

How did this case alter my approach to the care and treatment of my epilepsy patients?

p0300   Because of G, I too have arrived in a different place. I now know that while in my head I am a neurologist, in my heart I am a pediatrician. I recognize that too often treating epilepsy in children like G will not result in a cure and so for them my goals have to change.

p031   Treating chronic illness is not something I was taught by my professors during my training and I suspect it is rarely taught even today, except by children like G. To treat chronic illness effectively, we must listen to our patients' stories, their narratives.[1] We must not only treat diseases of the nervous system but also illnesses of the whole person.[7] Outcomes cannot be measured only by percentage of seizure reduction or even by quantitative measures of "health-related quality of life."[8] Rather, it is by listening to our patients, to their hopes and goals, that we can most help them live in "Holland."

p032C   I only hope that in my role as teacher and mentor, I can transmit to students and residents everything that G has taught me.

REFERENCES

1. Good BJ, Del Vecchio Good MJ. In the subjunctive mode: epilepsy narratives in Turkey. *Soc Sci Med* 1994;**38**:835–42.
2. Resnick T, Duchowny M, Jayakar P. Early surgery for epilepsy: redefining candidacy. *J Child Neurol* 1994;**9(suppl 2)**:S36–S41.
3. Juhasz C, Chugani DC, Muzik O, *et al.* Is epileptogenic cortex truly hypometabolic on interictal positron emission tomography? *Ann Neurol* 2000;**48**:88–96.
4. Chugani HT. Imaging: anatomic and functional. In: Wallace S, ed. *Epilepsy in children.* Cambridge: Chapman & Hall, 1995: 483–506.
5. Taylor DC, Neville BGR, Cross JH. New measure of outcome needed for the surgical treatment of epilepsy. *Epilepsia* 1997;**38**:625–30.
6. Crumrine PK. Vagal nerve stimulation in children. *Semin Pediatr Neurol* 2000;**7**:216–23.
7. Cassell E. Illness and disease. *Hastings Center Report* 1976;**6**:27–37.
8. Vickrey BG, Hays R, Engel J, *et al.* Outcome assessment for epilepsy surgery: the impact of measuring health-related quality of life. *Ann Neurol* 1995;**37**:158–66.

When Surgery Is Not Possible, All Hope Is Not Lost

Cassandra I Mateo and Brian Litt

HISTORY

A 31-year-old left-handed single white man was well until 1991, when he fell off a bunk and landed on a concrete floor. He experienced loss of consciousness and amnesia after the fall and had a generalized convulsive seizure 2 days later.

The patient began to have generalized convulsive seizures every other week, with occasional seizure-free periods of 2–3 weeks. There were also brief periods when he had flurries of seizures every other day. He denied auras. Soon after this time he began to experience complex partial seizures. During these events he was noticed to stare and look around with a blank stare on his face; sometimes he would get up and say the words "hike, hike" at the beginning of these events. Family members noted that he would tap on his legs and body with his hands at times. Complex partial seizures routinely lasted from between 15 s and 1 min. The patient was usually confused postictally and felt weak after the seizures. On average, complex partial seizures occurred approximately every other week. Of note, the patient was often able to speak, though unintelligibly, throughout his seizures.

Past medical history was not significant, other than his history of epilepsy. He was the normal product of a full-term gestation and was actually delivered 1 week postdate. The patient was delivered by caesarean section because of failure to progress. No hospital stay was required. The patient reached his motor and verbal milestones at appropriate ages and was a good student in school. There was no history of febrile convulsions, meningitis, or encephalitis during infancy.

He left school after the tenth grade and then pursued his graduate equivalency degree. He works as a cashier and lives alone. He has relatively few social contacts and has been primarily concerned with getting rid of his seizures so that he could improve his life situation and pursue more rewarding employment. There is no history of drug or alcohol use.

Prior medication trials included maximally tolerated doses of phenytoin, carbamazepine, valproate, lamotrigine, topiramate, and gabapentin. Medications at the time of the patient's initial visit were phenytoin and valproate.

EXAMINATION AND INVESTIGATIONS

The patient's general, cardiological, and neurological examinations were unremarkable. Previous routine EEGs demonstrated left temporal spikes. Magnetic resonance imaging showed no evidence of hippocampal sclerosis or focal lesion. The patient had been previously recorded in the epilepsy-monitoring unit at an outside hospital, where he experienced 13 seizures that were poorly localized, although it was suggested that seizures arose from the left hemisphere. Anterior to mid-temporal epileptiform discharges (at electrodes F7 and T3) were noted interictally. The patient then underwent epilepsy monitoring with intracranial electrodes, which did not define an operable ictal onset zone, owing to technical limitations of the procedure.

The patient was subsequently referred to our center for evaluation. He was admitted for scalp–sphenoidal monitoring, now 1 year after his phase II monitoring. This demonstrated frequent left anterior temporal spike discharges, maximum in amplitude at the left sphenoidal electrode. An ictal EEG showed poorly localized seizures, sometimes with bitemporal onset although usually with greater field seen over the left temporal region.

A positron emission tomography scan showed mild left temporal hypometabolism. Neuropsychological evaluation showed a full-scale IQ of 90, perceptual organization index 99 and verbal comprehension 86, demonstrating subtle language and verbal memory impairment that could be localized to the left temporal region. An amytal test demonstrated his speech to be in the left hemisphere and that the right hemisphere was capable of supporting memory.

The case was discussed in surgical conference and it was felt that the patient was an appropriate candidate for phase II evaluation with bilateral intrahippocampal depth electrodes and a large frontotemporal grid including subtemporal and subfrontal strips on the left side (Figure 83.1).

Depth electrodes were implanted without event. Seizures were recorded after medication taper. These demonstrated widespread onset in the left anterior frontal, lateral temporal, and posterior frontal regions (Figure 83.2).

DIAGNOSIS

Medically refractory partial seizures, poorly localized to left frontal and temporal lobes.

TREATMENT AND OUTCOME

Options for treatment were considered at our epilepsy conference. After careful review of the patient's comprehensive evaluation, it was concluded that the patient would not be a good surgical candidate. It was reasoned that any attempt at resection or subpial transection would have to be widespread, would have little chance of controlling the patient's seizures and might result in severe functional consequences, since both language and

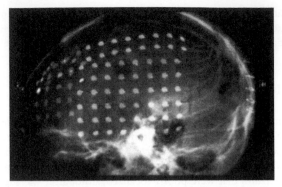

f0010   FIGURE 83.1   Plain postoperative X-ray of the subdural electrode grids placed over the frontal and temporal regions in this patient. Disc electrodes are embedded in a plastic sheet, with only the active side exposed to brain. Wires are embedded in silastic coverings, which are passed through the skull and scalp to make contact with digital EEG machines used for continuous monitoring.

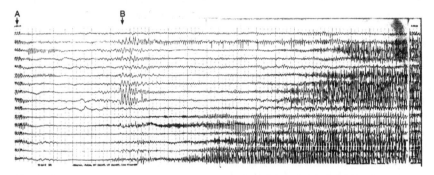

f002016   FIGURE 83.2   Sixteen channel intracranial EEG tracing demonstrating seizure onset from the patient's subdural grid placed over the frontal and temporal regions. The first burst of seizure activity is seen at the very beginning of the figure (arrow A). This is followed by another burst and then sustained seizure activity (arrow B). The top 9 channels are recording from the frontal lobe. The bottom 5 channels are recording from the temporal lobe. Note that seizure onset is not sufficiently localized for resective surgery to be a viable option.

verbal memory were found to reside in the region most appropriate for resection. Other options included newer antiepileptic drugs, an investigational antiepileptic drug, or vagus nerve stimulation.

After a long discussion, the patient chose a trial of levetiracetam as add-on therapy to his phenytoin. He reported less intoxication and tremor than with his previous combination therapy of phenytoin and valproate. Fortunately, the patient has remained seizure-free for the past 12 months on this new drug combination.

COMMENTARY

As epileptologists, we frequently encounter patients with medically refractory seizures. In such cases, epilepsy surgery is looked upon as the ultimate, most definitive therapeutic approach. Evaluation for epilepsy surgery includes a time consuming, comprehensive battery of tests, often culminating in surgical implantation of invasive electrodes, when scalp monitoring fails to identify the site of seizure onset. These evaluations are expensive, painful and involve risks to the patient.

There is great pressure to perform a definitive therapeutic procedure when this stage is reached. We are frequently put in the position of feeling as if we must do *something* after the patient has been implanted with depth electrodes, subdural strips and grids, even in the face of findings that suggest that this is not wise.

What did we learn from this case?

This case teaches that, despite these pressures, it is better to do nothing than to jeopardize the patient's well being in pursuit of overly aggressive or ill-advised treatment. This case had a "happy ending", although we have all seen many similar cases that end in disappointment and no improvement in the patient's condition despite enormous cost, effort, and personal sacrifice.

How did this case alter our approach to the care and treatment of our epilepsy patients?

We do not lose hope when surgery does not appear possible. We know now that failure to find a surgical solution, even in the face of extensive invasive monitoring, can still be followed by a good outcome. It may be that this outcome may be delayed, while new therapeutic approaches catch up with the desperate need of our patients.

This case also reminds us of the limitations of currently available techniques for localizing seizure onset and the inadequacy of our understanding of how cellular networks in the brain generate seizures. Our hope is that, as this understanding grows, there will be fewer and fewer cases like ours.

Sometimes Less Is More

R Eugene Ramsay and Flavia Pryor

HISTORY

A 32-year-old white woman presented with a history of "seizures" starting at the age of 8. These were diagnosed as "petit mal". At the age of 16 she began having "night seizures". These episodes were very dramatic – the patient would fall out of bed and scream, kick and move her arms as if fighting something. Frequency was between 2 and 20 episodes a night, and she would awake with injuries secondary to the events. She was seen by several neurologists and psychiatrists and was given a variety of diagnoses, including psychogenic seizures, parasomnia, anxiety, and substance abuse. Despite being treated with numerous medications the events continued unchanged.

The patient also has a significant history of physical and psychological abuse that she believes may have some influence on her seizures. She describes herself as "rather unstable" and has taken diazepam and alprazolam to obtain relief. In the past, the patient acknowledges occasional recreational use of cocaine and marijuana and, on some evenings, using alcohol in order to reduce her anxiety about having seizures.

In 1996 she was diagnosed as having "sleep terrors" and was treated with clonazepam. Later that year the diagnosis of myoclonic and absence epilepsy was made on the basis of the clinical description by the patient and her mother. She was switched from carbamazepine to divalproex without improvement.

EXAMINATION AND INVESTIGATION

In April 1997, EEG video-telemetry was carried out and multiple bizarre events were recorded. These events consisted of posturing of the upper extremity, gesturing and, on one occasion, a backward roll over the edge of the bed rail, which resulted in the patient falling out of bed. The EEG was normal during the events. Placebo induction was negative. After the induction, however, the patient became drowsy and fell asleep. The next day the patient reported having had an event.

DIAGNOSIS

On the basis of these clinical manifestations, the epilepsy service concluded that the patient had frontal lobe seizures with an interhemispheric focus that precluded epileptiform activity from being seen on the EEG.

TREATMENT AND OUTCOME

On May 26, 1998, the patient reported having frequent nocturnal seizures. Six days earlier she had a long series at night. Home video of a long nocturnal cluster revealed frequent myoclonic jerks that involved mainly the legs but occasionally would spread into the trunk and arms. These lasted only 1–2 s and occurred every 15–60 s. This pattern is quite different from what has been recorded in the past. Medications at the time included gabapentin 2400 mg/day and tiagabine 48 mg/day. It was decided that these seizures were different and most prominently appear to be myoclonic in nature. They were probably frontal lobe status with frequent myoclonic jerks. It was agreed to taper tiagabine while starting topiramate 25 mg/day and titrating the dose.

On September 30, 1998, the patient was noted to have had approximately 10 seizure clusters over the previous 2 months. These clusters consisted of microseizures occurring repeatedly over 1–2 h. The patient had not increased her topiramate as instructed last month because she was concerned that topiramate had increased her seizures. She had continued tiagabine 32 mg/day. The patient was reassured that topiramate was not likely to be worsening her seizures. In fact her seizures had improved and the topiramate was increased to 200 mg/day.

On December 17, 1998, the patient was reported to have done remarkably well. In the previous month she had only four of her typical frontal lobe seizures. Medications at this time were topiramate 300 mg/day and tiagabine 32 mg/day. Her menstrual periods had returned to normal, she was beginning to exercise and she reported feeling great. She also reported having a mild word-finding difficulty and a short temper. The other more important concern was that she found occasionally her knees buckled and she would fall to the ground. These were not seizure-related falls. She had a very significant abrasion above her left knee as a result of one of these falls. The word-finding difficulty was felt to be secondary to topiramate and the knee buckling to be secondary to tiagabine. This meant that an increase in the dose of either drug could result in more problems. It was agreed to maintain the present regimen and to see if symptoms would clear.

On October 28, 1999, the patient was noted to have had a number of medical problems in the past 10 months that resulted in increased seizure frequency. She had 12 seizures in the past month and the knee buckling had continued. It was agreed to taper and discontinue tiagabine since the maximum tolerated dose had been reached, and to increase topiramate to 400 mg/day.

On January 12, 2000, she was noted to have done very badly as the dose of tiagabine was reduced. Review of dosage changes and seizure occurrences revealed that side effects had resolved and seizures were controlled for the short time that she was on tiagabine 20 mg/day. This regimen was reinstated (topiramate 400 mg/day and tiagabine 20 mg/day).

On September 25, 2000, the patient was noted to have been seizure-free for 8 months on topiramate 400 mg/day and tiagabine 20 mg/day. This was really very

p0110

remarkable since she had in the past experienced 25–30 seizures in a day. She had no side effects from the medication and was doing very well.

COMMENTARY

s005

This patient initially presented with a very confusing clinical picture. Her spells were described as screaming, kicking, and moving her arms. Because of a strong family psychiatric history, the unusual character of her seizures, normal EEGs and coexisting anxiety disorder, she was thought by many to have non-epileptic seizures and sleep parasomnia syndrome. The epileptic etiology for her spells became apparent after video–EEG monitoring. Even though the ictal EEG was normal the clinical manifestations were those of frontal lobe motor association seizures. Subsequently, we felt more comfortable employing a more vigorous therapeutic approach, maximizing drug doses until side effects were encountered.

Frontal lobe seizures are notoriously difficult to control. At worst, this patient would experience 15–30 seizures a night. The seizures failed to improve with the older antiepileptic drugs. Although some improvement in seizure control was realized with the use of the newer antiepileptic drugs, complete control eluded us. High doses of tiagabine produced weakness (knee buckling), and increasing doses of topiramate caused some word-finding difficulty, which cleared as the tiagabine was decreased. Seizure control initially improved as the dose of topiramate was increased and monotherapy was achieved. Unfortunately, her seizures returned. Review of her seizure occurrences and medication changes revealed that she had been seizure-free for the 6 weeks when she had been on a combination of topiramate 400 mg/day and tiagabine 20 mg/day. Therefore, this regimen was reinstated and seizure control was again attained. The patient has now been seizure-free for 11 months on this combination.

What did we learn from this case?

s0060

This case illustrates two important clinical lessons. First, the definite diagnosis of epilepsy and particularly frontal lobe seizures was not clear until video–EEG monitoring was carried out. The second and perhaps more significant lesson is the importance of a careful review of a patient's response to medications. This patient had a partial response to several antiepileptic drugs in combination and in monotherapy; however, total control was achieved only by combined therapy with doses that were lower than those used in monotherapy.

How did this case alter our approach to the care and treatment of our epilepsy patients?

s0070

The careful tracking of seizures and medication changes in this case allowed us to realize that seizures came under control only when particular doses of tiagabine and topiramate were used together. We are now more carefully looking for other combinations with a similar synergistic efficacy.

FURTHER READING

Bourgeois BF. New antiepileptic drugs. *Arch Neurol* 1998;**55**:1181–3.

Brodie MJ. Drug interactions in epilepsy. *Epilepsia* 1992;**33(suppl 1)**:S13–S22.

Chez MG, Bourgeois BF, Pippenger CE, Knowles WD. Pharmacodynamic interactions between phenytoin and valproate: individual and combined antiepileptic and neurotoxic actions in mice. *Clin Pharmacol* 1994;**17**:32–7.

Datta PK, Crawford PM. Refractory epilepsy: treatment with new antiepileptic drugs. *Seizure* 2000;**9**:51–7.

Gatti G, Bonomi I, Jannuzzi G, Perucca E. The new antiepileptic drugs: pharmacological and clinical aspects. *Curr Pharm Des* 2000;**6**:839–60.

Ketter TA, Post RM, Theodore WH. Positive and negative psychiatric effects of antiepileptic drugs in patients with seizure disorders. *Neurology* 1999;**53(suppl 2)**:S53–S67.

Unexpected Benefit from an Old Antiepileptic Drug

Matti Sillanpää

HISTORY

A 30-year-old man had an uneventful previous history, except for moderate head trauma at the age of 3 years. Four years later, he started to have generalized convulsive seizures with abrupt loss of consciousness and some concomitant absence seizures. Most of the convulsions occurred on awakening; those few that did not occurred at random. There was no family history of epilepsy or febrile convulsions. At this time, the patient's sleep rhythm was irregular. He was awake late in the evenings and got up late in the mornings. According to his mother, he suffered from sleep deprivation. He was active in youth athletics but was somewhat hyperactive and restless. Antiepileptic drug therapy was initially unsuccessful but, at the age of 10 years, he was seizure-free.

After this, despite frequent discussions and advice, he continued his lifestyle with irregular and apparently inadequate nocturnal sleep. As an adult, he was well motivated to take his medication because of the risk of having his driving license revoked. He did not use alcohol.

EXAMINATION AND INVESTIGATIONS

Neurological examination was normal. His IQ was 80. The initial EEG showed massive 3–4 Hz bilateral symmetric spike-and-wave discharges, easily provocable by flicker light and hyperventilation. Eight years later, during a seizure-free period, EEG was normal in the waking state but during sleep there were a few right-sided spikes and spike-and-wave complexes, and flicker light and hyperventilation sensitivity had disappeared. Clinically, the patient's seizures were obviously primarily generalized without any warning, but the asymmetric spike-and-wave complexes on the EEG were interpreted by a neurophysiologist as a sign of a focal origin of the seizures. Not unexpectedly, however, a magnetic resonance imaging (MRI) scan of the brain was normal. A recent repeat MRI scan was also normal.

DIAGNOSIS

Generalized tonic–clonic seizures on awakening, and absence seizures.

TREATMENT AND OUTCOME

The patient was initially administered phenytoin but without success. Valproate up to 30 mg/kg per day replaced the phenytoin. Because of continued seizures, a daily dose of 50 mg phenobarbital was combined with the valproate and the seizures disappeared. After 3 years, phenobarbital was tapered off, and as a result of a complete seizure-free period of a further 4 years, valproate was slowly decreased to 25 mg/kg per day. However, a relapse occurred 6 months later. The dosage of valproate was increased to 40 mg/kg per day and later combined individually or in combination with pheno-barbital, primidone, carbamazepine, phenytoin, and lamotrigine, but without success. More than 1 year later, as a last resort, ethosuximide 750 mg/day in two divided doses was combined with valproate. Since the first dose of ethosuximide over 5 years ago, no seizures have occurred.

COMMENTARY

The early age of this awakening epilepsy and subnormal intelligence of the child initially did not lead to the correct epilepsy diagnosis. This case again shows the importance of an accurate and careful previous history in recognizing different types of epilepsy syndromes. The head trauma in the past history might argue for the Janz's hypothesis that the onset of this genetic epilepsy is precipitated by or predisposed by traumatic or ictogenic brain lesion.[1] Despite an asymmetric EEG, no abnormality was found on MRI.

Valproate is the first drug of choice in awakening epilepsy, but if it or lamotrigine does not work, one cannot reject the diagnosis *ex juvantibus*. The high frequency of relapses after reduction in dose or withdrawal of medication is well known, but the drug resistance in this case was embarrassing.

Still more striking was the beneficial effect of ethosuximide. It is still unclear why ethosuximide was beneficial. Its effect in both experimental and human studies has proved to be very selective against typical absences in young subjects. Ethosuximide might actually exacerbate, rather than prevent, generalized tonic–clonic seizures, even though this has not been proved. The clinical diagnosis of seizure was definitely ascertained by EEG in this case, so the diagnosis of seizures or epilepsy syndrome cannot be wrong. The mode of action of ethosuximide is still largely unknown. Although I cannot explain the effect, this case shows that one must never lose hope but must try even "impossible" antiepileptic medications in apparently hopeless cases.

What did I learn from this case?   s006

I learnt several things from this case. Even very young children may have generalized   p00*
tonic–clonic seizures on awakening. One must be able to differentiate between functional and lesional focal findings on the EEG to avoid misclassification of the origin
of seizures. The medication should not be changed if seizures stop. If the patient has
drug-resistant seizures, one should not lose hope but should try drugs that are not
supposed to work.

To my mind, this case again shows that whatever you say in medicine is correct in   p01(
no higher than 90% of cases. The importance of life habits and personal responsibility
for one's health should be emphasized to children. One should make them realize that
everyone is the molder of his or her own fortune and is also personally responsible for
his or her own health.

REFERENCE

1. Janz D. The grand mal epilepsies and sleep-waking cycle. *Epilepsia* 1962;**3**:69–109.

FURTHER READING

Janz D, Kern A, Mössinger HJ, Puhlmann HU. Rückfallprognose während und nach Reduktion der
    Medikamente bei Epilepsiebehandlung. In: Remschmidt H, Rentz R, Jungmann J, eds. *Epilepsia
    1981, Verlauf und Prognose, neuropsychologische und psychologische Aspekte.* Stuttgart: Thieme Verlag,
    1983: 17–24.
Wolf P. Epilepsy with grand mal on awakening. In: Roger J, Bureau M, Dravet C, Dreifuss FE, Perret
    A, Wolf P, eds. *Epileptic syndromes in infancy, childhood and adolescence.* London: John Libbey, 1992:
    329–41.

Status Epilepticus Responsive to Intravenous Immunoglobulin

c0086

Joseph I Sirven and Hoan Linh Banh

HISTORY

s0010

One week before admission, a healthy 30-year-old man developed flu-like symptoms. Four days later, he had three generalized tonic–clonic seizures, which began with focal left facial twitching. He had recovery of consciousness between the seizures. However, the night of seizure onset, he developed a cluster of generalized seizures with no recovery of consciousness.

p0010

He was admitted to an intensive care unit at a local community hospital. He was initially treated with phenytoin and phenobarbital, but his seizures failed to respond despite a phenytoin level of 20 μg/ml and phenobarbital level of 45 μg/ml. A magnetic resonance imaging (MRI) scan of the brain with gadolinium enhancement, a lumbar puncture, blood cultures, and cerebrospinal fluid cultures for fungal, bacterial, and viral organisms, and polymerase chain reaction for herpes virus were all normal. The patient was then given a continuous infusion of pentobarbital. Generalized tonic–clonic seizures were successfully terminated with phenytoin 300 mg intravenously every 6 h, valproate 750 mg intravenously every 6 h, and phenobarbital 90 mg intravenously every 8 h. When the pentobarbital was tapered, generalized tonic–clonic and myoclonic seizures returned, and these correlated with generalized polyspike-wave formations on the EEG. The patient subsequently relapsed into status epilepticus, both clinically and on EEG. He was then transferred to our institution for management of refractory status epilepticus.

p0020

EXAMINATION AND INVESTIGATIONS

s0020

Upon arrival, continuous pentobarbital infusion was continued, and phenytoin and phenobarbital were restarted to control his seizures. A brain MRI scan with gadolinium enhancement, a lumbar puncture, serum pyruvate and lactate levels, serum

p0030

electrolytes, liver enzymes, and blood and cerebrospinal fluid cultures were all normal. Despite titration of the pentobarbital infusion to suppress all electrographic activity completely, generalized convulsive and myoclonic seizures persisted. The myoclonic seizures became a prominent feature of the status epilepticus at this time in the clinical course. The myoclonus was both spontaneous and induced by tactile stimulation. The entire body was involved, but particularly the proximal muscles of the body and trunk. The EEG revealed generalized polyspike–wave activity during the myoclonic seizures.

s0030   ## DIAGNOSIS

p0040   Generalized tonic–clonic status epilepticus with myoclonic seizures secondary to an unidentified postinfectious etiology.

s0040   ## TREATMENT AND OUTCOME

p0050   Table 86.1 lists the antiepileptic drugs that were unsuccessful when tried as adjunctive therapy to the pentobarbital infusion.

p0060   Forty-five days after the initiation of pentobarbital, the infusion was terminated. The patient was not responsive to verbal stimuli and he developed both generalized myoclonus and occasional generalized tonic–clonic seizures. Cisatracurium (neuromuscular blockade) continuous infusion was used to control his severe generalized myoclonic twitching and to protect renal function against myoglobinuria.

p0070   Since the patient's myoclonus and seizures were not responding to antiepileptic drugs and his level of consciousness did not improve despite termination of pentobarbital, high-dose methylprednisolone was tried for 1 week. The patient awoke, but the myoclonus persisted. Because of the response to methylprednisolone, consideration of a potential underlying immune mechanism responsible for the status epilepticus was given. Thus, a decision was made to initiate intravenous immunoglobulin (IVIG) 30 g/ day (0.4 g/kg per day) for 7 days. Initially, no dramatic improvement in myoclonus was observed. However, on day 4 of IVIG therapy, the patient's myoclonic activity stopped and he was able to communicate with hand gestures. Four days after the completion of IVIG therapy, the patient became completely alert, awake, and verbally communicative.

p0080   Because of some breakthrough myoclonic jerking of the face, 5-hydroxytryptophan and carbidopa were initiated. The patient was transferred back to his local community hospital 2 weeks later on 5-hydroxy-L-tryptophan 200 mg every 8 h, phenobarbital 90 mg every 6 h, and lamotrigine 100 mg every 6 h. He was eventually transferred to a rehabilitation hospital and no further seizures were reported.

p0090   He has been subsequently discharged to home with minimal neurological deficits. All blood and cerebrospinal fluid cultures have remained negative for all organisms. No specific antibodies for herpes virus, western equine encephalitis, eastern equine encephalitis or St. Louis encephalitis were detected.

s0050   ## COMMENTARY

p0100   Our patient had a severe refractory myoclonic status epilepticus clinical syndrome that failed to respond to conventional management and management for refractory status t0010 TABLE 86.1 The Antiepileptic Drugs That Were Unsuccessfully Tried in This Patient as Adjunctive Therapy to Pentobarbital Infusion

Start (day number)	Stop (day number)	Drug	Dose	Comment
1	45	Pentobarbital	Infusion[a]	
52	59	Methylprednisolone	500 mg intravenously every 12 h	
0		Phenobarbital	90 mg intravenously every 8 h	
0	2	Valproate	750 mg/day intravenously	
0	60	Phenytoin	300 mg intravenously every 6 h	Drug fever developed secondary to phenytoin
1	6	Carbamazepine	200 mg by mouth every 6 h	
6	12	Carbamazepine	200 mg by mouth every 6 h	Suspected to be the cause of pancreatitis
12		Topiramate	Titrate to 100 mg by mouth every 12 h	
25		Lamotrigine	Titrate to 100 mg every 6 h (delivered per PEG tube)	
28	68	Clonazepam	3 mg by mouth every 8 h	
30	68	Cisatracurium	Infusion[b]	Given to control myoclonic seizures
59	63	Intravenous immunoglobulin	30 g/day	
68		5-hydroxy-L-tryptophan	200 mg by mouth every 8 h	

[a]10 mg/kg load followed by 1.5 μ/kg/h.
[b]1 μg/kg/min.

epilepticus. IVIG has been used for intractable seizures in children at a dose of 2 g/kg given over 7 days. The specific mechanism of action of IVIG in epilepsy is unclear, but it is clearly immunomodulatory. IVIG has many potential ways of modulating humoral and cellular immune responses. Anti-idiotype antibodies within IVIG could neutralize or counteract particular seizure-inducing antibodies. Perhaps IVIG has antibodies that down-regulate the production of epileptogenic antibodies. Additionally, IVIG may alter complement-mediated neuronal damage. Uncontrolled clinical observations suggest that IVIG may be effective in some patients with intractable epilepsy, especially children, and may be considered as a safe adjunctive therapy. Our patient clinically improved with IVIG and it was well tolerated.

p0110   The major limitations to this treatment are the severe national shortage of IVIG, its cost, and the risk of transmission of infectious diseases associated with blood derivatives.

s0060   What did we learn from this case?

p0120   We learned two major points from this case. In the absence of an etiology for refractory status epilepticus and no overt structural lesion on imaging, immune therapies such as corticosteroids and IVIG should be considered in the management of refractory status epilepticus and residual myoclonic activity. Although these are not clearly the treatments of choice for status epilepticus, one should at least consider their use when status epilepticus has persisted despite prolonged treatment with pentobarbital. The second major lesson was that patients can make a meaningful recovery despite prolonged duration of a protracted and serious status epilepticus.

s0070   How did this case alter our approach to the care and treatment of our epilepsy patients?

p0130   Because of this case, we are more optimistic about recovery from generalized status epilepticus in the absence of a clear catastrophic etiology. We are also willing to initiate corticosteroids in status epilepticus without a clear etiology.

p0140   We now know that one can never give up when treating status epilepticus regardless of its duration, criticisms from colleagues who advise discontinuing therapy, and the absence of the medical literature to guide treatment.

FURTHER READING

Ariizumi M, Shiihara H, Hibio S, et al. High dose gammaglobulin for intractable childhood epilepsy. Lancet 1998;2:162–3.

Baziel GM, van Engelen BG, Renier WO, et al. Immunoglobulin treatment in epilepsy: a review of the literature. Epilepsy Res 1994;19:181–90.

Duse M, Notarangelo D, Tiberti E, Menegati S, Plebani A, Ugazio AG. Intravenous immune globulin in the treatment of intractable childhood epilepsy. Clin Exp Immunol 1996;104(suppl 1):71–6.

Etzioni A, Jaffe M, Pollack S, et al. High dose intravenous gamma-globulin in intractable epilepsy. Eur J Pediatr 1991;150:681–3.

Fayed MN, Choueiri R, Mikati M. Landau–Kleffner syndrome: consistent response to repeated intravenous γ-globulin doses: a case report. Epilepsia 1997;38:489–94.

Imbach P, d'Appuzo V, Hirt A, *et al.* High dose intravenous gammaglobulin for idiopathic thrombocy-topenic purpura in childhood. *Lancet* 1998;**1**:1228–31.

Lagae LG, Silberstein J, Gillis L, Casaer PJ. Successful use of intravenous immunoglobulins in Landau–Kleffner syndrome. *Pediatr Neurol* 1998;**8**:165–8.

Van Engelen BG, Renier WO, Weemaes CM. Immunoglobulin treatment in human and experimental epilepsy. *J Neurol Neurosurg Psychiatry* 1995;**57(suppl)**:72–5.

c00087

Surgical Success in a Patient with Diffuse Brain Trauma

Brien J Smith

s0010

HISTORY

p0010

A 26-year-old right-handed man sustained a severe closed head injury 8 years before presentation. He was in a comatose state for 23 days and, on regaining consciousness, was severely impaired. He required retraining of language (speaking and writing), simple motor tasks (tying shoes, eating), and other basic skills during an 18-month inpatient rehabilitation. Residual deficits included a left hemiparesis, bilateral fourth nerve palsies, impaired reading comprehension, and difficulty in processing short-term memory.

p0020

During his rehabilitation, the patient began experiencing episodes of a "rising sensation" similar to a "rapid unexpected descent in an elevator." Initially these events were brief and infrequent. Subsequently, he began experiencing multiple events a day, with progression of symptoms to include difficulty in swallowing, gagging, drooling, and regurgitation. With most of these episodes he did not report an alteration in consciousness, but with longer events (duration 30–40 s) he reported "phasing out."

p0030

He was subsequently diagnosed with partial seizures and placed on carbamazepine. Despite treatment with various antiepileptic drugs, including valproate, phenytoin, gabapentin, and clonazepam in monotherapy and polytherapy, he continued to have daily seizures and significant side effects from medical therapy.

p0040

There was no history of birth complications, febrile seizures, meningitis, encephalitis, or other head trauma and there was no family history of seizure disorders.

p0050

Previous EEG studies reported sharp wave discharges over the left frontotemporal and left central head regions with intermixed slowing. A magnetic resonance imaging (MRI) scan of the brain 2 years earlier showed encephalomalacia of both frontal lobes and evidence of a remote parenchymal hemorrhage in the left frontal lobe (Figure 87.1). There was also evidence of progressive degenerative changes involving the body and splenium of the corpus callosum.

s0020

EXAMINATION AND INVESTIGATIONS

p0060

Neurological examination revealed dysconjugate eye position, mild left hemiparesis, hyperreflexia, and a positive Babinski sign on the left.

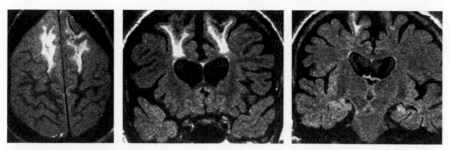

FIGURE 87.1   MRI scan of the brain (axial and coronal images) demonstrating atrophy, encephalomalacia, and bifrontal signal changes consistent with gliosis.

After an extensive discussion explaining the limitations and risks of surgical intervention, the patient wished to pursue the presurgical evaluation. Baseline EEG continued to show epileptiform discharges in the left frontotemporal and central head regions and bursts of delta-wave slowing. A repeat MRI scan showed no significant interval change with the exception of right ventral tegmental atrophy, suggestive of wallerian degeneration.

Inpatient monitoring with scalp and sphenoidal electrodes captured multiple typical simple partial seizures and some complex partial seizures. EEG ictal changes suggested left hemisphere lateralization but no clear-cut focal or regional pattern was evident. Ictal single photon emission computed tomography (SPECT) was completed 17 s after clinical onset and demonstrated focal increased uptake in the left temporal, left parietal, and left basal ganglia regions compared with the interictal study. The ictal and interictal SPECT studies both revealed hypoperfusion in both frontal lobes (concordant with the abnormalities on the MRI scan) and marked scattered heterogeneity in radiotracer distribution.

A battery of neuropsychological tests demonstrated short-term memory dysfunction and a full-scale IQ of 96 (verbal IQ 101, performance IQ 102). Language evaluation demonstrated anomia, and paraphasic and semantic errors, intracarotid amobarbital procedure (Wada study) was suggestive of left hemisphere language dominance and showed borderline memory scores after injection on each side.

Owing to the evidence of bihemispheric injury, the limited localizing value of non-invasive testing and the need to limit a potential cortical resection to a small, well-defined ictogenic zone, intracranial implantation was suggested. Widespread bilateral subdural coverage, more comprehensively on the left, demonstrated multiple seizures with a focal ictal pattern over the left anterior and midparahippocampal gyrus.

DIAGNOSIS

Medically refractory partial seizures arising from the left anterior and midparahippocampal gyrus secondary to head injury.

TREATMENT AND OUTCOME

Focal resection included the anterior temporal pole (2 cm), uncus, and parahippocampal gyrus (including the hippocampus up to 3 cm from the pes). The patient has had only seven simple partial seizures in more than 1-year follow-up, compared with at least three to five seizures a week before surgery. No significant change in language or memory function was noted in early postoperative testing.

s0050   ## COMMENTARY

p0130   Head trauma is a common risk factor for the development of partial epilepsy.[1,2] The option of epilepsy surgery for patients with refractory partial epilepsy secondary to a severe head injury is frequently pursued with reservation. This is, in part, because literature analyzing surgical outcome in post-traumatic epilepsy is limited[3–9] and also because the outcomes have been considered suboptimal[3,4] compared with the outcomes from surgery for other etiologies.

p0140   The approach to post-traumatic epilepsy is complicated by the variability of the clinical picture. Considerations include:

u0010   - the type of injury (penetrating or closed);
u0020   - the severity of the injury (mild, moderate, or severe);
u0030   - the mechanisms of neuronal injury (primary or secondary);[10]
u0040   - the potential sites of epileptogenicity (diffuse bilateral, unilateral, multilobar, hippocampal, or neocortical); and
u0050   - the age of the patient (pediatric or adult).

p0200   Moreover, the functional neurological reserve of a patient with previous severe brain injury is difficult to estimate when surgical resection is being considered.

p0210   Marks et al.[3] noted an association between head injury at an early age (less than 5 years) and mesial temporal sclerosis. Some patients with hippocampal atrophy on MRI scan, which was helpful in localization, had seizure-free outcomes. Other studies[4,5] have not found that the age at the time of the injury is a significant factor in determining the outcome. The seizures of patients without clear-cut focal lesions on MRI and of those with evidence of diffuse brain injury were difficult to localize and the patients had poor outcomes. In smaller series of patients with a focal or regional destructive lesion from penetrating injuries, patients have typically done better when complete resection of the site has been undertaken.[7–10]

p0220   Patients are often excluded from surgical consideration based on the presumption of a coup–contrecoup injury or bilateral frontotemporal polar injuries. These injuries have been demonstrated in neuropathology and imaging studies,[11] but they have never been clearly demonstrated to result in multifocal sites of epileptogenicity. At my center, we recognize that these patients may have multiple epileptogenic sites, but we do not routinely exclude them from surgical evaluation.

s0060   ### What did I learn from this case?

p0230   I learned that even in a patient with a severe closed head injury and diffuse changes on MRI, a small epileptogenic zone may be localized and successfully resected. The mechanisms of injury and subsequent development of epileptogenesis in post-traumatic brain injury is a complex process that has not been fully elucidated. MRI scanning may not have the same localizing value in these patients as it does in other patients because it may show no abnormalities or only diffuse changes. This case demonstrated atrophy that was more prominent on the right side, which was consistent with the acute neurological manifestations of the brain injury (left hemiparesis) but falsely localizing with regard to the seizures.

How did this case alter my approach to the care and treatment of my epilepsy patients?

I am now less likely to form a premature impression about surgical candidacy on the basis of a clinical history of severe head trauma or when viewing an MRI scan with diffuse bilateral changes. This case also reinforces the importance of obtaining a detailed history of the clinical semiology of seizures and of the frequency and severity of each seizure type, including the propensity to secondary generalization. In my experience with such patients, the history of frequent simple partial seizures or limited complex partial seizures with the same clinical semiology and no secondary generalization may actually be a positive prognostic factor.

REFERENCES

1. Annegers JF, Grabow JD, Grover RV, et al. Seizures after head trauma: a population study. *Neurology* 1980;**30**:683–9.
2. Rocca WA, Sharbrough FW, Hauser WA, et al. Risk factors for complex partial seizures: a population-based case–control study. *Ann Neurol* 1987;**21**:22–31.
3. Marks DA, Kim J, Spencer DD, Spencer SS. Seizure localization and pathology following head injury in patients with uncontrolled epilepsy. *Neurology* 1995;**45**:2051–7.
4. Schuh LA, Henry TR, Fromes G, et al. Influence of head trauma on outcome following temporal lobectomy. *Arch Neurol* 1998;**55**:1325–8.
5. Mathern GW, Pretorius JK, Babb TL. Influence of the type of initial precipitating injury and at what age it occurs on course and outcome in patients with temporal lobe seizures. *J Neurosurg* 1995;**82**:220–7.
6. Foerster O, Penfield W. The structural basis of traumatic epilepsy and results of radical operation. *Brain* 1930;**53**:99–119.
7. Kazemi NJ, So EL, Mosewich RK, et al. Resection of frontal encephalomalacias for intractable epilepsy: outcome and prognostic factors. *Epilepsia* 1997;**38**:670–7.
8. Cukiert A, Olivier A, Andermann F. Posttraumatic frontal lobe epilepsy with structural changes: excellent results after cortical resection. *Can J Neurol Sci* 1996;**23**:114–7.
9. Mathern GW, Babb TL, Vickrey BG, et al. Traumatic compared to non-traumatic clinical-pathologic associations in temporal lobe epilepsy. *Epilepsy Res* 1994;**19**:129–39.
10. Miller DJ, Piper JR, Jones PA. Pathophysiology of head injury. In: Narayan RK, Wilberger JE Jr., Povlishock JT, eds. *Neurotrauma.* New York: McGraw-Hill, 1996: 61–70.
11. Clifton GL, McCormick WF, Grossman RG. Neuropathology of early and late deaths after head injury. *Neurosurgery* 1981;**8**:309–14.

Dietary Treatment of Seizures from a Hypothalamic Hamartoma

c00

Vijay Maggio and James Wheless

HISTORY

s001

A 16-year-old male had a history of seizure onset at the age of 2 years. Initially, the seizures were brief and consisted of staring spells, occurring mainly at night during the transition from waking to sleep. They were refractory to medical treatment and increased in frequency with time. Neuroimaging studies revealed a hypothalamic hamartoma.

p001

The patient was evaluated at our institution at the age of 6½ years. During a typical event he would get a frightened look and complain of hearing or seeing scary things. He also perceived the room getting dark and fading away. These events were sometimes accompanied by facial grimacing (a smiling appearance). The events lasted for 15–20 s. There was no history of secondarily generalized tonic–clonic seizures except for one event that occurred after missing a medication dose. His longest seizure-free interval was 2 weeks. His partial seizure count was as high as 753 seizures in 1 month and 96 in 1 day; he typically averaged between 3 and 5 seizures a day.

p002

His birth history was unremarkable. His medical history was significant for behavioral problems consisting of obsessive–compulsive traits, attentional deficits, and perseveration. In addition, consecutive neuropsychological evaluations revealed progressive decline in intelligence and verbal memory skills and the development of a psychosis (Table 88.1).

p003

Medications tried alone or in combination included acetazolamide, carbamazepine, valproate, felbamate, gabapentin, phenytoin, phenobarbital, and lamotrigine. He

p004

t0010   TABLE 88.1   Neuropsychological Profile of the Patient on Assessment

Age (years)	IQ test	Full-scale IQ	Verbal IQ	Performance IQ	Other diagnoses
7.25	WISC-R	116	110	120	Attention disorder and poor right-hand dexterity
8.80	WISC-R	98	92	105	Attention disorder, poor right-hand dexterity, impaired expressive language, and reduction in affective tone
9.40	WISC-R	74	75	78	Attention disorder, poor right-hand dexterity, impaired expressive language, reduction in affective tone, marked disruption of memory abilities, and worsening of fine motor skills
11.5–14.2					Attention disorder, poor right-hand dexterity, impaired expressive language, reduction in affective tone, marked disruption of memory abilities, and worsening of fine motor skills
13.4 (began the ketogenic diet)					
15	PPVT-R	105	Average		

IQ, Intelligence quotient; PPVT-R, Peabody Picture Vocabulary Test – Revised; and WISC-R, Wechsler Intelligence Scale for Children – Revised.

had been treated with methylphenidate, amoxapine, and thioridazine for behavioral modification.

EXAMINATION AND INVESTIGATIONS

The patient's general examination was unremarkable. His neurological examination showed evidence of cognitive slowing, dysarthria, slowing of speech, and perseveration. His cranial nerve and motor examination revealed no focal deficits.

Multiple routine EEGs were normal. Magnetic resonance imaging of the brain revealed a hypothalamic mass 10–12 mm in diameter from the center of the hypothalamus, consistent with a hypothalamic hamartoma.

Video–EEG monitoring at the age of 13 years revealed a diffusely slow background (4.5–5 Hz with admixed delta activity in the waking state) without epileptiform discharges. Over 2 days he had 150 partial seizures. Most were simple partial seizures without EEG change; some were complex partial seizures with diffuse EEG attenuation.

DIAGNOSIS

Refractory seizures in a patient with hypothalamic hamartoma.

TREATMENT AND OUTCOME

All treatment options were discussed with the family, including surgical removal of the hamartoma, which was believed to be the only curative treatment for his condition. However, our patient did not want to risk the endocrine complications. He therefore agreed to a trial of the ketogenic diet, and then surgery if necessary.

The patient was initiated on the ketogenic diet and within days showed remarkable improvement. Within 1 year his antiepileptic drugs and the drugs used for behavioral therapy were withdrawn.

He has now been on the 4:1 ketogenic diet for 2 years and his urinary ketones are consistently 160 mg/dl. He is off all medications and only has one or two brief (5 s) simple sensory partial seizures a day. These are very mild and no one but the patient can tell when he has one.

The patient's neuropsychological examination was repeated 21 months after initiation of the ketogenic diet. There was improvement in his intelligence, which was now estimated to be in the average range with potential for further improvement. He was also found to be capable of making rapid academic progress. His executive functions were well developed.

He tolerates the ketogenic diet wonderfully and has had no complications. His lipid profile is normal. His dysarthria has showed significant improvement.

COMMENTARY

Hypothalamic hamartomas are congenital malformations that consist of masses of neuronal tissue in ectopic locations. They typically originate from one of the mamillary bodies and extend into the interpeduncular cistern.[1] The histological structure most often resembles that of normal posterior hypothalamus, containing neurosecretory granules. Extralesional abnormalities of cerebral structure may also be present.[2]

These malformations may be asymptomatic or they may cause cognitive decline, a seizure disorder, behavioral problems, or precocious puberty. The wide seizure spectrum associated with this condition is characterized by gelastic seizures, which are usually brief, repetitive, stereotyped attacks of laughter that begin in early childhood. Later, there may be complex partial seizures and a pattern of symptomatic generalized epilepsy with tonic, atonic, and other seizure types in association with slow spike–wave discharges.[3] Hypothalamic hamartomas are intrinsically epileptogenic.[2] There may be other epileptic foci in the presence of dysplastic cortex.

Seizures are often refractory to medical management. Abatement of seizures has been reported after surgical removal, but larger series imply that patients are unlikely to become seizure-free and extirpation of the hamartoma may be associated with significant morbidity, including diabetes insipidus and panhypopituitarism.[4] For patients with a midline hamartoma, surgery may mean a lifetime of endocrine replacement therapy. In a cognitively impaired child this can be difficult and, during acute illnesses, potentially life-threatening.

Other operative procedures include resection of epileptogenic cortex[5] and corpus callosotomy.[6] These surgical approaches have not been shown to have a favorable outcome in reducing seizures. We have seen seizure improvement with vagus nerve stimulation in some patients.[7]

What did we learn from this case?

We learned that the ketogenic diet might be efficacious in the management of refractory seizures in a patient with hypothalamic hamartoma. Additionally, this patient's progressive cognitive decline and psychosis were reversed.

How did this case alter our approach to the care and treatment of our epilepsy patients?

This case suggested that earlier institution of the ketogenic diet might have prevented the cognitive decline and the development of behavioral problems. As a result, we now offer the ketogenic diet early for seizures associated with hypothalamic hamartoma. We also offer vagus nerve stimulation as a treatment option. If these therapies are not successful we recommend direct surgical removal or gamma knife treatment.

REFERENCES

1. Diebler C, Ponsot G. Hamartomas of the tuber cinereum. *Neuroradiology* 1983;**25**:93–101.
2. Berkovic SF, Kuzniecky RI, Andermann F. Human epileptogenesis and hypothalmic hamartomas: new lessons from an experiment of nature. *Epilepsia* 1997;**38**:1–3.
3. Tasch E, Cendes F, Li LM, *et al.* Hypothalamic hamartomas and gelastic epilepsy: a spectroscopic study. *Neurology* 1998;**51**:1046–50.
4. Breningstall GN. Gelastic seizures, precocious puberty and hypothalamic hamartoma. *Neurology* 1985;**26**:509–27.
5. Cascino GD, Andermann F, Berkovic SF, *et al.* Gelastic seizures and hypothalamic hamartomas: evaluation of patients undergoing chronic intracranial EEG monitoring and outcome of surgical treatment. *Neurology* 1993;**43**:747–50.
6. Pallini R, Bozzini V, Coliccho G, Lauretti L, Scerrati M, Rossi GF. Callosotomy for generalized seizures associated with hypothalamic hamartoma. *Neurol Res* 1993;**15**:139–41.
7. Murphy JV, Wheless JW, Schmoll CM. Left vagal nerve stimulation in six patients with hypothalamic hamartoma. *Pediatr Neurol* 2000;**23**:167–8.

c0089

Can the Behavioral and Cognitive Effects of AEDs Be Predicted?

Kimford J Meador

s0010

HISTORY

p0180

SP sustained a closed head injury at the age of 17, when he was hit by a baseball while batting. He suffered a concussion and a right frontal skull fracture, but recovered quickly and returned to school. Three months later, he experienced his first generalized tonic–clonic seizure. He was placed on phenytoin and remained on it until 32 years of age. His blood levels were intermittently checked and were always within therapeutic ranges. Prior to his injury, SP had always been an excellent student and continued to make good grades through high school. Despite coming from a family of university researchers and having siblings with professional degrees, SP did not complete college for a decade after high school. Subsequently, he completed masters level training and worked as a social worker. Although he had several friends, SP never had a long-term intimate relationship.

p0190

Having been seizure-free on phenytoin for 15 years, SP was advised that he might be able to taper off anticonvulsant medication, which he did and remained seizure-free, off medications, for 3 years. After withdrawal of phenytoin, SP felt that his mind was much clearer and that his old personality had returned. He explained that prior to phenytoin therapy, he had an outgoing personality and was always energetic. During the years of phenytoin treatment, he felt that his mind was "foggy" and that he was "moody and lacked energy." SP was certain that the drug had affected his ability to achieve his personal life goals. During his drug-free period, SP was promoted and became engaged to be married.

p0200

Three years after coming off phenytoin, SP suffered two generalized tonic–clonic seizures within a month. During one of the seizures, he was noted to have left arm extension and head turning to the left prior to generalized motor activity. SP was placed back on phenytoin and has remained seizure-free. However, the same cognitive and behavioral side effects from phenytoin return. His physician switched him to valproate, but he continued to suffer similar symptoms. He withdrew from his friends, broke off his engagement, and felt that his job performance suffered. His physician told him that there were no other options that would make any difference and that SP would have to tolerate the drug side effects in order to maintain seizure freedom. SP came to our attention when he sought a second opinion on his own.

EXAMINATION AND INVESTIGATIONS

SP's general physical and neurological examinations were normal except that he appeared mildly depressed. When he suffered his recurrent seizures 3 years previously, an MRI was normal and an EEG revealed occasional sharp waves in the right frontal region. His only present medication was valproate, and recent blood levels were in the low therapeutic range.

DIAGNOSIS

SP has a focal seizure disorder with secondary generalization. His seizures were easily controlled with either phenytoin or valproate. Although his epilepsy was mild, it was having marked effects on his quality of life due to the side effects incurred by anticonvulsant medications.

TREATMENT AND OUTCOME

Various options and risks were explained to SP, and we decided to slowly titrate lamotrigine and then taper off valproate. SP remained seziure-free. He returned after completion of the conversion to lamotrigine monotherapy and stated that his cognitive side effects had disappeared once he was off the valproate. He felt that his personality and mood were back to normal.

COMMENTARY

As in this case, seizures may be well controlled, but the patient may suffer substantial behavioral/cognitive side effects, which impair their quality of life. Prediction of these side effects on an individual patient basis is very difficult, but the probability of such side effects can be estimated. Furthermore, such side effects can be anticipated and alternative therapeutic options considered.

Antiepileptic drugs (AEDs) can have positive effects on cognition by reducing seizures and interictal activity, but they can also have negative cognitive effects. AEDs can produce both positive and negative psychotropic effects. Prediction of these effects is inexact, especially on an individual patient basis. However, probability of positive or negative effects can be estimated.

Patients with epilepsy have lower cognitive performance as a group compared to healthy individuals, but cognitive capacity across individual patients varies widely. Most people with epilepsy have normal intelligence, but multiple factors may impair cognition in these patients[1] (see Table 89.1). These factors should be considered in evaluating cognitive complaints. Since AEDs are the major therapy for epilepsy and

:0010

TABLE 89.1   Factors Affecting Cognition in Patients with Epilepsy

- Underlying cause of seizures
- Cerebral lesions acquired prior to onset of seizures
- Seizure type
- Age at onset of epilepsy
- Seizure frequency
- Duration and severity of seizures
- Physiologic dysfunction (intraictal, interictal, or postictal) from seizures
- Structural cerebral damage due to repetitive or prolonged seizures
- Hereditary factors
- Psychosocial factors
- Untoward effects of treatments (e.g. antiepileptic drugs or surgery)

t0020

TABLE 89.2   Risks of AED-Induced Cognitive Side Effects

- Increase with higher dose and blood levels
- Increase with polytherapy
- Increase with rapid starting titration
- Reduce with time after drug initiation due to habituation
- Vary across different AEDs
- Vary across patients due to individual susceptibility

under the clinician's control, they are a factor that can potentially be modulated to reduce behavioral and cognitive side effects. Even modest neurocognitive effects from AEDs can affect quality of life. There is a high negative correlation between neuro-toxic symptoms and perception of quality of life, but seizure frequency is not related to quality of life unless a patient becomes seizure-free.[2,3]

Several factors can help predict risk for AED-induced cognitive side effects[1] (see Table 89.2). Recommended dosage ranges and standard therapeutic blood levels are guidelines which reflect dosages/levels that are likely to be at least minimally effective at the lower end and have increasing toxic side effects above the upper recommended ranges. The inverse relationship of cognition to AED blood level occurs primarily when levels are above the standard therapeutic range. Thus, risk of cognitive side effects increases with higher dosages/levels. Polytherapy is associated with increased risk of adverse cognitive effects. Even when blood levels for each of several AEDs in polytherapy are well within the therapeutic ranges, a patient may exhibit gross toxicity with ataxia and nystagmus. Clearly, more subtle neurotoxicity can occur in polytherapy even when dosages/levels are within recommended ranges. Adverse cognitive side effects are most likely to occur when starting a new AED. A rapid rate of titration on AED initiation can increase the prob-ability of cognitive side effects. This phenomenon is more pronounced for certain AEDs, but is present for all AEDs to some degree. Slowing titration is effective in reducing cognitive effects because it allows time for habituation to occur. The majority of habit-uation occurs in the first month after AED initiation. Habituation to the subjective

TABLE 89.3   Cognitive Effects of Newer AEDs versus Placebo in Healthy Volunteer Studies

t0030

AED	% tests with placebo better than AED
Tiagabine	0
Lamotrigine	1–17
Gabapentin	0–19
Levetiracetam	11
Oxcarbazepine	46
Topiramate	29–88

TABLE 89.4   Cognitive Effects of Newer AEDs versus Each Other in Healthy Volunteers

t0040

Less impact on cognition	More impact on cognition	% tests
Gabapentin	Carbamazepine	26
Lamotrigine	Carbamazepine	48
Levetiracetam	Carbamazepine	42
Oxcarbazepine	Phenytoin	0
Gabapentin	Topiramate	50
Lamotrigine	Topiramate	80

perception of cognitive effects frequently can be greater than actual habituation to objective cognitive effects.

Behavioral and cognitive effects of AEDs differ across individual drugs[4] (see Tables 89.3 and 89.4). There are no clinically significant differences in cognitive effects between carbamazepine, oxcarbazepine, phenytoin, and valproate. Topiramate is slightly worse than these AEDs. Risk of AED-induced cognitive effects is greatest for phenobarbital and benzodiazepines. AEDs with lowest potential for cognitive side effects are gabapentin, lamotrigine, levetiracetam, tiagabine, and vigabatrin. Well-controlled studies for other AEDs are inadequate.

Individual patients differ in susceptibility to AED-induced adverse behavioral and cognitive effects. Prediction of these effects is quite difficult on an individual basis although some risks can be inferred. Patients who have a history of sensitivity to drug-induced adverse cognitive effects are more likely to experience such side effects with future AEDs. Patients who require maximum attention, processing speed, and memory are more likely to suffer effects that affect their daily life. For example, patients with high cognitive abilities, especially if essential for their job or school, are more likely to have AED-induced cognitive problems than mentally retarded patients, who would be more likely to have behavioral than cognitive problems. Certain patient groups are at increased risk for cognitive side effects. The elderly have increased susceptibility to the central effects of drugs for both pharmacokinetic and pharmacodynamic reasons. At the other end of the age spectrum, chronic adverse effects of AEDs in children could be cumulative over the period of neurodevelopment. Additional research is needed to address this issue in children and the elderly.

Psychiatric disorders such as depression, anxiety, and psychosis are increased in patients with epilepsy. Further, rates of these comorbid disorders in epilepsy exceed rates in medical disorders of similar severity suggesting that they are due at least in part to dysfunction in networks related to the seizure disorder. AEDs can have positive or negative psychotropic effects. Carbamazepine, lamotrigine, and valproate are used routinely in bipolar disorder. In contrast, virtually all AEDs can produce adverse behavioral effects. Phenobarbital and other GABAergic agents have been implicated in precipitating depression. Gabapentin and lamotrigine can produce agitation in children, especially the mentally retarded. Levetiracetam and topiramate can produce irritability or even psychosis in some patients, especially if there is prior neuropsychiatric history.

Clinical assessment of AED-induced cognitive effects is primarily based on patient report. Evaluation of safety in regard to cognitive effects in clinical trials performed for FDA approval is based on patient report. However, patient perception of AED-induced cognitive effects is more related to mood than objective cognitive performance.[5] Presently, there is no standardized method of assessing AED cognitive effects. In the future, a technique combining electrophysiological indices with concomitant measures of neuropsychological function might offer a reliable expedient method to evaluate AED cognitive effects within an individual.[6] Such measures after initial AED dose might predict subsequent side effects on maintenance dose. Prospective controlled trials are needed to investigate and validate such approaches.

Prediction of AED-induced behavioral and cognitive side effects is difficult on an individual patient basis, and additional research is needed. Strategies to lower the risk of cognitive side effects include avoiding unnecessary polytherapy and slowing the initial titration to achieve the lowest effective dose in monotherapy, while keeping drug levels below upper limits of standard therapeutic ranges. However, these guidelines may not be applicable to all individuals with refractory epilepsy where seizure control is not achieved without using higher dosages or polytherapy. Overall, adverse cognitive and behavioral effects are more common with the older AEDs (especially barbiturates and benzodiazepines) than newer AEDs although there are exceptions.

REFERENCES

1. Meador KJ. Cognitive effects of epilepsy and of antiepileptic medications. In: Wyllie E, ed. *The treatment of epilepsy. Principles and practice*, 4th ed. Philadelphia, PA: Lippincott Williams & Wilkins, 2005: 1185–95.
2. Gilliam FG, Fessler AJ, Baker G, Vahle V, Carter J, Attarian H. Systematic screening allows reduction of adverse antiepileptic drug effects: a randomized trial. *Neurology* 2004;**62(1)**:23–7.
3. Vickrey BG, Hays RD, Rausch R, Sutherling WW, Engel J Jr., Brook RH. Quality of life of epilepsy surgery patients as compared with outpatients with hypertension, diabetes, heart disease, and/or depressive symptoms. *Epilepsia* 1994;**35(3)**:597–607.
4. Loring DW, Marino S, Meador KJ. Neuropsychological and behavioral effects of antiepilepsy drugs. *Neuropsychol Rev* 2007;**17(4)**:413–25.
5. Perrine K, Hermann BP, Meador KJ, Vickrey BG, Cramer JA, Hays RD, Devinsky O. The relationship of neuropsychological functioning to quality of life in epilepsy. *Arch Neurol* 1995;**52(10)**:997–1003.
6. Meador KJ, Gevins A, Loring DW, *et al.* Neuropsychological and neurophysiological effects of carbamazepine and levetiracetam. *Neurology* 2007;**69**:2076–84.

A Child with So-Called Nocturnal Paroxysmal Dystonia Whose Epilepsy Arose from Orbital Cortex

Cesare T Lombroso

INTRODUCTION

The nature of nocturnal paroxysmal abnormal motor events occurring in children has been the source of debate for decades and there are still some disagreements about their nosology and origins. Some of these hyperkinetic episodes arise during quiet sleep (NREM), the children suddenly exhibiting a series of often bizarre motor activities, such as dystonic posturing, choreoathetotic and repetitive body twisting, and ballistic flailings of limbs.

For some time, these events were thought to represent one of the non-epileptic sleep phenomena subsumed with the term of *parasomnias*. Their origin was attributed to one of the *arousal disorders* occurring during stages 2 and 3 of NREM sleep because of altered or delayed maturation of the chronobiological mechanisms leading to inability to maintain deep NREM sleep.[1–4]

Horner and Jackson were among the first to describe in some children attacks of involuntary dyskinetic movements occurring in sleep, with often familial incidence, that were not proven to be epileptic in nature.[5] Later, Lugaresi *et al.*, in the course of extensive clinical and electrographic evaluations in subjects exhibiting nocturnal episodes of motor behaviors, recognized that in several of these the patients displayed, while in NREM sleep, clusters of dystonic, athetoid posturing, and other abnormal movements. They considered these to constitute a distinct syndrome coined first as hypnagogic and later as *nocturnal paroxysmal dystonia* (NPD).[6–8] Although admitting a possible epileptic nature for these attacks, they stressed however that the evidence for epilepsy was largely circumstantial, in view of consistently normal EEGs between and during the episodes and the striking dystonic and other bizarre dyskinetic movements that are uncommon in nocturnal convulsive or complex partial seizures. Thus they concluded that NPD was more likely a parasomnia, an arousal disorder. Several other authors expressed similar doubts about the nature of NPD, still considering it to be a parasomnia.[9–20] A psychogenic hypothesis to explain and to treat this sleep disorder was also advanced[16] and the classification and nomenclature of sleep disorders still listed NPD as a movement disorder or parasomnia.[21]

As various expressions of frontal lobe epilepsy (FLE) began to be described,[22–27] several investigators started to incline toward the epileptic hypothesis about the nature of NPD.[17,18,28–33] Also those who had first described NPD as being likely a parasomnia, in continuing monitoring of subjects with nocturnal attacks of complex movements, reached the conclusion that NPD was likely an epileptic disorder with some of the characteristics described in frontal lobe seizures.[18,34–36] Soon NPD was stated to be one clinical manifestation of what was called *Nocturnal Frontal Lobe Epilepsy (NFLE)*.[37–39] However, NFLE has remained a source for diagnostic difficulties because of similarities with the vast repertoire of the NREM arousal parasomnias, and also because even in patients thought to suffer from NFLE, close to 40% have a personal or familial incidence of parasomnias.[18,38–41] Importantly, the origin in the brain for NPD, the main kind of seizure within the proposed syndrome of NFLE, remained unknown, and those who favored a specific brain locus could do so only on circumstantial evidence. All efforts to obtain on prolonged video–EEG monitoring any persuasive inter and ictal recordings with electrographic discharges in subjects displaying NPD attacks failed. The only exception was when following the attack the patient developed a generalized convulsion. In rare instances the frontal lobe origin was predicated on the basis of single photon emission computer tomography (SPECT). Many of those who favored the frontal lobe thought that the supplementary motor cortex (SMA) was a likely candidate.[27] Others suggested that NPD could arise from the temporal lobe,[22] from centro-parietal[32] or cingulated gyrus cortices[42]; and by using stereo video–EEG recording, it was concluded that NPD seizures may originate in the insula.[43] Perusal of the literature indicated that most of these hypotheses are not based on persuasive evidence.

During investigations of different kinds of paroxysmal dyskinesia, I studied three children whose frequent attacks had all the clinical and electrographic features characteristic for the syndrome of NPD arising from stage 2 NREM sleep. Here, I describe and discuss a patient who was first investigated more than 10 years ago and published in part in 2000.[44] To my knowledge this was the first demonstration of the NPD's ictal origin from a small area in the orbital cortex, with rapid spread to the supplementary sensory motorgyri. The patient was cured after surgical ablation of a small cortical dysplasia (CD) that had not been revealed by neuroimaging. This case also offers the possibility to critically analyze the still unresolved issues regarding the proposed syndromes of nocturnal FLE and of the autosomal dominant nocturnal FLE (see section on Discussion).

MATERIAL AND METHODS

A 9-year-old child was referred because of very frequent nightmares that had not been controlled by benzodiazepines or by behavioral psychology. His medical biography and family history were non-contributory. The neurological examination, the scalp EEGs (awake and asleep), and the CT and MRI scans were normal. On video–EEG polygraphy (LTM), several stereotypical events were captured: the child would wake up from stage 2 of NREM sleep displaying a complex series of activities that included dystonic, choreic, ballistic movements of all extremities with intermittent flailings of arms and legs (Figure 90.1). He appeared to be alert, but not responsive and without facial display of

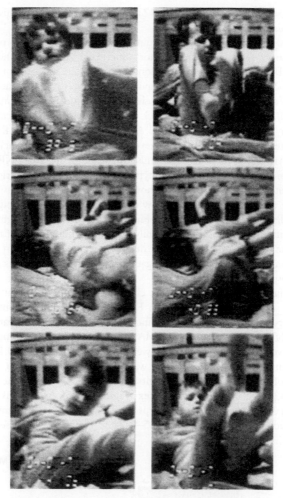

f0010

FIGURE 90.1   Shows a few features of one of the paroxysmal nocturnal seizures. Because these attacks occurred at night, only red light photography could be used, hence less optimal quality of the photos. Note, besides the varieties of motor activities, the lack of fearful facial expression.

fearful expression. There were no automatisms, vocalization, or incontinence. Tachycardia and brief apneas were present but without drops in blood oxygen saturation. The episodes lasted about 2–3 min, with sudden cessation of all motor activities and the child returning to sleep. The next morning, he had no recollection of awakening during sleep or of having had the event. He did not complain of having headaches, and was not dysarthric, but often he was somewhat sommolent during the day. The scalp EEG before and following the attack displayed normal NREM sleep patterns. During the episodes his movements and the EMG artifacts completely obliterated the underlying recordings. The characteristics of his frequent and only nocturnal attacks, the negative neurological examination, the negative neuroimaging and laboratory screenings with lack of improvement with benzodiazepines reproduced all the findings obtained in two previous patients in whom I had made a diagnosis of nocturnal paroxysmal dyskinesia. These children's attacks were helped by carbamazepine (CBZ) and it also afforded in this patient about 80% control of his nocturnal episodes.

The child was lost to follow up for about 2 years. When 11 years old, he was re-admitted because of relapsing frequent short nocturnal attacks that no longer were controlled by CBZ nor by valproate or clonazepam. Again he had not exhibited any paroxysmal episodes in daytime, but was having them five to eight times almost every night, with subsequently severely disrupted sleep architecture. All examinations (general and neurological), MRI, and interictal EEG were normal. During a scalp video–EEG monitoring, over 15 episodes were captured. Again artifacts masked the EEG during the spells and the interictal recordings did not reveal abnormalities. The attacks were identical to those he had displayed at his first admission, again arising from NREM sleep. An ictal SPECT scan demonstrated moderate hyperperfusion over the anterior right frontal lobe, where an interictal SPECT scan had shown hypoperfusion.

This time the child's attacks did not show improvement even with high blood levels of CBZ, benzodiazepines, valproate, and topiramate. Their frequent nightly occurrence was causing significant disruption for all family members and because of the child's progressive academic decline in school, it was decided to proceed with an invasive LTM, after full discussion of either positive or negative results with his parents and with consent from the hospital's Ethical Committee.

In view of the SPECT results and the clinical expression of the attacks, the right hemisphere was selected. Because the scalp EEG offered no clues about possible focal cortical origin, several areas were explored, including large portions of parietal and frontal lobes, the subfrontal (orbital) cortex, SMA, and first and second temporal lobe gyri (Figure 90.2). Several stereotypical episodes were captured (see Figure 90.1 and text), and all showed that these began while the child was in stage 2 NREM sleep, with an abrupt onset of a train of about 6–7 Hz spikes originating quite focally from the proximal contacts of the strip placed on the orbital cortex (Figure 90.3a). As the spikes increased in amplitude, about 3–4 s later low voltage sharps appeared focally in both anterior and posterior strips recording from the SMA. Some 5–8 s later (Figure 90.3b) these discharges had

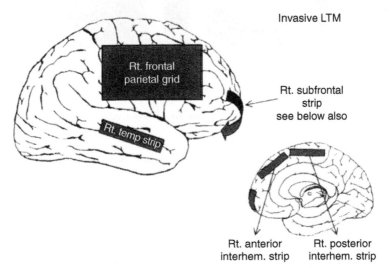

FIGURE 90.2   Shows a diagram of the subdural grid and strips for the invasive LTM.

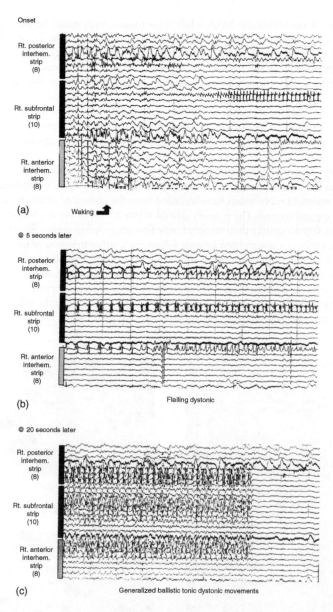

FIGURE 90.3   These figures illustrate three EEG epochs occurring in this and other typical clinical attacks. In (a) note the abrupt onset, during NREM sleep, of a train of about 6–7 Hz spikes originating very focally from the right orbital cortex where it remains for 5–6 s before invading focal areas in both inter-hemispheric strips (recording from SMA cortex). (b) The discharge now is more evident within the anterior and mid portions of the SMA cortex, while it continues within the orbital cortex with robust groups of polyspikes. (c) About 20 s later the discharge now involves adjacent areas of both orbital and SMA cortices, but without invading the convexity of the frontal lobe nor the parietal, temporal cortices (not shown here).

f0030

increased in voltage within the SMA, while it continued with robust bursts of polyspikes from the same focus in the orbital cortex. Figure 90.3c illustrates how, about 20 s later, the discharges had spread to larger areas of both SMA and orbital cortices, but without invading the strips placed over the frontal lobe convexity or over the parietal or temporal lobes (not shown here). Electrical stimulation (60 Hz, 25 mA, for 1–2 s) at the site where the initial train of spikes had begun produced 3–5 s long epochs of spikes without onset of clinical effects. These brief evoked responses were considered only in the absence of after discharges. This was not reproduced by stimulation of anterior and posterior frontal lobe cortex nor by stimuli applied to the SMA, or to the surface of the temporal lobe.

- *Surgery:* At surgery corticography revealed groups of spikes arising from a discrete area in the orbital cortex that became continuous after 25 mg of methohexital were injected i.v. No spikes were recorded from the convexity of the frontal or the temporal cortices. The surgeon ablated about 2.5 cm of the discharging orbital cortex. Corticography then recorded only few, single spikes arising from the borders of the excision; these did not increase following another injection of methohexital.

u0020
- *Pathology:* The surgical specimen showed features indicative of a focal cortical dysplasia (CD). There was no layering in this cortex. Neurons were of different sizes, some in clusters; there were some larger cells with paler cytoplasm, somewhat resembling balloon cells, mainly at the border with the white matter. In the latter were several ectopic neuronal cells (Figure 90.4).

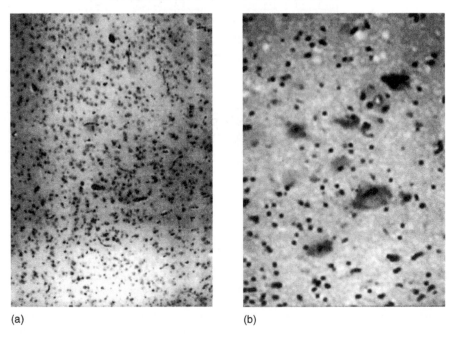

(a)   (b)

f0040   FIGURE 90.4   (a) Shows the disorganized, unlayered cortex, with neurons of different size and orientation, some occurring in clusters. The white matter contained an excessive number of ectopic neurons. (b) An example of the large cells with pale cytoplasm (balloon-like cells) present mainly at the border with the white matter.

- *Follow-up:* There were no post-surgical complications, nor evidence of neurological deficits. The child suffered two brief convulsions in sleep within 3 weeks after surgery, none of these recurred while on CBZ. There were no relapses of his nocturnal paroxysmal attacks or of diurnal seizures on follow-up visits for 7 years, being off CBZ for 4 years. Neurological examinations revealed no deficits; only some moderate cognitive delays were revealed by neuropsychological testing, but the fellow is now in regular high school.

DISCUSSION

One reason why episodes of NPD were generally thought to be parasomnias was because their dyskinetic, often bizarre motor activities generally are not seen in convulsions or in complex partial seizures occurring in sleep, while NREM arousal disorder can display similar phenomenologies. The lack of ictal or interictal electrographic concomitants, the normal neurological examinations and absent neuroimaging findings were other factors militating against an epileptic disorder. Once some intracerebral recordings, performed by surgeons in waking subjects, indicated that a few ictal discharges originating from frontal lobe cortices were associated with symptomatologies akin to some in NPD, the opinions expressed by some that the latter could be epileptic in nature were strengthened.[11,16–17,29–31,45] Also the clinicians who first described the NPD syndrome, after further investigations, now not only admitted its epileptic nature[34,35,46,47] but further subdivided the nocturnal episodes according to their clinical expressions, namely paroxysmal arousals (PA), NPD, and episodic nocturnal wanderings (ENW).[34–36,39,47] They further stated that these semiologically distinct phenotypes constituted what was termed the NFLE.[34,38]

This fragmentation became a source of nosological confusion, potentially increasing the difficulties facing clinicians in classifying nocturnal abnormal motor activities as being epileptic or parasomnia in nature. For example, while the intracerebral recording in a patient with refractory NFLE supported the notion that its minor motor activities (PA) were epileptic,[48] another intracerebral study on similar patients found that they were not epileptic but rather arousal disorders.[49] Interestingly, some investigators found that in their patients the typical NPD attacks were preceded by a non-epileptic brief motor phenomenon occurring as they aroused from NREM sleep.[50] Others described patients with paroxysmal dystonia whose attacks were triggered by sudden voluntary movements,[50–52] somewhat alike to what occurs in kinesiogenic paroxysmal choreoathetosis.[53] It is not surprising that in a recent paper, a careful analysis of video–EEG recordings of 66 subjects suspected of having NFLE, not only trainees but also experts could not reliably diagnose these subsets of NFLE.[54]

Emerging genetic discoveries

Nosological difficulties also arose when the Australian group first identified and described nocturnal frontal lobe seizures with clear autosomal dominant inheritance (ADNFLE).[55,56] Subsequently numerous investigations of several families revealed how ADNFLE can result from different mutations of genes encoding subunits of voltage-activated ion channels whose functions then are altered.[45,57–59,60–66] While these studies contributed to the seminal discoveries that some idiopathic epilepsies are caused by channelopathies (see for review Avanzini et al.[67]), they also added to nosological disarray when ADNFLE was stated to be a homogenous clinical syndrome distinct from NFLE.[55,56,65,66,68,69] In fact it became evident that ADNFLE, besides its genetic heterogeneity was also clinically heterogeneous, with both intra- and interfamilial semiological differences. These included ages of onset, evolutions, presence or absence of auras and of psychiatric disorders, responses to medication, occurrence of seizures also in daytime, as well as contrasting electrographic signatures and functional neuroimaging findings.[43,45,51,52,66,70–74] Thus, while in some papers it was stated that ADNFLE was a distinctive and clinically homogenous syndrome,[55–57] later the same group of investigators also recognized its clinical heterogeneity. They were confronted then by families with autosomal dominant nocturnal epilepsy that contained, besides members with seizures suggesting frontal lobe origin, also others whose seizures originated apparently from either temporal, centro-parietal or occipital lobes.[51,69,71,75,79] Hence a new syndrome was proposed: *Familial Partial Epilepsy with variable Foci (ADNFLE)*.[76] It was evidently surprising to find in such families, for example, individuals with cephalic aurae followed by complex partial seizures arising from temporal lobe and even patients with typical sylvian seizures arising from supra sylvian operculum in parietal lobe.[76–78] Therefore ADNFLE added further nosological confusion and, more dramatically, raised the question of how, in the absence of morphological lesions, a specific genetic defect might alone induce totally different seizures arising from such different regions of the brain.

s0050

Are NFLE and ADNFLE distinct syndromes?

p0160

The authors who had proposed the syndrome of NFLE and those who had proposed the syndrome of ADNFLE at first stated that these were two entirely distinct clinical syndromes. However, a careful perusal of the literature reveals that this distinction appears nebulous.[34,38,45,55,68,79] On the one hand it seems clear that ADNFLE families contain subjects exhibiting classical NPD attacks, the principal phenotypic expression of NFLE.[43,45,51,56,61,65,68,69,71,74–76,80,81] On the other hand, while ADNFLE contains the distinction of the genetic leit-motif, a genetic factor also occurs in NFLE. Besides the more common sporadic cases, familial cases have been described in many articles dealing with cohorts of subjects with NPD or with episodic sleep wandering.[6,11,29,34,37,38,43,47]

p0170

Hence it was suggested by some that ADNFLE is a genetic variant of NFLE.[39,50,51,62,71,74,75,81,82] In parallel, in a classical review of paroxysmal motor disorders of sleep, the Australian authors use the term "sporadic or familial NLFE," rather than the term ADNFLE.[40]

p0180

Both these proposed syndromes share the puzzling question of how a distinct epileptogenic condition or a gene defect in the brain might cause seizures that are so different in phenotypes and that originate from quite different regions of the brain. Logically some additional factors and mechanisms have to be involved. There is another problem shared by these proposed syndromes. They contend to be the only kind of sleep-related epilepsies occurring in the frontal lobes, thus ignoring those arising from the supplementary motor areas (SMAs), or from the anterior convexity or the pre-rolandic cortices, and even those originating within the temporal lobe regions. It is true that the complex dyskinetic features of NPD, the main type of NFLE, generally should help in differentiating it from the ictal phenomenologies arising from other areas of the brain, particularly from the usual SMA-related seizures.[19,25,27,29,71,83,91] However, sleep-related dyskinetic features may occur in seizures originating within the temporal lobe,[84–87] adding to the problem presented by the potential overlap with the parasomnias.[18,40,41,88–90]

Therefore, as a corollary of the problems mentioned in the section 'Discussion' and of those listed in this section it seems logically justifiable to abandon both the terms NFLE and ADNFLE in favor of a nosologically inclusive term. Tentatively such a simplified term might be: *Nocturnal Sporadic or Familial Epileptic Dyskinetic Seizures.* This would also eliminate the confusion generated by the parcellation of a single epileptic clinical event according to its possible various phases, namely into a PA, an NPD, or an ENW. Likewise it is also time to abandon these terms, including that of NPD, since it perpetuates the ambiguity of it possibly being an arousal disorder instead of an epileptic seizure. Thus, it should also be abandoned in favor of: *Nocturnal Epileptic Dyskinesia.*

Why has demonstration of the epileptic nature of this nocturnal bizarre dyskinesia proved to be such a hard task?

As mentioned in the section 'Introduction', ever since Lugaresi *et al.* described the episodes of dystonic and dyskinetic movements occurring out of NREM sleep (NPD), whether they were arousal disorders (parasomnias) or epileptic seizures has been controversial. In favor of the former were: first, the intriguing lack of clear EEG discharges between and during attacks; second, the occasional coexistence of the most striking event (NPD) with phenomenologies whose semiology could be considered more akin to parasomnias;[1–4,15,49,90] third, the frequent positive family history of various kinds of parasomnias; and fourth, the normal neurological examinations and neuroimaging studies. In favor of the epileptic hypothesis were: first, the occurrence at times of similar diurnal attacks, or of generalized convulsions; second, the often favorable response to CBZ; third, the generally greater severity of the bizarre repertoire of "motor activities," their stereotypy and clustering of short episodes in one night, their occurrence during earlier stages of NREM sleep; and fourth, often some recollection of episodes in the morning. Although prolonged video–scalp EEG monitoring can offer some diagnostic clues, often it may not be possible to reach a diagnosis of epilepsy or of parasomnia. Even most of those who suggested a specific locus for the ictogenesis of NPD collectively agreed that scalp derived EEGs could not reliably be of assistance either inter- or intra-ictally.[17,28–30,32,42,43,45,76,91–94] Some investigators resorted to functional neuroimaging (SPECT, PET scans) since routine MRIs, as the EEGs, were of no help unless there was a demonstrable and occasional lesion.[32,43,44,68,73,93,94,99] But the results of functional neuroimaging studies also failed to reveal the true epileptogenic zone in the brain since SPECT and PET scans pointed to quite disparate loci, and it is often difficult to know if what they show is the primary zone or is the result of the ictal spread from another region.

Further analysis of available literature thus indicated, on the one hand, a striking disparity of opinions and hypotheses regarding the epileptogenic zone of NPD and, on the other hand, a general paucity of persuasive data supporting them. It is fair to state that there has been scarce electroencephalographic support for any of the suggested zones in the brain that might be the primary locus for the epileptogenesis of NPDs. Papers reporting that a few subjects displayed some EEG abnormalities, as reviewed in the literature, are not persuasive. Sometimes "epileptiform features" were mentioned, but these were not better qualified; these most often were without localizing value, and some actually were normal EEG features related to different stages of NREM sleep, such as K-complexes, for example[6,11,16,18,29–32,34,36,37,40,41,46,50,51,55,83,90,93]

p0220   The most potent boost to drive the pendulum toward the epileptic hypothesis came when neurosurgeons, using intracerebral techniques, recorded from mesial frontal cortex or from the inferior surface of the frontal pole, ictal EEG seizures that could not be detected via scalp recordings. Importantly, some of these electrical discharges were accompanied by symptomatologies that had features similar to those occurring in subjects with NPD attacks.[24–27,32,42,43,48,49,95,96,98]

p0230   Therefore, the issue arose about considering invasive monitoring as the procedure more likely to resolve such diagnostic dilemmas. However, an invasive video–EEG polygraphy is hardly justifiable in patients with sleep-related disorders that do not impinge seriously on their quality of life, like the PA disorders such as night terror, somnambulism or panic attack. But at times the major events, dubbed as NPDs, if not medically controllable, can severely disrupt a patient's well-being, and cause cognitive and behavioral problems. These patients should become candidates for intracranial techniques, in conjunction with functional neuroimaging findings. These are now the only available means to reveal the presence of an occult lesion or of an epileptogenic cortical area amenable to surgical ablation.

s0070   **Such was the situation that arose in the child presented here**

p0240   His spells of complex, bizarre motor phenomenology arising in early stages of NREM were the hallmark for a tentative diagnosis of the so-called NPD but with otherwise non-contributive video scalp-derived EEG or neuroimaging. When these episodes became pharmacologically uncontrolled and he showed evidence of cognitive decline, it was decided to proceed with an invasive video-EEG polygraphy. The problem then was what areas of his brain should be monitored in the hope of discovering the cortical source of the NPD. The perusal of the literature had shown that there are quite discordant opinions and very few data regarding the epileptogenic locus for such seizures. A majority of the authors had favored the frontal lobe as the generator of NPD attacks, but without specifying in which region of the lobe it might be located.[31,34,37,41,45,46,68,75,99,100,101] Some did focus on specific cortices, mentioning the SMA as the possible site for the epileptogenesis of NPDs but without confirmations by either interictal or ictal electrographic data.[17,28–30,40,91] Others instead favored at times the temporal lobe, also on only a circumstantial basis.[11,28,46,76,86] A few, using invasive techniques, chose the cingulate gyri as the best candidates for the origin of the NPD,[42,93–95] while pre-rolandic lesions were thought by others to be its epileptogenic source.[32,76] Recently, a stereo-encephalographic study on patients with nocturnal hypermotor seizures suggested that these might be generated within the antero-superior insular cortex.[43]

p0250   Thus these few reports using invasive techniques, in spite of unequivocally confirming the epileptic nature of sleep-related hypermotor paroxysms, again failed to agree about the brain's zone responsible for their ictogenesis. Another small number of invasive studies were performed, but these dealt with rather peripheral issues. As mentioned, two of them were directed to establish if the minor events of these nocturnal episodes were also epileptic in nature and these studies reached opposite conclusions.[48,49] Others were done to show the outcome of surgical ablations in patients in whom the stereo–EEG was said to provide localizing information. However, 20 of 21 such subjects had focal CD likely to guide where best to locate the recording electrodes.[85]

What did the invasive study in this child show?

As stated in the results and illustrated in the figures, invasive monitoring of this patient confirmed the epileptic nature of the nocturnal dyskinetic episode (NPD); (2) established that its epileptogenic locus resided in a very limited area of the orbital cortex, corresponding, in this child, to an occult small dysplastic lesion; (3) the ictal discharge in the orbital cortex spread after several seconds (4–7) to the SMA without invading any of the monitored areas in the frontal, parietal, or temporal lobes; (4) the clinical phenomenologies became apparent only when both anterior and posterior SMA were invaded by the discharge; (5) the epileptic phenotypes usually arising from the SMA did not resemble those events captured by the video in this child; and (6) the electrical stimulations induced an ictal discharge only when applied to the two electrodes from where the spontaneous electrical seizures were recorded, and never when other areas of frontal, parietal, or temporal lobes were tested. The ablation of the small lesion, minimally including the surrounding cortex brought full seizure control, now for over 6 years, on no medication for 4 years.

There have been a few previous papers regarding seizures said to arise from fronto-orbital cortex with electrical–clinical correlation. To my knowledge the first was from Tharp who wrote about an "orbito-frontal seizure syndrome" in three children. Clinically there were prominent autonomic symptoms together, at times, with "disorganized motility." While interictally the scalp EEG contained spike discharges, unfortunately an electrical–clinical correlation was vitiated because no electrical or clinical seizures were recorded when a "depth electrode" was inserted into the orbital cortex of one child. Also, the surgical ablation of the structural lesion present in the child largely crossed the limits of the orbital cortex.[103] An earlier paper[102] mentioned seizures of "probable orbito-frontal origin" but this was based only on finding interictal discharges without obtaining a clinical and electrical seizure. Another paper described some patients with episodic somnambulism who responded to antiepileptic drugs, suggesting an epileptic origin. However, there was again no clinico-electrical correlation.[10] Williamson et al.,[24] in describing clinical criteria to distinguish "frontal-pole seizures" from the CPS of temporal lobe origin, mentioned that in those originating from the frontal pole the patients frequently displayed motor automatisms and often violent and bizarre behaviors, akin to those exhibited by my patient. They also state that these attacks may be misdiagnosed as "hysterical" episodes because inter- and intraictal scalp EEG were often misleading. However, clear clinical electrical correlation was again lacking. A somewhat similar phenomenon occurred during the extensive investigations by Munari and Bancaud.[103] They found that in patients with uncontrollable epilepsy of frontal lobe origin, when an electrical seizure remained in the orbital cortex without spreading, there were no clinical symptoms. However, they also state that a majority of discharges originating in the orbital cortex spread to other frontal and extra-frontal regions. When discharges reached the SMA cortex for a few seconds there were again no clinical manifestations. However, when SMA or cingulated gyrus were invaded, some patients would engage in "complex gestural automatisms." From such observations Munari wrote "the ictal discharges starting in the orbital cortex" without spreading elsewhere are "asymptomatic." This is what was found in my patient. Namely, the ictal discharges recorded from the more proximal electrodes placed on the orbital cortex were clinically asymptomatic until they invaded both the anterior and the posterior portions of the SMA. At about this time, the bizarre and complex motor phenomenology began (see figures).

However, as mentioned before, the phenotypes of seizures originating from the SMA are generally notably different from the very complex hypermotor seizures occurring in this syndrome. The SMA discharges also tend to invade other frontal lobe areas.[29,83,90,91] It is therefore tempting to hypothesize that the discharge originating from orbital cortex, then invading SMA, will not spread from SMA to other frontal areas but rather spread downward to nuclei of the striatum, as has been shown to occur in kinesiogenic dyskinesias.[53] Rich efferent and afferent connections of the SMA with various basal ganglia nuclei have been shown in several studies.[104–106] Obviously, such downward spread of ictal discharges from orbital cortex to striatum remains hypothetical.

s0090   REFERENCES

1. Broughton R. Sleep disorders: disorders of arousal. *Science* 1968;**158**:1070–8.
2. Gastaut H, Broughton R. A clinical and polygraphic study of episodic phenomena during sleep. *Recent Advances in Biological Psychiatry* 1965;**7**:197–221.
3. Guilleminault C, Palombini L, Pelayo R. Chervin RD. Sleepwalking and sleep terrors in prepubertal children: what triggers them? *Pediatrics* 2003;**111**:e17–e25.
4. Sheldon SH. Disorders of development and maturation of sleep, and sleep disorders of infancy, childhood and cerebral palsy. In: Culebras A, ed. *Sleep disorders and neurological disease*. New York: Marcel Dekker, 2000: 59–82.
5. Horner FJ, Jackson LC. Familial paroxysmal choreoathetosis. *Amsterdam: Excerpta Medica* 1969:745–57.
6. Lugaresi E, Cirignotta F. Hypnogenic paroxysmal dystonia: epileptic seizure or a new syndrome? *Sleep* 1981;**4**:129–38.
7. Lugaresi E, Cirignotta F. Two variants of nocturnal paroxysmal dystonia with attacks of short and long duration. In: Degen R, Niedermeyer E, eds. *Epilepsy. Sleep and sleep disorders*. Elsevier Science Publisher BV, 1984: 169–72.
8. Lugaresi E, Cirignotta F, Montagna P. Nocturnal paroxysmal dystonia. *J Neurol Neurosurg Psychiatry* 1986;**49**:375–80.
9. Boller F, Wright DG, Cavalieri R, Mitsumoto H. Paroxysmal nightmares. *Neurology* 1975;**25**:1026–8.
10. Pedley TA, Guilleminault C. Episodic nocturnal wandering responsive to anti-convulsant drug therapy. *Ann Neurol* 1979;**2**:30–5.
11. Goodbout R, Montplaisir J, Rouleau I. Hypnogenic paroxysmal dystonia: epilepsy or sleep disorder? *Clin Electroenceph* 1985;**16**:135–42.
12. Lee BI, Lessor RP, Pippinger CE, *et al.* Familial paroxysmal hypnogenic dystonia. *Neurology* 1985;**35**:1357–60.
13. DiMario FJ, Emery ES. The natural history of night terrors. *Clinical Pediatrics* 1987;**26**:505–11.
14. Silvestri R, Di Domenico P, Xerra A, Di Perri R. Hypnogenic paroxysmal dystonia: a new type of parasomnia? *Funct Neurol* 1988;**3**:95–103.
15. Maselli RA, Rosenberg RS, Spire JP. Episodic nocturnal wanderings in nonepileptic young patients. *Sleep* 1988;**11**:156–61.
16. Berger HJ, Berendsen-Versteeg TM, Joosten EM. Hypnogenic paroxysmal dystonia: epilepsy or a new syndrome? *Ned Tijdschr Geneeskd* 1984;**128**:1697–8.
17. Meierkord H, Fish Dr, Smith SJM, *et al.* Is nocturnal paroxysmal dystonia a form of frontal lobe epilepsy? *Mov Disord* 1992;**7**:38–42.
18. Riggio S, Harner R, Privitera M. Frontal lobe epilepsy: difficulties with diagnosis and a proposal for classification. *Epilepsia* 1990;**31**:626–7.
19. Roberts R. Differential diagnosis of sleep disorders, non-epileptic attacks and epileptic seizures. *Curr Opin Neurol* 1998;**11**:135–9.
20. Maccario M, Lustmap LI. Paroxysmal nocturnal dystonia presenting as excessive daytime somnolence. *Arch Neurol* 1990;**41**:291–4.
21. Thorpy MJ. Classification and nomenclature of sleep disorders. In: Thorpy MJ, ed. *Handbook of sleep disorders*. New York: Marcel Dekker, 1990: 155–76.

22. Fegersten L, Roger A. Frontal epileptogenic foci and their clinical correlations. *Electroenceph Clin Neurophysiol* 1961;**13**:905–13.
23. Talairach J, Bancaud J. Stereotactic approach to epilepsy: methodology of anatomofunctional stereotaxic investigations. *Prog Neurol Surg* 1973;**5**:294–354.
24. Williamson PS, Spencer DD, Spencer SS, Novelly RA, Mattson RH. Complex partial seizures of frontal lobe origin. *Ann Neurol* 1985;**18**:497–504.
25. Delgado-Escueta AV, Swartz BE, Maldonado HM, *et al*. Complex partial seizures of frontal lobe origin. In: Wieser HG, Elger CE, eds. *Presurgical evaluation of epileptics*. Berlin, Heidelberg: Springer-Verlag, 1987.
26. Munari C, Giallonardo AT, Brunet P, Broglin D, Bancaud J. Stereotactic investigations in frontal lobe epilepsies. *Acta Neurochir* 1989;**46**:9–12.
27. Waterman K, Purves SJ, Kosaka B, Strauss E, Wada SA. An epileptic syndrome caused by mesial frontal lobe seizure foci. *Neurology* 1987;**37**:577–82.
28. Sellai F, Hirsch E, Maquet P, Salmon E, *et al*. Postures and abnormal paroxysmal movements during sleep: hypnogenic paroxysmal dystonia or partial epilepsy? *Neurol (Paris)* 1991;**147**:121–8.
29. Vigevano F, Fusco L. Hypnic tonic seizures in healthy children provide evidence for a partial epileptic syndrome of frontal lobe origin. *Epilepsia* 1993;**39**:110–9.
30. Hirsch E, Sella F, Maton B, Rumbach L, Marescaux C. Nocturnal paroxysmal dystonia: a clinical form of focal epilepsy. *Neurophysiol Clin (Paris)* 1994;**24**:207–17.
31. Fish DR, Marsden CD. Epilepsy masquerading as a movement disorder. In: Marsden CD, Fahn S, eds. *Movement disorders 3*. Boston, Oxford: Butterworth-Heinemann 1994: 346–58.
32. Arroyo S, Santamaria J, Setoain JF, *et al*. Nocturnal paroxysmal dystonia related to a pre-rolandic dysplasia. *Epilepsy* 1998;**11**:301–5.
33. Chavel P, Kliemann F, Vignal JP, Chodkiewicz JP, Talairach J, Bancaud J. The clinical signs and symptoms of frontal lobe seizures: phenomenology and classification. In: Jasper HH, Riggio S, Goldman-Rakic, eds. *Epilepsy and the functional anatomy of the frontal lobe*. New York: Raven Press, 1995: 115–26.
34. Tinuper P, Cerullo A, Cirignotta F, *et al*. Nocturnal paroxysmal dystonia with short-lasting attacks: three cases with evidence for an epileptic frontal lobe origin of seizures. *Epilepsia* 1990;**31**:349–56.
35. Montagna P, Sforza E, Tinuper P, Cirignotta E, Lugaresi E. Paroxysmal arousals during sleep. *Neurology* 1990;**40**:1063–6.
36. Provini F, Plazzi G, Lugaresi E. From nocturnal paroxysmal dystonia to nocturnal frontal lobe epilepsy. *Clin Neurophysiol* 2000;**111**:S2–S8.
37. Montagna P. Nocturnal paroxysmal dystonia and nocturnal wandering. *Neurology* 1992;**42**:61–7.
38. Provini F, Plazzi G, Montagna P, Lugaresi E. The wide clinical spectrum of nocturnal frontal lobe epilepsy. *Sleep Med Rev* 2000;**4**:375–86.
39. Provini F, Plazzi G, Montagna P, Lugaresi E. Nocturnal frontal lobe epilepsy: a wide spectrum of seizures. *Mov Disord* 2000;**15**:1264.
40. Derry CP, Duncan JS, Berkovic SF. Paroxysmal motor disorders of sleep: the clinical spectrum and differentiation from epilepsy. *Epilepsia* 2006;**47**:1775–91.
41. Ferini-Strambi L, Zucconi M. REM sleep behavior disorder. *Clin Neurophysiol* 2000;**11**:S136–S140.
42. Rajna P, Kundra O, Halasz P. Vigilance level-dependent tonic seizures-epilepsy or sleep disorders? *Epilepsia* 1983;**24**:725–33.
43. Ryvlin P, Minotti L, Demarquay G, Hirsch E, *et al*. Nocturnal hypermotor seizures, suggesting frontal lobe epilepsy, can originate in the insula. *Epilepsia* 2006;**47**:755–65.
44. Lombroso CT. Nocturnal paroxysmal dystonia due to a subfrontal cortical dysplasia. *Epileptic Disord* 2000;**2**:15–20.
45. Oldani A, Zucconi M, Ferini-Strambi L, Bizzozero D, Smirne S. Autosomal dominant nocturnal frontal lobe epilepsy: electroclinical picture. *Epilepsia* 1996;**37**:964–76.
46. Provini F, Plazzi G, Tinuper P, Vandi S, Luggaresi E, Montagna P. Nocturnal frontal lobe epilepsy. A clinical and polygraphic overview of 100 consecutive cases. *Brain* 1999;**122**:1017–31.
47. Plazzi G, Provini F, Tinuper P, *et al*. Nocturnal frontal lobe epilepsy (NFLE): clinical, videopolysomnographic and genetic data in 100 cases. *Neurology* 1998;**50**:1467.

48. Nobili L, Francione S, Mai R, et al. Nocturnal frontal lobe epilepsy: intracerebral recordings of paroxysmal motor attacks with increasing complexity. Sleep 2003;**26**:883–6.
49. Terzaghi M, Sartori I, Mai R, et al. Sleep-related minor events in nocturnal frontal lobe epilepsy. Epilepsia 2007;**48**:335–41.
50. Pardal Fernández JM, López-Agreda JM, Carrillo-Yague R. Nocturnal paroxysmal dystonia, movement disorder and epilepsy. Rev Neurol 2002;**34**:940–4.
51. Ito M, Kobayashi K, Okuno T, et al. Electroclinical picture of autosomal dominant nocturnal frontal epilepsy in a Japanese family. Epilepsia 2000;**41**:52–8.
52. de Saint-Martin A, Badinand N, Picard F, et al. Diurnal and nocturnal paroxysmal dyskinesia in young children: a new entity? Rev Neurol (Paris) 1997;**153**:262–7.
53. Lombroso CT. Paroxysmal choreoathetosis: an epileptic or non-epileptic disorder? Ital J Neurol Sci 1995;**16**:271–7.
54. Vignatelli L, Bisulli F, Provini F, et al. Interobserver reliability of video recording in the diagnosis of nocturnal frontal lobe seizures. Epilepsia 2007;**48**:1506–11.
55. Scheffer IE, Bhatia KP, Lopes-Cendes I, et al. Autosomal dominant frontal lobe epilepsy misdiagnosed as sleep disorder. Lancet 1994;**343**:515–7.
56. Scheffer IE, Bhatia KP, Lopes-Cendes I, et al. Autosomal dominant nocturnal frontal lobe epilepsy. A distinctive clinical disorder. Brain 1995;**188**:61–73.
57. Phillips HA, Scheffer IE, Berkovic SF, et al. Localization of a gene for autosomal dominant nocturnal frontal lobe epilepsy to chromosome 20q 13.2. Nat Genet 1995;**10**:117–8.
58. Steinlein OK, Mulley JC, Propping P. A missense mutation in the neuronal nicotinic acetylcholine receptor alpha 4 subunit is associated with autosomal dominant nocturnal frontal lobe epilepsy. Nat Genet 1995;**11**:201–3.
59. Berkovic SF, Phillips HA, Scheffer IE, et al. Genetic heterogenicity in autosomal dominant frontal lobe epilepsy. Epilepsia 1995;**36**:147–8.
60. Steinlein OK. New insights into the molecular and genetic mechanisms underlying idiopathic epilepsies. Clin Genet 1998;**54**:169–75.
61. Picard F, Chauvel P. Autosomal dominant nocturnal frontal lobe epilepsy: the syndrome. J Allerg Clin Immunol 1999;**155**:445–9.
62. Hirose S, Iwata H, Akiyoshi HA. A novel mutation of CHRNA 4 responsible for autosomal dominant nocturnal frontal lobe epilepsy. Neurology 1999;**53**:1749–53.
63. Gambardella A, Annesi G, DeFusco M, et al. A new locus for autosomal dominant nocturnal frontal lobe epilepsy maps to chromosome 1. Neurology 2000;**55**:1467–71.
64. Sutor B, Zolles G. Neuronal nicotinic acetylcholine receptors and autosomal dominant frontal lobe epilepsy. Pflugers Arch 2001;**64**:73–4.
65. McLellan A, Phillips HA, Rittey C, et al. Phenotypic comparison of two Scottish families with mutations in different genes causing autosomal dominant nocturnal frontal lobe epilepsy. Epilepsia 2003;**44**:613–7.
66. De Marco EV, Gambardella A, Annesi F, et al. Further evidence of genetic heterogeneity in families with autosomal dominant nocturnal frontal lobe epilepsy. Epilepsy Res 2007;**74**:70–3.
67. Avanzini G, Franceschetti S, Mantegazza M. Epileptogenic channelopathies: experimental models of human pathologies. Epilepsia 2007;**48**:51–64.
68. Hayman M, Scheffer IE, Chinvarun Y, Berlangieri SU, Berkovic SF. Autosomal dominant nocturnal frontal lobe epilepsy: demonstration of focal frontal onset and intrafamilial variation. Neurology 1997;**49**:969–75.
69. Berkovic SF, Scheffer IE. Genetics of the epilepsies. Epilepsia 2001;**42(supp 5)**:S15–S23.
70. Mochi M, Provini F, Plazzi G, et al. Genetic heterogeneity in autosomal dominant nocturnal frontal lobe epilepsy. Ital J Neurol Sci 1997;**18**:183.
71. Oldani A, Zucconi M, Asselta R, et al. Autosomal dominant nocturnal frontal lobe epilepsy. A video-polysomnographic and genetic appraisal of 40 patients and delineation of the epileptic syndrome. Brain 1988;**121**:205–23.
72. Xiong L, Labuda M, Li DS, et al. Mapping of a gene determining familial partial epilepsy with variable foci to chromosome 22q11-q12. Am I Hum Genet 1999;**65**:1698–710.

73. Schmidt D. Editorial note. 'Nocturnal paroxysmal dystonia related to a prerolandic dysplasia'. *Epilepsy Res* 2001;**43**:1–9.

74. Callenbach PM, van den Maagdenberg AM, Hottenga JJ, *et al*. Familial partial epilepsy with variable foci in a Dutch family: clinical characteristics and confirmation of linkage to chromosome 22q. *Epilepsia* 2003;**44**:1298–305.

75. Combi R, Ferini-Strambi L, Montruccoli A, *et al*. Two new putative susceptibility loci for ADNFLE. *Brain Res Bull* 2005;**67**:257–63.

76. Berkovic SF, Serratosa JM, Phillips HA, *et al*. Familial partial epilepsy with variable foci: clinical features and linkage to chromosome 22q12. *Epilepsia* 2004;**45**:1054–60.

77. Lombroso CT. Lingual seizures and mid-temporal spike foci in children. *6th International Congress on EEG and Clinical Neurophysiology Proceedings* 1965;**16**:271–7.Vienna.

78. Lombroso CT. Sylvian seizures and mid-temporal spike foci in children. *Arch Neurol* 1967; **17**:52–9.

79. Scheffer IE. Autosomal dominant nocturnal frontal lobe epilepsy. *Epilepsia* 2000;**41**:1059–60.

80. Steinlein OK. Nicotinic acetylcholine receptors and epilepsy. *Curr Drug Targets CNS Neurol Disord* 2002;**1**:443–8.

81. Di Corcia G, Blasetti A, De Simone M, Verrotti A, Chiarelli F. Recent advances on autosomal dominant nocturnal frontal lobe epilepsy: understanding the nicotinic acetylcholine receptor (nAChR). *Eur J Paediatr Neurol* 2005;**9**:59–66.

82. Zucconi M, Oldani A, Ferini-Strambi L, Bizzozero D, Smirne S. Nocturnal paroxysmal arousals with motor behaviors during sleep: frontal lobe epilepsy or parasomnia? *J Clin Neurophysiol* 1997;**14**:513–22.

83. Morris HH 3rd, Dinner DS, Luders H, Wyllie E, Kramer R. Supplementary motor seizures: clinical and electroencephalographic findings. *Neurology* 1988;**38**:1075–82.

84. Swartz BE. Electrophysiology of bimanual-bipedal automatisms. *Epilepsia* 1994;**35**:264–74.

85. Nobili L, Francione S, Cardinale F, Lo Russo G. Epileptic nocturnal wanderings with a temporal lobe origin: a stereo-electroencephalographic study. *Sleep* 2002;**15(25)**:669–71.

86. Nobili L, Cossu M, Mai R, *et al*. Sleep-related hyperkinetic seizures of temporal lobe origin. *Neurology* 2004;**62**:482–5.

87. Silvestri R, Bromfield E. Recurrent nightmares and disorders of arousal in temporal lobe epilepsy. *Brain Res Bull* 2004;**30(63(5))**:369–76.

88. Schenck CH, Boyd JL, Marowald MW. A parasomnia overlap disorder involving sleepwalking, sleep terrors, and REM sleep behavior disorder in 33 polysomnographically confirmed cases. *Sleep* 1997;**20**:972–81.

89. Vaughn BV. Differential diagnosis of paroxysmal nocturnal dystonia in adults. In: Bazil CW, Malow BA, Sammaritano MR, eds. *Sleep and epilepsy*, Amsterdam: Elsevier Science, 325–38.

90. Niedermeyer E, Lopes da Silva F. *Electrencephalography: basic principles, clinical applications and related fields*. Elsevier Saunders, 2004: 7.

91. Connolly MB, Langill L, Wong PF, Farrell K. Seizures involving the supplementary sensorimotor area in children: a video-EEG analysis. *Epilepsia* 1995;**36**:1025–32.

92. Scheffer IE, Phillips HA, O'Brien CE, *et al*. Familial partial epilepsy with variable foci: a new partial epilepsy syndrome with suggestion of linkage to chromosome 2. *Ann Neurol* 1998;**44**:890–9.

93. Schindler K, Gast H, Bassetti C, *et al*. Hyperperfusion of anterior cingulate gyrus in a case of paroxysmal nocturnal dystonia. *Neurology* 2001;**57**:917–20.

94. Vetrugno R, Mascalchi M, Vella A, *et al*. Paroxysmal arousal in epilepsy associated with cingulate hyperperfusion. *Neurology* 2005;**64**:356–8.

95. Geier S, Bancaud J, Talairach J, *et al*. The seizures of frontal lobe epilepsy. A study of clinical manifestations. *Neurology* 1977;**27**:951–8.

96. Tharp BR. Orbital frontal seizures. A unique electrical encephalographic and clinical syndrome. *Epilepsia* 1972;**13**:627–42.

97. Rougier A, Loiseau P. Orbital frontal epilepsy: a case report. *J Neurol Neurosurg Psychiatry* 1988;**51**:146–7.

98. Harvery AS, Hopkins IJ, Bowe IM, *et al*. Frontal lobe epilepsy: clinical seizure characteristics and localization with ictal 99mTc-HMPAO SPECT. *Neurology* 1993;**43**:1166–90.

99. Schlaug G, Antke C, Holthausen H, *et al.* Ictal motor signs and interictal regional cerebral hypometabolism. *Neurology* 1997;**49**:341–50.

100. Thomas P, Picard F, Hirsch E, Chatel M, Marescaux C. Autosomal dominant nocturnal frontal lobe epilepsy. *Rev Neurol (Paris)* 1998;**154**:228–35.

101. Phillips HA, Marini C, Scheffer IE, *et al.* A de novo mutation in sporadic nocturnal frontal lobe epilepsy. *Ann Neurol* 2000;**48**:264–7.

102. Ludwig B, Ajmone-Marsan C, Van Buren J. Cerebral seizures of probable orbitofrontal origin. *Epilepsia* 1975;**16**:141–58.

103. Munari C, Bancaud J. Electroclinical symptomatology of partial seizures of orbital frontal origin. *Adv Neurol* 1992;**57**:257–65.

104. Jurgens U. The efferent and afferent connections of the supplementary motor area. *Brain Res* 1984;**300**:63–81.

105. Lehericy S, Ducros M, Krainik A, *et al.* 3-D diffusion tensor axonal tracking shows distinct SMA and pre-SMA projections to the human striatum. *Cereb Cortex* 2004;**14**:1302–9.

106. Leh SE, Pitto A, Chakravarty MM, Strafella AP. Fronto-striatal connections in the human brain: a probabilistic diffusion tractography study. *Neurosci Lett* 2007;**419**:113–8.

The Night Mom Didn't Come Back

Jane Boggs

HISTORY

The patient was a 39-year-old Caucasian woman with a 20-year history of complex partial seizures with rare generalization. She had her first seizure while a senior in college, described as staring, clenching her fists, and odd movements of her left hand. She rarely had a generalized convulsion, and typically would be lethargic for 10–15 min after a seizure. She never had status epilepticus but usually had a cluster of several seizures in a day. No definite etiology or trigger was identified by her neurologist. Her seizures remained poorly controlled with clusters of seizures nearly daily for 15 years. She was treated with monotherapy in maximally tolerated doses of all marketed medications for epilepsy, but to no avail. Her medication serum levels varied from the usual therapeutic to the supratherapeutic range and overall she tolerated the medications well with the exception of mild sedation. She fastidiously optimized her lifestyle, exercising and avoiding sleep deprivation and taking medications scrupulously according to directions. She took care of her household well, with the unfortunate result of injuring several toes (during a seizure) while she mowed their lawn. Her husband, who witnessed her typical seizure on their first date in college, provided exceptional emotional support and they had a healthy child when she was 27 (she later admitted this was the only time in her life she was noncompliant, trying to protect her unborn child. Tapering and stopping her medications had no effect on her seizure frequency). At age 34, she sought one of many second opinions from one of the foremost epileptologists of our time, Dr. Fritz Dreifuss, who recommended surgical evaluation.

SURGERY

Not only did this remarkable young woman prepare for epilepsy surgery, but agreed to a recording of the entire procedure, in the hope that it would not only increase awareness of epilepsy, but might also dispel some of the fears of epilepsy surgery. She (or rather her brain) became the cover for a 1995 issue of *National Geographic*. A feature article documented everything from shaving her head to the exposure and resection of the offending area of dysplastic cortex. She was in favor of the article with the exception of admitting that the stereotactic frame "hurt" because she did not want to frighten other patients with epilepsy from undergoing the necessary procedures. She was an excellent candidate for the procedure, with a surgically identifiable lesion by video–EEG and MRI, and good bilateral memory and language representation on Wada. She underwent right lateral temporal resection of the apparently localized cortical lesion and had no post-op seizures for 2 months.

POST-OP COURSE

She returned to her usual neurologic baseline, and resumed all previous activities, including helping with her son's Boy Scout troop, working on church projects for the homeless and engaging in a daily exercise routine. Her seizures recurred, though not as "severe" as in the past, and less frequent. She now had clusters of three to four every month, and typically of only a minute duration. Previously she had longer seizures and longer post-ictal periods. Thus, her surgery had effected an improvement, though not a meaningful enough one to allow her to drive. She once confided to her neurologist that her husband had allowed her to drive with him occasionally around the empty church parking lot. Those were the only times she drove after college.

She maintained this pattern, confirmed to be true epileptic seizures, with no evidence of non-epileptic seizures, by repeated epilepsy monitoring, for 4 years. She became the leader of the local epilepsy support group and participated in the Red Cross. Newer antiepileptic drugs appeared as investigational and eventually on the market: felbamate, gabapentin, topiramate, lamotrigine, tiagabine. She had no improvement with any medication combination tried, but more sedation with polytherapy. She and her family viewed her seizures as "something to deal with, but not a burden."[1] She remained on monotherapy with long-acting carbamazepine for over 1 year with stable seizure frequency at serum levels of 8–10. Adjunctive agents and alternate monotherapies did not improve or worsen control, but lower levels resulted in more frequent clusters. The only other medication she took was a standard multivitamin.

One typical Tuesday night, she and her family said their prayers and went to bed. Half an hour later, she had a typical seizure, with left body tonicity followed briefly by bilateral hand clenching. Her husband witnessed this and gently positioned her on her side, as usual, as the seizure ended and she entered into her usual post-ictal breathing pattern with a slight shudder. He expected her to become restless after a minute or two, with gradual awareness returning after no more than 5 min. When she did not, he reached over to try to rouse her. He realized at that instant that she was not breathing and immediately began CPR (cardiopulmonary resuscitation) and called 911. She was taken to the local hospital, not 10 min away, and could not be resuscitated. She underwent full advanced cardiac life support (ACLS) resuscitation efforts, including intubation with successful aeration with no recovery from asystole in slightly over 40 min. The medical examiner was notified but no autopsy performed.

COMMENTARY

Sudden unexpected death is unquestionably the most horrifying potential consequence of epilepsy. Epidemiologic studies have estimated a risk of at least 1–2 per 1000 patient-years,[2] though refractory patients' rates are 3–9 per 1000 patient-years.[3]

This case is unusual for this book as the original diagnosis is not in question, especially since she underwent definitive evaluation and treatment by the eminent Dr. Dreifuss. Failed surgery is not uncommonly encountered in patients with SUDEP (sudden unexpected death in epilepsy), but is more likely related due to refractoriness of seizures than the surgery itself. She had undergone multiple adequate medication trials and had incomplete seizure control after an apparently well-delineated resection. Multiple concomitant medications and frequent regimen changes have been associated with a higher risk of SUDEP.[4] Also, this woman's surgery occurred in the era pre-dating high-resolution MRIs or MEG. It is possible that another area of dysplasia could have been identified with these newer technologies, leading to a second or more extensive surgery, possibly removing a residual seizure nidus. Whether surgery which rendered her seizure-free could have reduced her risk of SUDEP is, however, unknown, as the long duration of her epilepsy would not have been changed.

She also passed away before the newest generation of automated external defibrillators (AEDs) and neurostimulators came to the market. Given the failure of her multiple previous treatments, it is unlikely that further medications changes would have drastically improved her seizure control. Certainly, responsive neurostimulation offers a completely different paradigm for seizure management, and may prove to be a much-needed solution to the psychological complications affecting many patients after removal of brain tissue. Fortunately, this intelligent and charming woman had no evidence of ill effects of her surgery, and went on to do much good for the community afterward.

Finally, one must wonder whether she had definitive SUDEP or not. Without an autopsy to eliminate other potential, unsuspected causes of death, she can only be considered a highly probable case of SUDEP, though certainly a better documented one than in many instances. Witnessed SUDEP is exceedingly rare, with few cases in the literature.[5] She did, however, fit one published profile of longstanding refractory epilepsy, age between 20 and 40 years, and multiple medication regimen changes[4]. Then why, exactly, does the accumulated ictal burden of a lifetime increase one's risk for SUDEP? Hypotheses implicate the autonomic nervous system with ultimate failure of central nervous system control of cardiac conduction, respiratory regulatory mechanisms, or both. Patients have been observed after prolonged seizures and status epilepticus to die with abrupt bradycardia–asystole as well as ventricular fibrillation unresponsive to cardioversion.[6] Some of these patients have been found to have scattered microscopic areas of myocardial damage, similar to that seen in catecholamine excess states.[7] A lifelong high ictal burden is analogous to the excessive, sudden seizure activity of status epilepticus, and can be proposed to result in disrupted responses of the neurocardiac plexus, thereby contributing to sudden death. Pre-existing compromise of cardiopulmonary function will, of course, increase the risk that any ictal or even interictal discharge will be lethal. Lack of autopsy in her case, as in many others who are presumed to have SUDEP, makes it impossible to know if some other underlying factor contributed to her death. Although the family requested no autopsy should be performed, coroners may deem medical examination unnecessary when SUDEP appears probable. Unfortunately, it is just such cases which may be able to provide us with important pathologic information that can ultimately reduce the risk of SUDEP.

REFERENCE

1. Quote "The Night Mom Didn't Come Back", *The Roanoke Times* 1998; **22**: A2.

2. Nashef L, Fish DR, Sander JW, Shorvon SD. Incidence of sudden unexpected death in an adult out-patient cohort with epilepsy at a tertiary referral centre. *JNNP* 1995;**58**:462–4.
3. Tomson T, Walczak T, Sillanpaa M, Sander JW. Sudden unexpected death in epilepsy: a review of incidence and risk factors. *Epilepsia* 2005;**46(suppl 11)**:54–61.
4. Nilsson L, Farahmand BY, Persson PG, Thiblin I, Tomson T. Risk factors for sudden unexpected death in epilepsy: a case control study. *Lancet* 1999;**353(9156)**:888–93.
5. Langan Y, Nashef L, Sander JWA. Sudden unexpected death in epilepsy: a series of witnessed deaths. *JNNP* 2000;**68(2)**:211–3.
6. Boggs JG, Marmarou A, Agnew JP, *et al.* Hemodynamic monitoring prior to and at the time of death in status epilepticus. *Epilepsy Res* 1998;**31(3)**:199–209.
7. Manno EM, Pfeifer EA, Cascino GD, Noe KH, Wijdicks EF. Cardiac pathology in status epilepticus. *Ann Neurol* 2005;**58(6)**:954–7.

The EEG – Not
the EEG Report – Makes
the Difference

Jane Boggs

The patient is a 48-year-old African-American man who works as a delivery driver. He was brought to the local hospital emergency department after crashing his vehicle in a parking lot, sustaining a right femoral fracture and bruising. Although there was no evidence of a head injury, he was dazed on presentation and had no recollection of the crash. The neurologist on call was consulted and the possibility of seizure or syncope as the cause of his event was entertained. He had a normal noncontrast head CT, and a normal head MRI prior to having open reduction with internal fixation of his right femur that evening. The following morning he was in his usual normal mental state but still could not recall the accident. A routine EEG was performed, according to the hospital laboratory standards on a digital machine for 20 min, with photic stimulation and hyperventilation. The consulting neurologist reviewed the EEG the next day with the following conclusions:

> This EEG is performed in the awake and drowsy state and shows shifting asymmetries with variable frequencies represented bilaterally and intermittently. There are periods of distortion which arise during drowsiness which contain some occasional slower morphologies of questionable significance. There appear to be no waveforms that are pathognomonic of definitive epileptiform activity.

The patient was then referred to a cardiologist for evaluation of possible syncope due his multiple risk factors for cardiovascular disease, including hypertension, hypercholesterolemia, and family history of coronary artery disease. His cardiac workup, including nuclear stress test, echocardiogram, cardiac catheterization, and electrophysiology studies revealed no additional risks, and he was continued on his regimen of aspirin, ACE inhibitor, and statin. His wife reported that he had been intermittently noncompliant, and so it was concluded he only needed reinforcement of the need to take his medications. He followed up once with the neurologist, who told him he had no evidence of a neurological problem and to see his primary care physician in the future unless things changed. He resumed driving as soon as his orthopedic injury allowed.

Three months later, his wife saw him getting into his car and then sit inside it for several minutes. She went out to see what was wrong and discovered he was leaning across the steering wheel with his eyes and head deviated to the right. He was making gurgling noises and had bitten his tongue on the left. She called 911 and observed him having several vigorous clonic movements before starting to breathe loudly in a snoring fashion. When the rescue squad arrived, he was becoming alert and appeared restless but answered questions. He had no memory of getting into his car that morning, and complained of a headache.

He was admitted to the same hospital as the last time. The emergency physician started him on phenytoin, ordered an EEG and consulted a neurologist (a different physician was on call that day). An EEG was again performed, and was normal in the awake, drowsy, and asleep states. The neurologist requested the previous EEG and was initially given the above report. Unable to determine what the first EEG report meant, she asked for the actual EEG to be loaded on a review station from the archived data storage.

The EEG from 3 months prior indeed contained "periods of distortion," but they were unquestionably significant. In fact, four recorded electrographic seizures occurred in the 20 min recording, ranging from 30 s to 2 min in duration. During the first one, shown in Figure 92.1, the technologist performing the recording noted on the EEG that the patient was "staring" and had "NR" (no response) when asked questions. After the event, the technologist also noted the patient complained of a headache. The second neurologist initiated oxcarbazepine, obtained an MRI (which showed multiple old strokes) and advised the patient that he had epilepsy, likely due to cerebrovascular disease, which also needed to be evaluated. She also advised him that by state law he must not drive for a minimum of 6 months, and that he could not drive with a commercial license until at least 2 years seizure-free on stable therapy.

COMMENTARY

This patient illustrates two important principles in making a diagnosis of epilepsy. First, one should never rely on a summary as a substitute for reviewing the actual EEG waveforms and MRI images. All physicians, at one time or another, will be pushed for time or have difficulty finding both old and new records. Transcription errors may change key meanings (e.g. "a symmetric pattern" can become "asymmetric pattern"). Unfortunately, to review only the report and not the EEG can perpetuate an initially wrong interpretation, and delay appropriate diagnosis and treatment. Although there are reports in the literature of overinterpreting minor sharp waveforms into epilepsy, no reports could be found of the opposite problem.[1] The second neurologist realized that the clinical story associated with the second event was strongly indicative of a seizure witnessed by the wife, and pursued the first EEG in hope of corroborating a suspected cerebral focality. As it turned out, the first MRI, unlike the first EEG, was correctly interpreted as normal. Unfortunately, it was of poor quality, as it was done on an open MRI (which had only a 0.3 T magnet) compared to the second, closed MRI (which had a 1.5 T magnet).

Second, not all neurologists are equally able to interpret an EEG. Although the first neurologist was a board-certified neurologist from a prominent university neurology program, his fellowship training was not in EEG, but in another subspecialty. He had undergone the usual 3 months training in EEG as a resident, 14 years previously. The ACGME and ABPN require training in epilepsy and EEG as part of a neurology residency, but individual program requirements usually determine the length and technical content of the rotations. Although this neurologist read between 100 and 200 EEGs every year at

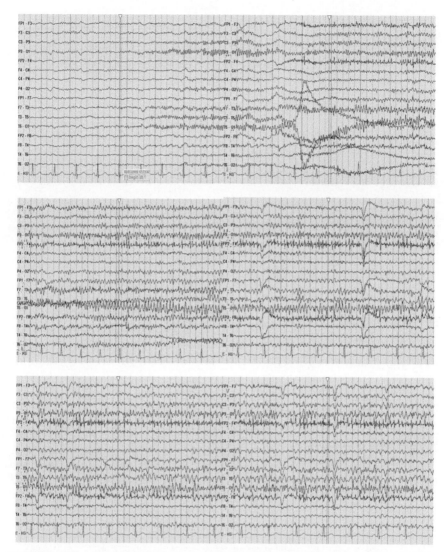

FIGURE 92.1   Example of one of the recorded focal seizures in this case, with onset at T5 as rhythmic 6–7 Hz apiculate activity, distinct from preceding background. This pattern gradually increases in amplitude and involves the surrounding electrical field. Postictal slowing manifests first locally on the left, then spreads to affect the right electrodes as well.

a large regional medical center, no one reviewed any of his interpretations for accuracy. In fact, the only requirement to be allowed to read EEGs independently at the hospital was to be "proctored" by the chief of neurology (who also had no subspecialty training in EEG) for his first 10 EEG readings. This otherwise excellent neurologist cannot be faulted for being unable to properly interpret EEGs, but he should be faulted for stretching beyond his fund of knowledge and skill. The vague description and inconclusive conclusions, even had they been correct, should be a "red flag" that this neurologist not only did not know what he was looking at, but also had no idea how to describe it.

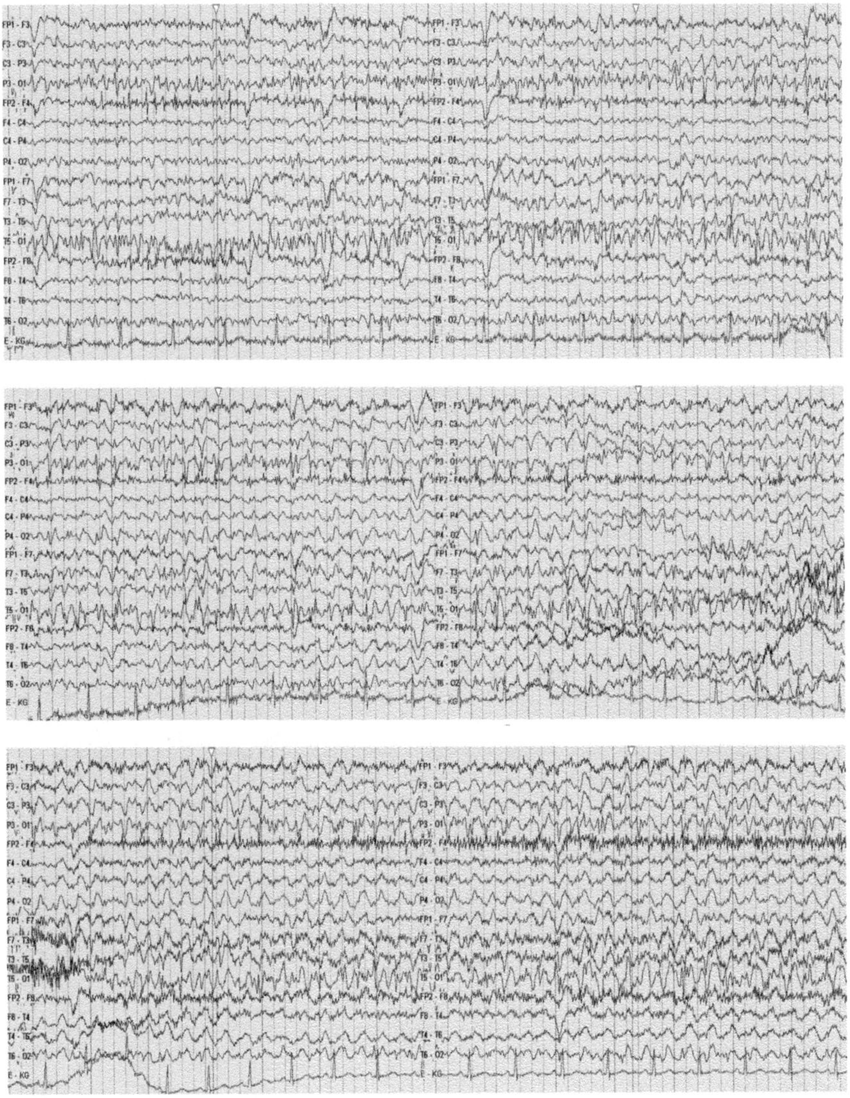

FIGURE 92.1   (*Continued*)

Completing a neurology residency and passing one's boards do not necessarily imply one is equally capable in all aspects of neurology. Certainly technical procedures which are subject to technology advances (such as EEG, EMG, sleep, and intraoperative monitoring) warrant additional board certification and ongoing honing of interpretation skills with qualified teachers. The extraordinary variety of normal variants, epilepsy and coma patterns, as well as the ubiquitous biologic and electrical artifacts, inadvertent, and purposeful adjustments of the recording by technologists (who also have variable skills) makes a mere 3 months of EEG insufficient training. Finally, the need to convey a meaningful interpretation is crucial, especially as studies may be reported to non-neurologists. The American Clinical Neurophysiology Society has published guidelines

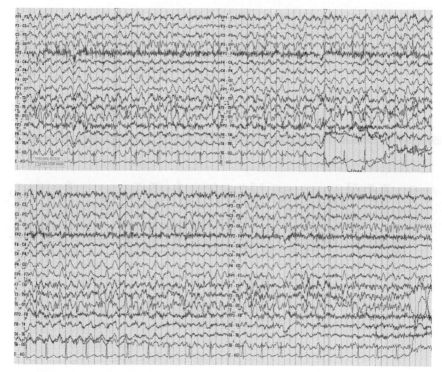

FIGURE 92.1   (*Continued*)

that address the qualifications of EEG interpretation and report generation.[2] Unfortunately, these guidelines are not mandated in many hospitals or practices. Worse, there is no supervising body to educate and improve performance of those who choose to read (or misread) EEGs. Medicare, hospitals, and practices set low or no standards for obtaining interpreting privileges for some procedures, including EEG. Whether this is because of misplaced trust in training program content, financial motives, or simply ignorance of appropriate quality standards and guidelines is unclear.

This patient and the first neurologist were fortunate that the misinterpretation of his initial EEG did not result in a fatal motor vehicle accident. Since multiple seizures were identified in a mere 20 min recording, he certainly must have continued to have unwitnessed seizures over the next 3 months. In addition, if the correct diagnosis had been made initially, the patient quite likely would not have been subjected to so many thousands of dollars of cardiac workup. This case should warn all neurologists: graduation and board certification of neurology residents may not provide adequate training to read EEGs correctly, misinterpretation of EEGs is likely commonplace, and patients are placed at risk as a result.

REFERENCES

1. Benbadis S. Misinterpretation of EEG. *Prac Neurol* 2007;**7(Oct)**:323–5.
2. The American Clinical Neurophysiology Society. Guideline 7: guidelines for writing EEG reports. *J Clin Neurophysiol* 2006;**23(2)**:118–21.

PART VI

Where Clinical Knowledge and Preclinical Science Meet

EDITORS' NOTE

In Part VI, each case is accompanied by one or two companion comments. These comments are intended to discuss preclinical or clinical implications and considerations raised by the case.

c00093

The Double-Hit Hypothesis: Is It Clinically Relevant?

Sookyong Koh and Kent Kelley

s0010

HISTORY

p0020

The patient is a 16-year-old right-handed young woman with a history of normal development, benign focal epilepsy of childhood with centrotemporal spikes (BECTs)/rolandic epilepsy, and malrotation of the left hippocampus, who later developed left temporal lobe epilepsy with complex partial seizures.

p0030

She initially presented at the age of 8 years when she had a nocturnal seizure with "fumbling" facial movements during which she was unable to call out to her parents. Her EEG showed rolandic spikes and she was treated with phenytoin, but developed a rash. She was then switched to carbamazepine. She became seizure-free and the rolandic spikes resolved by 10 years of age and carbamazepine was weaned.

p0040

After the onset of puberty at 12½ years of age, she then experienced a new type of seizure that occurred while awake. This seizure type was initially described as beginning with the sensation of "panic," increased heart rate, and a metallic taste "like sucking on a quarter." She has at times also seen colored dots. The aura was then followed by right hand movements, an interruption of language and loss of awareness that have rarely been followed by secondary generalization. For example, she reported a convulsion while playing the violin in the orchestra. Once in Mississippi while volunteering in the aftermath of hurricane Katrina, she had three seizures. These clusters of seizures, as often happened, occurred during her menstrual period and she experienced an unpleasant smell and taste of fruit, blacked out and then woke up after 30–45 s. Her parents and friends report that during her seizures, she is unable to talk and has right hand and leg trembling movements.

p0050

Her medical history is significant only for a history of appendicitis in 8th grade. She does not have a history of febrile seizures, head trauma, or meningitis. She currently is an honor roll student and is taking advanced placement classes. She is active in student government and has a good group of friends.

EXAMINATION AND INVESTIGATIONS

Her neurological examination is normal. Family history is significant for a maternal grandmother with absence seizures, who reportedly died in the shower from a convulsion.

Her EEG shows left temporal slow waves and sharp discharges. Extended video–EEG monitoring has not captured any seizures. MRI is normal except for a malrotation of the left hippocampus. Functional MRI shows normal motor activation and left temporal language representation.

DIAGNOSIS

Benign Childhood Epilepsy with Centrotemporal Spikes (BECTs). Malrotation of the left hippocampus. She then developed left temporal lobe epilepsy with complex partial seizures that were initially refractory to treatment and she later developed a catamenial seizure pattern.

TREATMENT AND OUTCOME

She was treated with a variety of anticonvulsants, which were either not effective or intolerable. She was first treated for her temporal lobe epilepsy with lamotrigine, which did not work and she developed a rash. Levetiracetam did not work at a low dose. High-dose oxcarbazepine produced double vision. Zonisamide was not tolerated because of stomachache and irritability. Pregabalin was also not tolerated because of irritability. She is currently treated with levetiracetam (2500 mg/day) and intermittent acetazolamide for a catamenial pattern of seizure exacerbation. She has been seizure free for 1 year. She wants to become a psychologist.

COMMENTARY

Our patient has malrotation of the left hippocampus, benign rolandic epilepsy and a family history of epilepsy; she subsequently develops temporal lobe epilepsy. It is highly unusual for patients with BECTs to later develop other seizure types.[1] In this case, one wonders whether her abnormal left hippocampal formation and BECT represent an example of "a double-hit" that led to later development of temporal lobe epilepsy.

The double-hit hypothesis of epileptogenesis provides a useful conceptual framework to understand the contribution of early-life events in the future development of epilepsy. The impetus for developing a "two-hit" animal model was to incorporate the clinical observation that prolonged early childhood convulsions often precede mesial temporal sclerosis and medically intractable temporal lobe epilepsy in later life. In the original model,[2] the first hit was seizures induced by a chemoconvulsant, kainic acid (KA), in rats during the second week of life (roughly corresponding to 1–2 years old in human), followed by the second hit of KA seizures in adulthood. Early-life seizures, even in the absence of cell death, render the developing brain more vulnerable to seizures and to seizure-induced neuronal damage in adulthood. Such susceptibility caused by early-life seizures has been observed in different animal models involving seizures induced by flurothyl, hyperthermia, or hypoxia.[3-5] Further, intrauterine toxin-induced neuronal migration defects (simulating congenital brain malformation) can act as the first hit and predispose the brain to the damaging effect of seizures later in life.[6] During early brain development, synaptic activity is critical for the process of refinement of connections between axons and their appropriate targets. A prolonged seizure, via intense synchronized neuronal activation, could have a permanent effect at this critical time of afferent-dependent synaptic remodeling.

In complex multifactorial disorders such as epilepsy, depression, or cancer, it is conceivable that both genetic susceptibility and injury (seizures, stressful life events, trauma, or insults) are necessary for disease manifestation. The concept of a "two-hit" hypothesis originated in cancer research by Nordling and Knudson who proposed that multiple "hits" to DNA are necessary to cause cancer. Similarly, the polygenic heterogeneity model of epileptogenesis predicts that the combination of a sufficient number of mutations or polymorphisms in epilepsy susceptibility genes within the human gene pool will result in the manifestation of idiopathic epilepsy.[7] A more encompassing concept of a double-hit hypothesis for disease expression beyond multiple gene mutations is perhaps best illustrated in a recent epidemiological study of depression. Childhood maltreatment was predictive of adult depression among the individuals with genetic susceptibility of carrying a less efficient serotonin transporter gene (short allele-5HTT), while no such association was found among long allele-5HTT gene carriers.[8] It is the combination of diathesis (gene) and stress (environment), or the interaction of "nature and nurture," that may cause an individual to succumb to a major depressive episode. Likewise, abnormal hippocampal shape and position can be found in healthy persons, however, such abnormalities are found in a significantly greater proportion of patients with partial epilepsy either from cortical malformation or of temporal lobe origin, suggesting increased vulnerability.[9]

This case illustrates the additive effect of several contributing factors associated with chronic epilepsy that is often seen in the clinic. The two-hit hypothesis of epileptogenesis may be clinically relevant to understanding the overlap of the relatively common syndrome of BECTS or early-life prolonged febrile convulsions with the underlying temporal malrotation and the expression of later-life refractory temporal lobe epilepsy in this case.

REFERENCES

1. Bouma PA, Bovenkerk AC, Westendorp RG, et al. The course of benign partial epilepsy of childhood with centrotemporal spikes: a meta-analysis. *Neurology* 1997;**48(2)**:430–7.
2. Koh S, Storey TW, Santos TC, et al. Early-life seizures in rats increase susceptibility to seizure-induced brain injury in adulthood. *Neurology* 1999;**53(5)**:915–21.
3. Koh S, Jensen FE. Topiramate blocks perinatal hypoxia-induced seizures in rat pups. *Ann Neurol* 2001;**50(3)**:366–72.
4. Dube C, Chen K, Eghbal-Ahmadi M, et al. Prolonged febrile seizures in the immature rat model enhance hippocampal excitability long term. *Ann Neurol* 2000;**47(3)**:336–44.
5. Schmid R, Tandon P, Stafstrom CE, et al. Effects of neonatal seizures on subsequent seizure-induced brain injury. *Neurology* 1999;**53(8)**:1754–61.
6. Germano IM, Sperber EF, Ahuja S, et al. Evidence of enhanced kindling and hippocampal neuronal injury in immature rats with neuronal migration disorders. *Epilepsia* 1998;**39(12)**:1253–60.
7. Heron SE, Khosravani H, Varela D, et al. Extended spectrum of idiopathic generalized epilepsies associated with CACNA1H functional variants. *Ann Neurol* 2007;**62**:560–8.
8. Caspi A, Sugden K, Moffitt TE, et al. Influence of life stress on depression: moderation by a polymorphism in the 5-HTT gene. *Science* 2003;**301(5631)**:386–9.

9. Bernasconi N, Kinay D, Andermann F, *et al*. Analysis of shape and positioning of the hippocampal formation: an MRI study in patients with partial epilepsy and healthy controls. *Brain* 2005;**128(Pt 10)**:2442–52.

10. Bethmann K, Brandt C, Loscher W. Resistance to phenobarbital extends to phenytoin in a rat model of temporal lobe epilepsy. *Epilepsia* 2007;**48(4)**:816–26.

c0020

The Double-Hit Hypothesis: Is It Clinically Relevant?

David Henshall

s0070

INTRODUCTION

p0150

Unlike primary generalized epilepsies, localization-related epilepsy of temporal lobe type or temporal lobe epilepsy (TLE) has rather unimpressive heritability and is thought to develop in three stages. A CNS insult leads to a period of epileptogenesis involving an insult- and age-dependent interplay of factors including cell death, gliosis, neuronal plasticity and changes to channel function, and finally the emergence of spontaneous seizures.[1] The double-hit hypothesis posits that disease expression (i.e. epileptic seizures or hippocampal sclerosis) in some individuals requires a predisposing factor.[2,3] Seizure episodes in childhood are normally considered first "hits" in this scenario. The insult is insufficient to precipitate epilepsy but predisposes to seizures or damage vulnerability, which in conjunction with a later life insult breaches a threshold for hippocampal sclerosis or emergence of TLE.

p0160

Benign childhood epilepsy with centrotemporal spikes (BCECTS) may result from out-of-phase development of excitation and inhibition within brain regions such as the perirolandic region in the upper sylvian bank.[4] Remission is normal by adolescence and is not associated with brain injury or development of TLE.[4-7] While certainly an unusual case, TLE development in the patient of Koh *et al.* may be due to a double-hit, but which factor(s) such as early-life seizures, hippocampal malrotation or medication are also plausible.

s0080

Influence of early-life seizures

p0170

The availability of several animal models has enabled the double-hit hypothesis to be tested.[2,8-11] The hypothesis is clearly relevant for early-life seizures and later-life development of TLE. Even single early-life seizures can have long-lasting effects on inhibitory tone and cell vulnerability, in the absence of neuronal death.[12,13] Febrile seizures modeled in immature rats by raised body temperature cause enduring changes in γ-aminobutyric acid (GABA) systems and other ion channels.[14-17] Altered channel properties favor increased probability of rebound depolarization and sporadic seizures which may underlie the lowered threshold for seizure development when re-challenged at adulthood.[8,18] After a second insult at adulthood, rats subject to early-life seizures are predisposed to earlier seizure onset, increased susceptibility to status epilepticus and more extensive hippocampal injury.[2,8] Repeated seizures also exacerbate cognitive defects induced by early-life status epilepticus.[10]

Experimental early-life seizures can also directly provoke spontaneous seizures by adulthood.[19–21] This rather questions the necessity of a double hit to explain the pathogenesis of epilepsy after early-life seizures. A pre-existing cerebral abnormality (cortical "freeze" lesion) further raises the proportion of rats developing epilepsy after febrile seizures from 35% to 86%.[11,21] That epilepsy only develops in a subpopulation despite a controlled precipitating injury in genetically homogeneous inbred rats highlights the challenge with explaining patient outcomes. Disparities in seizure and damage thresholds are also seen for common mouse strains.[22]

Taken together, experimental modeling largely supports a double-hit influence of early-life seizures. However, a double seizure "hit" is not epileptogenic under all conditions. Seizure onset can become increasingly protracted with multiple kainic acid treatments of immature rats[23] and epileptic "tolerance" has been reported where experimental non-harmful seizures confer protection against damage resulting from subsequent status epilepticus.[24,25]

Influence of hippocampal abnormality

Hippocampal changes have long been implicated as the primary pathogenic substrate in TLE and this is supported by experimental modeling.[26,27] Experimentally induced hippocampal or cortical dysgenesis also predisposes to febrile seizure development.[28] Hippocampal abnormalities in which neuronal loss is not prominent may also be pathogenic in human TLE. Invaginations of hippocampal granule cell layer organization in mainly non-lesional resected human hippocampi from TLE patients may contribute to development of febrile seizures in affected patients or TLE in the absence of overt neuropathology.[29] Hippocampal malrotation is characterized by incomplete inversion of the hippocampus with an abnormally round shape and may be associated with blurred internal structure.[30] A pathogenic role here is plausible given the influence of even non-lesional hippocampal abnormalities on TLE or seizure predisposition, and such has been suggested.[31] However, hippocampal malrotation is uncommon and not overrepresented in patients with TLE.[30,32] More clinical data or the advent of an animal model will be important to understand whether lateralization of seizure focus with hippocampal malrotation is coincidental or pathogenic for TLE.

Influence of anticonvulsants

It is unlikely that the use of phenytoin or carbamazepine contributed a first hit. Anticonvulsants are prescribed for other conditions (e.g. pain) and are not associated with development of seizures in those populations. Prospective studies following children from first seizure to epilepsy show antiepileptic drug (AED) treatment of first seizures does not influence recurrence in later life.[33,34] Nevertheless, AED exposure in childhood can be detrimental to IQ[35] and experimental models suggest AEDs influence memory function and GABA systems.[13] Phenytoin at therapeutically relevant doses causes widespread neuronal apoptosis in immature rat pups, including in the subiculum.[36] The clinical relevance of these findings remains to be firmly corroborated.

s0110 ## Genetic "hit"

p0220 The double-hit hypothesis is most challenged by our poor understanding of the relevance of the underlying genetic architecture of the patient to sporadic epilepsy including TLE. Autosomal dominant inheritance has been suggested for BCECTS but other genetic and environmental factors are likely involved.[4] A genetic contribution is certainly possible for hippocampal malrotation but has not been formerly explored. While a clear genetic component has been identified and quantified for common forms of epilepsy,[37] the first multi-institutional, large-population study into genetic factors that might underlie sporadic epilepsy, although illustrating the genetic component, failed to identify clear, individual risk factors in 279 biologically plausible candidate genes.[38] While genetic "load" is likely to be influential, we are some way from understanding the spectrum of effects in individual cases such as that presented here.

s0120 ## Summary and final perspectives

p0230 The double-hit hypothesis is experimentally supportable as a conceptual framework to explain localization-related epilepsy development in some individuals. Each "hit" discussed here could act to elevate damage and seizure susceptibility, or precipitate epilepsy where it would not otherwise be expressed. Its ubiquity is uncertain and it may not apply to primary generalized epilepsies. Moreover, we should not exclude that the patient had TLE from the start with the centrotemporal spikes referred from the abnormal hippocampus, then with increasing seizures becoming more clearly of temporal lobe onset. Finally, the concept is over-simplistic in accounting for predisposing factors within a patient's genetic architecture. Revision of the hypothesis might mean restricting its use to acquired focal epilepsies and thinking in terms of three or more "hits" where a patient's underlying genetic susceptibility, early-life trauma and their inter-relationship with age/developmental programming are fully accounted.

s0130 ## ACKNOWLEDGEMENTS

p0240 The author thanks Colin Doherty, Michael Farrell, Gianpiero Cavalleri, and Roger Simon for helpful discussion of the manuscript.

REFERENCES

1. Pitkanen A, Kharatishvili I, Karhunen H, *et al.* Epileptogenesis in experimental models. *Epilepsia* 2007;**48(suppl 2)**:13–20.
2. Koh S, Storey TW, Santos TC, Mian AY, Cole AJ. Early-life seizures in rats increase susceptibility to seizure-induced brain injury in adulthood. *Neurology* 1999;**53**:915–21.

3. Lewis DV. Losing neurons: selective vulnerability and mesial temporal sclerosis. *Epilepsia* 2005;**46(suppl 7)**:39–44.

4. Wirrell EC, Camfield CS, Camfield PR. Idiopathic and benign partial epilepsies of childhood. In: Wyllie E, ed. *The treatment of epilepsy*. Philadelphia, PA: Lippincott, Williams & Wilkins, 2006: 373–89.

5. Bouma PA, Bovenkerk AC, Westendorp RG, Brouwer OF. The course of benign partial epilepsy of childhood with centrotemporal spikes: a meta-analysis. *Neurology* 1997;**48**:430–7.

6. Guerrini R. Epilepsy in children. *Lancet* 2006;**367**:499–524.

7. Boxerman JL, Hawash K, Bali B, Clarke T, Rogg J, Pal DK. Is Rolandic epilepsy associated with abnormal findings on cranial MRI? *Epilepsy Res* 2007;**75**:180–5.

8. Dube C, Chen K, Eghbal-Ahmadi M, Brunson K, Soltesz I, Baram TZ. Prolonged febrile seizures in the immature rat model enhance hippocampal excitability long term. *Ann Neurol* 2000;**47**:336–44.

9. Mellanby J, Milward AJ. Do fits really beget fits? The effect of previous epileptic activity on the subsequent induction of the tetanus toxin model of limbic epilepsy in the rat. *Neurobiol Dis* 2001;**8**:679–91.

10. Hoffmann AF, Zhao Q, Holmes GL. Cognitive impairment following status epilepticus and recurrent seizures during early development: support for the "two-hit hypothesis". *Epilepsy Behav* 2004;**5**:873–7.

11. Scantlebury MH, Gibbs SA, Foadjo B, Lema P, Psarropoulou C, Carmant L. Febrile seizures in the predisposed brain: a new model of temporal lobe epilepsy. *Ann Neurol* 2005;**58**:41–9.

12. Ben-Ari Y, Holmes GL. Effects of seizures on developmental processes in the immature brain. *Lancet Neurol* 2006;**5**:1055–63.

13. Marsh ED, Brooks-Kayal AR, Porter BE. Seizures and antiepileptic drugs: does exposure alter normal brain development? *Epilepsia* 2006;**47**:1999–2010.

14. Chen K, Baram TZ, Soltesz I. Febrile seizures in the developing brain result in persistent modification of neuronal excitability in limbic circuits. *Nat Med* 1999;**5**:888–94.

15. Chen K, Aradi I, Thon N, Eghbal-Ahmadi M, Baram TZ, Soltesz I. Persistently modified h-channels after complex febrile seizures convert the seizure-induced enhancement of inhibition to hyperexcitability. *Nat Med* 2001;**7**:331–7.

16. Brewster A, Bender RA, Chen Y, Dube C, Eghbal-Ahmadi M, Baram TZ. Developmental febrile seizures modulate hippocampal gene expression of hyperpolarization-activated channels in an isoform- and cell-specific manner. *J Neurosci* 2002;**22**:4591–9.

17. Tsai ML, Leung LS. Decrease of hippocampal GABA B receptor-mediated inhibition after hyperthermia-induced seizures in immature rats. *Epilepsia* 2006;**47**:277–87.

18. Dube CM, Brewster AL, Richichi C, Zha Q, Baram TZ. Fever, febrile seizures and epilepsy. *Trends Neurosci* 2007;**30**:490–6.

19. Sankar R, Shin DH, Liu H, Mazarati A, Pereira de Vasconcelos A, Wasterlain CG. Patterns of status epilepticus-induced neuronal injury during development and long-term consequences. *J Neurosci* 1998;**18**:8382–93.

20. Sankar R, Shin D, Mazarati AM. Epileptogenesis after status epilepticus reflects age- and model-dependent plasticity. *Ann Neurol* 2000;**48**:580–9.

21. Dube C, Richichi C, Bender RA, Chung G, Litt B, Baram TZ. Temporal lobe epilepsy after experimental prolonged febrile seizures: prospective analysis. *Brain* 2006;**129**:911–22.

22. Schauwecker PE. Complications associated with genetic background effects in models of experimental epilepsy. *Prog Brain Res* 2002;**135**:139–48.

23. Sarkisian MR, Tandon P, Liu Z, et al. Multiple kainic acid seizures in the immature and adult brain: ictal manifestations and long-term effects on learning and memory. *Epilepsia* 1997;**38**:1157–66.

24. Borges K, Shaw R, Dingledine R. Gene expression changes after seizure preconditioning in the three major hippocampal cell layers. *Neurobiol Dis* 2007;**26**:66–77.

25. Hatazaki S, Bellver-Estelles C, Jimenez-Mateos EM, et al. Microarray profile of seizure damage-refractory hippocampal CA3 in a mouse model of epileptic preconditioning. *Neuroscience* 2007;**150**:467–77.

26. Sloviter RS. Decreased hippocampal inhibition and a selective loss of interneurons in experimental epilepsy. *Science* 1987;**235**:73–6.

27. Zappone CA, Sloviter RS. Translamellar disinhibition in the rat hippocampal dentate gyrus after seizure-induced degeneration of vulnerable hilar neurons. *J Neurosci* 2004;**24**:853–64.

28. Germano IM, Zhang YF, Sperber EF, Moshe SL. Neuronal migration disorders increase susceptibility to hyperthermia-induced seizures in developing rats. *Epilepsia* 1996;**37**:902–10.

29. Sloviter RS, Kudrimoti HS, Laxer KD, *et al.* "Tectonic" hippocampal malformations in patients with temporal lobe epilepsy. *Epilepsy Res* 2004;**59**:123–53.

30. Barsi P, Kenez J, Solymosi D, *et al.* Hippocampal malrotation with normal corpus callosum: a new entity? *Neuroradiology* 2000;**42**:339–45.

31. Vigliano P, Duca S, Isocrono A, Silengo M. Hippocampal malrotation in a supernumerary der(22) syndrome and epilepsy: a case report. *J Pediatr Neurol* 2003;**1**:39–42.

32. Lehéricy S, Dormont D, Sémah F. Developmental abnormalities of the medial temporal lobe in patients with temporal lobe epilepsy. *Am J Neuroradiol* 1995;**16**:617–26.

33. Camfield PR, Camfield CS, Dooley JM, Tibbles JA, Fung T, Garner B. Epilepsy after a first unprovoked seizure in childhood. *Neurology* 1985;**35**:1657–60.

34. Shinnar S, Berg AT, Moshe SL, *et al.* Risk of seizure recurrence following a first unprovoked seizure in childhood: a prospective study. *Pediatrics* 1990;**85**:1076–85.

35. Farwell JR, Lee YJ, Hirtz DG, *et al.* Phenobarbital for febrile seizures – effects on intelligence and on seizure recurrence. *N Engl J Med* 1990;**322**:364–9.

36. Bittigau P, Sifringer M, Genz K, *et al.* Antiepileptic drugs and apoptotic neurodegeneration in the developing brain. *Proc Natl Acad Sci USA* 2002;**99**:15089–94.

37. Turnbull J, Lohi H, Kearney JA, *et al.* Sacred disease secrets revealed: the genetics of human epilepsy. *Hum Mol Genet* 2005;**14**:2491–500.

38. Cavalleri GL, Weale ME, Shianna KV, *et al.* Multicentre search for genetic susceptibility loci in sporadic epilepsy syndrome and seizure types: a case-control study. *Lancet Neurol* 2007; **6**:970–80.

94

Atypical Evolution in a Case of Benign Childhood Epilepsy with Centrotemporal Spikes

Natalio Fejerman

)

HISTORY

p0020 This girl was 5.7 years old at her first visit. She was born to healthy parents and had three healthy siblings. Her neuropsychologic development was normal.

30   Her first seizures occurred at 3 years of age and were brief focal motor seizures affecting her left hand. After several months free of seizures, she presented motor facial seizures (on the left side) plus sialorrhea while awake lasting 10–60 s. She had been medicated with carbamazepine and free of seizures for 6 months. She came for a second opinion because of reappearance of motor seizures with persistent anarthria and inhibitory seizures in lower limbs causing gate disturbance. Carbamazepine was switched to valproic acid but improvement lasted only 1 month, and the new episodes with head-drops and myoclonic jerks in upper limbs occurred. At the same time several episodes with dysarthria and aphasic features were seen and frank dysgraphia was noted in her schoolwork. In Figure 94.1a–c we can see the deterioration of her writing abilities in the course of one and a half months. Incidentally, this girl attended a bilingual school including Spanish and Slovenian. Sulthiame 300 mg/day was added and since 2 days later she has been seizure-free until her last visit at 14.7 years of age.

EXAMINATION AND INVESTIGATIONS

40 Neurological examination was normal. Routine laboratory examinations were normal. Brain MRI was normal. The EEG she had at the onset of the disease showed left centrotemporal spikes, more frequent during sleep. The EEG we took during worsening of her clinical picture showed electrical status epilepticus with continuous spike–wave activity during slow sleep (Figure 94.2).

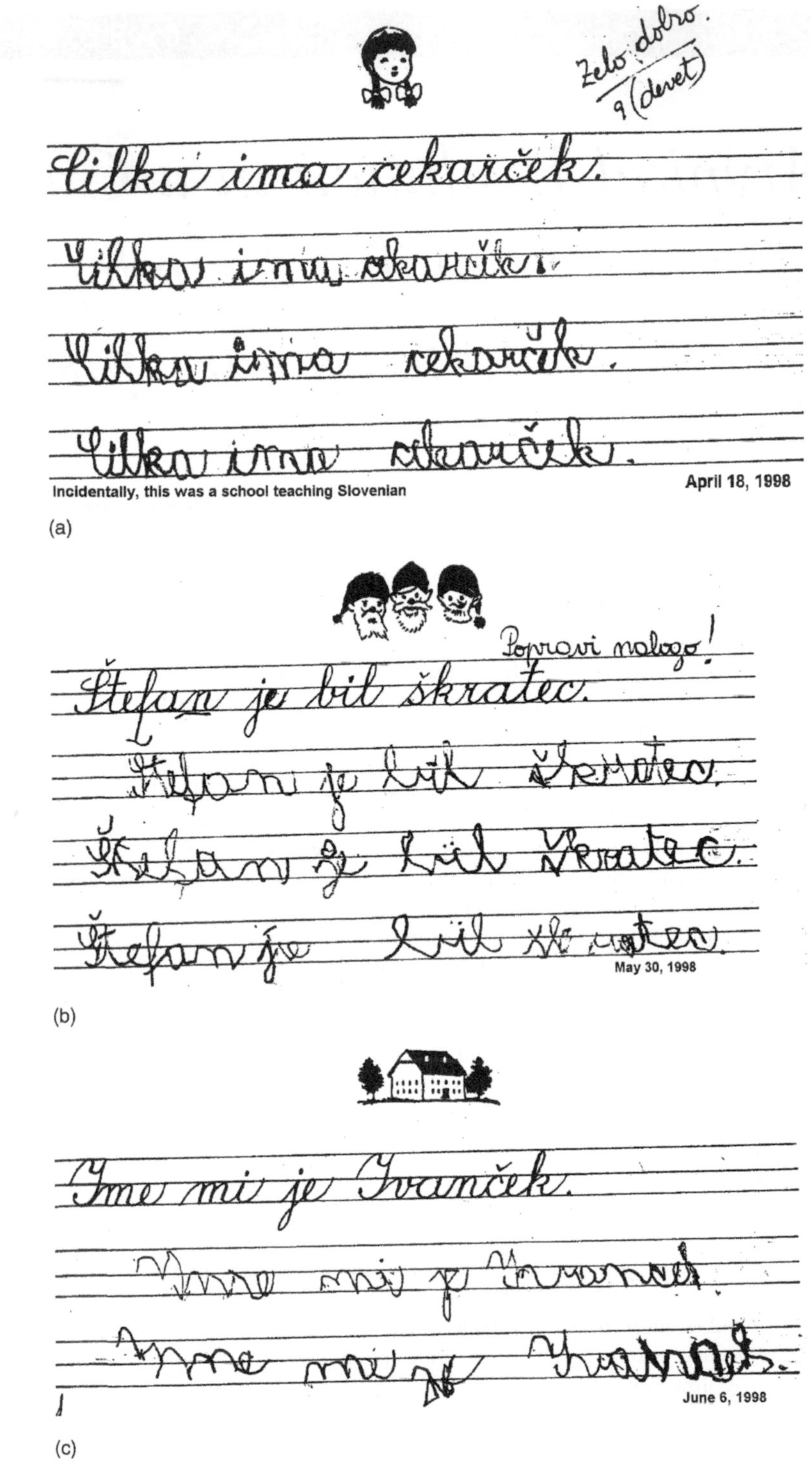

Zelo dobro.
9 (devet)

Tilka ima cekarček.

Tilka ima cekarček.

Tilka ima cekarček.

Tilka ima cekarček.

Incidentally, this was a school teaching Slovenian

April 18, 1998

(a)

Popravi nalogo!

Štefan je bil škratec.

Štefan je bil škratec.

Štefan je bil škratec.

Štefan je bil škratec.

May 30, 1998

(b)

Ime mi je Ivanček.

Ime mi je Ivanček.

Ime mi je Ivanček.

June 6, 1998

(c)

FIGURE 94.1   (a–c) Dysgraphia appearing after normal writing abilities in a 5.9-year-old girl.

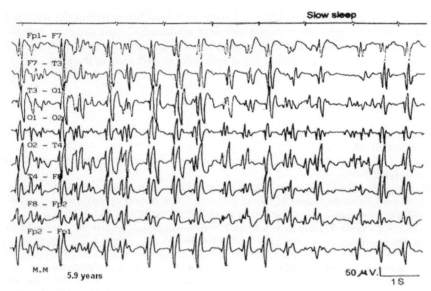

FIGURE 94.2   Sleep EEG with continuous spike and waves during slow sleep.

TREATMENT AND OUTCOME

We already mentioned the sequence of antiepileptic drugs (AEDs) used in her treatment and she kept taking sulthiame until age 13, when the EEG became normal. She is now a good student in high school.

DIAGNOSIS

In summary, the diagnosis at onset corresponds to a benign childhood epilepsy with centrotemporal spikes (BECTS) syndrome with some atypical features (age of onset, frequency of seizures). During the evolution of her disorder, the girl presented manifestations of atypical benign partial epilepsy of childhood (ABPEC) (inhibitory seizures, myoclonic seizures, learning difficulties) plus episodes of status epilepticus of BECTS (SEBECTS) (sialorrhea during 2h, prolonged anarthria), plus some symptoms of Landau–Kleffner syndrome (LKS; language deterioration). All three groups of symptoms and signs were associated with electrical status epilepticus during slow sleep (ESES). This EEG pattern is considered to be the result of secondary bilateral synchronies elicited after the appearance of focal spikes (left centrotemporal in this case). Association of this phenomenon with the use of certain AEDs has been proven in several cases, but we did not attempt to prove the association in this case by adding the first AED back again.

COMMENTARY

This case exemplifies the risk of atypical evolutions of benign focal epilepsies in childhood (BFEC). She presented mixed features of ABPEC, SEBECTS, and LKS. All these conditions are associated with ESES and there are mixed forms within the spectrum of the continuous spike-waves during slow sleep syndrome. Certain drugs are particularly indicated in cases of BFEC presenting atypical features such as early onset, frequent seizures, and increased frequency of epileptiform discharges in the EEG.

FURTHER READING

Aicardi J, Chevrie JJ. Atypical benign partial epilepsy of childhood. *Dev Med Child Neurol* 1982;**24**:281–92.

Chahine LM, Mikati MA. Benign pediatric localization-related epilepsies. *Epileptic Disord* 2006;**8(4)**:243–58.

Dalla Bernardina B, Sgró V, Fejerman N. Epilepsy with centrotemporal spikes and related syndromes. In: Roger J, Bureau M, Dravet CH, Genton P, Tassinari CA, Wolf P, eds. *Epileptic syndromes in infancy, childhood and adolescence*, 3rd ed. Eastleigh: John Libbey, 2002: 181–202.

Fejerman N, Caraballo R, Tenembaum S. Atypical evolutions of benign localization-related epilepsies in children: are they predictable? *Epilepsia* 2000;**41(4)**:380–90.

Fejerman N, Engel J. Landau Kleffner syndrome. In: Engel J, Fejerman N, eds. *MedLink neurology (section of epilepsy)*. San Diego: MedLink Corporation, 2008. Available at www.medlink.com.

Fejerman N. Benign childhood epilepsy with centrotemporal spikes. In: Engel J, Pedley TA, eds. *Epilepsy: a comprehensive textbook*. Philadelphia, PA: Lippincott Williams & Wilkins, 2008: 2369–77.

Fejerman N, Caraballo RH, Dalla Bernardina B. Atypical evolutions of benign focal epilepsies in childhood (BFEC). In: Fejerman N, Caraballo RH, eds. *Benign focal epilepsies in infancy, childhood and adolescence*. Eastleigh: John Libbey, 2007: 179–219.

Hahn A, Pistohl J, Neubauer BA, Stephani U. Atypical "benign" partial epilepsy or pseudo-Lennox syndrome. Part I: symptomatology and long-term prognosis. *Neuropediatrics* 2001;**32(1)**:1–8.

Tassinari CA, Rubboli G, Volpi L, Billard C, Bureau M. Electrical status epilepticus during slow sleep (ESES or CSWS) including acquired epileptic aphasia (Landau-Kleffner syndrome). In: Roger J, Bureau M, Dravet CH, Genton P, Tassinari CA, Wolf P, eds. *Epileptic syndromes in infancy, childhood and adolescence*, 4th ed. Montrouge: John Libbey Eurotext Ltd., 2005: 295–314.

Does Kindling in Humans Occur? Comments Based on the Previous Case Study

Dan McIntyre

Typical benign epilepsy of childhood with focal discharges in the central or rolandic midtemporal area (BECT) is a common form of epilepsy in childhood. The clinical symptoms normally indicate disturbed neuronal behavior in the lower rolandic area, innervating the face and throat. The natural history of this disorder is also indicative of a familial predisposition, where as many as 40% of close relatives manifest some variety of a seizure disorder. However, as many as 50% of children who manifest the EEG signature of BECT do not actually express clinical seizures, and are described as asymptomatic but *seizure-prone*. Because of its age dependency in onset/offset (between the ages of 3 and 13 years), it is considered to be maturation-dependent and sensitive to genetic factors. The unique neocortical expression of abnormal rolandic activity in BECT patients indicates a local low threshold for hyperexcitability during this age window, a window that ultimately closes in the early teens. The hyperexcitability also appears to be circadian, as ~80% of the seizures occur during sleep, where some become intractable and develop into bouts of status epilepticus. Many of the ensuing behavioral seizures are hemiconvulsive, and can secondarily generalize with a loss of consciousness. In older children, the convulsive expression is usually more restricted than in younger children, and treatment with carbamazepine can trigger an *atypical* presentation in the child that is drug dependent, that is, terminates with drug removal.[1]

The case report of Dr. Fejerman is described as *atypical* BECT, because of its early age of onset (3 years), development of inhibitory seizures with gait disturbance, and frank episodes of status epilepticus during sleep. These latter episodes were likely triggered by carbamazepine. The behavioral problems, including dysarthria, and aphasia with clear dysgraphia occurred following periods of nocturnal status epilepticus. All of these features eventually resolved, and the patient appears to be normal today, similar to typical BECT patients.

Kindling, of course, is defined as a progressive and relatively permanent increase in seizure expression as a result of repeated daily provocation.[2] The relationship of this atypical BECT case to traditional demonstrations of kindling is not clear. The most obvious similarity between the two would be in the progression of symptoms, where the patient case evolved from mild partial to secondarily generalized seizures with varieties of convulsive expression. The most obvious difference between the two is the lack of relative permanence in the patient case.

p0110   Like this patient case, however, kindling is also decidedly sensitive to genetic considerations, since rats have been selectively bred to be seizure-prone versus seizure-resistant.[3,4] The rat selection was for differential rates of amygdala kindling to secondarily generalized convulsions and not amygdala after-discharge thresholds; this selection resulted in seizure-prone rats (called fast rats) and seizure-resistant rats (slow rats). The clear ease of recruitment during amygdala kindling in fast rats is likely precipitated by the rapid involvement of the adjacent piriform and perirhinal cortices, areas that support and direct convulsive expression via their projections to and recruitment of frontal motor networks.[5-7] This is important because the piriform and perirhinal cortices in fast rats have exquisitely low-seizure thresholds compared to slow rats. These low-cortical thresholds are perhaps similar to the many BECT examples, where the cortical focus in the rolandic area in both typical and atypical cases has a pathologically low threshold for activation. However, in the present atypical case, the low-threshold partial seizures often generalized from the focal area, which suggests easy recruitment of additional ipsilateral or bilateral neural networks, like the naturally seizure-prone fast kindling rats.

p0120   Kindling stimulation studies also tell us that neocortical thresholds for triggering focal seizure activity are normally quite high (e.g., Ref. [4]). Importantly, kindling is known to reduce those thresholds, facilitating subsequent provocation.[8] It is also known that neocortical kindling is relatively slow by comparison to various limbic sites like the amygdala or adjacent limbic cortices. The slowness of progressive neocortical kindling is likely based in part on its high threshold but also because the daily triggered discharges are relatively non-progressive. Although the neocortical discharges do not progress over many applications in adult rats, sufficient repetitions eventually will induce progression into more advanced forms with secondary generalization. Whether this slowness of adult neocortical kindling happens in young rats has not been tested. It is clear, however, that young rats are far more seizure-prone than adult rats, similar to the maturational phenomenology of BECT.

p0130   In addition to the basic slowness of neocortical kindling in rats, an important difference between humans and rats in seizure progression may result from the belief that there is far less inhibition in the rat brain capable of constraining partial seizures and preventing generalization than in humans; as a consequence, in the case of kindling, rats are far more able than humans of manifesting reliable generalization from triggered focal seizures, and, perhaps, generalized spontaneous seizures after the latent period in models of status epilepticus.

p0140   In addition, the *frequency* of seizure activity is also critical in the progression and permanence of kindling. Kindling progresses much more rapidly with infrequent provocation. Frequent provocation in the amygdala of adult rats results in only a slight progression in fast rats and absolutely no progression in slow rats.[9-11] As to whether this is also true of neocortex remains untested. Thus the repeated triggering of seizures in rat paradigms (massed versus distributed kindling) does not necessarily result in permanent changes in the excitability of neural networks; the changes depend upon which networks are involved and the genetic background of the animal.

p0150   Does the human brain kindle? Almost certainly it does, depending upon where in the brain, and when and how. It would be unreasonably arrogant of us to suggest that we are the only animal "tested" so far that does not show kindling.[12] In that context, however, the exact network (e.g. cortical and subcortical), age and genetic background under question are likely critical to both the progressive development of seizure activity and its relative permanence.

REFERENCES

1. Lerman P. Benign childhood epilepsy with centrotemporal spikes (BECT). In: Engel J, Pedley TA, eds. *Epilepsy: a comprehensive textbook.* Philadelphia, PA: Lippincott-Raven Publishers, 1997: 2307–14.
2. Goddard GV, McIntyre DC, Leech CK. A permanent change in brain function resulting from daily electrical stimulation. *Expl Neurol* 1969;**25**:295–330.
3. Racine RJ, Steingart M, McIntyre DC. Development of kindling-prone and kindling-resistant rats: selective breeding and electrophysiological studies. *Epilepsy Res* 1999;**35**:183–95.
4. McIntyre DC, Kelly ME, Dufresne C. FAST and SLOW amygdala kindling rat strains: comparison of amygdala, hippocampal, piriform and perirhinal cortex kindling. *Epilepsy Res* 1999;**35**:197–209.
5. McIntyre DC, Kelly ME, Staines WA. Efferent projections of the anterior perirhinal cortex in the rat. *J Comp Neurol* 1996;**369**:302–18.
6. Kelly ME, Battye RA, McIntyre DC. Cortical spreading depression reversibly disrupts convulsive motor seizure expression in amygdala kindled rats. *Neuroscience* 1999;**91**:305–13.
7. Kelly ME, Staines WA, McIntyre DC. Secondary generalization of hippocampal kindled seizures: role of the piriform cortex. *Brain Res* 2002;**957**:152–61.
8. Löscher W, Horstermann D, Honack D, Rundfeldt C, Wahnschaffe U. Transmitter amino acid levels in rat brain regions after amygdala-kindling or chronic electrode implantation without kindling: evidence for a pro-kindling effect of prolonged electrode implantation. *Neurochem Res* 1993;**18**:775–8.
9. McIntyre DC, Rajala J, Edson N. Suppression of amygdala kindling with short interstimulus intervals: effect of norepinephrine depletion. *Exp Neurol* 1987;**25**:391–402.
10. Elmér E, Kokaia M, Kokaia Z, McIntyre DC, Lindvall O. Epileptogenesis induced by rapidly recurring seizures in genetically fast but not slow kindling rats. *Brain Res* 1998;**789**:111–7.
11. Shin RS, McIntyre DC. Differential noradrenergic influence on seizure expression in genetically fast and slow kindling rat strains during massed trial stimulation of the amygdala. *Neuropharmacol* 2007;**52**:321–32.
12. Coulter DA, McIntyre DC, Löscher W. Animal models of limbic epilepsy: what can they tell us? *Brain Pathol* 2002;**12**:240–57.

Does Kindling in Humans Occur? Comments Based on the Previous Case from a Preclinical Perspective

Andreas Draguhn

p0160   The case reported by Dr. Fejerman describes a combination of BECTS with additional features, leading to the diagnosis of ABPEC. Complicating issues included episodes of electrographic status epilepticus, learning difficulties and, most importantly, the development of pharmacoresistance toward carbamazepine and valproic acid. BECTS belong to a family of "benign" epileptic syndromes and typically show remission during adolescence.[1] The present case highlights several features of this disease which are interesting from a basic science point of view.

p0170   First, the syndrome starts at about 3–5 years of age and shows spontaneous remission in most cases. Second, a considerable number of cases (though not the present one) show cortical lesions in imaging studies (these are then classified as "pseudo-BECTS"[2]). Thus, structural alterations in the developing cortex might play a role.[3] Third, the girl had been successfully treated with two different AEDs which both lost efficacy after a relatively short period of time. Fourth, and in line with previous reports,[4,5] successful therapy involved sulthiame, an inhibitor of carbonic anhydrase.[6,7] These characteristics raise several scientific issues which have been addressed experimentally during past years. I will highlight some relevant recent results concerning cortical maturation with respect to pharmacoresistance, and the role of carbonic anhydrase in epilepsy, not pretending, though, that these concepts can already easily be translated into clinical applications.

p0180   The layered organization of the human neocortex involves complex steps of migration, cell differentiation, apoptosis of transiently occurring Cajal–Retzius cells, cell proliferation, and cell lineage differentiation. Irregular activity or external noxious stimuli may disturb these processes and lead to cortical malformations which, later on, can be the focus of epileptic syndromes.[8] Interestingly, the increasing power of imaging technology, together with refined electrophysiological methods and histopathological analysis of surgically removed tissue, reveal an increasing number of "cryptogenic" epilepsies with circumscribed cortical malformations.[9] Thus, developmental abnormalities are a major candidate mechanism causing epileptic syndromes in early childhood, and are potentially underlying many cases of benign childhood epilepsy.[2,3] Development of cortical and sub-cortical networks is dependent on electrical activity which is present even before birth (Refs. [10, 11]; see also below). This opens the possibility that altered electrical activity (as, e.g. during seizures) can disrupt normal development of the respective brain circuits.

Most experimental studies on epilepsy are being performed in rodents. It should be noted that mice and rats are born in a relatively immature state, corresponding to the beginning of the last trimester in humans.[12] Following pioneering work by Dreyfus-Brisac and Larroche,[13] recent DC–EEG recordings from prematurely born humans show that early cortical electrical activity shares many features of the spontaneous network events seen in all mammalian species tested.[14] The long-term sequelae of altered early activity in humans are not known, but it is suspicious that many patients with BECTS have a history of neonatal or infantile seizures.[15]

Immature neurons and networks have unique functional properties. A prominent feature is that the mature chloride gradient (low intracellular versus high extracellular concentration) is not present at early stages.[16] This yields GABAergic potentials depo-larizing and can turn GABAergic "inhibition" into an excitatory signal. At later stages, increased expression of the outwardly directed chloride transporter KCC-2 lowers intracellular chloride levels, leading to hyperpolarizing inhibitory postsynaptic poten-tials.[17] This developmental program can be reversed by seizures, probably by down-regulating KCC-2 expression via the BDNF–TrkB pathway.[18,19] Such developmental regression may be typical for chronic epilepsy and may underlie the depolarizing GABAergic potentials found in adult human epileptic tissue.[20,21] Chloride dysregula-tion might be aggravated by a parallel increase in expression of the inwardly directed chloride transporter NKCC-1, especially in juvenile tissue.[22] Reversal of developmen-tal programs and altered expression of receptors and ion channels may well contribute to the development of pharmacoresistance, as observed in the present case (see, e.g. Refs. [23, 24]). In addition, altered expression of drug transporters (with considerable genetic variability) contributes to this adverse development.[25]

There is a plethora of further differences between early and mature network activity. For our understanding of epilepsy, it is important to note that neuronal communication undergoes fundamental changes during cortical development. Electrical synapses (gap junctions) are far more widespread in early networks, mediating direct, fast transmission of electrical and metabolic signals from neuron to neuron.[26] A recent study has revealed that early postnatal cortical network oscillations in mice are synchronized by gap junc-tions, whereas later juvenile stages express similar patterns by NMDA (N-Methyl-D-Aspartate) receptor-mediated glutamatergic transmission.[27] Gap junctions might be crucially involved in the generation of hypersynchronized activity and aberrant regula-tion of these signaling molecules may contribute to cortical hyperexcitability, especially at young ages.[28–30] Without going into further detail, these findings show that imma-ture cortical networks have unique properties which may make them especially prone to seizure generation. Normal cortical development can be severely disrupted (or even reversed) by hypersynchronous electrical activity.[31]

The successful application of sulthiame in the case reported by Fejerman points toward another interesting feature of seizure generation, which may be related to the mecha-nisms outlined above: sulthiame is an inhibitor of carbonic anhydrase which catalyzes the conversion of CO_2 and water into H^+ and HCO_3^-. Therefore, the enzyme is critical for pH regulation, especially under conditions of enhanced metabolic rates. Block of the carbonic anhydrase by sulthiame leads to an acidification of neurons.[7] This might negatively regulate gap junctions and contribute to the cessation of seizures.[32] At the same time, the intracellularly located, and developmentally upregulated, carbonic anhydrase Type VII contributes to the generation of large GABA-induced network bursts which occur upon hypersynchronous discharge of interneurons and might contribute to epileptic seizures.[19] Therefore, gap junctions, intracellular pH regulation and abnormal GABAergic signaling might well be crucial elements of ictogenesis in the immature brain.

p0230   These mechanistic considerations are by no means complete and their relationship with the complicated case of BECTS is rather loose. We can, however, derive several urgent needs for further research: (i) the pharmacology of gap junctions is poorly developed and specific drugs which interfere with certain subtypes of connexins are needed; (ii) special attention should be paid to the development of subtle cortical abnormalities upon altered electrical activity in the maturing brain; and (iii) the precise mechanisms of pH regulation in normal and pathological brain tissue have to be dissected. Most of all, we need more knowledge about the functional maturation of the human cortex and to compare it with homologous time-scales in species which serve as model systems for epilepsy. The emerging power of functional imaging and refinements in electrodiagnostics give hope that we will soon learn more about the lesions underlying complicated cases of BECTS and related syndromes.

s0060   ## ▪REFERENCES

1. Chahine LM, Mikati MA. Benign pediatric localization-related epilepsies. Syndromes in infancy. *Epileptic Disord* 2006;**8**:169–83.
2. Shevell MI, Rosenblatt B, Watters GV, O'Gorman AM, Montes JL. "Pseudo-BECRS": intracranial focal lesions suggestive of a primary partial epilepsy syndrome. *Pediatr Neurol* 1996;**14**:31–5.
3. Doose H, Baier WK. Benign partial epilepsy and related conditions: multifactorial pathogenesis with hereditary impairment of brain maturation. *Eur J Pediatr* 1989;**149**:152–8.
4. Rating D, Wolf C, Bast T. Sulthiame as monotherapy in children with benign childhood epilepsy with centrotemporal spikes: a 6-month randomized, double-blind, placebo-controlled study. Sulthiame Study Group. *Epilepsia* 2000;**41**:1284–8.
5. Doose H, Baier WK, Ernst JP, Tuxhorn I, Volzke E. Benign partial epilepsy – treatment with sulthiame. *Dev Med Child Neurol* 1988;**30**:683–4.
6. Tanimukai H, Nishimura T, Sano I. N-(4'Sulfamyphenyl)- Butansultam (1-4) (Ospolot) as carbonic anhydrase inhibitor in the brain. *Klin Wochenschr* 1964;**42**:918–20.
7. Leniger T, Wiemann M, Bingmann D, Widman G, Hufnagel A, Bonnet U. Carbonic anhydrase inhibitor sulthiame reduces intracellular pH and epileptiform activity of hippocampal CA3 neurons. *Epilepsia* 2002;**43**:469–74.
8. Bentivoglio M, Tassi L, Pech E, Costa C, Fabene PF, Spreafico R. Cortical development and focal cortical dysplasia. *Epileptic Disord* 2003;**5**:S27–S34.
9. Bast T, Ramantani G, Seitz A, Rating D. Focal cortical dysplasia: prevalence, clinical presentation and epilepsy in children and adults. *Acta Neurol Scand* 2006;**113**:72–81.
10. Katz LC, Crowley JC. Development of cortical circuits: lessons from ocular dominance columns. *Nat Rev Neurosci* 2002;**3**:34–42.
11. Katz LC, Shatz CJ. Synaptic activity and the construction of cortical circuits. *Science* 1996;**274**:1133–8.
12. Khazipov R, Luhmann HJ. Early patterns of electrical activity in the developing cerebral cortex of humans and rodents. *Trends Neurosci* 2006;**29**:414–8.
13. Dreyfus-Brisac C, Larroche JC. Discontinuous electroencephalograms in the premature newborn and at term. *Electro-anatomo-clinical correlations Rev Electroencephalogr Neurophysiol Clin* 1971;**1**:95–9.

14. Vanhatalo S, Tallgren P, Andersson S, Sainio K, Voipio J, Kaila K. DC-EEG discloses prominent, very slow activity patterns during sleep in preterm infants. *Clin Neurophysiol* 2002;**113**:1822–5.

15. Wirrell EC. Benign epilepsy of childhood with centrotemporal spikes. *Epilepsia* 1998;**39**:S32–S41.

16. Ben-Ari Y, Cherubini E, Corradetti R, Gaiarsa JL. Giant synaptic potentials in immature rat CA3 hippocampal neurones. *J Physiol* 1989;**416**:303–25.

17. Payne JA, Rivera C, Voipio J, Kaila K. Cation-chloride co-transporters in neuronal communication, development and trauma. *Trends Neurosci* 2003;**26**:199–206.

18. Rivera C, Li H, Thomas-Crusells J, Lahtinen H, et al. BDNF-induced TrkB activation down-regulates the K + -Cl- cotransporter KCC2 and impairs neuronal Cl- extrus ion. *J Cell Biol* 2002;**159**:747–52.

19. Rivera C, Voipio J, Kaila K. Two developmental switches in GABAergic signalling: the K + -Cl- cotransporter KCC2 and carbonic anhydrase CAVII. *J Physiol* 2005;**562**:27–36.

20. Cohen I, Navarro V, Clemenceau S, Baulac M, Miles R. On the origin of interictal activity in human temporal lobe epilepsy in vitro. *Science* 2002;**298**:1418–21.

21. Cohen I, Navarro V, Le Duigou C, Miles R. Mesial temporal lobe epilepsy: a pathological replay of developmental mechanisms? *Biol Cell* 2003;**95**:329–33.

22. Dzhala VI, Talos DM, Sdrulla DA, et al. NKCC1 transporter facilitates seizures in the developing brain. *Nat Med* 2005;**11**:1205–13.

23. Schaub C, Uebachs M, Beck H. Diminished response of CA1 neurons to antiepileptic drugs in chronic epilepsy. *Epilepsia* 2007;**48**:1339–50.

24. Coulter DA. Epilepsy-associated plasticity in gamma-aminobutyric acid receptor expression, function, and inhibitory synaptic properties. *Int Rev Neurobiol* 2001;**45**:237–52.

25. Loscher W. Drug transporters in the epileptic brain. *Epilepsia* 2007;**48(suppl 1)**:8–13.

26. Sutor B. Gap junctions and their implications for neurogenesis and maturation of synaptic circuitry in the developing neocortex. *Results Probl Cell Differ* 2002;**39**:53–73.

27. Dupont E, Hanganu IL, Kilb W, Hirsch S, Luhmann HJ. Rapid developmental switch in the mechanisms driving early cortical columnar networks. *Nature* 2006;**439**:79–83.

28. Li J, Shen H, Naus CC, Zhang L, Carlen PL. Upregulation of gap junction connexin 32 with epileptiform activity in the isolated mouse hippocampus. *Neuroscience* 2001;**105**:589–98.

29. Carlen PL, Skinner F, Zhang L, Naus C, Kushnir M, Perez Velazquez JL. The role of gap junctions in seizures. *Brain Res Brain Res Rev* 2000;**32**:235–41.

30. Traub RD, Michelson-Law H, Bibbig AE, Buhl EH, Whittington MA. Gap junctions, fast oscillations and the initiation of seizures. *Adv Exp Med Biol* 2004;**548**:110–22.

31. Ben-Ari Y, Holmes GL. Effects of seizures on developmental processes in the immature brain. *Lancet Neurol* 2006;**5**:1055–63.

32. de Curtis M, Manfridi A, Biella G. Activity-dependent pH shifts and periodic recurrence of spontaneous interictal spikes in a model of focal epileptogenesis. *J Neurosci* 1998;**18**:7543–51.

33. Rivera C, Voipio J, Thomas-Crusells J, et al. Mechanism of activity-dependent downregulation of the neuron-specific K-Cl cotransporter KCC2. *J Neurosci* 2004;**24**:4683–91.

c0095

Does Status Epilepticus Represent a Different Pathophysiology than Epilepsy? A Patient with Recurrent Status Epilepticus as the Single Manifestation of Her Epilepsy

Christoph Baumgartner and Paolo Gallmetzer

s0010

HISTORY

p0020

This is a 40-year-old right-handed white woman with epilepsy since 3 years of age. The patient is the product of a normal pregnancy and delivery. Psychomotor development was normal. History is negative for meningitis, encephalitis, significant head trauma, or febrile convulsions. Family history is positive – the mother's brother experienced several alcohol-related seizures. The patient experienced her first seizure while playing; the patient suddenly became unresponsive, stared, and then threw her toys across the room at 3 years of age. Since then the patient continued to suffer from seizures which never remitted for longer than 1 month.

p0030

Seizures were preceded by prodromal symptoms of listlessness, dysphoria, and a strange feeling (which could not be specified more accurately by the patient) lasting for minutes to hours. The patient distinguished three types of seizures: Seizure type 1 consisted of a tingling sensation in both arms and feet which ascended within seconds to the trunk. Seizure type 2 started identical as seizure type 1, but evolved further to a tonic contraction of all four extremities, consciousness was preserved during these episodes, the patient could hear everything, but was unable to speak. Seizure type 3 evolved from seizure types 1 and 2 to secondary generalized tonic–clonic seizures.

Seizure frequency was described as follows: The patient would experience seizures at least every 2 weeks. All seizures would occur in series and eventually evolve into status epilepticus consisting of type 2 seizures (asymmetric tonic seizures) usually lasting several hours. Status would not stop spontaneously and had to be stopped by the application of intravenous antiepileptic drugs. Notably, status epilepticus never could be stopped by benodiazepines alone, but required additional administration of phenytoin and/or valproic acid. Furthermore, status proved to be refractory to these measures several times a year. These episodes of refractory focal or generalized status epilepticus therefore necessitated intensive care treatment including intubation and thiopental narcosis. The patient's seizures were refractory to all currently available antiepileptic drugs in monotherapy and various combination therapies. Dosage was increased to toxicity on several occasions without achieving longer seizure-free periods.

EXAMINATIONS AND INVESTIGATIONS

The patient underwent an extensive presurgical evaluation for possible surgical treatment of her medically refractory seizures. Neurological examination was normal. During intensive video–EEG monitoring, several episodes of status epilepticus could be recorded. Clinical seizure semiology consisted of an aura of tingling in all extremities, then the patient would elevate her left arm and say that she was experiencing

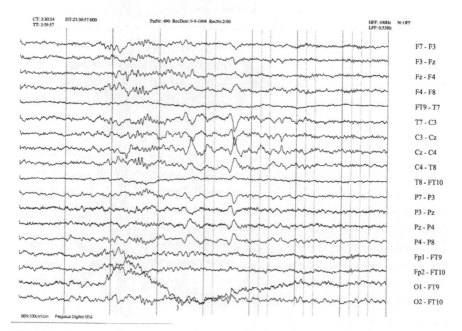

FIGURE 95.1a   Interictal scalp-EEG. Interictal spikes showed a maximum at electrodes C3, CZ and C4.

a seizure. Subsequently, seizures would evolve into tonic contractions of all four extremities predominating on the left side and vocalizations which always evolved into seizure series or status epilepticus. Seizures were classified as asymmetric tonic seizures.[1] Seizures never stopped spontaneously, but always had to be terminated by intravenous antiepileptic drugs. Intravenous lorazepam alone never could stop the seizures – the patient always required additional high doses of phenytoin or valproic acid. On interictal EEG, spikes with a maximum at electrodes C3, CZ, and C4 could be recorded (Figure 95.1a). Ictal EEG was obscured by muscle artifacts – nevertheless a rhythmic theta activity over the vertex could be appreciated (Figure 95.1b). MRI scans performed on several occasions including several studies on a 3T machine were normal. Interictal FDG-PET and Tc-HMPAO-SPECT were normal. Ictal Tc-HMPAO-SPECT showed questionable hyperperfusions in the supplementary sensorimotor area (no lateralization was possible on the basis of the SPECT images) and in the right insular regions. Based on the clinical seizure semiology and the findings of scalp-EEG, we performed an invasive evaluation with chronically indwelling subdural grid electrodes covering the interhemispheric fissure and the right frontal convexity (Figure 95.2a). Invasive EEG documented a seizure onset in the right supplementary sensorimotor area (Figure 95.2b).

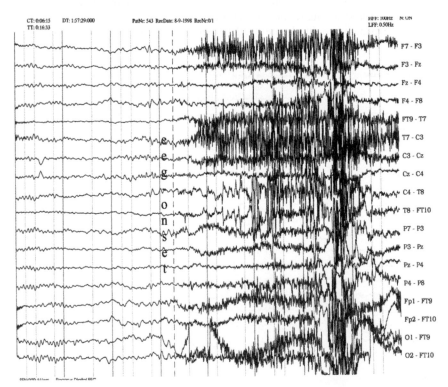

FIGURE 95.1b Ictal scalp-EEG. After initial muscle artifacts a rhythmic theta activity with a maximum over the vertex can be appreciated.

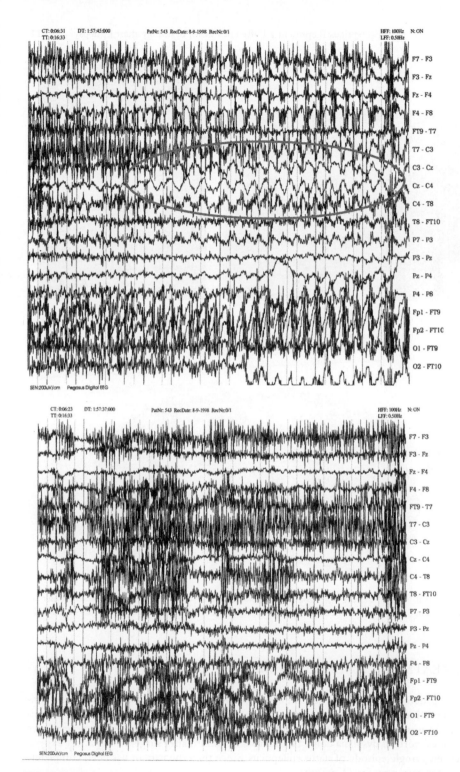

FIGURE 95.1b (*Continued*)

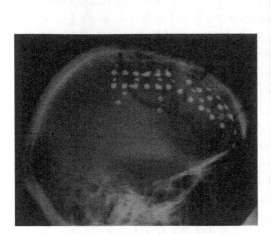
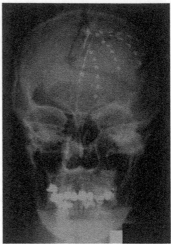

FIGURE 95.2a   Lateral and anterior-posterior x-rays showing the chronically indwelling subdural grid electrodes covering the interhemispheric fissure and the right lateral convexity.

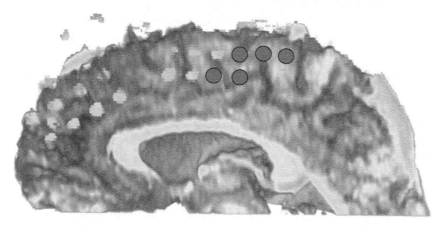

f0020   FIGURE 95.2b   Seizure onset zone on intracranial EEG – electrodes involved at seizure onset are denoted in dark grey circles (reconstruction and projection of interhemispheric electrodes onto MRI).

s0030   # TREATMENT AND OUTCOME

p0060   The patient underwent a resection of the EEG-defined seizure onset zone under continuous intraoperative monitoring of the leg motor function. The neurological examination was normal after the operation. Histology was normal, specifically no evidence of focal cortical dysplasia could be found. One month after surgery the patient experienced a single episode of status epilepticus. Since then the patient has been completely seizure-free, now for 11 months.

DIAGNOSIS

Our patient represents a case of non-lesional, medically refractory frontal lobe epilepsy with seizures originating in the right supplementary sensorimotor area. Virtually all seizures evolved into focal or secondary generalized status epilepticus which could be stopped only by intravenous application of antiepileptic drugs other than benzodiazepines. Refractory status epilepticus occurred several times a year necessitating intubation and barbiturate narcosis. Seizures could be controlled by epilepsy surgery although histology revealed no abnormalities.

COMMENTARY

This case is remarkable for several reasons. First, this patient demonstrates the deleterious effects of a failure of seizure-terminating mechanisms.[2] From our clinical experience we are confident that most seizures will stop spontaneously without medical intervention.[3,4] The development of status epilepticus in patients with chronic epilepsy actually is a rare event, usually is ascribed to special circumstances including non-compliance with antiepileptic medication, alcohol intake, or acute illness, and usually can be controlled easily.[5] Under controlled conditions like in an intensive video–EEG monitoring unit where patients receive intravenous medications immediately once seizures do not terminate the occurrence of status epilepticus fortunately is extremely rare.[6] Our patient developed status epilepticus even under these conditions indicating a profound failure of seizure-terminating mechanisms.

Second, seizures usually could not be stopped by the sole application of intravenous benzodiazepines. Instead high doses of phenytoin or valproic acid and on many occasions barbiturate narcosis was necessary to stop seizures. This observation corroborates experimental findings indicating that seizures during status epilepticus rapidly become resistant to benzodiazepines due to a decrease of $GABA_A$ receptors.[7]

Third, patients with frontal lobe epilepsy seem to be particularly prone to develop recurrent seizure series or status epilepticus. This could possibly be explained by alterations of excitation and inhibition unique to the frontal lobes.[8,9]

Finally, although we expected to find some abnormalities on pathological examination (specifically, signs of focal cortical dysplasia), histology was normal in our patient. The excellent outcome in our patient documents that we indeed removed the epileptogenic zone.[10] Therefore, we believe that the occurrence of recurrent status epilepticus is not restricted to a single pathological entity.

REFERENCES

1. Bleasel AF, Morris HH. Supplementary sensorimotor area seizures. In: Wyllie E, ed. *The treatment of epilepsy: principles and practice*, 2nd ed. Baltimore: Williams & Wilkins, 1997: 432–41.
2. Chen JW, Wasterlain CG. Status epilepticus: pathophysiology and management in adults. *Lancet Neurol* 2006;**5**:246–56.
3. Lowenstein DH, Bleck T, Macdonald RL. It's time to revise the definition of status epilepticus. *Epilepsia* 1999;**40**:120–2.
4. Jenssen S, Gracely EJ, Sperling MR. How long do most seizures last? A systematic comparison of seizures recorded in the epilepsy monitoring unit. *Epilepsia* 2006;**47**:1499–503.

5. Lowenstein DH, Alldredge BK. Status epilepticus. *N Engl J Med* 1998;**338**:970–6.
6. Velis D, Plouin P, Gotman J, da Silva FL. Recommendations regarding the requirements and applications for long-term recordings in epilepsy. *Epilepsia* 2007;**48**:379–84.
7. Kapur J. Status epilepticus in epileptogenesis. *Curr Opin Neurol* 1999;**12**:191–5.
8. Jobst BC, Siegel AM, Thadani VM, Roberts DW, Rhodes HC, Williamson PD. Intractable seizures of frontal lobe origin: clinical characteristics, localizing signs, and results of surgery. *Epilepsia* 2000;**41**:1139–52.
9. Bonelli SB, Lurger S, Zimprich F, Stogmann E, Assem-Hilger E, Baumgartner C. Clinical seizure lateralization in frontal lobe epilepsy. *Epilepsia* 2007;**48**:517–23.
10. Rosenow F, Luders H. Presurgical evaluation of epilepsy. *Brain* 2001;**124**:1683–700.

Does Status Epilepticus Represent a Different Pathophysiology than Epilepsy? A Preclinical Perspective

Hana Kubova

Epilepsy is a common episodic neurological condition which is heterogeneous in clinical presentation and is characterized by recurrent paroxysmal episodes. Epileptic seizures occur suddenly and nearly always terminate spontaneously, without a need of pharmacological intervention. The cessation of epileptic activity at the end of an ordinary epileptic seizure is remarkable. All mechanisms participating in seizure termination are not fully understood, but sophisticated synaptic and ionic mechanisms rather than energetic failure are responsible for stopping epileptic seizures. In contrast, status epilepticus (SE) is a unique pathological state during which seizures are unremitting and tend to become self-sustained. SE may occur in epileptic patients for various reasons, but frequently it develops in patients with no previous history of epilepsy. In fact, epilepsy can follow SE in some patients. Thus, SE might be a precipitating factor for epileptogenesis, even though it is frequently impossible to decide whether epilepsy develops due to SE-induced cerebral damage or to the underlying cause. Causes of SE are enormously variable, and they include various brain insults (head trauma, cerebrovascular disease, hypoxia), central nervous system infections, focal cerebral abnormalities, tumors, drug addiction or withdrawal and many others.

Recent information about the molecular or cellular pathophysiology of SE, development of time-related pharmacoresistance and the consequences of SE is from experimental models in which SE is induced in healthy experimental animal. This is clear evidence that SE can be induced in naïve brain with no previous experience with epileptic seizures and also without presence of additional pathologies. Almost exclusively, models of convulsive SE, which is induced either chemically or by electrical stimulation of various temporal structures, are used to study features of SE. Data on non–convulsive SE or SE due to other pathologies commonly seen in clinics (brain abnormalities, metabolic cause, neuroinfection, etc.) are very limited or not available. Thus, this commentary focuses exclusively on features of major, convulsive SE induced in healthy animals, which represents the main source of our recent knowledge.

s0060   ## TRANSITION FROM THE ISOLATED SEIZURE TO STATUS EPILEPTICUS

p0140   The pathophysiological processes which initiate status epilepticus are very similar to those initiating isolated seizures and there is close electrophysiological and clinical resemblance between seizures at the SE onset and a single attack. In experimental animals, intensity or duration of the epileptogenic stimulus (i.e. duration of electrical stimulation or dose of convulsive drug) clearly determines whether SE or an individual seizure occurs, suggesting that SE and seizures have a common substrate of initiation. However, there is good experimental evidence that after 15–30 min, repeated or continuous seizures become self-sustained (i.e. they continue after discontinuation of the epileptogenic stimulus). Thus the main difference between SE and an individual seizure is more likely related to the failure of seizure-termination ability than with seizure onset. What are the mechanisms responsible for transformation from an isolated seizure to SE? The appearance of a prolonged seizure has been presumed to represent excessive excitation, a failure of inhibition, or their combination. Experimental studies show that progressive decline of inhibition is one of the most important features of progressing SE. Recent data support the critical role of reduced inhibition mediated by GABA, the most common inhibitory neurotransmitter in the brain, in transition from an isolated seizure into SE. Reduction of GABA inhibition seems to be related to a decrease in the potency and efficacy of GABA rather than insufficient GABA levels, because an increase of GABA levels above basal values was documented in several brain regions at the intervals when SE becomes self-sustained.[1] This hypothesis is supported by the fact that during 1 h of SE, the number of GABA$_A$ receptors (measured per dentate granule synapse) decreases by 50%.[2] Early decrease of GABA$_A$ receptors is due to receptor endocytosis – a process in which receptors are inactivated by internalization, that is, by transfer into lysosomes for destruction or into Golgi apparatus from where they are recycled. At the same time, AMPA and NMDA receptors move to the synaptic membrane, where they form additional excitatory receptors which further increase excitability. Other mechanisms also seem to participate in transformation of isolated seizures to SE and in maintaining seizure activity. Among them, inhibitory modulatory systems (e.g. adenosinergic[3]) seem to play an important role. Increased expression of proconvulsant neuropeptides such as substance P, neurokinin B, or proconvulsant tachykinins together with depletion of predominantly inhibitory peptides (dynorphins, galanin, and other), which were described in the hippocampus of animals during SE, may play a role in the shift of balance between excitation and inhibition (for more detailed information see Ref. [4] or [5]).

s0070   ## TIME-DEPENDENT PHARMACORESISTANCE

p0150   Time-related changes of pharmacological sensitivity of self-sustained SE represent another unique feature. In models of isolated seizures, enhancement of GABA inhibition can prevent seizure development and drugs which potentiate the GABAergic system are used as antiepileptics. In the early phases, SE can be easily stopped by GABAergic drugs such as benzodiazepines, but anticonvulsant potency of these drugs can decrease by 20 times within 30 min of self-sustaining SE.[6] In contrast, administration of NMDA or AMPA/kainate antagonists can block established self-sustained SE (see Ref. [5]).

Detailed description of all differences between a single brief seizure and status epilepticus is far beyond the scope of this commentary, which highlights the recent progress made in our understanding of the nature of SE in animal models. Recently published data on SE clearly suggest that, despite certain similarities, SE represents a unique pathophysiology. Differences between features of individual seizures and SE demonstrate the need for developing specific treatment strategies and new drugs for SE.

REFERENCES

1. Walton NY, Gunawan S, Treiman DM. Brain amino acid concentration changes during status epilepticus induced by lithium and pilocarpine. *Exp Neurol* 1990;**108**:61–70.
2. Naylor DE, Liu H, Wasterlain CG. Trafficking of GABA(A) receptors, loss of inhibition, and a mechanism for pharmacoresistance in status epilepticus. *J Neurosci* 2005;**24(25)**:7724–33.
3. Dragunow M. Endogenous anticonvulsant substances. *Neurosci Biobehav Rev* 1986;**10**:229–44.
4. Chen JW, Wasterlain CG. Status epilepticus: pathophysiology and management in adults. *Lancet Neurol* 2006;**5**:246–56.
5. Chen JW, Naylor DE, Wasterlain CG. Advances in the pathophysiology of status epilepticus. *Acta Neurol Scand* 2007;**115**:7–15.
6. Macdonald RL, Kapur J. Acute cellular alterations in the hippocampus after status epilepticus. *Epilepsia* 1999;**40(suppl 1)**:S9–S20.

Does Status Epilepticus Represent a Different Pathophysiology than Epilepsy? A Clinical Perspective

Gerhard Bauer and Eugen Trinka

p0170   The pathophysiology of status epilepticus (SE) was extensively studied in animal experiments (for summary see comments of Kubova (above); Ref. [1]). Most experiments were performed in SE with generalized tonic–clonic seizures. To what extent the results apply to other forms of SE and to SE in humans cannot be decided. Kubova commented on the factors responsible for the transition of a single seizure into SE encompassing endocytosis of $GABA_A$ – receptors, movements of excitatory receptors to the synaptic surface, and changes in peptides. These processes may support early treatment with non-GABAergic antiepileptic drugs (AEDs).[2] However, it is not clear why these mechanisms do not happen with shorter self-limited seizures. Moreover, with GABAergic drugs, such as lorazepam, more than 60% of cases of generalized convulsive SE (GCSE) are successfully treated and even in the refractory stages treatment with GABAergic drugs (midazolam, barbiturates) may still be successful after initial failure of benodiazepines and phenytoin.[3] In general, seizure initiation and spread are similar in single seizures and in SE.[4] SE represents the failure of seizure-terminating mechanisms,[5] which are only partially understood. The EEG signals increase in their complexity at the end of a seizure,[6,7] the endogenous cannabinoid system may modulate neuroexcitation[8] and activity-dependent intracellular acidification can terminate nonsynaptic neuronal synchronization.[9] Why these seizure terminating mechanisms fail in SE is not clear.

p0180   Besides these considerations in basic mechanisms, Christoph Baumgartner's case report raises several clinical questions. How long do most seizures last? Jenssen et al.[10] investigated the duration of seizures systematically with continuous video and scalp EEG. Considerable differences have been found between the types of seizures. Gastaut[11] defined SE "a term used whenever a seizure persists for a sufficient length of time or is repeated frequently enough to produce a fixed or enduring epileptic condition." This classical definition was widely accepted and a time limit of 30–60 min was suggested to diagnose status. Later classical experimental work by Meldrum and coworkers[12,13] demonstrated that seizure-related neuronal damage occurs after prolonged seizure activity. Repetitive seizures become self-sustaining and pharmacoresistant within 15–30 min and can lead to neuronal injury at about the same time (reviewed in Ref. [1]). The duration of what is accepted as convulsive status epilepticus has been shrinking progressively to an operational definition of 5 min of continuous or intermittent seizure activity.[14] This definition does not take into account the different seizure types in humans and a duration of 30 min of nonconvulsive seizure activity is still accepted as required to diagnose nonconvulsive SE. In many cases it even lasts much longer until a so-called confusional state is diagnosed as nonconvulsive SE.[15] Though seizure-related MRI changes are well recognized, it is not clear whether they reflect permanent neuronal damage and cell loss or are a transient phenomenon.[16] Time limits for diagnosing SE and start of AED treatment are not stringent. The imminent danger of SE depends on its type, the underlying pathophysiology, and – for acute symptomatic cases – on etiology.

Baumgartner reports a patient with recurrent status epilepticus as the single manifestation of her epilepsy. This is quite unique and one is tempted to ask if it is due to the withdrawal of AEDs during epilepsy monitoring. Seizure clustering and status epilepticus are increased during presurgical workup.[17,18,33,34] However, in the present case the unique feature of repeated SE was observed from the ages of 3 to 40. To our knowledge, SE as the single manifestation of a chronic epilepsy was never reported. In chronic epilepsies, repeated episodes of SE besides less prominent single seizures have been described in Panayiotopoulos syndrome[19,35] and in epilepsies associated with ring chromosome 20.[20,36]

Baumgartner's patient suffered a nonlesional frontal lobe epilepsy. Epileptic patients with frontal lobe lesions are well known to be at an increased risk of SE. This was already documented by Janz in the early 1960s.[21,22,37,38] The presented case expands these observations to nonlesional frontal lobe epilepsies. One might speculate that the complex organization and interconnectivity of the frontal lobe underlies the danger of self-sustaining epileptic seizures.

REFERENCES

1. Chen JWY, Naylor DE, Wasterlain CG. Advances in the pathophysiology of status epilepticus. *Acta Neurol Scand* 2007;**115(S 186)**:7–15.
2. Chen JWY, Wasterlain CG. Status epilepticus: pathophysiology and management in adults. *Lancet Neurol* 2007;**5**:246–56.
3. Claassen J, Hirsch LJ, Emerson RG, Mayer SA. Treatment of refractory status epilepticus with pentobarbital, propofol, or midazolam: a systematic review. *Epilepsia* 2002;**43**:146–53.
4. Engel J. Report of the ILAE classification core group. *Epilepsia* 2006;**47**:1558–68.
5. Wasterlain CG, Treiman DM. *Status epilepticus: mechanisms and management.* Boston: MIT Press, 2006.
6. Elger CE, Lehnertz K. Seizure prediction by non-linear time series analysis of brain electrical activity. *Eur J Neusosci* 1998;**10**:786–9.
7. Bergey GK, Franaszczuk PJ. Epileptic seizures are characterized by changing signal complexity. *Clin Neurophysiol* 2001;**112**:241–9.

8. Wallace MJ, Blair RE, Falenski KW, Martin BR, Delorenzo RJ. The endogenous cannabinoid system regulates seizure frequency and duration in a model of temporal lobe epilepsy. *J Pharmacol Exp Therap* 2003;**307**:129–37.

9. Xiong Z-Q, Saggau P, Stringer JL. Activity-dependent intracellular acidification correlates with the duration of seizure activity. *J Neurosci* 2000;**20**:1290–6.

10. Jenssen S, Gracely EJ, Sperling MR. How long do most seizures last? A systematic comparison of seizures recorded in the epilepsy monitoring unit. *Epilepsia* 2006;**47**:1499–503.

11. Gastaut H. A propos d'une classification symptomatologique des etats de mal epileptiques. In: Gastaut H, Roger J, Lob H, eds. *Les etats de mal epileptiques*. Paris: Masson, 1967: 1–8.

12. Meldrum BS, Brierley JAN. Prolonged epileptic seizures in primates: ischemic cell change and its relation to ictal physiological events. *Arch Neurol* 1973;**28**:10–7.

13. Meldrum BS, Horton RW. Physiology of status epilepticus in primates. *Arch Neurol* 1973;**28**:1–9.

14. Lowenstein DH, Bleck T, Macdonald RL. It's time to revise the definition of status epilepticus. *Epilepsia* 1999;**40**:120–2.

15. Bauer G, Aichner F, Mayr U. Nonconvulsive status epilepticus following generalized tonic-clonic seizures. *Eur Neurol* 1982;**21**:411–9.

16. Bauer G, Gotwald T, Dobesberger J, et al. Transient and permanent magnetic resonance imaging abnormalities after complex partial status epilepticus. *Epilepsy Behav* 2006;**8**:666–71.

17. Haut SR, Swick C, Freeman K, Spencer S. Seizure clustering during epilepsy monitoring. *Epilepsia* 2002;**43**:711–5.

18. Rose AB, McCabe PH, Gilliam FG, et al. Consortium for research in epilepsy: occurrence of seizure clusters and status epilepticus during inpatient video-EEG monitoring. *Neurology* 2003;**60**:975–8.

19. Ferrie CD, Caraballo R, Covanis A, et al. Autonomic status epilepticus in Panayiotopoulos syndrome and other childhood and adult epilepsies: a consensus view. *Epilepsia* 2007;**48**:1165–72.

20. Inoue Y, Fujiwara T, Matsuda K, et al. Ring chromosome 20 and nonconvulsive status epilepticus. A new epileptic syndrome. *Brain* 1997;**120**:939–53.

21. Janz D. Status epilepticus und Stirnhirn. *Deutsche Zeitschrift für Nervenheilkunde* 1960;**180**:562–94.

22. Janz D. Status epilepticus and frontal lobe lesions. *J Neurol Sci* 1964;**1**:446–57.

Why Do Some Patients Seem to Develop Tolerance to AEDs? Development of Antiepileptic Drug Tolerance in a Patient with Temporal Lobe Epilepsy

Bassel Abou-Khalil

HISTORY

This 50-year-old woman first presented to our clinic in February 2000, at age 43. She gave a history of seizures first recognized at age 30 when she drove through a red light and crashed her car without being aware. However, she believes that seizures may have started as early as 15 years of age, because she remembers her aura of tingling rising from the abdomen to the neck and head, and a taste in her mouth.

Complex partial seizures (CPS) were usually preceded by an aura, then altered awareness, lip smacking, right extremity automatisms, and well-formed verbal automatisms. She estimated 50 CPS in the preceding year with up to 3 per day and about 10 isolated auras per month.

She reported that she was first treated with phenytoin which made her seizure-free for over 6 months. When seizures recurred, divalproex was added. It also stopped the seizures for 3–6 months, but they returned. Carbamazepine caused a rash and she could not tolerate phenobarbital. Each time a new antiepileptic drug (AED) was started, seizures stopped for weeks to months, but then started again. AED dose escalation also stopped seizures temporarily. In October 1999, lamotrigine was added, and CPS as well as isolated auras stopped completely. However, she experienced excessive drowsiness and cognitive dysfunction on the regimen of divalproex sodium 2500 mg/day, phenytoin 400 mg alternating with 500 mg/day, and lamotrigine 25 mg/day. She requested to be evaluated for epilepsy surgery because she did not trust that her seizure control would last.

Puzzling Cases of Epilepsy

p0130   Past medical history revealed no clear risk factors for epilepsy. She was not aware of any febrile seizures in infancy. Family history was negative for epilepsy or febrile seizures. She had a college education and worked as a bookkeeper.

s0020   # EXAMINATION AND INVESTIGATIONS

p0140   Neurological examination was normal. Complete blood count and comprehensive metabolic profile (including liver enzymes) were normal. Valproate level was 97 µg/ml, total phenytoin level was 15.5 µg/ml, and free phenytoin level 2.5 µg/ml. She was advised to titrate lamotrigine slowly to 100 mg bid in preparation for conversion to lamotrigine monotherapy in the epilepsy monitoring unit (EMU). Upon admission to the EMU, all AEDs were stopped, but no seizures were recorded in 5 days of monitoring. The interictal electroencephalogram (EEG) showed occasional right temporal sharp waves and intermittent delta activity, both predominant in the inferomesial temporal region. Brain MRI (magnetic resonance imaging) revealed right hippocampal sclerosis.

s0040   # DIAGNOSIS

p0170   The diagnosis is right temporal lobe epilepsy secondary to hippocampal sclerosis. The onset of epilepsy was as early as the second decade of life and it is presumed that the process of epileptogenesis was complete before her initial presentation. The pattern of transient seizure control after initiating a new AED or increasing its dose is consistent with development of tolerance to AEDs.

s0030   # TREATMENT AND OUTCOME

p0150   After discharge from the EMU in May 2000, she was treated with lamotrigine monotherapy at a dose of 150 mg bid. However, she had recurrent isolated auras and CPS even though the dose of lamotrigine was later increased to 200 mg bid. She developed insomnia, which was partially helped by taking the last dose at noon. In the month of June she had 4 days of clustered isolated auras and three CPS. On June 19, 2000, levetiracetam was added at a dose of 500 mg bid. She had no seizures for 4 months after that, but developed very brief isolated auras 2–3 times a week in October 2000. In January 2001, levetiracetam was increased to 1500 mg/day. However, isolated auras continued and became nearly daily, and CPS resumed in June 2001. In July 2001, she became free of CPS on lamotrigine 500 mg every morning and levetiracetam 1500 mg/day. When she returned in June 2003 she reported only isolated auras in 2 years, with no more than 8 in 6 months. Lamotrigine level was 15 µg/ml and levetiracetam level 33 µg/ml. However, shortly after her visit auras recurred and increased in frequency despite increasing lamotrigine to 600 mg/day. After increasing levetiracetam to 2500 mg/day she reported no auras for a few weeks. However, isolated auras recurred and their frequency increased to an average of 12 per month, and in June 2005, CPS recurred with a frequency of 2 per week. Increasing levetiracetam to 3000 mg/day did not help and she could not tolerate further increases in lamotrigine. She demanded epilepsy surgery.

p0160   Video–EEG recorded four CPS with ictal onset in the right inferomesial temporal region. Frequent right inferomesial temporal sharp waves and irregular slow activity were noted interictally. She had a right selective amygdalohippocampectomy on June 9, 2006. She has been free of seizures and auras since then. She reduced her AED doses to lamotrigine 300 mg in the morning and levetiracetam 500 mg in the morning and 1000 mg at bedtime, uneventfully.

COMMENTARY

AED tolerance refers to the loss of initial efficacy of an AED over time. AED tolerance may be associated with rebound worsening of seizures upon withdrawal, as well as transient improvement in efficacy after a drug holiday. AED tolerance is a well-recognized phenomenon in animal models of epilepsy, demonstrated for several AEDs. In patients with epilepsy, AED tolerance is recognized mainly for benzodiazepines and barbiturates. However, there are suggestions that this phenomenon may occur with other AEDs in some individuals. Rebound seizures upon withdrawal and improved efficacy with reinstitution were observed for carbamazepine in patients admitted to the EMU. It may be hard to prove that loss of efficacy in the clinical setting is due to tolerance, because there are many confounding seizure precipitating factors such as stress, sleep deprivation, and missing medication doses. There is also the possibility that the process of epileptogenesis may still be progressing. The case above shows a consistent pattern of transient improvement in seizure control in relation to adding a new AED or increasing the AED dose. This pattern is most likely a result of AED tolerance.

FURTHER READING

Avanzini G. Is tolerance to antiepileptic drugs clinically relevant? *Epilepsia* 2006;**47**:1285–7.

Barcs G, Halasz P. Effectiveness and tolerance of clobazam in temporal lobe epilepsy. *Acta Neurol Scand* 1996;**93**:88–93.

Doyle WK, Devinsky O, Luciano D, Perrine K, Dogali M. Decreased seizure frequency after withdrawal and reinstitution of antiepileptic drug therapy. *Seizure* 1994;**3**:61–5.

Frey HH. Tolerance to antiepileptic drug effects. Experimental evidence and clinical significance. *Pol J Pharmacol Pharm* 1987;**39**:495–504.

Laowattana S, Abou-Khalil B, Fakhoury T, Ashmead D. Brief antiepileptic drug withdrawal prolongs interval to next seizure. *Neurology* 1999;**53**:1736–41.

Löscher W, Rundfeldt C, Honack D, Ebert U. Long-term studies on anticonvulsant tolerance and withdrawal characteristics of benzodiazepine receptor ligands in different seizure models in mice. I. Comparison of diazepam, clonazepam, clobazam and abecarnil. *J Pharmacol Exp Ther* 1996;**279**:561–72.

Löscher W, Schmidt D. Experimental and clinical evidence for loss of effect (tolerance) during prolonged treatment with antiepileptic drugs. *Epilepsia* 2006;**47**:1253–84.

Malow BA, Lynch B, Blaxton TA, Mikati MA. Relationship of carbamazepine reduction rate to seizure frequency during inpatient telemetry. *Epilepsia* 1994;**35**:1160–4.

Marciani MG, Gotman J, Andermann F, Olivier A. Patterns of seizure activation after withdrawal of antiepileptic medication. *Neurology* 1985;**35**:1537–43.

Schmidt D, Kupferberg HJ, Yonekawa W, Penry JK. The development of tolerance to the anticonvulsant effect of phenobarbital in mice. *Epilepsia* 1980;**21**:141–7.

Singh A, Guberman AH, Boisvert D. Clobazam in long-term epilepsy treatment: sustained responders versus those developing tolerance. *Epilepsia* 1995;**36**:798–803.

Vajda FJ, Lewis SJ, Harris QL, Jarrott B, Young NA. Tolerance to the anticonvulsant effects of clonazepam and clobazam in the amygdaloid kindled rat. *Clin Exp Neurol* 1987;**23**:155–64.

Zhou D, Wang Y, Hopp P, et al. Influence on ictal seizure semiology of rapid withdrawal of carbamazepine and valproate in monotherapy. *Epilepsia* 2002;**43**:386–93.

c0020

Why Do Some Patients Seem to Develop Tolerance to AEDs? A Preclinical Discussion

Wolfgang Löscher

p0190

Tolerance is defined as the progressive reduction in response to a drug during prolonged administration.[1] Development of tolerance is an adaptive response of the body to prolonged exposure of chemical substances that are foreign to the body, and AEDs are no exception. Thus, there is a reduction in adverse CNS effects during prolonged administration of most AEDs in patients with epilepsy.[2,3] However, the risk for development of tolerance to antiepileptic efficacy is generally considered small. The only AEDs for which tolerance to efficacy is generally accepted are the benzodiazepines (BZDs). BZDs, however, are no exception, but tolerance to antiepileptic effect occurs with most old and modern AEDs, although only in a subgroup of patients.[3] In apparent contrast to patients, tolerance to AED efficacy can be easily demonstrated in animal models of seizures or epilepsy.[3] What are the reasons for this apparent difference in occurrence of tolerance in animal models versus epilepsy patients?

p0200

Different experimental approaches have been used to study occurrence and degree of tolerance to AEDs in laboratory animals.[2,3] In one widely used approach, groups of mice or rats are treated over a prolonged period with an AED and antiepileptic efficacy is determined at the onset and end of the treatment period. The degree of tolerance is usually proportional to the degree of drug exposure. In other words, the higher the dose and the longer the period of treatment, the higher is the likelihood that tolerance will develop. Often, doses of AEDs that are tested in rodents are considerably higher than clinically used doses, which will favor development of tolerance. In animal models, a reduction in antiepileptic efficacy was demonstrated for most clinically used AEDs (Table 96.1).[3] This tolerance was generally of the functional or pharmacodynamic type, i.e. due to adaptive changes at the level of molecular brain targets of AEDs during prolonged AED exposure. Pharmacokinetic or metabolic tolerance, which is due to induction of AED-metabolizing enzymes, only occurred with old, enzyme-inducing AEDs, and was less important for loss of efficacy than functional tolerance.[3]

TABLE 96.1   Evidence for Loss of Antiepileptic Efficacy (i.e. Tolerance) during Prolonged Treatment with AEDs in Animal Models or Patients with Epilepsy. Animal data are from kindled rats and/or electrical or chemical seizure models in mice or rats. In patients, diminished seizure control, as caused by functional tolerance, was operationally defined as a shift from responder status (showing 50% or more reduction versus baseline at visit 1) to a return to below 50% reduction during subsequent visits in an individual patient. This responder-to-nonresponder shift is shown in percentage of responders in brackets.

AED	Evidence for functional tolerance to antiepileptic efficacy	
	Animal models	Clinical studies (responder-to-nonresponder shift in % of responders)
First generation AEDs		
Benzodiazepines	Yes	Yes (27–48%)
Carbamazepine	Yes	Yes (4%)
Ethosuximide	No	No data available
Phenobarbital	Yes	Yes (11%)
Phenytoin	Yes	Yes (7%)
Primidone	Yes	No data available
Valproate	Yes	Yes (21–58%)[a]
Second and third generation AEDs		
Felbamate	No (only one study)	Yes (11%)
Gabapentin	No data available	Yes (7–80%)
Lamotrigine	Yes	Yes (1–15%)
Levetiracetam	Yes	Yes (5–27%)
Oxcarbazepine	No (only one study)	Yes (14%)
Pregabalin	No data available	Yes (32%)
Tiagabine	No (only one study)	No data available
Topiramate	No data available	Yes (20–47%)
Vigabatrin	Yes	Yes (12–33%)
Zonisamide	Yes	Yes (23%)

Source: For details see Ref. [5].
[a]But also one study in which no tolerance was observed.

Because of diverse confounding factors, detecting tolerance in patients with epilepsy is more difficult but can be done with careful assessment of AED efficacy during long-term individual patient response.[3] After excluding confounding factors, tolerance to antiepileptic effect for most modern and old AEDs can be shown in subgroups of responders (Table 96.1). The percentage of responders affected from a responder-to-nonresponder shift between visits ranges widely from <10% to 58%, and one outlier of 80% (Table 96.1). Thus, as shown in Table 96.1, there seems to be no qualitative difference in the occurrence of tolerance to AED efficacy between animal models and epilepsy patients, when clinical data are based on individual responder analysis. Instead, group-response analysis (i.e. the number of responders between two visits to the clinic) is not a reliable tool to assess tolerance in the clinic, which is one major reason that clinicians often fail to detect tolerance unless it causes dramatic loss of group net effect, as is the case with BZDs.[3] Group response between visits detects net loss of response but may miss tolerance in a subgroup, if response improves over time in other patients.

p0220   Group-response analysis is the common method to study tolerance in animal models. So the major difference between experimental and clinical studies on tolerance is that group-response analysis is suitable to detect tolerance in animal models, whereas individual responder analysis is better suited to measure tolerance in patients with epilepsy. There are several reasons for this important methodological difference in identifying tolerance in animals versus patients. These reasons, which are discussed in the following, also explain why tolerance is much easier to identify in animal models than in patients.

o0090   1. For studying tolerance in animal models, groups of mice or rats are treated with doses of AEDs that are known to exert significant antiepileptic effects after single-dose administration. Thus, per definition, a significant group response is seen after the very first dosing and usually this response does not increase during further drug administration. This is different in patients, in which antiepileptic efficacy may take some time to develop, so that a nonresponder-to-responder shift may occur in several patients during visits. This may conceal loss of efficacy in other patients when analysis is based on group responses.

o0100   2. During prolonged drug administration in animals, the doses of AEDs are not adjusted according to effect but are kept constant throughout the period of treatment. In other words, if antiepileptic efficacy decreases during treatment, the dosage is not increased but kept constant throughout the period of treatment. In contrast, clinicians are accustomed to repeatedly increasing and adapting the dosage of AEDs until adequate seizure control is achieved. This fact alone may explain why a loss of efficacy that can be counteracted by increasing the dosage may not be recognized as tolerance by clinicians.

o0110   3. During long-term efficacy studies with AEDs in animals, an AED is usually given alone. In contrast, particularly in efficacy studies with novel AEDs, these drugs are co-administered together with other AEDs, which may conceal development of tolerance in epilepsy patients.

o0120   4. For animal studies, a seizure type is chosen which is particularly sensitive to the AED that will be examined during prolonged exposure. Furthermore, at the doses chosen for treatment, usually most if not all animals will be responders to the AED at onset of treatment. Consequently, a group-response analysis will easily identify loss of antiepileptic efficacy during prolonged treatment. This is completely different in patients, particularly in the case of add-on studies, where patient groups consist of both responders and nonresponders, and may comprise different etiologies of epilepsies.

o0130   5. In contrast to animal studies, in which most variables can be controlled, various confounding factors complicate the identification of tolerance in patients.[3] Such confounding factors may either mimic or conceal development of tolerance. Confounding factors that may mimic tolerance include lack of compliance, inclusion biases, disease progression, lowering of comedication, and natural fluctuation of seizure frequency. A major confounding factor that conceals tolerance is the fact that failure to maintain efficacy after reaching a maintenance dosage is routinely compensated by dose increments in clinical studies.

6. Animal studies are usually performed in one strain and gender of rodents, e.g. male Sprague–Dawley rats, so that genetic variation between group members is relatively low. Furthermore, all animals per group are of the same age. This, again, is strikingly different in patients, who differ in sex, age, and various genetic factors that may affect AED response.

Despite these differences between animal and clinical studies on AED efficacy, the fact that tolerance to efficacy occurs with most AEDs in both animal models and patients with epilepsy (Table 96.1) strongly indicates that functional tolerance is an important reason for drug failure, at least in a subgroup of patients who initially responded. The individual factors that determine whether a patient will develop tolerance upon prolonged administration of an AED are not sufficiently understood, but most likely include genetic factors. Furthermore, the time course of tolerance development may differ among patients. A temporary response with high initial efficacy ("honeymoon effect") during the first months followed by a loss of effectiveness has been described for adjunctive treatment with several AEDs, including levetiracetam, in subgroups of patients with partial epilepsy,[4,5] whereas in other patients a reduction in the response to AEDs may develop more gradually during prolonged treatment and lead to a condition of intractable epilepsy.[6] As shown by various preclinical studies, the tolerance induced by a specific drug may also affect responsiveness to other AEDs, which is termed cross-tolerance.[3] Tolerance would not present any serious problem if it could generally be overcome by increasing dosage of the AED. However, although it is generally believed that tolerance is relative, i.e. the initial efficacy can be regained by increasing drug dosage, there are examples indicating that "absolute tolerance" exists, i.e. the loss of efficacy cannot be counteracted by increasing dosage because of qualitative changes in drug activity.[3] If this is the case, then tolerance and cross-tolerance may lead to intractable epilepsy. Thus, strategies for preventing tolerance or restoring drug efficacy once tolerance has developed need to be assessed. Strategies that have been proposed, such as intermittent treatment, drug holidays, or the use of receptor antagonists, are impracticable or of unproved efficacy.[6]

REFERENCES

1. O'Brien CP. Drug addiction and drug abuse. In: Hardman JG, Limbird LE, eds. *Goodman & Gilman's The pharmacological basis of therapeutics*, 10th ed. New York: McGraw-Hill, 2001: 621–44.
2. Frey H-H, Fröscher W, Koella WP, Meinardi H. *Tolerance to beneficial and adverse effects of antiepileptic drugs.* New York: Raven Press, 1986.
3. Löscher W, Schmidt D. Experimental and clinical evidence for loss of effect (tolerance) during prolonged treatment with antiepileptic drugs. *Epilepsia* 2006;47:1253–84.
4. Boggs JG, Nowack WJ, Drinkard CR. Analysis of the "honeymoon effect" in adult epilepsy patients. *Epilepsia* 2000;41(suppl 7):222.
5. Kinirons P, McCarthy M, Doherty CP, Delanty N. Predicting drug-resistant patients who respond to add-on therapy with levetiracetam. *Seizure* 2006;15:387–92.
6. Avanzini G. Is tolerance to antiepileptic drugs clinically relevant? *Epilepsia* 2006;47:1285–7.

How Can We Detect the Development of Tolerance (Loss of Effect) to AEDs in Patients with Epilepsy? A Clinical Discussion

Dieter Schmidt

p0300 Development of tolerance, i.e. the reduction in response to a drug after repeated administrations, is an adaptive response of the body to prolonged exposure to the drug, and tolerance to AEDs is no exception. Tolerance may lead to attenuation of side effects but also to loss of efficacy of AEDs and is reversible after discontinuation of drug treatment. This commentary addresses the question of how we can detect tolerance in patients with epilepsy. In contrast to findings in experimental animals where there is convincing experimental evidence that almost all first, second, and third generation AEDs lose their antiepileptic activity during prolonged treatment, although to a different extent, tolerance has been reported in a minority of patients as reviewed in detail elsewhere.[1] Before we try to answer this specific question, it may be useful to review the two major types of tolerance that exist in patients with epilepsy. One is pharmacokinetic tolerance, i.e. loss of effect caused by a drop in the serum or brain concentration of the drug. The other is pharmacodynamic tolerance, caused by functional changes at the receptor site while serum or brain concentrations of the drug remain unaffected. However, both pharmacokinetic and pharmacodynamic tolerance may co-exist in the same patient.

p0310 Pharmacokinetic tolerance is well recognized for the first generation, enzyme-inducing AEDs. By far the most important mechanism of pharmacokinetic tolerance to effect are pharmacokinetic interactions in patients receiving add-on medication. Most commonly involved are pharmacokinetic interactions involving cytochrome P450 isoenzymes in hepatic metabolism.[2] Among older generation AEDs, carbamazepine, phenytoin, phenobarbital, and primidone induce the activity of several enzymes involved in drug metabolism, leading to decreased plasma concentration and reduced pharmacological effect of drugs which are substrates of the same enzymes (e.g. tiagabine, valproic acid, lamotrigine, and topiramate). In some cases, these interactions have small clinical consequences because the loss of efficacy caused by the decreased concentration of the affected drug is compensated for by the independent anticonvulsant effect of the enzyme-inducing agent.[2] In other cases, however, the decrease in plasma concentration of the affected drug has adverse effects on seizure control, and an increase in dose is then indicated.[2] However, the clinical impact of pharmacokinetic tolerance is small as it is routinely compensated for by up-titration of dose during treatment. In addition, pharmacokinetic tolerance is of no concern for most newer AEDs such as gabapentin, lamotrigine, levetiracetam, tiagabine, topiramate, vigabatrin, and zonisamide, which have been developed specifically to be free of enzyme-inducing properties. Among the first generation AEDs, pharmacokinetic tolerance is of little importance in single drug treatment, except perhaps for CBZ where autoinduction occurs.[2] In addition to drug-metabolizing enzyme induction, the possibility of efflux transporter induction by AEDs deserves mention.

Functional tolerance to effects of AEDs is not as obvious as shown in animal experiments, for reasons that will be discussed below. It is not an uncommon clinical experience that seizures return in patients seizure-free for several months without a change in treatment and despite good compliance. Long-term clinical trials have shown that, mainly through recurrence of seizures, the number of patients remaining seizure-free declines with prolonged treatment.[3,4] For example, in a monotherapy trial of first generation AEDs, analysis of outcome for the 167 children with newly diagnosed partial epilepsy in the study showed that the percentage of seizure-free patients gradually declined from 38% at 6 months to 20% at 36 months of follow-up.[4] These outcomes are similar to those of a study by the same group of investigators in adults, in which the percentage of seizure-free patients declined to 23% by 3 years of follow-up.[3] In both studies, in addition to seizure recurrence, adverse effects or other reasons may have required withdrawal of seizure-free patients from the study, so the decline may have other causes than loss of efficacy during prolonged treatment. In addition, competing causes for seizure recurrence other than tolerance need to be considered. In fact, several confounding factors hamper the attribution of loss of efficacy to the development of tolerance. These confounding factors will be discussed in the next section.

CONFOUNDING FACTORS FOR DETECTION OF TOLERANCE

Because of diverse confounding factors, detecting tolerance in patients with epilepsy is more difficult but can be done with careful assessment of decline during long-term individual patient response. Several investigators have examined the importance of the individual confounding factors that mimic the development of tolerance (Table 96.1). Following add-on treatment with LEV, loss of efficacy was reported in 32 of 107 patients with 50% or more reduction of seizure frequency.[5] The authors attributed the loss of efficacy to the following causes: lower co-medication in 17 patients, natural fluctuation of seizure frequency in 8 patients, poor compliance in 4 patients, and tolerance in 5 patients, which represents 5% of 107 responders, and 16% of 32 patients with a loss of efficacy.[5] Among 131 cases from a series in Switzerland with reported loss of efficacy of CBZ, the most common confounding factor was ill-advised use of the drug, for example, in patients with absence seizures where it is not efficacious or may even aggravate seizures (43% of patients).[6] In addition, a transient increase in seizures was noted in 12%, followed by progression of underlying brain disease in 5%, and seizure aggravation with correct use of CBZ in 3%.[6] Otherwise unexplained failure that could be attributed to functional tolerance was documented in 5% of patients.[6] Together with pharmaco-kinetic tolerance in an additional 21%, a total of 26% of patients had developed either functional or pharmacokinetic tolerance during prolonged treatment with CBZ.[6]

p0340   One further important confounding factor is that in clinical practice, in contrast to a pharmacological experiment, failure to maintain efficacy after reaching a maintenance dosage is routinely compensated by dose increments. If seizures return shortly after the steady state of the target dose has been reached, the dosage may have been sim-ply too low, alternatively, tolerance to effect may have developed quickly. If, however, seizures return after several months of stable seizure control, tolerance may be a more likely explanation. Whatever the reason, the physician tries to regain seizure control by increasing the dose. Tolerance may remain undetected, again in contrast to a pharma-cological experiment, during clinical treatment of epilepsy for another reason. In case the drug concentration required for seizure protection rises due to the development of tolerance but remains below the achieved steady-state concentration, epilepsy remains controlled by the dosage chosen, and tolerance remains undetected by the clinician. However, pharmacologists who are able to elicit seizures at will and to assess protection or development of tolerance at very low serum concentrations may be able to detect tolerance more often. This may, at least in part, explain the discrepancy between the experimental evidence which demonstrates tolerance to effect in most or all animals tested and for almost all AEDs studied, as discussed earlier, and the reports in the clinical literature where, as will be shown, tolerance is seen in only a subgroup of responders.

p0350   Although it has not been systematically studied how often control can be regained with dose increments when seizures occur in patients with good compliance and sta-ble maintenance dose and serum concentration, it would seem not to be uncommon. For example, in a randomized controlled comparison of PHT and VPA in previously untreated adults with epilepsy who were followed for 12 months, 4 patients (17%) on VPA had further seizures at 3–9 months after the initiation of therapy and required an increase in dosage. Three patients were controlled at the first dosage increment of VPA (1.2 g/day) for periods of 6 and 18 months. One patient had a further seizure 3 months after the first dosage increment of VPA and required a second increment to 2.1 g/day, but has been followed for 9 months without further seizures.[7] Six patients (21%) ran-domized to PHT required an increase in PHT dosage because of further seizures occur-ring 1–6 months (mean 4.6) after the start of therapy. Two patients remained seizure-free after the first dosage increment of PHT for periods of 9 and 12 months, respectively. Four patients required a second increment of PHT because of further seizures which occurred between 1 and 6 months (mean 2.8) after the first increment. Three of these patients have subsequently been followed for a further 12 months without seizures, but one has continued to have seizures at AED doses sufficient to cause acute intoxication.[7]

p0360   One further important confounding factor which makes detection of tolerance, if it exists, very difficult is that – in contrast to most studies in experimental animals – clini-cally detectable loss of effect does not affect all patients treated but is restricted to a sub-group of patients, if it occurs. Furthermore, tolerance may not lead to a complete loss of effect. Theoretically, genetic susceptibility to develop tolerance may differ between individual patients. Whatever the reason for tolerance in one subgroup, if another sub-group of patients shows concurrent improvement of seizure control during prolonged treatment, a study focusing on the proportion of responders and not evaluating out-come shift of individual responders may not be able to detect the development of tol-erance. One important confounding factor is that the development of tolerance may be due in some cases to the progression or exacerbation of the underlying disease. More specifically, a spontaneous increase of seizure frequency by 100% or more compared to baseline which has been observed in 3–9% of patients entering the placebo arm of add-on trials[8] or regression to the mean may be mistaken for the development of tolerance. To evaluate the contribution, if any, of spontaneous changes in seizure frequency, it is important to assess if tolerance does occur to placebo response. In consideration of the described confounding factors, methods to identify tolerance to efficacy, if it exists, will be discussed in the next section.

CLINICAL METHODS TO DETECT TOLERANCE

Several methods have been described to assess the existence of functional tolerance to efficacy (Table 96.2). Any method needs to show loss of efficacy and ideally exclude confounding factors as outlined earlier. One approach, which has been used in the literature to demonstrate that tolerance has not occurred, is measuring group response, i.e. the number of responders between two visits to the clinic. For example, in a study of add-on treatment with LEV, the proportion of responders during the first 3 months of treatment was 39%. This proportion remained stable during the second, consecutive 3-month period. However, a total of 7% of patients were nonresponders during the first 3 months and shifted to become responders during the following 3-month period. A loss of response was described in 8% of patients who were responders during the first 3 months and shifted to become nonresponders during the following 3 months.[9] As a result, the observed outcome shift with loss of effect would not have been detected if the study would have relied only on measurement of group response and not included the individual patient response shift, which clearly showed loss of response in a subgroup of patients. This is why group response analysis is not a reliable tool to assess tolerance in the clinic. In fact, reliance on group analysis is one reason why clinicians fail to detect tolerance unless it caused dramatic loss of group net effect as is the case with BZDs and perhaps VGB. Instead, individual responder analysis, which detects an outcome shift from responder to nonresponder status in individual patients between visits, is a much more reliable method to detect tolerance even if it only occurs in a subgroup of patients.

In fact, individual responder analysis is hardly a new method. When Alfred Hauptmann described his discovery of PB as an AED in his seminal paper in 1912, he discussed one patient with what he called at the time "habituation" who returned to previous seizure frequency after a few months of treatment.[10] One advantage of individual responder analysis is that it can measure complete or partial loss of response between visits. Although individual responder analysis is useful, there are shortcomings to the procedure. One, individual responder analysis is vulnerable, as any procedure to

TABLE 96.2   Confounding Factors: Reasons Other than Tolerance for Decreased Seizure Control or Loss of Effect

---

- Pharmacokinetic changes leading to lower serum concentration of AEDs including dose reduction, change in comedication, drug interactions, and poor adherence to the prescribed drug regimen
- Aggravating factors (alcohol, stress, sleep loss)
- Progression of the epilepsy
- Natural fluctuations of seizure frequency
- Acquired drug resistance mediated by mechanisms other than tolerance

---

Source: From Ref. [1].

measure efficacy, to the hazards of uncontrolled observations, and two, providing evidence for tolerance requires reasonable exclusion or control of confounding factors as discussed earlier.

p0390   After excluding confounding factors, tolerance to antiepileptic effect for most modern and old AEDs can be shown in small subgroups of responders by assessing individual or group response (Table 96.3). Development of tolerance to the antiepileptic activity of an AED may be an important reason for failure of drug treatment. Knowledge of tolerance to AED effects as a mechanism of drug resistance in previous responders is important for patients, physicians, and scientists (Table 96.4).

t0030   TABLE 96.3   Methods to Identify Tolerance in the Clinic

o0060   – *Group response* between visits detects net loss of response but may miss tolerance in a subgroup, if response improves over time in other patients.
o0070   – *Individual responder analysis* between visits shows decline of response but fails to detect improved control in earlier nonresponders.
o0080   – *Individual patient response* in constant cohort over visits. Detects patients shifting from responder to nonresponder status and vice versa between visits, is a much more reliable method to detect tolerance, even if it occurs in only a subgroup of patients.

Source: From Ref. [1].

t0040   TABLE 96.4   Clinical Evidence for Tolerance to Effect During Prolonged Administration of Antiepileptic Drugs. Given is the shift from responder to nonresponder in percentage and (mostly very small) numbers of responders for the individual drugs in each study.

Antiepileptic drug	Responder to nonresponder shift in percentage of responders (*n/n*)
Acetazolamide	15% (3/20), 55% (5/9)
Benzodiazepines	36% (clobazam), 27% (4/15) (clonazepam), 48% (82/170) (clorazepate)
Carbamazepine	4% (2/48)
Felbamate	11% (6/56)
Gabapentin	7% (2/27), 8% (1/12), 80% (12/15)
Lamotrigine	1% (1/127), 15% (4/26)
Levetiracetam	5% (5/107), 19% (68/362), 27% (4/15)
Oxcarbazepine	14% (51/356)
Methsuximide	38% (3/8)
Phenytoin	7% (1/15)
Phenobarbital	11% (2/18)
Pregabalin	32% (66/205)
Stiripentol	16% (15/94)
Sulthiame	19% (5/26)
Topiramate	20% (2/10), 47% (7/15)
Valproate	58% (7/12, p), 21% (6/28 a), 0 (0/115, IGE)
Vigabatrin	12% (12/100), 33% (5/15)
Zonisamide	23% (8/35)

Abbreviations: a, absence seizures; IGE, idiopathic generalized epilepsy; and p, partial epilepsy.
Source: Individual references see Ref. [1].

REFERENCES

1. Löscher W, Schmidt D. Experimental and clinical evidence for tolerance (loss of effect) during treatment with antiepileptic drugs. *Epilepsia* 2006;**47(8)**:1253–84.
2. Patsalos PN, Perucca E. Clinically important drug interactions in epilepsy: general features and interactions between antiepileptic drugs. *Lancet Neurol* 2003;**2**:347–56.
3. Heller AJ, Chesterman P, Elwes RD, *et al*. Phenobarbitone, phenytoin, carbamazepine, or sodium valproate for newly diagnosed adult epilepsy: a randomised comparative monotherapy trial. *J Neurol Neurosurg Psychiatry* 1995;**58**:44–50.
4. de Silva M, Macardle B, Mcgowan M, *et al*. Randomised comparative monotherapy trial of phenobarbitone, phenytoin, carbamazepine, or sodium valproate for newly diagnosed childhood epilepsy. *Lancet* 1996;**347**:709–13.
5. Meencke HJ, Meinke-Jäggi D. Ursachen für sekundären Wirkungsverlust sorgsam differenzieren. *PharmaFokus ZNS* 2004;**1**:30–3.
6. Jain KK. Investigation and management of loss of efficacy of an antiepileptic medication using carbamazepine as an example. *J R Soc Med* 1993;**86**:133–6.
7. Turnbull DM, Rawlins MD, Weightman D, Chadwick DW. A comparison of phenytoin and valproate in previously untreated adult epileptic patients. *J Neurol Neurosurg Psychiatry* 1982;**45**:55–9.
8. Somerville ER. Aggravation of partial seizures by antiepileptic drugs: is there evidence from clinical trials? *Neurology* 2002;**59**:79–83.
9. Ben Menachem E, Edrich P, Van Vleymen B, Sander JW, Schmidt B. Evidence for sustained efficacy of levetiracetam as add-on epilepsy therapy. *Epilepsy Res* 2003;**53**:57–64.
10. Hauptmann A. Luminal bei Epilepsie. *Münch Med Wschr* 1912;**35**:1907–9.
11. Schmidt D, Kupferberg HJ, Yonekawa W, Penry JK. The development of tolerance to the anticonvulsant effect of phenobarbital in mice. *Epilepsia* 1980;**21**:141–7.

c00097

Why Is There a Similar Ceiling Effect for the Efficacy of Most If Not All Antiepileptic Drugs in Adult Epilepsy? Reaching the Ceiling or Hitting the Wall?

Jane Boggs

The patient is a 35-year-old Caucasian man who initially presented at age 20 with a generalized tonic–clonic seizure at a restaurant, which was witnessed by his girlfriend. She did not see the onset of his seizure, and so could not state whether it had a focal onset. The emergency physician initiated phenytoin 300 mg qhs and referred him to a neurologist. He had a routine outpatient EEG, which was normal. No further seizures were reported for 3 months, and there was consideration that this may have been an isolated event. A second seizure occurred while he was in a college classroom, and a variety of observers agreed that he had mumbled and turned his head prior to convulsing. He had been scrupulously compliant, as he was anxious to resume driving, and his phenytoin level at the time of the seizure was 18 mg/l with no drug-related complaints.

His neurologist concluded that phenytoin was simply not an effective agent for him, and referred him to an epileptologist. A repeat prolonged EEG showed multiple spike and sharp waves in the left temporal region, and an magnetic resonance imaging (MRI) failed to demonstrate any pathology. Although his initial dose of phenytoin had been increased to 400 mg daily, and his level rose to 25, he only had minimal increased sedation. He had several other mumbling episodes, and his epileptologist added lamotrigine with an appropriately slow titration to 200 mg bid. No further events ensued for 3 months, and he agreed to taper his phenytoin by 50 mg per week to attain monotherapy with lamotrigine.

He had one complex partial seizure without secondary generalization in the sixth week of downward titration of phenytoin. This event was felt to represent possible withdrawal effect as his level had precipitously dropped in the previous week. He continued on with no further seizures for 2 months after complete elimination of phenytoin.

He then had a day with two complex partial seizures, the second of which secondarily generalized and resulted in a fractured finger. The emergency physician resumed his phenytoin at 400 mg daily and his epileptologist saw him urgently the next morning. Because he complained of sedation on phenytoin–lamotrigine duotherapy, he was then started on levetiracetam and titrated over 2 weeks up to 1500 mg bid. The phenytoin was not continued.

He did well for 5 months, and then had a complex partial seizure. His lamotrigine was increased gradually to his maximal tolerance at 400 mg bid. Fortunately, his epileptologist had become concerned that he should refrain from driving until he was a full year seizure-free. This time his seizures recurred after 7 months.

Subsequently, he underwent a phase I pre-surgical evaluation at a comprehensive epilepsy center, and he was found to have a positive ictal single photon emission computed tomography (SPECT) in the left posterior temporal lobe and a possible area of polymicrogyria on 3T MRI. At this point he was 4 years after presentation. Wada testing indicated that his language and memory had inadequate bilateral representation and the lesion was likely quite close to eloquent cortex. He declined surgery and returned to his epileptologist.

He then pursued a sequence of 3- to 6-month trials of various duo- and triotherapies, including the following:

Oxcarbazepine and lamotrigine
Oxcarbazepine and levetiracetam
Levetiracetam and divalproex
Topiramate and divalproex
Topiramate, divalproex and levetiracetam

None of these combinations resulted in any change in his usual frequency of 1–2 complex partial seizures every 3–5 months. He did, however, stop having convulsive events whenever on levetiracetam. Otherwise, no meaningful conclusions could be made about his response to therapies. At his request, he tried LEV monotherapy up to 2000 mg bid but still had complex partial seizures every 3 months. He remained on LEV 1500 mg bid and oxcarbazepine 900 mg bid as his "optimal" therapy to minimize seizures and side effects. He has not driven for 8 years and moved to an area with good public transportation to maintain his employment in an engineering firm.

COMMENTARY

Pharmacoresistant epilepsy is more prevalent among, but not restricted to, localization-related cases. What determines pharmacoresistance, and when, in a particular case, further treatment adjustments become moot, is an elusive question. Considered another way, there is no evidence that explains why a particular patient has a ceiling for overall seizure control, or when the treating epileptologists 'hit the wall' in finding useful therapeutic options.

Outcome studies in adults have indicated that 59.2% of patients ultimately achieve long-term remission of seizures.[1] This outcome does not appear to be markedly influenced by epilepsy syndrome or choice of drugs (as long as not inappropriate for the seizure type). Over half of these good responses were achieved by the first drug selected.[2]

The Standard And New Antiepileptic Drug (SANAD) study indicated that there was little difference in success in localization-related epilepsy seizure freedom for the initial 12 months of therapy with carbamazepine (29% with 95% CI 24–34%), lamotrigine (25% with 95% CI 18–32%), oxcarbazepine (27% with 95% CI 17–36%), or topiramate (25% with 95% CI 18–33%).[3] Although immediate response was greatest for sodium valproate (36% with 95%CI 29–42%) in the idiopathic generalized epilepsy subjects, topiramate (32% with 95% CI 23–42%) and lamotrigine (26% with 95% CI 17–35%) were comparable, especially when the overlap of confidence intervals was considered.[4] Levetiracetam (LEV) was not utilized in SANAD, but a comparative study between levetiracetam and controlled release CBZ-CR showed similar 1-year seizure freedom rates of about 50% in new epilepsy patients.[5] Thus, at least for the first year, efficacy may not be strikingly different among antiepileptic drugs (AEDs) appropriate for seizure type.

p0180   Those patients whose seizures do not remit with the first selected AED have a progressively worse chance of seizure freedom with every subsequent drug attempted. Failing the first drug portended a 27% chance of poor ultimate control, while failing the second and third options lowered the chance of remission to 10% and 3%, respectively.[6] Considering the converse, patients who did not become seizure-free with their second AED had a 90% chance of continuing to have seizures despite any medication.

It is usually when a patient's seizures fail to improve with two to three appropriate choices of AEDs that consideration of more complex therapies begins. Whether there is also a ceiling effect with neurostimulation and surgical options is not clear, as these therapies are more commonly performed in patients who are already felt to be refractory to AEDs. The duration of seizure freedom in the post-surgical population is particularly difficult to analyze, due to both continued use and tapering of AEDs, as well as the potential for evolution of the causative lesion.

Patients with refractory epilepsy often seek help from epileptologists and comprehensive epilepsy centers. When such patients have a singularly good response to an agent, the result is notable. Of course, the question remains whether this response is simply a transient response or one that may be longer lasting than the duration of the study. Thus, the patient with refractory epilepsy justifies study extensions to determine long-term prognosis and late adverse effects.

On a personal perspective, the patients with refractory and difficult-to-control seizures are the lifeblood, the bane and the brass ring of the epileptologist's existence. Without them, we would be superfluous. With them, we and our patients have to endure repeated failures toward the goal of "no seizures". Careful and successful analysis of patients who never become seizure-free will hopefully further our knowledge of pharmacodynamics as well as the emerging field of pharmacogenomics. If we can identify the genetic patterns that determine resistance to seizure freedom, then we may be able to raise the ceiling on epilepsy.

REFERENCES

1. Mohanraj R, Brodie MJ. Outcomes in newly diagnosed localization-related epilepsies. *Seizure* 2005;**14**:318–23.
2. Mohanraj R, Brodie MJ. Diagnosing refractory epilepsy: response to sequential treatment schedules. *Eur J Neurol* 2006;**13**:277–82.

3. Marson AG, Al-Kharusi AM, Alwaidh M, *et al.* The SANAD study of the effectiveness of carbamazepine, gabapentin, lamotrigine, oxcarbazepine, or topiramate for treatment of partial epilepsy: an unblended randomized controlled trial. *Lancet* 2007;**369**:1000–15.
4. Marson AG, Al-Kharusi AM, Alwaidh M, *et al.* The SANAD study of the effectiveness of valproate, lamotrigine, or topiramate for generalized and unclassifiable epilepsy: an unblended randomized controlled trial. *Lancet* 2007;**369**:1016–26.
5. Brodie MJ, Perucca E, Ryvlin P, Ben-Menachem E, Meencke H-J for the Levetiracetam Monotherapy Study Group. Comparison of levetiracetam and controlled release carbamazepine in newly diagnosed epilepsy. *Neurology* 2007;**68**:402–8.
6. Mohanraj R, Brodie MJ. Diagnosing refractory epilepsy: response to sequential treatment schedules. *Eur J Neurol* 2006;**13**:277–82.

Why Is There a Similar Ceiling Effect for the Efficacy of Most If Not All Antiepileptic Drugs in Adult Epilepsy? A Clinical Perspective

Rajiv Mohanraj and Martin J Brodie

s0080

OUTCOMES DATA REVIEW

p0320

Data from outcome studies in adults with newly diagnosed epilepsy suggest patterns of response to AEDs that can be observed consistently across a range of epilepsy syndromes. In a series of 780 patients starting on their first AED over a 20-year period at the Western Infirmary in Glasgow, Scotland, 31.4% responded immediately to treatment, suffering no further seizures after taking the first drug dose.[1] These immediate responders constituted more than half of the 59.2% of patients who subsequently achieved long-term remission. The prognosis for immediate response was not markedly influenced by syndrome classification or choice of drugs.[2] Indeed, many patients were controlled on a modest or moderate AED dose.[3] A smaller proportion (5.4% overall) showed a transiently good response, achieving seizure freedom for more than 12 months before suffering relapse of seizures and subsequently developing refractory epilepsy.[1] The remaining 35.4% of this population never achieved seizure freedom for any consecutive 12–month period despite treatment with a range of AEDs.

p0330

Similar patterns of response to treatment were observed in the recently concluded SANAD study. In the localization-related epilepsy arm, 29% (95% CI 24–34%) of patients starting on CBZ–CR achieved 12 months of seizure freedom by the end of the first year on treatment. This immediate responder rate was significantly different only for gabapentin [20% (95% CI 13–26%)], with lamotrigine [25% (95% CI 18–32%)], oxcarbazepine [27% (95% CI 17–36%)] and topiramate [25% (95% CI 18–32%)] producing similar seizure-free rates in the per protocol analysis.[4] In the idiopathic generalized epilepsy arm, the immediate responder rate for sodium valproate was 36% (95% CI 29–42%). Lamotrigine [26% (95% CI 17–35%)] and topiramate [32% (95% CI 23–42%)] produced comparable immediate responder rates.[5]

These observations have been supported by a recent double-blind, randomized trial in newly diagnosed epilepsy comparing controlled-release CBZ–CR with LEV.[6] No difference in outcome was found between the drugs. One year seizure-free rates of around 50% were observed with both agents using the intention-to-treat analysis. These figures were almost identical to those reported from Glasgow.[1] In addition, the vast majority of responders (89% taking CBZ–CR versus 86% on LEV) did so at low dosage, that is, CBZ–CR 200 mg or LEV 500 mg twice daily, again mirroring the modest doses that were effective in many Scottish patients.[3]

A number of studies have demonstrated that early treatment with AEDs, while preventing seizure recurrence in the short term, did not alter long-term outcomes.[7-8] On the other hand, failure to respond to the first AED does herald a poorer prognosis.[9-11] In the Glasgow series, only 27% of those patients failing their first AED due to lack of efficacy subsequently demonstrated a good outcome.[1] Those who did not become seizure-free with two or three AED schedules because of lack of efficacy had a less than 10% and 3% chance, respectively, of ever achieving remission. This last group could, therefore, be considered to have refractory epilepsy.

Given the lack of influence of timing and choice of AED, the prognosis for patients with epilepsy has been considered to be an inherent property of the epilepsy syndrome. This is certainly the case for a range of epilepsies in infancy and childhood. There is a less clear link between pathological substrates underlying some adult epilepsies and treatment outcomes.[12,13] In addition, people with the same syndrome do not all respond to AEDs in a uniform manner. In our analysis of 343 patients with newly diagnosed localization-related epilepsy, no significant differences were found in remission rates between patient populations with cryptogenic and symptomatic epilepsies. Immediate responder and remission rates were also comparable with some patients with the same syndrome doing well and others doing badly despite taking similar AED therapy.[2] This also applied to small groups of patients with newly diagnosed epilepsy thought to be secondary to mesial temporal sclerosis or cortical dysplasia. Although, overall, patients with newly diagnosed idiopathic generalized epilepsies were more likely to achieve remission than those with localization-related epilepsies, again some teenagers with, for instance, juvenile myoclonic epilepsy appeared to be refractory de novo.[14]

Relevance to clinical practice

The vast majority of adults who respond to pharmacotherapy will do so with their first AED. The more regimens required to be tried, the more likely will the epilepsy prove to be refractory with only a handful of individuals doing well after failing three drug schedules. Initial response to treatment in adult newly diagnosed epilepsy appears to be largely independent of seizure or syndrome classification and choice of AED. Thus, the prognosis for many patients with newly diagnosed epilepsy, whether good or bad, will become apparent within a few months of starting treatment.

What unanswered questions still remain for clinical researchers

The majority of epilepsy syndromes encountered in adults display the complete gamut of responsiveness to AED treatment from immediate control of seizures to refractoriness from the outset. This raises an important question – does clinical classification of epilepsy syndromes reflect the pathophysiological mechanisms responsible for seizure generation and drug responsiveness? Studies of monogenic epilepsies suggest a great deal of genetic heterogeneity underlying well-defined phenotypes.[15] The same is likely to be true of acquired epilepsies. There are likely to be differences in molecular, cellular and network alterations that underpin clinically homogenous epilepsy syndromes. Elucidating these is crucial to our understanding of drug resistance in human epilepsies.[16]

There is no published evidence to suggest that the advent of newer AEDs with novel mechanisms of action has resulted in better treatment outcomes. It is reasonable, therefore, to postulate a common mechanism limiting the effectiveness of AEDs. This may relate to the expression throughout the brain of drug-resistance proteins, such as P-glycoprotein.[17] Pharmacokinetic and pharmacodynamic tolerance to AEDs may also play a role in patients who show initial response to AEDs before becoming treatment resistant.[18]

Alterations in the structure, expression levels and function of drug transporter proteins, metabolizing enzymes and drug targets caused by genetic variations have the potential to affect the response to AEDs. However, the design, execution and data analysis in pharmacogenetic studies are not straightforward.[19] Treatment response is a complex outcome, brought about by a combination of genetic and environmental factors. This will limit the predictive power of any single genetic marker. Pharmacogenomic studies can be considered analogous to genetic association studies of complex disorders in this respect, and an approach utilizing the concept of multiple susceptibility single-nucleotide polymorphisms may be more informative. Perhaps we need to examine the complete genotype before we understand the individual basis for pharmacoresistance.

Determining phenotypes is also complicated, as a uniform definition of responders and nonresponders can be difficult to identify. A pragmatic approach might be to limit comparisons initially to immediate responders and those who remain refractory from the outset. The short answer to the question posed in the title is that the adult epilepsy population largely divides into two with most responders doing well on a modest dose of any therapeutic agent while those with refractory epilepsy usually tend to be pharmacoresistant *de novo* to all available AEDs used singly or in combination.

REFERENCES

1. Mohanraj R, Brodie MJ. Diagnosing refractory epilepsy: response to sequential treatment schedules. *Eur J Neurol* 2006;**13**:277–82.
2. Mohanraj R, Brodie MJ. Outcomes in newly diagnosed localization-related epilepsies. *Seizure* 2005;**14**:318–23.
3. Mohanraj R, Brodie MJ. Pharmacological outcomes in newly diagnosed epilepsy. *Epilepsy Behav* 2005;**6**:382–7.

4. Marson AG, Al-Kharusi AM, Alwaidh M, *et al.* The SANAD study of effectiveness of carbamaze-pine, gabapentin, lamotrigine, oxcarbazepine, or topiramate for treatment of partial epilepsy: an unblinded randomised controlled trial. *Lancet* 2007;**369**:1000–15.

5. Marson AG, Al-Kharusi AM, Alwaidh M, *et al.* The SANAD study of effectiveness of valproate, lamotrigine, or topiramate for generalised and unclassifiable epilepsy: an unblinded randomised controlled trial. *Lancet* 2007;**369**:1016–26.

6. Brodie MJ, Perucca E, Ryvlin P, Ben-Menachem E, Meenche H-J for the Levetiracetam Monotherapy Study Group. Comparison of levetiracetam and controlled-release carbamazepine in newly diagnosed epilepsy. *Neurology* 2007;**68**:402–8.

7. Musicco M, Beghi E, Solari A, Viani F. Treatment of first tonic-clonic seizure does not improve the prognosis of epilepsy. First Seizure Trial Group (FIRST Group). *Neurology* 1997;**49**:991–8.

8. Marson A, Jacoby A, Johnson A, Kim L, Gamble C, Chadwick D; Medical Research Council MESS Study Group. Immediate versus deferred antiepileptic drug treatment for early epilepsy and single seizures: a randomised controlled trial. *Lancet* 2005;**365**:2007–13.

9. Camfield PR, Camfield CS, Gordon K, Dooley JM. If a first antiepileptic drug fails to control a child's epilepsy, what are the chances of success with the next drug? *J Pediatr* 1997;**131**:821–4.

10. Kwan P, Brodie MJ. Early identification of refractory epilepsy. *N Engl J Med* 2000;**342**:314–9.

11. Dlugos DJ, Sammel MD, Strom BL, Farrar JT. Response to first drug trial predicts outcome in childhood temporal lobe epilepsy. *Neurology* 2001;**57**:2259–64.

12. Semah F, Picot MC, Adam C, *et al.* Is the underlying cause of epilepsy a major prognostic factor for recurrence? *Neurology* 1998;**51**:1256–62.

13. Stephen LJ, Kwan P, Brodie MJ. Does the cause of localization-related epilepsy influence the response to antiepileptic drug treatment? *Epilepsia* 2001;**42**:357–62.

14. Mohanraj R, Brodie MJ. Outcomes of newly diagnosed idiopathic generalized epilepsy syndromes in a non-pediatric setting. *Acta Neurol Scand* 2007;**115**:204–8.

15. Scheffer IE, Berkovic SF. The genetics of human epilepsy. *Trends Pharmacol Sci* 2003;**24**:428–33.

16. Kwan P, Brodie MJ. Potential role of drug transporters in the pathogenesis of medically intractable epilepsy. *Epilepsia* 2005;**46**:224–35.

17. Löscher W, Schmidt D. Experimental and clinical evidence for loss of effect (tolerance) during pro-longed treatment with antiepileptic drugs. *Epilepsia* 2006;**47**:1253–84.

18. Depondt C, Shorvon SD. Genetic association studies in epilepsy pharmacogenomics: lessons learnt and potential applications. *Pharmacogenomics* 2006;**7**:731–45.

19. Brodie MJ. Response to antiepileptic drug therapy: winners and losers. *Epilepsia* 2006;**46(suppl 10)**:31–2. .

What Clinical Observations on the Epidemiology of Antiepileptic Drug Intractability Tell Us About the Mechanisms of Pharmacoresistance

Michael A Rogawski

In the past several years, there have been important advances in the clinical epidemiology of antiepileptic drug resistance, as reviewed by Mohanraj and Brodie in the preceding commentary. It would appear that by and large, intractability is independent of the choice of AED. Many patients will become seizure-free on the first agent tried, irrespective of which one their physician decides to pick. Nonresponders to the first drug are in a different category: It is likely that they will continue to have seizures no matter which medicine or combination of medicines is tried. This simple clinical observation puts important constraints on the possible biological mechanisms for pharmacoresistance. In this essay, I consider the clinical implications of the new research on the neurobiological mechanisms of AED intractability.

AEDS HAVE MANY DISTINCT CELLULAR MECHANISMS OF ACTION

Clinicians have a wide range of AEDs to choose from. There are 23 distinct chemical entities marketed worldwide for epilepsy therapy. Some of these agents are known to be useful for a limited range of seizure types. For example, ethosuximide is largely exclusively used in childhood absence. Tiagabine, vigabatrin, phenytoin, carbamazepine, and oxcarbazepine are mainly useful for partial and primarily generalized seizures.

The other agents, including valproate, topiramate and levetiracetam, have broader utility. With very few exceptions, each AED acts in a mechanistically distinct way. This is not the situation in other therapeutic areas. For example, the triptans used to abort migraine attacks all act in a similar fashion as agonists of serotonin 5-HT$_{1B}$ and 5-HT$_{1D}$ receptors; the selective serotonin reuptake inhibitors used to treat depression all block the serotonin transporter; the many statins are all HMG-CoA reductase inhibitors; and the proton pump inhibitors all have the same molecular target. In contrast, each AED generally acts on a unique set of molecular targets. Even when they share the same molecular target, as is the case for AEDs that act on voltage-activated sodium channels, the biophysical details for each drug are sufficiently different that the mechanisms must be considered distinct.[1] For example, there may be important differences in binding rate, binding affinity,[2] the ability to block open channels[3] or effects on persistent sodium current[4], or effects on other ion channels, as is the case for lamotrigine, where modulation of voltage-activated calcium channels may be relevant to its therapeutic activity. Another major class of AED actions relates to interactions with GABA-mediated inhibition. Some drugs, most notably benzodiazepines and phenobarbital, but also felbamate and topiramate, positively modulate GABA$_A$ receptors. The specific actions of these agents are distinct. For example, benzodiazepines and phenobarbital modulate GABA$_A$ receptors at distinct sites and in different ways. Unlike benzodiazepines, phenobarbital, felbamate and topiramate act on targets other than GABA$_A$ receptors that likely contribute to therapeutic activity. Vigabatrin inhibits GABA transaminase, whereas tiagabine blocks the GAT-1 GABA transporter; each of these agents affects the dynamics of inhibitory function in dramatically different ways. Other AEDs exert their anticonvulsant action through novel targets. For example, LEV acts through SV2A, a ubiquitous synaptic vesicle protein, whereas gabapentin and pregabalin act through $\alpha_2\delta$, a novel presynaptic protein associated with voltage-activated calcium channels.[5,6]

INADEQUACY OF THE TARGET HYPOTHESIS

A number of hypotheses have been proposed to explain AED pharmacoresistance.[7] One major hypothesis is that alterations in the structure or function of the molecular targets through which AEDs act lead to reduced drug activity. However, since diverse AEDs act in so many different ways and on different sets of molecular targets, this so-called target hypothesis seems incompatible with the clinical evidence that certain patients are resistant to all available drugs. It is unlikely that all of the targets would become changed in such a way to produce pan pharmacoresistance. There are two forms to the target hypothesis and this argument applies equally well to both. In the conventional form of the target hypothesis, the molecular target − most commonly voltage-activated sodium channels − loses pharmacological sensitivity to AEDs during the acquisition of pharmacoresistance.[8–10] However, in the studies supporting this hypothesis, the sensitivity to drugs that act on other molecular targets, notably valproate and lamotrigine, was unaffected. The mechanism of action of valproate is poorly understood but is unlikely to relate largely to an interaction with sodium channels. Lamotrigine has a different spectrum of activity than other AEDs and, as noted, acts on calcium channels in addition to sodium channels. Clearly, this resistance mechanism could only apply to AEDs that act largely on the specific target affected. Other challenges to the target hypothesis are discussed by Schmidt and Löscher.[7] A second form of the target hypothesis posits that there are genetically determined polymorphisms in an AED target that alter

AED responsiveness. Indeed, Tate *et al.*[11] identified a polymorphism in the SCNA1 sodium channel gene that appeared to confer resistance to carbamazepine and phenytoin, although they subsequently did not replicate the association.[12] Whether or not a sodium channel polymorphism is associated with pharmacoresistance to drugs that act on sodium channels, clinical AED intractability, in which there is a failure to adequately respond to all available agents, is not explained.

QUESTIONS REGARDING THE TRANSPORTER HYPOTHESIS

A leading hypothesis regarding drug resistance in epilepsy is the so-called transporter hypothesis which postulates that drug efflux transporters located in the apical membrane of capillary endothelial cells that form the blood–brain barrier limit AED availability to their molecular targets in the brain.[13] The best-studied transporter is P-glycoprotein (P-gp) but other transporters, including multidrug-resistance-associated proteins (MRPs), could also play a role in pharmacoresistance to AEDs. Reports that P-gp and members of the MRP family are overexpressed in experimentally induced seizure foci and brain tissue specimens removed during surgery of patients with pharmacoresistant epilepsy have raised the possibility that localized overexpression of transporter proteins accounts for the inability to overcome resistance by increasing the drug dose, since other brain regions would then be exposed to supratherapeutic (toxic) drug concentrations.[14–16] In addition to the observation of increased transporter expression, which could be due to the epileptic process itself or the occurrence of seizures, it has been proposed that genetic polymorphisms in a transporter gene could account for increased functional transporter activity. However, none of the proposed associations between transporter genotype and clinical drug response have been replicated.[17–19] In any case the genetic form of the transporter hypothesis seems unlikely since a generalized upregulation of transporter activity could be overcome by increasing the AED dose.

The major weakness of the multidrug transporter hypothesis is the lack of evidence that AEDs are substrates for P-gp or any other human efflux transporter.[20,21] While there is evidence in experimental animals that several commonly used AEDs are transported to some extent by both P-gp and MRPs,[13,22] recent experiments employing transfected cell lines expressing rodent and human efflux transporters have cast doubt that the drugs are truly substrates for the human forms of the transporters.[23] Even in mice, the extent to which AEDs are transported by P-gp must be very small as genetic deletion of P-gp does not influence brain uptake of many AEDs.[24] Indeed, it is apparent that AEDs are not efficiently extruded from brain since all AEDs exhibit CNS side effects, even if they fail to confer adequate seizure protection. Finally, the fact that most AEDs show linear uptake into the brain over a wide range of concentrations calls into question the existence of a saturable transport system that influences the dynamics of AED transport across the blood–brain barrier.[25]

DOES "INHERENT SEVERITY" ACCOUNT FOR PHARMACORESISTANCE?

A variety of clinical factors are known to be associated with intractability. The most important and well validated of these factors is the frequency of seizures in the period immediately after diagnosis. Several early studies demonstrated that frequent seizures are associated with bad prognosis[26] and that high initial seizure frequency during the period after presentation is an important predictor of seizure intractability.[27–29] A recent study confirmed the prognostic implications of high early seizure frequency and also identified several other factors associated with intractability including family history of epilepsy, febrile seizures, traumatic brain injury, recreational drug use and a history of depression.[30] These results suggest that neurobiological factors related to the occurrence of frequent seizures are associated with intractability. This observation seems logical: If the epilepsy is of a nature that seizures are easy to trigger, the seizures may be more difficult to prevent. AEDs probably do not act as a switch to turn off the possibility of seizure occurrence; rather, they make it more difficult to trigger a seizure. That is, they raise the threshold for a seizure-inducing stimulus. In most (but not all) animal models in which seizures are induced by a pharmacological or electrical stimulus, raising the intensity of the trigger can overcome the seizure protection conferred by a given dose of an AED. As is the case with a triggered seizure, if seizure susceptibility is inherently high, it may not be possible to prevent seizure occurrence with any nontoxic drug dose. This leads to the concept that there is a degree of inherent severity in any individual epilepsy patient that does not necessarily depend upon the underlying etiology. Rather, for syndromes of similar etiology, the severity can range from mild to severe, just as diabetes or cystic fibrosis can range in disease severity. Indeed, it appears that disease severity can depend upon specific modifier genes, as in the case of a movement disorder in mice linked to a mutation in the $Na_V1.6$ voltage-activated sodium channel.[31] Mice homozygous for the $Na_V1.6$ mutation (med^J/med^J) exhibit a highly variable phenotype ranging from slowly progressive tremor and dystonia and lifespan >1.5 years to paralysis and death at 1 month of life. Disease severity has been found to depend upon the genetic background, specifically to an unlinked gene ($Scnm1$) that influences the splicing of the mRNA that encodes $Na_V1.6$. This modifier gene dramatically alters the severity of the neurological syndrome. It seems likely that there are similar modifier effects that alter the severity of epilepsy and overall drug responsiveness.

The concept of genetically determined epilepsy severity implies that seizures in severely affected patients are difficult to control from the time of their first seizure and that the occurrence of uncontrolled seizures over time is not the cause of the intractability. Indeed, the wealth of evidence suggests that most cases of epilepsy are not progressive and do not worsen over time as a result of uncontrolled seizures.[32,33] Finally, I note that disease severity need not necessarily be static, but may fluctuate in response to internal factors and environmental influences. For example, in perimenstrual catamenial epilepsy, severity (and drug intractability) is dependent on hormonal fluctuations occurring at the time of menstruation.[34]

CONCLUSIONS

What implications does the "inherent severity" hypothesis have for the development of strategies to overcome pharmacoresistance? While it will always be challenging to treat more severely affected patients, it should not be assumed that seizure freedom is unattainable in such patients. The inherent severity model proposes that there is a continuum in severity so that new AEDs acting on novel molecular targets may offer protection for such patients. Recent data is compatible with this optimistic view. Thus, Callaghan et al.[35] found that drug refractory patients who have not responded to at least two AEDs do achieve remission at a rate of about 5% per year. In the majority of cases, the remission was associated with the addition or increase in dose of an

AED, most commonly lamotrigine or levetiracetam. While insufficient data was available for these authors to conclude that these drugs are more likely to induce remission than other AEDs, it seems plausible that the availability of a broader range of AEDs accounts for the fact that these authors obtained better rates of seizure remission in their patients with previously refractory seizures than has previously been observed. A variety of new AEDs are currently in development, some of which act in new ways on old targets and others that act on entirely new targets.[36] We can expect that these new drugs will further benefit patients by having improved side effect profiles, improved pharmacokinetic properties, reduced propensity for drug interactions, less teratogenic potential, an improved spectrum of activity and, most importantly, by their ability to induce seizure remission in some patients previously considered to have intractable seizures. In the future, if modifier genes can be identified that influence severity in human epilepsies, it may be possible to specifically target the biological mechanisms accounting for greater severity, making seizure control feasible for patients with difficult-to-control seizures.

s0070   # REFERENCES

1. Rogawski MA, Löscher W. The neurobiology of antiepileptic drugs. *Nat Rev Neurosci* 2004;**5**:553–64.
2. Kuo C-C. A common anticonvulsant binding site for phenytoin, carbamazepine, and lamotrigine in neuronal Na$^+$ channels. *Mol Pharmacol* 1998;**54**:712–21.
3. Yang Y-C, Kuo C-C. Inhibition of Na$^+$ current by imipramine and related compounds: different binding kinetics as an inactivation stabilizer and as an open channel blocker. *Mol Pharmacol* 2002;**62**:1228–37.
4. Stafstrom CE. Persistent sodium current and its role in epilepsy. *Epilepsy Curr* 2007;**7**:15–22.
5. Rogawski MA, Taylor CP. Ion channels. In: Löscher W, Schmidt D. New horizons in the development of antiepileptic drugs: Innovative strategies. *Epilepsy Res* 2006;**69**:183–272.
6. Meldrum BS, Rogawski MA. Molecular targets for antiepileptic drug development. *Neurotherapeutics* 2007;**4**:18–61.
7. Schmidt D, Löscher W. Drug resistance in epilepsy: putative neurobiologic and clinical mechanisms. *Epilepsia* 2005;**46**:858–77.
8. Vreugdenhil M, Wadman WJ. Modulation of sodium currents in rat CA1 neurons by carbamazepine and valproate after kindling epileptogenesis. *Epilepsia* 1999;**40**:1512–22.
9. Remy S, Gabriel S, Urban BW, et al. A novel mechanism underlying drug resistance in chronic epilepsy. *Ann Neurol* 2003;**53**:469–79.
10. Ellerkmann RK, Remy S, Chen J, et al. Molecular and functional changes in voltage-dependent Na$^+$ channels following pilocarpine-induced status epilepticus in rat dentate granule cells. *Neuroscience* 2003;**119**:323–33.
11. Tate SK, Depondt C, Sisodiya SM, et al. Genetic predictors of the maximum doses patients receive during clinical use of the anti-epileptic drugs carbamazepine and phenytoin. *Proc Natl Acad Sci USA* 2005;**102**:5507–12.
12. Tate SK, Singh R, Hung CC, et al. A common polymorphism in the SCN1A gene associates with phenytoin serum levels at maintenance dose. *Pharmacogenet Genomics* 2006;**16**:721–6.
13. Löscher W, Potschka H. Drug resistance in brain diseases and the role of drug efflux transporters. *Nat Rev Neurosci* 2005;**6**:591–602.
14. Tishler DM, Weinberg KI, Hinton DR, Barbaro N, Annett GM, Raffel C. MDR1 gene expression in brain of patients with medically intractable epilepsy. *Epilepsia* 1995;**36**:1–6.
15. Dombrowski SM, Desai SY, Marroni M, et al. Overexpression of multiple drug resistance genes in endothelial cells from patients with refractory epilepsy. *Epilepsia* 2001;**42**:1501–6.
16. Aronica E, Gorter JA, Ramkema M, et al. Expression and cellular distribution of multidrug resistance-related proteins in the hippocampus of patients with mesial temporal lobe epilepsy. *Epilepsia* 2004;**45**:441–51.

17. Soranzo N, Kelly L, Martinian L, *et al.* Lack of support for a role for RLIP76 (RALBP1) in response to treatment or predisposition to epilepsy. *Epilepsia* 2007;**48**:674–83.

18. Leschziner GD, Andrew T, Pirmohamed M, Johnson MR. ABCB1 genotype and PGP expression, function and therapeutic drug response: a critical review and recommendations for future research. *Pharmacogenomics J* 2007;**7**:154–79.

19. Leschziner GD, Jorgensen AL, Andrew T, *et al.* The association between polymorphisms in RLIP76 and drug response in epilepsy. *Pharmacogenomics* 2007;**8**:1715–22.

20. Rogawski MA. Does P-glycoprotein play a role in pharmacoresistance to antiepileptic drugs? *Epilepsy Behav* 2002;**3**:493–5.

21. Löscher W, Sills GJ. Drug resistance in epilepsy: Why is a simple explanation not enough? *Epilepsia* 2007;**48**:2370–2.

22. van Vliet EA, van Schaik R, Edelbroek PM, *et al.* Inhibition of the multidrug transporter P-glycoprotein improves seizure control in phenytoin-treated chronic epileptic rats. *Epilepsia* 2006;**47**:672–80.

23. Crowe A, Teoh YK. Limited P-glycoprotein mediated efflux for anti-epileptic drugs. *J Drug Target* 2006;**14**:291–300.

24. Sills GJ, Kwan P, Butler E, de Lange EC, van den Berg DJ, Brodie MJ. P-glycoprotein-mediated efflux of antiepileptic drugs: preliminary studies in mdr1a knockout mice. *Epilepsy Behav* 2002;**3**:427–32.

25. Anderson GD, Shen DD. Where is the evidence that P-glycoprotein limits brain uptake of antiepileptic drug and contributes to drug resistance in epilepsy? *Epilepsia* 2007;**48**:2372–4.

26. Brorson LO, Wranne L. Long-term prognosis in childhood epilepsy: survival and seizure prognosis. *Epilepsia* 1987;**28**:324–30.

27. Collaborative Group for the Study of Epilepsy. Prognosis of epilepsy in newly referred patients: a multicenter prospective study of the effects of monotherapy on the long-term course of epilepsy. *Epilepsia* 1992;**33**:45–51.

28. Sillanpää M. Remission of seizures and predictors of intractability in long-term follow-up. *Epilepsia* 1993;**34**:930–6.

29. MacDonald BK, Johnson AL, Goodridge DM, Cockerell OC, Sander JW, Shorvon SD. Factors predicting prognosis of epilepsy after presentation with seizures. *Ann Neurol* 2000;**48**:833–41.

30. Hitiris N, Mohanraj R, Norrie J, Sills GJ, Brodie MJ. Predictors of pharmacoresistant epilepsy. *Epilepsy Res* 2007;**75**:192–6.

31. Buchner DA, Trudeau M, Meisler MH. SCNM1, a putative RNA splicing factor that modifies disease severity in mice. *Science* 2003;**30**:967–9.

32. Berg AT, Shinnar S. Do seizures beget seizures? An assessment of the clinical evidence in humans. *J Clin Neurophysiol* 1997;**14**:102–10.

33. Shorvon S, Luciano AL. Prognosis of chronic and newly diagnosed epilepsy: revisiting temporal aspects. *Curr Opin Neurol* 2007;**20**:208–12.

34. Rogawski MA. Progesterone, neurosteroids, and the hormonal basis of catamenial epilepsy. *Ann Neurol* 2003;**53**:288–91.

35. Callaghan BC, Anand K, Hesdorffer D, Hauser WA, French JA. Likelihood of seizure remission in an adult population with refractory epilepsy. *Ann Neurol* 2007;**62**:382–9.

36. Rogawski MA. Diverse mechanisms of antiepileptic drugs in the development pipeline. *Epilepsy Res* 2006;**69**:273–94.

c00098

Difficult-to-Treat Idiopathic Generalized Epilepsy in a Young Woman

Mar Carreño

s0010

HISTORY

p0020

S. S. C. is a left-handed lady first seen in our clinic in 2005, when she was 30. Her seizures had started apparently at the age of 18, when she noticed frequent myoclonic jerks happening mainly in the morning (about once or twice a week), more frequent and intense in relation to sleep deprivation or alcohol intake. In addition, she presented rare episodes when she lost awareness for a very brief period of time (seconds), making her lose track of conversations (once a month). During those, she apparently had blank staring without blinking or automatisms.

p0030

She remained without treatment until the age of 22, when she was diagnosed with "petit mal" and started on valproic acid (500 mg bid). On valproic acid she gained weight (around 5 kg) and complained of hair loss and epigastralgia. The patient admitted that from the ages of 23 to 25 she was noncompliant with her medication, and she often missed the morning dose. She continued to have frequent myoclonic jerks and occasional absences.

p0040

At the age of 25, she had her first generalized motor seizure at work, consisting of sudden loss of awareness not preceded by blank staring or myoclonic jerks, generalized stiffening and bilateral clonic jerks lasting several minutes, with tongue biting and postictal confusion. At that time, lamotrigine (LTG) was added to valproate (VPA) and she was encouraged to take her medication properly.

p0050

In spite of apparent good compliance with the medication, she continued to have generalized tonic–clonic seizures (once every 6 months, approximately) and frequent myoclonic jerks (several every week).

p0060

Because of inefficacy and adverse effects, at the age of 28, VPA was switched to topiramate (TPM). Since TPM was started, myoclonic jerks disappeared but occasionally (once every 6–7 months) she had generalized tonic–clonic seizures. Most commonly, generalized tonic–clonic seizures happened after some type of precipitating event (sleep deprivation or emotional upset).

EVOLUTION AND TREATMENT

When she was first seen in our clinic, she was taking TPM (200 mg a day) and LTG (400 mg a day), with good tolerance to the medications.

At that times no changes were made in her medications. A complete metabolic profile, LTG level, sleep-deprived 1 h EEG, and a 3T MRI with specific epilepsy protocol were ordered.

The patient missed the follow-up visit 4 months later. She was seen again 1 year later, when she stated that the frequency of generalized tonic–clonic convulsions had increased; in the previous 2 months she had six generalized tonic–clonic seizures. In addition, she complained of frequent myoclonic jerks in the morning and had two long confusional episodes where she was 'in and out' of reality for several hours. She denied sleep deprivation or alcohol intake. She continued to take TPM (200 mg a day) and LTG (400 mg a day); she had lost 7 kg, was feeling weak and reported psychomotor slowing and difficulty with word finding. Blood cell count and biochemistry were normal. LTG level was 5.9 μg/ml.

At that time, TPM was switched to levetiracetam (LEV) (2000 mg a day). Four months later, she continued to have generalized tonic–clonic seizures (once a month) and frequent myoclonic jerks.

Zonisamide was added to the treatment. Six months later, on LEV (2000 mg/day), zonisamide (200 mg/day), and LTG (400 mg/day), she was seizure-free. Myoclonic jerks, absences, and generalized tonic–clonic seizures had disappeared. She did not report any relevant side effects from medication. LEV discontinuation is planned.

PAST MEDICAL HISTORY

She is the product of a normal pregnancy and delivery, without history of CNS infection or significant head trauma, and had normal psychomotor development. Family history is negative for epilepsy or febrile convulsions. She works as a professional make-up artist.

EXAMINATION AND INVESTIGATIONS

Neurological examination was normal. Complete blood count and metabolic profile (including liver enzymes) have been repeatedly normal. LTG levels were 4.9 μg/ml on her first visit and 5.3 μg/ml 1 year later.

EEG performed shortly after the first visit showed generalized polyspikes and generalized spike and wave discharges at 4–5 Hz, mainly during drowsiness.

A 3T MRI with a specific epilepsy protocol was normal.

DIAGNOSIS AND COMMENTS

The patient has juvenile myoclonic epilepsy (JME), with three seizure types: myoclonic seizures, absence seizures, and generalized tonic–clonic seizures. The case illustrates a common phenomenon in this syndrome, namely the delay in diagnosis (she started to have myoclonic jerks and absences when she was 18 but was not diagnosed with epilepsy until the age of 22).

Evidence-based treatment for JME includes the limited data from well-controlled trials as initial monotherapy in this particular epilepsy syndrome, a deficiency noted in various evidence-based guidelines for epilepsy.[1,2] Based on open-label studies and clinical experience, VPA is widely regarded as the drug of choice in JME. In a recent randomized, pragmatic trial that included patients with generalized or unclassified epilepsies, VPA was considered the most effective drug.[3] However, suitability of VPA for specific populations such as young women in childbearing age has not been addressed in controlled trials, although reliable reports of increased teratogenicity are available,[4] which indeed should be taken into account by the clinician prescribing the drug. Young women may also be prone to develop some specific side effects of VPA, including weight gain and reproductive dysfunction, all of which has to be considered when choosing the initial monotherapy, as there is a need for prolonged treatment in the majority of patients.[5] Adverse effects are associated with poor compliance and worsened quality of life. Another option to treat JME in patients whose seizures are not fully controlled on VPA or who develop intolerable side effects is LTG. Controlled trials have demonstrated its efficacy in primary generalized tonic–clonic seizures[6] and, less compellingly, in absence seizures.[7,8] Open label studies have specifically addressed its efficacy in JME;[9–12] myoclonic seizures seem to be less responsive to LTG than generalized tonic–clonic seizures and absence seizures, and may even worsen in some patients.[13,14] LTG appears to have a synergistic effect when combined with VPA to treat complex partial seizures,[15] and is often used in association with VPA in idiopathic generalized epilepsies,[5] but the evidence regarding its synergistic effect in IGE is scarce.[9] Apart from LTG, other treatment options are also available. LEV has shown effectiveness against refractory myoclonic and primary generalized tonic–clonic seizures in controlled studies providing class I evidence even for the strict criteria of the ILAE, and is usually well tolerated. TPM is effective against generalized tonic–clonic seizures.[16,17] It seems to be effective also against myoclonic seizures and may be effective against absences.[10,18] Some patients on TPM develop troublesome cognitive side effects. In the absence of controlled trials, clinical experience with the drug suggests that ZNS may be effective against GTC, myoclonic seizures, and absence seizures.[19–21] To choose the right drug for the right patient, the clinician has to consider the data regarding general efficacy and tolerability of different antiepileptic drugs (AEDs) for the epilepsy syndrome and the different types of epileptic seizures the patient has. The specific profile of the patient (age, sex, concomitant medications, childbearing potential) has to be taken into account, together with the individual response to previously tried drugs.[22]

REFERENCES

1. French JA, Kanner AM, Bautista J, et al. Efficacy and tolerability of the new antiepileptic drugs I: treatment of new onset epilepsy: report of the Therapeutics and Technology Assessment Subcommittee and Quality Standards Subcommittee of the American Academy of Neurology and the American Epilepsy Society. *Neurology* 2004;**62(8)**:1252–60.
2. Glauser TA. Following catastrophic epilepsy patients from childhood to adulthood. *Epilepsia* 2004;**45(Suppl 5)**:23–6.
3. Marson AG, Al Kharusi AM, Alwaidh M, et al. The SANAD study of effectiveness of valproate, lamotrigine, or topiramate for generalised and unclassifiable epilepsy: an unblinded randomised controlled trial. *Lancet* 2007;**369(9566)**:1016–26.

4. Kalviainen R, Tomson T. Optimizing treatment of epilepsy during pregnancy. *Neurology* 2006;**67(12 Suppl 4)**:S59–S63.

5. Thomas P, Genton P, Gelisse P, Wof P. Juvenile myoclonic epilepsy. In: Roger J, Bureau M, Dravet C, Genton P, Tassinari C, Wolf P, eds. *Epileptic syndromes in infancy, childhood and adolescence.* John Libbey, 2005: 372–88.

6. Biton V, Sackellares JC, Vuong A, Hammer AE, Barrett PS, Messenheimer JA. Double-blind, placebo-controlled study of lamotrigine in primary generalized tonic-clonic seizures. *Neurology* 2005;**65(11)**:1737–43.

7. Frank LM, Enlow T, Holmes GL, *et al.* Lamictal (lamotrigine) monotherapy for typical absence seizures in children. *Epilepsia* 1999;**40(7)**:973–9.

8. Coppola G, Auricchio G, Federico R, Carotenuto M, Pascotto A. Lamotrigine versus valproic acid as first-line monotherapy in newly diagnosed typical absence seizures: an open-label, randomized, parallel-group study. *Epilepsia* 2004;**45(9)**:1049–53.

9. Buchanan N. The use of lamotrigine in juvenile myoclonic epilepsy. *Seizure* 1996;**5(2)**:149–51.

10. Morris GL, Hammer AE, Kustra RP, Messenheimer JA. Lamotrigine for patients with juvenile myoclonic epilepsy following prior treatment with valproate: results of an open-label study. *Epilepsy Behav* 2004;**5(4)**:509–12.

11. Nicolson A, Appleton RE, Chadwick DW, Smith DF. The relationship between treatment with valproate, lamotrigine, and topiramate and the prognosis of the idiopathic generalised epilepsies. *J Neurol Neurosurg Psychiatry* 2004;**75(1)**:75–9.

12. Prasad A, Kuzniecky RI, Knowlton RC, *et al.* Evolving antiepileptic drug treatment in juvenile myoclonic epilepsy. *Arch Neurol* 2003;**60(8)**:1100–5.

13. Biraben A, Allain H, Scarabin JM, Schuck S, Edan G. Exacerbation of juvenile myoclonic epilepsy with lamotrigine. *Neurology* 2000;**55(11)**:1758.

14. Carrazana EJ, Wheeler SD. Exacerbation of juvenile myoclonic epilepsy with lamotrigine. *Neurology* 2001;**56(10)**:1424–5.

15. Pisani F, Oteri G, Russo MF, Perri Di R, Perucca E, Richens A. The efficacy of valproate-lamotrigine comedication in refractory complex partial seizures: evidence for a pharmacodynamic interaction. *Epilepsia* 1999;**40(8)**:1141–6.

16. Biton V, Montouris GD, Ritter F, *et al.* A randomized, placebo-controlled study of topiramate in primary generalized tonic-clonic seizures. Topiramate YTC Study Group. *Neurology* 1999; **52(7)**: 1330–7.

17. Biton V, Bourgeois BF. Topiramate in patients with juvenile myoclonic epilepsy. *Arch Neurol* 2005;**62(11)**:1705–8.

18. Levisohn PM, Holland KD. Topiramate or valproate in patients with juvenile myoclonic epilepsy: a randomized open-label comparison. *Epilepsy Behav* 2007;**10(4)**:547–52.

19. Kothare SV, Valencia I, Khurana DS, Hardison H, Melvin JJ, Legido A. Efficacy and tolerability of zonisamide in juvenile myoclonic epilepsy. *Epileptic Disord* 2004;**6(4)**:267–70.

20. O'Rourke D, Flynn C, White M, Doherty C, Delanty N. Potential efficacy of zonisamide in refractory juvenile myoclonic epilepsy: retrospective evidence from an Irish compassionate-use case series. *Ir Med J* 2007;**100(4)**:431–3.

21. Wilfong A, Schultz R. Zonisamide for absence seizures. *Epilepsy Res* 2005;**64(1-2)**:31–4.

22. French JA. Can evidence-based guidelines and clinical trials tell us how to treat patients? *Epilepsia* 2007;**48(7)**:1264–7.

Can We Predict a Drug's Efficacy in a Specific Epilepsy Syndrome? A Preclinical Discussion.

Emilio Perucca

The case presented by Dr. Carreño is remarkable in at least two aspects: (i) the refractoriness to several AEDs of a syndrome that usually responds well to treatment and (ii) the fact that seizure control was eventually achieved on a complex polytherapy, although it remains unclear whether the same effect could have been achieved by stabilizing the patient on zonisamide alone.

From a preclinical perspective, a question relevant to this case is whether experimental tools are available that allow us to predict a drug's efficacy in a specific epilepsy syndrome. The two primary screening tests for efficacy in animal models continue to be the maximal electroshock (MES) test, which measures the ability to prevent seizure spread, and the subcutaneous pentylenetetrazole (PTZ) test, which provides an estimate of the ability to raise seizure threshold. Although compounds active in the MES test are likely to be clinically effective against partial and generalized tonic–clonic seizures, and compounds active in the PTZ test may display efficacy against absence and possibly myoclonic seizures, the predictive value of this paradigm is less than perfect.[1] For example, although Dr. Carreño's case and other lines of evidence suggest that zonisamide has clinical efficacy against absence and myoclonic seizures, zonisamide is ineffective in the PTZ test.[2]

Preclinical characterization of the potential spectrum of efficacy of a candidate AED is best obtained by testing it in a variety of other models. For example, activity against amygdaloid-kindled seizures has good reliability in predicting efficacy against partial-onset seizures, whereas the Generalized Absence Epilepsy Rat from Strasbourg (GAERS), the lethargic mouse or the WAG/Rij rat are superior to the PTZ model in predicting efficacy against absence seizures.[3,4] Although no single animal model has 100% specificity and sensitivity in identifying clinical efficacy,[2,5] assessment of a drug's activity in different models is essential to predict the spectrum of efficacy in the clinic. Other useful information relates to knowledge of mechanisms of actions[6] and of blood levels at which activity is obtained in experimental models.[7]

Pharmaceutical companies that develop potential AEDs often perform extensive pre-clinical testing in models that predict efficacy in partial seizures (or models with little predictive value for effects on specific seizure types), and they neglect testing their candidate compounds in spontaneous generalized seizure models, which are of great value in identifying potential activity in human generalized epilepsies. This is regrettable, because the spectrum of activity of a drug in generalized seizure types is an important feature of the overall pharmacology profile, and can be used to guide exploratory studies in the clinical setting. In many generalized epilepsy syndromes, including JME, some AEDs are known to induce paradoxical aggravation of seizures,[8] and animal models of absence seizures are relatively sensitive in identifying the potential for such aggravation.[1,9] These preclinical data are important to anticipate clinically relevant safety issues in the clinic.

The models discussed above are useful to predict the spectrum of efficacy of an AED against different seizure types and, consequently, potential clinical usefulness in syndromes which, like JME, are associated with multiple seizure types. However, the ability to generalize from preclinical data is limited by the fact that we do not have models that reproduce all the pathophysiological features (and drug responsiveness) of human epilepsy syndromes. Moreover, preclinical pharmacology data cannot be used to identify subjects refractory to an AED that is usually efficacious in a given syndrome. Potential mechanisms for drug resistance have been identified, but their contribution to treatment failure in individual cases cannot be ascertained. In the case of JME, resistance to specific AEDs might be related to genetic heterogeneity (and possibly mechanistic heterogeneity) underlying this syndrome.[10]

In the absence of reliable tools to predict individual drug responses, the clinical management of epilepsy has to rely on a trial-and-error strategy, as in Dr. Carreño's case. In this setting, AED selection should be guided primarily by available evidence about clinical efficacy and tolerability of individual drugs in the syndrome of interest.[11] However, predictions based on preclinical data should also be taken into account, particularly when there are reasons to consider use of AEDs for which clinical experience is lacking or minimal. Whether preclinical information should be taken into account in selecting specific AED combinations (e.g. by combining preferentially AEDs with different mechanisms of action) is open to discussion. Experimental models can identify AED combinations with a superior protective index due to synergistic "efficacy" or infra-additive neurotoxicity.[12] However, the generalizability of these findings to the clinical situation is uncertain,[6] and therapeutic decisions should be based whenever possible on evidence from well-conducted clinical studies.[13]

REFERENCES

1. Hosford DA, Wang Y. Utility of the lethargic (lh/lh) mouse model of absence seizures in predicting the effects of lamotrigine, vigabatrin, tiagabine, gabapentin, and topiramate against human absence seizures. *Epilepsia* 1997;**38**:408–14.

2. White HS, Woodhead JH, Stables JP, Kupferberg HJ, Wolf HH. Discovery and preclinical development of antiepileptic drugs. In: Levy RH, Mattson RH, Meldrum BS, Perucca E, eds. *Antiepileptic Drugs*. Philadelphia: Lippincott Williams and Wilkins, 2002: 36–48.

3. Löscher W, Leppik IE. Critical re-evaluation of previous preclinical strategies for the discovery and the development of new antiepileptic drugs. *Epilepsy Res* 2002;**50**:17–20.

4. Rogawski MA. Molecular targets versus models for new antiepileptic drug discovery. *Epilepsy Res* 2006;**68**:22–8.
5. Kamin M, Cazzaniga EK, Raina MK, Shank RP. The utility of the lh/lh mutant mouse as an animal model of human absence epilepsy. *Epilepsia* 1998;**39**:232–3.
6. Deckers CL, Czuczwar SJ, Hekster YA, *et al.* Selection of antiepileptic drug polytherapy based on mechanisms of action: the evidence reviewed. *Epilepsia* 2000;**41**:1364–74.
7. Bialer M, Twyman RE, White HS. Correlation analysis between anticonvulsant ED50 values of antiepileptic drugs in mice and rats and their therapeutic doses and plasma levels. *Epilepsy Behav* 2004;**5**:866–72.
8. Perucca E, Gram L, Avanzini G, Dulac O. Antiepileptic drugs as a cause of worsening seizures. *Epilepsia* 1998;**39**:5–17.
9. Gurbanova AA, Aker R, Berkman K, Onat FY, Rijn van CM, Luijtelaar van G. Effect of systemic and intracortical administration of phenytoin in two genetic models of absence epilepsy. *Br J Pharmacol* 2006;**148**:1076–82.
10. Annesi F, Gambardella A, Michelucci R, *et al.* Mutational analysis of EFHC1 gene in Italian families with juvenile myoclonic epilepsy. *Epilepsia* 2007;**48**:1686–90.
11. Perucca E. An introduction to antiepileptic drugs. *Epilepsia* 2005;**46(Suppl 4)**:31–7.
12. Luszczki JJ, Czuczwar SJ. Gabapentin synergistically interacts with topiramate in the mouse maximal electroshock seizure model: an isobolographic analysis. *Pharmacol Rep* 2006;**58**:944–54.
13. Perucca E. Current trends in antiepileptic drug therapy. *Epilepsia* 2003;**44(Suppl 4)**:41–7.

Bridging the Gap between Evidence-Based Medicine and Clinical Practice

Jacqueline French

The case outlined by Dr. Carreño exemplifies the major frustrations that clinicians face when approaching patients with epilepsy. A number of AEDs have been identified that are effective in certain types of patients (e.g. those with partial seizures, or those with JME). Unfortunately, there is no clear scientific basis by which to choose from among the drugs that might be effective in a given patient. In this example, three "appropriate" drugs (VPA, TPM, LEV) were tried, without success, before zonisamide was initiated, and proved successful. There are several excellent reasons why clinical trials are poor measures of individual response. Some of these are discussed below, in turn.

1. *Many trials of new AEDs are performed not head-to-head, but versus placebo.* This provides the information that the new AED is "better than nothing", but does not indicate that it is a particularly effective treatment for the seizure type under study. For example, recent studies of TPM, LTG and LEV demonstrated that these drugs, respectively, are effective in the treatment of refractory generalized tonic–clonic seizures, but it is not clear if any are superior, or even equivalent to older drugs such as VPA, or how they stack up against each other.[1–3] In these trials, only a small portion of patients (up to 16%) became completely seizure-free. In another study of absence seizures, LTG was proven superior to placebo, but only in a population that had already been pre-selected as responders in a preceding open-label experience.[4] It is very difficult to assess from such a study how LTG should fit into the treatment armamentarium.

2. *We often test drugs against some, but not all seizure types within a trial.* In the studies mentioned above, a specific seizure type was selected for the primary outcome measure, usually because it was the most countable. However, it is difficult to determine, for each study, what the outcome was for other seizure types

experienced by the same patient. In the LTG and TPM studies mentioned above, generalized tonic–clonic seizures were used as the primary seizure type for study, and the only other outcome reported was "all generalized seizures", making it difficult to tease out the specific outcomes for the different seizure types. Similarly, three studies using patients with the Lennox–Gastaut syndrome focused on "major" seizures (tonic, tonic–clonic, and/or atonic), with little specific data available on other seizure types.[5−7] Thus, a clinician who is facing a patient with multiple seizure types would not be substantially helped by randomized trial data.

3. *Trials do a very poor job of identifying tolerability and safety issues, which may be very important in drug selection.* Clinical trials are well equipped to identify dose-related adverse events (dizziness, ataxia, sleepiness). However, these adverse events are not subdivided for even the most basic populations (e.g. males versus females, those taking VPA versus those taking enzyme inducers, fat versus thin). Also, most studies exclude populations of great interest, such as those with a history of psychiatric disturbance, or those of childbearing potential. Thus, physicians cannot identify individual potential for risk or benefit within their patient population. Most studies that address these issues in more detail are poorly controlled. Finally, infrequent or rare serious adverse events, for which some populations may have an increased risk, are typically not identified in clinical trials at all.

4. *Trials can only identify population outcomes, not individual outcomes.* Once again, specific patient characteristics are not explored within randomized controlled trials. The most basic information (the cause of the patient's epilepsy; whether it is temporal or extratemporal, lesional or non-lesional) is not available, and therefore physicians cannot optimize drug selection in any but the most basic way (e.g. partial versus generalized).

5. *Head-to-head trials can be biased, particularly if the outcome measure is a "mixture" of efficacy and toxicity.* Based on the discussion above, one might conclude that head-to-head trials would be preferable to placebo-controlled trials for uncovering the "best" drug in a particular situation. Unfortunately, head-to-head trials are fraught with potentials for confounding and bias. When two or more drugs are compared, one can only compare them *as they were used in the trial*. How drugs are used in a trial can drive the outcome in very significant ways. Some examples of this are quite obvious; if one drug is tried at a sub-therapeutic dose, and the other at a therapeutic dose, most people would agree that it is not a "fair fight". Since most studies are done with fixed, rather than flexible dosing, someone must choose the doses, and bias can be introduced. Perhaps more subtle, but not less concerning, are issues of titration rate, overdosing, and formulation. For example, in a large head-to-head comparison study of LTG versus carbamazepine in newly diagnosed epilepsy, the comparator (carbamazepine) was administered BID, although it is known to be a drug with a short half-life.[8] What is even more surprising is that the investigators chose to administer it in uneven doses, with 200 mg in the morning, and 400 mg at night. This may be quite adequate for some patients, but may increase both the likelihood of seizure breakthrough (after the smaller dose) and side effects (after the larger dose) in others. Many similar examples exist. Even for the best designed head-to-head trials, clinicians cannot use the outcomes to drive their own prescribing practices, unless their habits match those used in the study.[9]

Clinical trials can provide a substantial amount of useful data, but they should not be over-interpreted or used incorrectly. In the future, it is the responsibility of researchers to consider prediction of individual patient outcomes when designing trials.

REFERENCE

1. Biton V, Sackellares JC, Vuong A, Hammer AE, Barrett PS, Messenheimer JA. Double-blind, placebo-controlled study of lamotrigine in primary generalized tonic-clonic seizures. *Neurology* 2005;**65**:1737–43.
2. Biton V, Montouris GD, Ritter F, *et al.* A randomized, placebo-controlled study of topiramate in primary generalized tonic-clonic seizures. Topiramate YTC Study Group. *Neurology* 1999;**52**:1330–7.
3. Berkovic SF, Knowlton RC, Leroy RF, Schiemann J, Falter U. Placebo-controlled study of levetiracetam in idiopathic generalized epilepsy. *Neurology* 2007;**69**:1751–60.
4. Frank LM, Enlow T, Holmes GL, *et al.* Lamictal (lamotrigine) monotherapy for typical absence seizures in children. *Epilepsia* 1999;**40**:973–9.
5. Efficacy of felbamate in childhood epileptic encephalopathy (Lennox-Gastaut syndrome). The Felbamate Study Group in Lennox-Gastaut Syndrome. *N Engl J Med* 1993;**328**:29–33.
6. Sachdeo RC, Glauser TA, Ritter F, Reife R, Lim P, Pledger G. A double-blind, randomized trial of topiramate in Lennox-Gastaut syndrome. Topiramate YL Study Group. *Neurology* 1999;**52**:1882–7.
7. Motte J, Trevathan E, Arvidsson JF, Barrera MN, Mullens EL, Manasco P. Lamotrigine for generalized seizures associated with the Lennox-Gastaut syndrome. Lamictal Lennox-Gastaut Study Group. *N Engl J Med* 1997;**337**:1807–12.
8. Brodie MJ, Richens A, Yuen AW. Double-blind comparison of lamotrigine and carbamazepine in newly diagnosed epilepsy. UK Lamotrigine/Carbamazepine Monotherapy Trial Group. *Lancet* 1995;**345**:476–9.
9. French JA. Can evidence-based guidelines and clinical trials tell us how to treat patients? *Epilepsia* 2007;**48**:1264–7.

c0099

Psychogenic Non-Epileptic Seizures "Redux"

Gregory Krauss

s0010

HISTORY

p0020

The following cautionary tale illustrates a challenge faced by clinicians trying to distinguish between epileptic and psychogenic non-epileptic seizures (PNES): sometimes patients have both ... and they may occur at different times.[1]

p0030

A patient was first seen in an epilepsy clinic 10 years ago, when he was 27 years old. He was having daily seizures. These began when he was 21 and had increased in frequency over the past several months, despite treatment with five different AEDs. The seizures consisted of sudden onset of confusion and limb shaking, followed by rapid recovery. He was referred for 5 days of video–EEG monitoring. His phenytoin, valproic acid, and gabapentin were discontinued and he had eight seizures, consisting of altered awareness with "spacey," spinning sensations. During one seizure, he had spinning sensations followed by violent convulsive behavior. The EEG during all these episodes was normal including clearly recorded waking EEG during the convulsive episode. The patient also had a convulsive-like episode induced by hyperventilation with normal EEG. His interictal EEG was normal and he was diagnosed with PNES. A psychiatric consultant noted that the patient had a history of substance abuse with several major drug overdoses and family difficulties, which contributed to abnormal coping and PNES. Since all his observed episodes were PNES, including a hyperventilation-induced episode, and his EEG was normal, he was not restarted on AEDs. He had outpatient counseling with a psychologist and had no seizures at a follow-up visit.

p0040

The patient was next seen in the epilepsy clinic 10 years later. He had been seizure-free for 4 years and then began having one to two seizures per month. He re-entered counseling for presumed PNES, but his seizures continued. During these episodes, he said he had a warning feeling during which he lost track of time, then typically screamed and stiffened, with his eyes rolling back followed by convulsive shaking. The episodes lasted approximately 3 min followed by moaning, confusion, and slurred speech. He then recovered in 15 min. The episodes were often triggered by stress, anxiety, or sleep deprivation and frequently resulted in injuries. Two years ago, the patient fell off a 20-foot ladder during a seizure. He was hospitalized with multiple fractures and required a tracheotomy. He was now married, has a tenth grade education, and operates a cleaning company. He does not drive and has his workers drive him to jobs.

He has four children. He smokes one pack of cigarettes per day. He no longer drinks alcohol.

EXAMINATION AND INVESTIGATIONS

The patient's physical examination was normal at his follow-up examination including his neurological examination, except for a tracheotomy scar. He was referred for additional video–EEG monitoring. During the monitoring he had three seizures: two were associated with auras, brief behavioral arrest, and confusion. During a third seizure, he had behavioral arrest followed by generalized tonic–clonic movements. At seizure onset, he had high-voltage bi-frontal 3–5 per second polyspike and slow wave complexes, with spike amplitudes recorded maximally over the right frontal area. He also had a several-hour period during which he felt "funny," but was fully responsive. During this time, he had frequent bi-frontal spike and wave bursts on EEG. Hyperventilation induced a complex partial seizure with behavioral arrest and brief bursts of 3–4 per second generalized spike and slow waves. Interictally, he had occasional right hemisphere polyspike-wave complexes.

DIAGNOSES

- Complex partial and secondary generalized epileptic seizures with probable frontal lobe onset. Right hemisphere interictal spikes and a hyperventilation-induced complex partial seizure.
- Previous psychogenic PNES with behaviors similar to his epileptic seizures. Normal interictal EEG and a hyperventilation-induced non-epileptic seizure.

TREATMENT AND OUTCOME

The patient was started on oxcarbazepine at discharge from the epilepsy monitoring unit. He, however, had several seizures on oxcarbazepine 600 mg BID and was drowsy on 900 mg BID. He was switched to levetiracetam, but had four generalized seizures and was quite irritable. He fought with his wife and warned that he wanted to drive their car into a tree. He stopped levetiracetam, was restarted on oxcarbazepine 600 mg TID, and during the past 4 months has had no seizures.

COMMENTARY

Patients who have both epilepsy and psychogenic PNES can be extremely difficult to identify because their non-epileptic episodes are often modeled on their epileptic seizures. Similarities in PNES and epileptic seizure behaviors may mislead physicians and cause them to conclude that epileptic seizures are continued PNES. Roy noted that for patients with both epilepsy and PNES "the nature of the hysterical fits closely resembled the type of epileptic fit the patient had".[2] He reported five patients with tonic–clonic seizures who had PNES resembling convulsions, whereas four patients with complex partial seizures had PNES which resembled complex partial, more than convulsive, seizures.

In this patient's case, similarities in his epileptic and PNES contributed to a delayed diagnosis of his frontal lobe epilepsy. He suffered a major injury and had several years of uncontrolled seizures before repeated video–EEG monitoring identified frontal lobe seizures. In retrospect, one clue that the patient may have had seizures earlier in life was that he reported a previous seizure episode associated with severe tongue biting. Epileptic seizures usually precede PNES, often by many years, for patients with both conditions.[3]

Important clues that patients with PNES may also have epileptic seizures include: seizures much earlier in life, several patterns of seizures, presence of interictal epileptiform activity on EEG, and a history of brain injury. None of these indicators were present in our patient's case during the time he was diagnosed with PNES. Although our patient's EEGs were initially normal, 70% of patients with epileptic seizures and PNES have epileptiform abnormalities.[4] EEG epileptiform abnormalities are uncommon in patients with PNES alone (Figure 99.1). It is important, however, not to "over-read" the EEG. Patients with PNES frequently have wicket rhythms and other drowsy patterns which are misclassified as epileptiform activity by neurologists.[5] It is important to obtain and "re-read" previous abnormal EEGs for patients with PNES.

Roy observed that patients with epilepsy tend to develop PNES "at times of stress, when they use their knowledge of epileptic seizures to develop pseudoseizures as a signal of distress".[6] Most patients with epileptic seizures and PNES, in addition to EEG epileptiform abnormalities, have signs of brain injuries on MRI and neuropsychological testing. This suggests that brain dysfunction contributes to the patients' seizures and to their abnormal coping reactions. Most patients with PNES and epilepsy benefit from parallel treatment with psychiatric evaluation and psychotherapy and AEDs. Our patient

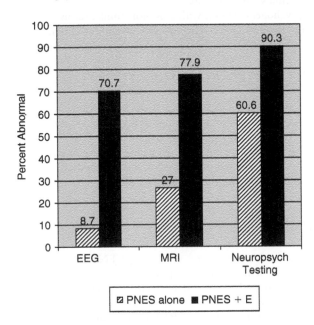

FIGURE.   EEG epileptiform abnormalities distinguish patients with PNES alone and patients with PNES and epilepsy. Adapted from Reuber, 2002.

was unusual in that PNES was diagnosed 10 years before epilepsy was confirmed. Psychotherapy helped him cope with family stresses and substance abuse and his PNES ceased. Four years later, he required AED treatment for uncontrolled epileptic seizures, but was emotionally stable and no longer required psychiatric care.

REFERENCES

1. Krumholz A, Ting T. Coexisting epilepsy and nonepileptic seizures. In: Kaplan P, Fisher R, eds. *Imitators of epilepsy*, 2nd ed. New York, NY: Demos Medical Publishing, 2005: 261–76.
2. Roy A. Identification and hysterical symptoms. *Br J Med Psychol* 1977;**50**:317–18.
3. Devinsky O, Sanchez-Villasenor F, Vazquez B, Kothari M, Alper K, Luciano D. Clinical profile of patients with epileptic and nonepileptic seizures. *Neurology* 1996;**46(6)**:1530–3.
4. Reuber M, Fernandez G, Helmstaedter C, Qurishi A, Elger CE. Evidence of brain abnormality in patients with psychogenic nonepileptic seizures. *Epilepsy Behav* 2002:249–54.
5. Krauss G, Abdallah A, Lesser R, Thompson RE, Niedermeyer E. Clinical and EEG features of patients with EEG wicket rhythms misdiagnosed with epilepsy. *Neurology* 2005;**64**:1879–84.
6. Roy A. Pseudoseizures: a psychiatric perspecitve. *J Neuropsychiatr* 1989;**1(1)**:69–71.

FURTHER READING

Ramsay RE, Cohen A, Brown MC. Coexisting epilepsy and non-epileptic seizures. In: Rowan AJ, Gates J, eds. *Non-epileptic seizures*. Stoneham, MA: Butterworth-Heinemann, 1993: 47–54.

c0020

Is There a Neurobiological Basis to Stress-induced, Non-epileptic Behaviors that Mimic Seizures?

Stephen C Heinrichs

p0140   Sudden, irregular movements of the face, limb, or whole body mimicking epileptic seizures can be readily induced in normal, non-human animals without presupposing either a history of or genetic predisposition for convulsive behaviors. The fact that stressor exposure is a reliable trigger in animals for non-epileptic convulsions allows such noxious stimuli to be employed in the modeling of the psychogenic seizure phenomenon, and to serve as effective tools for probing the neural mechanisms of non-recurrent seizure-related behaviors.

s0060   ## EVIDENCE FROM BASIC SCIENCE EXPERIMENTS

p0150   Three specific lines of compelling pre-clinical evidence suggest that there are indeed neurobiological bases for stress-induced, non-epileptic seizures (Table 99.1): (1) stressor exposure evokes hippocampal plasticity, (2) stressor exposure induces noradrenergic neurotransmission, and (3) stressor exposure activates corticotropin-releasing factor signaling in the brain. A stress-exposed organism appears to be at higher risk of seizure onset in the event of hippocampal imbalance, adrenergic loss of function or corticotropin-releasing factor overabundance.

s0070   ### Hippocampal plasticity

p0160   Hippocampal nuclei mediate stress-induced seizures as a primary neural substrate for morphological, neuroendocrine, and functional adaptations triggered by persistent exposure to noxious stimuli.[1] Stress suppresses neurogenesis of hippocampal dentate gyrus granule neurons, and repeated stress causes atrophy of dendrites in the CA3 region.

TABLE 99.1   Three stressor reactivity mechanisms: Neurological implications

Brain mechanism	Reactivity to stressors	Impact on seizures	Predicted neurological deficit
Hippocampal plasticity	Stressor exposure exerts neuronal remodeling and negative feedback at dentate glucocorticoid receptors	Forebrain and kindled seizures are propagated via the hippocampus	Hippocampal atrophy and dendritic pruning[2]
Noradrenergic neurotransmission	Stressor exposure triggers noradrenaline release	Noradrenergic activation attenuates seizures; inactivation promotes seizures	Locus ceruleus impairment[8]
Corticotropin-releasing modulation	Stressor exposure triggers corticotropin-releasing factor release	Corticotropin-releasing factor administration is pro-convulsive	Neuronal injury accompanying corticotropin-releasing factor excess[24]

Structural remodeling of the hippocampus is mediated by hormones working in concert with excitatory amino acid receptors, which are involved in pyramidal neuronal death caused by seizures.[2] In addition to morphological changes, stress-sensitive hippocampal nuclei play a key role in regulating pituitary-adrenocortical negative feedback, a formative process in seizure onset.[3] In particular, a hippocampal stress circuit composed of "resonator" neurons sensitive to noxious stimuli is hypothesized to respond to normal input with an abnormally large discharge that triggers a seizure.[4] These results suggest that tonic inhibitory functions of the hippocampus can be supplanted by stress-induced excitation and synaptic reorganization accompanying the development of seizures.[5]

Noradrenergic neurotransmission

In animal models the hindbrain locus ceruleus plays a major role in stressor reactivity,[6] synaptic plasticity,[7] and the expression of seizures.[8] Norepinephrine systems emanating from the locus ceruleus have long been hypothesized to be involved in mediating behaviors associated with alertness, arousal, and stress.[6] The locus ceruleus provides adrenergic inputs to cerebral cortex and hippocampus[9] such that increased activity in the locus ceruleus acts in a seizure prophylactic manner.[8] In particular, dense noradrenergic innervation of the hippocampus delays the development of seizures produced by hippocampal kindling.[10] Similarly, genetically epilepsy-prone rats exhibit deficits in adrenergic neurotransmission arising from abnormalities in the locus ceruleus[11] and administration of adrenergic receptor agonists inhibits seizures in epilepsy-prone mice.[12] Most convincingly, locus ceruleus lesions convert sporadic seizures into limbic status epilepticus.[13] Taken together, these findings suggest that adrenergic neurotransmission is a stress-sensitive brain mechanism well constituted for seizure attenuation.

Corticotropin-releasing factor modulation

There is strong evidence that stressors which trigger seizures increase glucocorticoid levels which in turn lower the threshold for seizure induction.[14] For example, glucocorticoids are reported to significantly facilitate the development of cocaine-induced kindled seizures[15] and to increase the severity of handling-induced convulsions during ethanol withdrawal.[16] Neural circuits that mediate the pro-convulsant actions of glucocorticoids likely include brain stress neuropeptide pathways that initiate pituitary-adrenocortical activation. In particular, available evidence implicates the excitatory stress neuropeptide, corticotropin-releasing factor, as a seizure trigger during the post-natal period of development.[17] In adult rodents, low doses of corticotropin-releasing factor given intracerebroventricularly arouse electrographic activity,[18] whereas higher doses induce electrographic and behavioral signs of seizure activity indistinguishable from those which occur following electrical kindling of the amygdala.[19] If one postulates that persistent neuroadaptations arise in the brains of stressed organisms, then the emergence of seizure pathology can be viewed as an expected consequence of accumulated stressor exposure in the context of genetic vulnerability according to the "diathesis-stress" hypothesis.[20]

POSSIBLE RELEVANCE TO CLINICAL PRACTICE

Each of the three mechanisms for stress-induced non-epileptic seizure induction discussed above translates readily into clinical practice. First, the hippocampal locus of neuropathological and pituitary-adrenocortical adaptation following seizure-related stress exposure provides a potential anatomical basis for psychogenic seizures. Hippocampal stress-reactivity deficits contributing to seizure susceptibility could be explored in clinical practice using brain-imaging techniques together with an assessment of pituitary-adrenocortical status. Second, adrenergic and corticotropin-releasing factor mechanisms for modulating neuronal excitability following seizure-related stressor exposure provide potential neurochemical bases for psychogenic seizures. Anomalies in stress-related neurotransmission, specifically adrenergic insufficiency or corticotropin-releasing factor overflow, could be explored in clinical practice via emerging pharmacotherapeutic strategies which target these brain signaling systems.[21] Moreover, all three putative neurobiological mechanisms for psychogenic seizure induction elicit symptomatic markers of clinical interest: learning/memory impairment with hippocampal deficits, alterations in sleep/wake cycle with adrenergic deficits, and affective disorders with corticotropin-releasing factor excess.

UNANSWERED QUESTIONS WHICH STILL REMAIN FOR BASIC RESEARCHERS

In many ways, sensory, chemical, and electrically induced convulsions in normal animals are suitable as models for the psychogenic seizure phenomenon because of the direct, causal link between stress-related trigger stimuli and the resulting seizure-related behaviors. Nonetheless, numerous basic research questions remain to be answered. Most importantly, as stressor exposure is a routine, daily event for all living organisms, why do only a minority of such exposures lead to seizure-related pathology in a selected group of individuals? Perhaps a modified version of the "two-hit" hypothesis relating multiple stressor exposure to developmental seizure induction[22] could be proposed to account for the etiology of psychogenic seizures. Another unanswered basic research question is how to discount the many non-specific biological consequences of stressor exposure unrelated to seizure induction in order to focus on those mechanisms that are homologous for non-human animal and human pathology. The near certainty of obtaining a significant difference on some dependent measure in animal experiments involving stressor exposure mirrors a problem faced in contemporary gene expression studies: how to identify the seminal biological antecedent(s) against a background of alternative events which are secondary or spurious? The most compelling approach for animal modelers at the present time may be a systematic, albeit laborious, stressor-reactivity phenotyping effort.[23]

REFERENCES

1. McEwen BS. Plasticity of the hippocampus: adaptation to chronic stress and allostatic load. *Ann NY Acad Sci* 2001;**933**:265–77.
2. McEwen BS, Magarinos AM. Stress and hippocampal plasticity: implications for the pathophysiology of affective disorders. *Human Psychopharmacology* 2001;**16(suppl 1)**:S7–S19.
3. Baram TZ, Hatalski CG. Neuropeptide-mediated excitability: a key triggering mechanism for seizure generation in the developing brain. *Trends Neurosci* 1998;**21(11)**:471–6.
4. Eggers AE. Temporal lobe epilepsy is a disease of faulty neuronal resonators rather than oscillators, and all seizures are provoked, usually by stress. *Med Hypotheses* 2007;**17**:45–56.
5. Drage MG, Holmes GL, Seyfried TN. Hippocampal neurons and glia in epileptic EL mice. *J Neurocytol* 2002;**31(8–9)**:681–92.
6. Koob GF. Corticotropin-releasing factor, norepinephrine, and stress. *Biol Psychiatry* 1999;**46(9)**:1167–80.
7. Walling SG, Harley CW. Locus ceruleus activation initiates delayed synaptic potentiation of perforant path input to the dentate gyrus in awake rats: a novel beta-adrenergic- and protein synthesis-dependent mammalian plasticity mechanism. *J Neurosci* 2004;**24(3)**:598–604.
8. Giorgi FS, Ferrucci M, Lazzeri G, *et al*. A damage to locus coeruleus neurons converts sporadic seizures into self-sustaining limbic status epilepticus. *Eur J Neurosci* 2003;**17(12)**:2593–601.
9. Brown RA, Walling SG, Milway JS, Harley CW. Locus ceruleus activation suppresses feedforward interneurons and reduces beta-gamma electroencephalogram frequencies while it enhances theta frequencies in rat dentate gyrus. *J Neurosci* 2005;**25(8)**:1985–91.
10. Barry DI, Wanscher B, Kragh J, *et al*. Grafts of fetal locus coeruleus neurons in rat amygdala-piriform cortex suppress seizure development in hippocampal kindling. *Exp Neurol* 1989;**106(2)**:125–32.
11. Ko KH, Dailey JW, Jobe PC. Evaluation of monoaminergic receptors in the genetically epilepsy prone rat. *Experientia* 1984;**40(1)**:70–3.
12. Tsuda H, Ito M, Oguro K, *et al*. Age- and seizure-related changes in noradrenaline and dopamine in several brain regions of epileptic El mice. *Neurochem Res* 1993;**18(2)**:111–17.
13. Giorgi FS, Mauceli G, Blandini F, *et al*. Locus coeruleus and neuronal plasticity in a model of focal limbic epilepsy. *Epilepsia* 2006;**47(suppl 5)**:21–5.
14. Anisman H, Zaharia MD, Meaney MJ, Merali Z. Do early-life events permanently alter behavioral and hormonal responses to stressors? *Int J Dev Neurosci* 1998;**16(3–4)**:149–64.
15. Kling MA, Smith MA, Glowa JR, *et al*. Facilitation of cocaine kindling by glucocorticoids in rats. *Brain Res* 1993;**629(1)**:163–6.
16. Roberts AJ, Crabbe JC, Keith LD. Corticosterone increases severity of acute withdrawal from ethanol, pentobarbital, and diazepam in mice. *Psychopharmacology (Berl)* 1994;**115(1–2)**:278–84.
17. Baram TZ, Hatalski CG. Neuropeptide-mediated excitability: a key triggering mechanism for seizure generation in the developing brain. *Trends Neurosci* 1998;**21(11)**:471–6.

18. Ehlers CL, Henriksen SJ, Wang M, Rivier J, Vale W, Bloom FE. Corticotropin releasing factor produces increases in brain excitability and convulsive seizures in rats. *Brain Res* 1983;**278(1–2)**:332–6.

19. Weiss SR, Post RM, Gold PW, *et al.* CRF-induced seizures and behavior: interaction with amygdala kindling. *Brain Res* 1986;**372(2)**:345–51.

20. McEwen BS. Allostasis, allostatic load, and the aging nervous system: role of excitatory amino acids and excitotoxicity. *Neurochem Res* 2000;**25(9–10)**:1219–31.

21. McCarthy JR, Heinrichs SC, Grigoriadis DE. Recent advances with the CRF1 receptor: design of small molecule inhibitors, receptor subtypes and clinical indications. *Curr Pharm Des* 1999;**5(5)**:289–315.

22. Koh S, Storey TW, Santos TC, Mian AY, Cole AJ. Early-life seizures in rats increase susceptibility to seizure-induced brain injury in adulthood. *Neurology* 1999;**53(5)**:915–21.

23. Groticke I, Hoffmann K, Loscher W. Behavioral alterations in the pilocarpine model of temporal lobe epilepsy in mice. *Exp Neurol* 2007;**207(2)**:329–49.

24. Brunson KL, Eghbal-Ahmadi M, Baram TZ. How do the many etiologies of West syndrome lead to excitability and seizures? The corticotropin releasing hormone excess hypothesis. *Brain Develop* 2001;**23(7)**:533–8.

Evidence for a Neurobiological Basis for Non-epileptic Seizures

Siddhartha S Nadkarni, Kenneth Alper and Orrin Devinsky

> *We must recollect that all of our provisional ideas in psychology will*
> *presumably one day be based on an organic substrate.*
>
> –Sigmund Freud, *On Narcissism*

PNES fall into the category of dissociative or conversion phenomena, wherein a presumed unconscious motivator creates a paroxysmal behavior that shares clinical characteristics and appearances with epileptic seizures. By definition, PNES do not show epileptiform changes on EEG during the behavior, and are *judged* to be of psychogenic origin. The behavior is thought to be an unconscious and dissociative response to emotional or psychic content that would overwhelm the individual should it be experienced consciously. The neural mechanism which orchestrates such responses is neither known nor well studied. We will review the data, scant as it is, and mostly correlative, that exists for the neurobiological underpinnings of PNES.

PNES: A BRIEF HISTORY

The first description of PNES as a conversion phenomenon in the West was made by Moreau de Tours, whose term *desagregation* described isolation of certain notions in "hysterics."[1] In the late 1800s, Gilles de la Tourette and contemporaries started using the idea of a "dissociated consciousness."[2] Charcot referred to all conversion symptoms that were not seizures as "minor hysteria," and to hysterical seizures as "major hysteria."[2] Pierre Janet solidified a notion of dissociation that still has bearing today.[2,3] His theory is that memories and emotions that are not accessible to conscious recall are not necessarily deleted. Rather they are held in a separate state of consciousness and can generally be recalled, if unconsciously. He noted that these elements could influence people without them being aware of it, and termed these emotions and memories "psychologic automatisms." Further, these psychologic automatisms were split off, or dissociated, from conscious control under circumstances of trauma, and they could return and hold sway during a conversion phenomenon still outside conscious awareness of the patient.[4] Freud modified this theory into one of repression of inappropriate incestuous urges and wishes for fulfillment of inappropriate fantasies (thus removing the element of trauma) creating psychological conflict that was *converted* into somatic symptoms: hence, the term conversion.[5-7] All of these theories speak to a notion of consciousness that is disparate and partitioned, not unitary. Our ability to study this consciousness is crude and lacking, but some findings do suggest a correlation with demonstrable brain dysfunction in PNES patients.

NEUROIMAGING IN PNES

Recent studies looking at functional neuroimaging (PET, SPECT, and fMRI) have highlighted changes seen in patients with various conversion symptoms. One such study looking at unilateral loss of motor function and conversion parkinsonism implicated the prefrontal and parietal cortices, anterior cingulate cortex, thalamus, and basal ganglia.[8] Vuilleumier and colleagues studied psychogenic hemi-sensorimotor loss with brain SPECT. Seven patients were tested with passive vibratory stimulation in both arms during a SPECT scan. In all seven patients hypoperfusion was seen in the basal ganglia and thalamus contralateral to the psychogenic deficit. Two to four months later, after the symptoms had resolved, this deficit on SPECT was gone in all the patients.[9] Functional neuroimaging has revealed correlative deficits in multiple conversion syndromes, including decreased activity of frontal and subcortical circuits in psychogenic paralysis, decreased parietal cortical activity in conversion anesthesia or decreases in visual cortex activity during "hysterical" blindness.[10] Increased activation in certain limbic structures such as the cingulate or orbitofrontal cortex may occur in conversion syndromes as well.[10,11]

Neuroimaging and functional neuroimaging studies in PNES are rare. Spanaki *et al.* studied 11 patients (3/11 also had epilepsy and 5/11 were on anti-epileptic drugs) with both ictal and interictal SPECT scans. On visual analysis alone 9/11 patients had either increased (6/9) or decreased (3/9) localized blood flow; however, when quantitative methods were applied to measure blood flow, no abnormalities were seen.[12] In 2001 we published data from our center on 79 consecutive patients with PNES. Sixty (76%) of these patients had unilateral cerebral abnormalities on neuroimaging, 85% of which were structural. Among the 60 patients, 22 had PNES alone and 38 had PNES and epilepsy. Of the 22 who had PNES alone 19 had abnormal CAT scans or MRIs. Fifteen of these 22 had a right-sided cerebral abnormality either on neuroimaging or EEG.[13] We hypothesized that right brain dysfunction predisposed to the fragmentation of consciousness required for dissociative events, a hypothesis that is consistent with conventional thinking of the right brain as arbiter of both conscious and unconscious bilateral awareness. A study in 2002 by Reuber *et al.* catalogued brain abnormalities in 329 patients with PNES with and without concomitant epilepsy. Seventy-four patients with PNES alone had MRI scans and 20 (27%) of these scans were abnormal. Ten of the 20 had bilateral or global abnormalities, 6 had right-sided abnormalities and 4 had left-sided abnormalities. One was noted to have a frontal lesion and 8 had temporal lesions. These percentages increase significantly when the patients with

PNES and epilepsy are included; however, the presence of epilepsy clearly confounds the data.[14]

EEG IN PNES

In Reuber's study mentioned above all 329 patients had EEGs. Of all the patients, 206 had PNES alone, and only 18 (8.7%) had evidence of EEG abnormality. Four had a right-sided EEG abnormality, 6 left sided, and 10 bilateral.[14] In the study from our center at NYU, 9/22 (41%) patients had abnormalities on interictal EEG that went beyond mild generalized slowing of the background. Another study by Reuber highlights even more robust evidence of EEG abnormality in patients with PNES. Patients with PNES only (130) were divided into patients who had a reason for an abnormal EEG (head trauma, stroke, developmental delay, etc. =80) and those who had no reason for abnormal EEG (50). Patients with PNES and epilepsy were also included. The patients with PNES and reason for abnormal EEG had an abnormal EEG 55% of the time (50% had non-specific abnormalities and 15% had epileptiform discharges). Of the 50 patients without reason for EEG abnormalities 52% had abnormal EEGs. Among these 50, 50% had non-specific abnormalities and 8% had epileptiform abnormalities. Of these, 22% had right-sided EEG abnormality, 44% had left sided, and 33% had bilateral. [15]

NEUROPSYCHOLOGICAL FINDINGS IN NES

In one study 20/33 patients with PNES alone had evidence of neuropsychological deficits. Two of these had right-sided deficits, 9 had left-sided deficits, and 9 had bilateral deficits.[14] Drane et al. looked at neurocognitive profiles of patients with PNES and with epilepsy. On a measure of symptom validity, the Word Memory Test, patients with PNES had a much higher failure rate than those with epilepsy. After correcting for this deficiency in effort or motivation, the patients with PNES scored substantially better on their testing compared to those with epilepsy.[16] Bailles et al. found in a cohort of 30 patients with PNES in Spain that there were high rates of Axis I psychopathology, but no clear consistent characterologic substrate predisposing to PNES, based on MMPI (Minnesota Multiphasic Personality Inventory).

CONCLUSIONS

PNES is a varied illness with protean manifestations and difficulties at each step: understanding the pathophysiology, diagnosis, and treatment. It appears to be a dissociative disorder, unconscious in nature (rarely arising either out of sleep or at the moment of arousal[18]), and manifesting somatically. The precise mechanism of the conversion of unconscious elements into physical manifestations is unknown, but there appears to be a much higher rate of cerebral abnormalities in patients with PNES than the general population. Only after understanding the machinery of conscious and unconscious processing as well as the intricacies of memory, emotions, and trauma, will we be able to dissect this difficult disorder. Our crude tools of neuroimaging, electroencephalography, and neuropsychological testing already point in the direction of Freud's "organic substrate."

s0170   REFERENCES

1. Moreau de Tours JJ. *De la folie hysterie et de quelque phenomenes nerviux propres a l'hysterie (convulsive) a l'hysterie-epilepsie et a epilepsie.* Paris:Victor Masson et Fils, 1865.
2. Vieth I. *Hysteria. The history of a disease.* Chicago: University of Chicago, 1965. pp. 2–10.
3. Bowman ES. Why conversion seizures should be classified as a dissociative disorder. *Psychiatr Clin N Am* 2006;**29**:185–211.
4. Janet P. *L'automatisme psychologique.* Paris: Felix Alcan, 1889.
5. Freud S. My views on the part played by sexuality in the etiology of the neuroses. In: Strachey J, ed. *The standard edition of the complete works of Sigmund Freud*, vol. 7. London: Hogarth, 1953: 269–79. [Strache J, trans.; original work published in 1906.].
6. Freud S. The etiology of hysteria. In: Strachey J, ed. *The standard edition of the complete works of Sigmund Freud*, vol. 3. London: Hogarth, 1953: 189–221. [Strache J, trans.; original work published in 1906.].
7. Freud S. Three essays on the theory of sexuality. In: Strachey J, ed. *The standard edition of the complete works of Sigmund Freud*, vol. 7. London: Hogarth, 1953: 125–243. [Strache J, trans.; original work published in 1906.]
8. Montoya A, Price BH, Lepage M. Neural correlates of 'functional' symptoms in neurology. *Funct Neurol* 2006;**21(4)**:193–7.
9. Vuilleumier P, Chicherio C, Assal F, Schwartz S, Slosman D, Landis T. Functional neuroanatomical correlates of hysterical sensorimotor loss. *Brain* 2001;**124(Pt 6)**:1077–90.
10. Vuilleumier P. Hysterical conversion and brain function. *Prog Brain Res* 2005;**150**:309–29.
11. Mailis-Gagnon A, Giannoylis I, Downar J, et al. Altered central somatosensory processing in chronic pain patients with 'hysterical' anesthesia. *Neurology* 2003;**60(9)**:1501–7.
12. Spanaki MV, Spencer SS, Corsi M, MacMullan J, Seibyl J, Zubal IG. The role of quantitative ictal SPECT analysis in the evaluation of nonepileptic seizures. *J Neuroimaging* 1999;**9(4)**:210–6.
13. Devinsky O, Mesad S, Alper K. Nondominant hemisphere lesions and conversion nonepileptic seizures. *J Neuropsychiatry Clin Neurosci* 2001;**13**:367–73.
14. Reuber M, Fernández G, Helmstaedter C, Qurishi A, Elger CE. Evidence of brain abnormality in patients with psychogenic nonepileptic seizures. *Epilepsy Behav* 2002;**3**:249–54.
15. Reuber M, Fernández G, Bauer J, Singh DD, Elger CE. Interictal EEG abnormalities in patients with psychogenic nonepileptic seizures. *Epilepsia* 2002;**43(9)**:1013–20.
16. Drane DL, Williamson DJ, Stroup ES, et al. Cognitive impairment is not equal in patients with epileptic and psychogenic nonepileptic seizures. *Epilepsia* 2006;**47(11)**:1879–86.
17. Baillés E, Pintor L, Fernandez-Egea E, Torres X, et al. Psychiatric disorders, trauma, and MMPI profile in a Spanish sample of nonepileptic seizure patients. *Gen Hosp Psychiatry* 2004;**26**:310–5.
18. Orbach D, Ritaccio A, Devinsky O. Psychogenic, nonepileptic seizures associated with VEEG-verified sleep. *Epilepsia* 2004;**44(1)**:64–8.

Why Does VNS Take So Long to Work?

Paul Boon, Veerle De Herdt and Kristl Vonck

HISTORY

This right-handed 38-year-old female with a history of mild mental retardation developed severe refractory epilepsy with complex partial seizures (CPSs) and secondary generalization at the age of 2. From 1985 to 1998 she had been treated with various combinations of antiepileptic drugs (AEDs) including phenytoin, valproate, carbamazepine, gabapentin, primidone, and clonazepam. Routine electroencephalogram (EEG) showed a slow background activity and bilateral, nonsynchronous, diffuse interictal epileptiform discharges. When lamotrigine was included in 1998, seizure frequency improved. The patient was admitted to the hospital the same year because of ataxia and nystagmus, related to a pharmacodynamic interaction between carbamazepine and lamotrigine. Carbamazepine dosage was decreased, resulting in an increase of seizures. AEDs were changed to valproate, topiramate, and lamotrigine without success. She had CPSs at least two times per week, and convulsions occurred at least once per month, often during the night. Habitual seizures were often preceded by an epigastric aura. A seizure consisted of loss of contact followed by automatisms on the left or right side of the upper extremities. The patient's husband reported frequent falls and a prolonged postictal period with confusion and aggressiveness.

EXAMINATIONS AND INVESTIGATIONS

Presurgical evaluation with an optimum MRI in 1999 showed bilateral mesiotemporal sclerosis, more pronounced on the left side. Video–EEG monitoring was performed: five CPS were recorded. Ictal EEG showed recruitment with rhythmical theta activity in the left temporal electrodes in three seizures; during two CPS there was early right temporal rhythmicity. Interictal EEG showed independent frequent left and right frontotemporal spiking and independent left frontal spike–wave activity. Because of the clear-cut bilateral involvement, it was decided at the multidisciplinary epilepsy

Puzzling Cases of Epilepsy

surgery meeting that the patient was not a suitable candidate for resective surgery, but rather a candidate for vagus nerve stimulation (VNS). At that time, she was treated with valproate 2000 mg/day, topiramate 150 mg/day, and lamotrigine 300 mg/day.

s0030 ## DIAGNOSIS

p0040 Drug-resistant bitemporal lobe epilepsy

s0040 ## TREATMENT AND OUTCOME

p0050 In July 2001 she was implanted with VNS. The perioperative period was uneventful. The AED regimen remained unchanged. During the ramping-up period, mild hoarseness was reported. The output current was gradually increased to 1.75 mA over a 3-month period, without a clear reduction in seizure frequency. The patient was unsatisfied with the situation but she did report prevention of seizures when using the magnet in case of an aura. A second video–EEG monitoring was performed to reevaluate the patient's seizures. Identical results to the initial hospital admission were found. AED drug levels were therapeutic. During the hospitalization, the output current of the VNS was set to 2.0 mA using a stimulation frequency of 20 Hz. Two months later the patient reported a marked decrease in CPS and one full month without generalized convulsions. She still complained of mild intermittent hoarseness but stimulation parameters could slowly be increased to an output current of 2.5 mA. Three months later the patient reported a CPS frequency of <1 per month. After 2 years of follow-up, the patient reports occasional CPS, about once every 3 months with a markedly reduced postictal period. She also reports occasionally using the magnet when she experiences an aura with a frequency of about one per month. Secondary generalized convulsions have not reoccurred. Side effects have fully resolved.

s0050 ## COMMENTARY

p0060 In this patient with a long history of medically refractory epilepsy, the efficacy of VNS became evident only after about 5 months of treatment. Large patient series have shown that one-third of patients treated with VNS are nonresponders. This had been discussed with the patient prior to VNS but she was however very disappointed with the initial lack of seizure control. She did report efficacy of the magnet in attempts to acutely prevent a seizure following an aura. We discussed with the patient the fact that VNS may act in a neuromodulatory way and that establishment of efficacy may take time. Also there was still an option to further increase the output current if she could tolerate this.

s0060 ## WHAT DID I LEARN FROM THIS CASE?

p0070 Changing treatment of patients with refractory epilepsy from drugs to implantation with a device increases their expectations with regard to seizure control. Patients need to be clearly informed about the potential efficacy and the nonresponder rates of VNS. It is important to explain that VNS is currently an add-on treatment and that the treatment needs time to be ramped-up and efficacy may not appear until months after the implantation procedure.

Even after several months of treatment, further attempts to increase stimulation output current should be made. By that time patients usually present with less side effects and if not, stimulation frequency or pulse width should be decreased to allow output current increases.

However difficult it is to objectively evaluate magnet efficacy, patients who report early efficacy of the magnet often become responders and this may be a good indicator to further push the treatment.

HOW DID THIS CASE ALTER MY APPROACH TO THE CARE AND TREATMENT OF MY EPILEPSY PATIENTS?

I have learned to fully inform patients about the potential benefits of VNS and also that patience is needed when this type of treatment is involved. Years of established refractory epilepsy cannot be switched off by switching on a biomedical device. However, I have learned to have patience myself and not classify patients as nonresponders after 3 months of treatment. I also learned that pushing the treatment by making use of the potential to change the other parameters may be successful. Every patient with refractory epilepsy is clearly different and may require an individualized stimulation paradigm.

Commentary: Why Does VNS Take So Long to Work?

Steven Schachter

s0080

PRECLINICAL PERSPECTIVE

p0110

Early preclinical studies of VNS provided the scientific rationale for proceeding to human studies in epilepsy by demonstrating acute and prophylactic anticonvulsant effects. However, the results of these studies did not predict the later clinical observations of a delay in the onset of efficacy in some patients treated with VNS or improved efficacy over time in others.

p0120

For example, early mechanistic studies in which the vagus nerve was repetitively stimulated in anesthetized animals showed acute synchronization or desynchronization of brain electrical activity as seen on the EEG.[1-3] Likewise, low-intensity repetitive stimulation of rat vagus nerve ($100\,\mu A$, $30\,Hz$, $500\,\mu s$, $20\,s$ on time) was found to acutely hyperpolarize pyramidal neurons of the parietal association cortex.[4] A recently published study in rats demonstrated that VNS acutely increased the expression of brain-derived neurotrophic factor and fibroblast growth factor in hippocampus and cerebral cortex, decreased hippocampal nerve growth factor mRNA and increased norepinephrine concentration in prefrontal cortex (supporting earlier work suggesting a role for the locus coeruleus in the mechanism of action of VNS),[5] raising the question of what happens to these effects over extended periods of treatment with VNS.[6]

p0130

The in vivo effects of VNS on seizures were studied in several acute animal models of induced seizures.[7-10] In other studies, the prophylactic effect of VNS was evaluated,[11,12] which is more relevant to its use in human epilepsy, but these studies were not designed to evaluate possible changes in efficacy over prolonged periods of continued VNS treatment.

p0140

Consequently, the evolution of effects of VNS on brain function that could be the basis for improved clinical efficacy over time has not been well studied to date in the laboratory. While such work may pose technical challenges, it could lead to findings with clinical implications for maximizing the benefit of VNS to patients with epilepsy.

CLINICAL SCIENCE PERSPECTIVE

The VNS Therapy System^{TM} (Cyberonics, Inc.) was approved by the FDA in 1997 as adjunctive therapy for adults and adolescents over 12 years of age whose partial-onset seizures were refractory to AEDs, becoming the first FDA-approved nonpharmaco-logical treatment for epileptic seizures. VNS treatment is generally offered to patients with medically refractory partial-onset seizures who are either opposed to intracranial surgery for seizure control or not candidates.[13]

Clinical relevance

As observed in the case of Boon et al., the results of long-term trials as well as anec-dotal experience suggest that the onset of efficacy from VNS may be delayed in some patients, while other patients appear to have progressive improvement in seizure con-trol over a period of months of ongoing VNS treatment. These observations are in contrast to the typical temporal pattern of efficacy with AEDs, which is generally characterized by a relatively early response that is maintained or decreases over time.

In clinical practice, patients undergoing VNS implantation should be counseled, as was this patient, that the therapeutic benefit may be delayed in onset, unlike their usual experiences with AEDs. In our practice, we generally provide at least 6 months of VNS therapy before concluding it is ineffective and often wait 12 months or more. Once we reach that circumstance, we turn the stimulator off. If seizures worsen in fre-quency or severity then we continue stimulation, otherwise the generator is explanted after discussion with the patient.

The clinical evidence in randomized trials and relevant clinical observations

The clinical studies leading up to FDA approval were short term and therefore not designed to evaluate the possibility of progressive changes in seizure frequency over time.[14–20] In the pivotal trials (E03 and E05), the primary measure of efficacy was the percentage change in seizure frequency during the entire VNS treatment period compared to the preimplantation baseline. Thus while both studies showed that high stimulation was more effective than low stimulation, they did not specifically evaluate efficacy as a function of duration of VNS treatment.

The results of several long-term prospective and retrospective population studies up to 12 years postimplantation suggest that VNS efficacy is maintained over time, or even increases over months to years.[17,21–29] However, because VNS treatment is unblinded during long-term treatment, and stimulation parameters and AED dosages are adjusted as clinically necessary, these results do not definitively prove a delayed or progressive benefit to VNS. In one suggestive study, albeit retrospective, 269 patients whose AEDs were kept constant for one year after VNS implantation were found to have a median 45% reduction of seizure frequency at 3 months postimplantation, compared to preim-plantation baseline, and 58% reduction at 12 months.[30]

A retrospective analysis of on-demand magnet activation suggested an association between acute anticonvulsant effects from magnet-induced stimulation and overall prophylactic effects of intermittent VNS.[31] Interestingly, the patient described by Boon *et al.* reported an acute response to the magnet well in advance of evidence for prophylactic benefit, suggesting the possibility that the mechanisms underlying acute seizure suppression may have a different time course for their development than those associated with seizure prophylaxis.

Prospective studies in patients treated with VNS for epilepsy offer the potential for identifying surrogate markers of progressive efficacy. For example, Marrosu and colleagues measured gamma aminobutyric acid (GABA(A)) receptor density (GRD) in cortex prior to and 1 year after VNS treatment in 10 subjects with drug-resistant partial epilepsy using SPECT with the benzodiazepine receptor inverse agonist [^{123}I]iomazenil.[32] VNS therapeutic responses significantly correlated with normalization of GRD, whereas a control group failed to show significant GRD variations after 1 year of stable drug therapy. These results suggest that VNS modulates the plasticity of GABA(A) receptor density and therefore cortical excitability. Similar work that adds additional time points for measurement of GABA(A) receptor density, for example after 1, 3, and 18 months of treatment may provide additional insights. Further, in a limited series of patients whose seizures responded to VNS, Marrosu *et al.* found normalization of impaired neuronal inhibition,[32] and in 11 other patients, the same group showed decreased synchronization of theta frequencies and increased gamma power spectrum and synchronization.[33] Likewise, a study of transcranial magnetic stimulation in five patients initially treated with VNS and after 1 month of therapy ($n = 1$) for epilepsy showed significantly increased cortical inhibition associated with stimulation without any evidence of an effect on cortical excitability.[34] Obtaining serial measures over more extended periods and correlating those changes with seizure outcome using each of these methodological approaches should be pursued.

What can experimental researchers learn from the clinical data?

The evidence for a delayed or progressive anticonvulsant effect of VNS is intriguing, though not conclusive, and merits further research at the bench to elucidate the possible underlying mechanisms and in the clinic to find surrogate markers and determine ways to accelerate improvements in seizure frequency and severity for patients treated with VNS. Published mechanistic studies provide a starting point. It will also be interesting to determine if similar temporal patterns of efficacy are seen with other forms of electrical brain stimulation that are currently under development for the treatment of epilepsy or being planned.

REFERENCES

1. Chase MH, Sterman MB, Clemente CD. Cortical and subcortical patterns of response to afferent vagal stimulation. *Exp Neurol* 1966;**16**:36–49.
2. Chase MH, Nakamura Y, Clemente CD, Sterman MB. Afferent vagal stimulation: neurographic correlates of induced EEG synchronization and desynchronization. *Brain Res* 1967;**5**:236–49.
3. Chase MH, Nakamura Y, Clemente CD, Sterman MB. Cortical and subcortical EEG patterns of response to afferent abdominal vagal stimulation: neurographic correlates. *Physiol Behav* 1968;**3**:605–10.

4. Zagon A, Kemeny AA. Slow hyperpolarization in cortical neurons: a possible mechanism behind vagus nerve simulation therapy for refractory epilepsy? *Epilepsia* 2000;**41**:1382–9.

5. Krahl SE, Clark KB, Smith DC, Browning RA. Locus coeruleus lesions suppress the seizure–attenuating effects of vagus nerve stimulation. *Epilepsia* 1998;**39**:709–14.

6. Follesa P, Biggio F, Gorini G, *et al.* Vagus nerve stimulation increases norepinephrine concentration and the gene expression of BDNF and bFGF in the rat brain. *Brain Res* 2007;**1179**:28–34.

7. McLachlan RS. Suppression of interictal spikes and seizures by stimulation of the vagus nerve. *Epilepsia* 1993;**34**:918–23.

8. Woodbury DM, Woodbury JW. Effects of vagal stimulation on experimentally induced seizures in rats. *Epilepsia* 1990;**31(suppl 2)**:S7–S19.

9. Woodbury JW, Woodbury DM. Vagal stimulation reduces the severity of maximal electroshock seizures in intact rats: use of a cuff electrode for stimulating and recording. *Pacing Clin Electrophysiol* 1991;**14**:94–107.

10. Zabara J. Inhibition of experimental seizures in canines by repetitive vagal stimulation. *Epilepsia* 1992;**33**:1005–12.

11. Lockard JS, Congdon WC, DuCharme LL. Feasibility and safety of vagal stimulation in monkey model. *Epilepsia* 1990;**31(suppl 2)**:S20–S26.

12. Takaya M, Terry WJ, Naritoku DK. Vagus nerve stimulation induces a sustained anticonvulsant effect. *Epilepsia* 1996;**37**:1111–6.

13. Schachter SC. Vagus nerve stimulation: where are we? *Curr Opin Neurol* 2002;**15**:201–6.

14. Penry JK, Dean JC. Prevention of intractable partial seizures by intermittent vagal stimulation in humans: preliminary results. *Epilepsia* 1990;**31(suppl 2)**:S40–S43.

15. Ben-Menachem E, Manon-Espaillat R, Ristanovic R, *et al.* Vagus nerve stimulation for treatment of partial seizures: 1. A controlled study of effect on seizures. *Epilepsia* 1994;**35**:616–26.

16. Ramsay RE, Uthman BM, Augustinsson LE, *et al.* Vagus nerve stimulation for treatment of partial seizures: 2. Safety, side effects, and tolerability. *Epilepsia* 1994;**35**:627–36.

17. George R, Salinsky M, Kuzniecky R, *et al.* Vagus nerve stimulation for treatment of partial seizures: 3. Long-term follow-up on first 67 patients exiting a controlled study. *Epilepsia* 1994;**35**:637–43.

18. The Vagus Nerve Stimulation Study Group. A randomized controlled trial of chronic vagus nerve stimulation for treatment of medically intractable seizures. *Neurology* 1995;**45**:224–30.

19. Handforth A, DeGiorgio CM, Schachter SC, *et al.* Vagus nerve stimulation therapy for partial-onset seizures: a randomized active-control trial. *Neurology* 1998;**51**:48–55.

20. Labar D, Murphy J, Tecoma E. Vagus nerve stimulation for medication-resistant generalized epilepsy. E04 VNS Study Group. *Neurology* 1999;**52**:1510–2.

21. Michael JE, Wegener K, Barnes DW. Vagus nerve stimulation for intractable seizures: one year follow-up. *J Neurosci Nurs* 1993;**25**:362–6.

22. Salinsky MC, Uthman BM, Ristanovic RK, Wernicke JF, Tarver WB. Vagus nerve stimulation for the treatment of medically intractable seizures. Results of a 1-year open-extension trial. *Arch Neurol* 1996;**53**:1176–80.

23. DeGiorgio CM, Schachter SC, Handforth A, *et al.* Prospective long-term study of vagus nerve stimulation for the treatment of refractory seizures. *Epilepsia* 2000;**41**:1195–200.

24. Sirven JI, Sperling M, Naritoku D, *et al.* Vagus nerve stimulation therapy for epilepsy in older adults. *Neurology* 2000;**54**:1179–82.

25. Uthman BM, Reichl AM, Dean JC, *et al.* Effectiveness of vagus nerve stimulation in epilepsy patients: A 12-year observation. *Neurology* 2004;**63**:1124–6.

26. Spanaki MV, Allen LS, Mueller WM, Morris GL 3rd. Vagus nerve stimulation therapy: 5-year or greater outcome at a university-based epilepsy center. *Seizure* 2004;**13**:587–90.

27. Vonck K, Thadani V, Gilbert K, *et al.* Vagus nerve stimulation for refractory epilepsy: a transatlantic experience. *J Clin Neurophysiol* 2004;**21**:283–9.

28. Kuba R, Brazdil M, Novak Z, Chrastina J, Rektor I. Effect of vagal nerve stimulation on patients with bitemporal epilepsy. *Eur J Neurol* 2003;**10**:91–4.

29. Majoie HJM, Berfelo MW, Aldenkamp AP, Renier WO, Kessels AGH. Vagus nerve stimulation in patients with catastrophic childhood epilepsy, a 2-year follow-up study. *Seizure* 2005;**14**:10–8.

30. Labar D. Vagus nerve stimulation for 1 year in 269 patients on unchanged antiepileptic drugs. *Seizure* 2004;**13**:392–8.
31. Morris GL III. A retrospective analysis of the effects of magnet-activated stimulation in conjunction with vagus nerve stimulation therapy. *Epilepsy Behav* 2003;**4**:740–5.
32. Marrosu F, Serra A, Maleci A, Puligheddu M, Biggio G, Piga M. Correlation between GABA(A) receptor density and vagus nerve stimulation in individuals with drug-resistant partial epilepsy. *Epilepsy Res* 2003;**55**:59–70.
33. Marrosu F, Santoni F, Puligheddu M, *et al.* Increase in 20–50 Hz (gamma frequencies) power spectrum and synchronization after chronic vagal nerve stimulation. *Clin Neurophysiol* 2005;**116**: 2026–36.
34. Di Lazzaro V, Oliviero A, Pilato F, *et al.* Effects of vagus nerve stimulation on cortical excitability in epileptic patients. *Neurology* 2004;**62**:2310–2.

If at First You Don't Succeed ...

Andrew N Wilner

HISTORY

F came to the office for his first visit when he was 40 years old. His mother's pregnancy was unremarkable, but he was premature by 6 weeks and blue at birth. He did not walk until 16 months of age or speak until 3 years of age.

F's first convulsion occurred at 15 months of age. He also had brief spells where he appeared afraid and ran to his mother. Despite phenobarbital and phenytoin, he continued to have seizures. After his physician switched him to primidone at the age of 12 years, F became violent and attacked a neighbor with a hatchet. He required institutionalization until he was aged 18.

While taking valproate 2 years ago he again became aggressive and was said to have a "psychotic reaction". His behavior improved when he began phenytoin. However, he continues to have seizures three times a month, although they can occur as often as nine times a day. According to his parents, he has right hand jerks, which sometimes proceed to a generalized convulsion. He also has other spells where he smacks his lips and stares. His seizures have failed to improve with acetazolamide, carbamazepine, chlordiazepoxide, clorazepate, diazepam, and ethosuximide. He had an episode of status epilepticus when an intercurrent illness resulted in protracted nausea and vomiting.

His past medical history includes hyperthyroidism and hypertension, which he treats with medications. As a result of his seizures, he has fractured both wrists and his right foot and has suffered numerous lacerations on his face and scalp. He has no allergies and does not abuse drugs; nor does he drink alcohol or smoke. F is the only one in his family with epilepsy. His social life is very limited because of his seizures and limited cognitive and social skills. His mother is overprotective. His stepfather mostly ignores him. A prior evaluation included a normal electroencephalogram (EEG) and a normal magnetic resonance imaging (MRI) study. He takes phenytoin (100 mg four times daily) and primidone (250 mg four times daily).

EXAMINATION AND INVESTIGATIONS

F answers questions slowly, but appropriately. His Mini Mental State Examination score is 25/30. His physical examination is normal and his neurological examination is non-focal.

Puzzling Cases of Epilepsy

Video–EEG monitoring of eight seizures failed to reveal lateralization or localization (because of muscle artifact produced by grimacing and chewing at the onset of each seizure). Depth electrode monitoring revealed that 12 of 13 seizures originated from his right temporal lobe. The origin of the remaining seizure was unclear.

p0240   F's repeat MRI scan demonstrated right hippocampal atrophy with increased T2-weighted signal consistent with mesial temporal sclerosis. Positron emission tomography was normal. Neuropsychological testing did not lateralize or localize. The IQ was 83. A Wada test determined that he was left hemisphere dominant for language. Using his left hemisphere, he was able to remember 11 of 12 items. Using his right hemisphere, F could not answer any questions correctly.

s0030 ## DIAGNOSIS

p0250   Intractable epilepsy caused by partial complex seizures and partial seizures with secondary generalization from the right temporal lobe.

s0040 ## TREATMENT AND OUTCOME

p0260   F had a right anterior temporal lobectomy without complication. Postoperatively, primidone was discontinued and he had two breakthrough seizures. I restarted the medication and he remains seizure-free on two antiepileptic drugs. He attended adult education classes and passed his high-school equivalency exam. He has been to vocational rehabilitation and found some part-time work. He also volunteers at the local hospital. He has learned to drive and can do errands, but he continues to live at home. He has made some friends at the epilepsy support group and has a girlfriend. He went fishing with his stepfather for the first time.

s0050 ## COMMENTARY

p0270   F presented with seizures that failed to respond to treatment. His stepfather considered him little more than a nuisance, and his mother worried about him daily. At the age of 40, there seemed little hope that he would ever live independently or become seizure-free. However, after a new and extensive evaluation, I was able to define an epileptic syndrome that was amenable to surgical treatment.

p0280   Many patients who appear "hopeless" can be helped, whether by new antiepileptic drugs, vagus nerve stimulation or epilepsy surgery. In F's case, a right temporal lobectomy resulted in a 99% reduction of his seizures and a significant improvement in his quality of life.

s0060 ### What did I learn from this case?

p0290   First, I learned that although witnessed reports of seizures can be valuable, they pale in comparison to ictal videotapes. F's convulsions beginning with "right hand jerks" reported by his family suggested Jacksonian seizures from a left frontal lobe lesion, unlikely to be amenable to seizure surgery. But video–EEG monitoring revealed that F's seizures consisted primarily of chewing and bouncing movements, with additional automatisms of right hand trembling, swinging, and kicking of the right leg.

Second, I learned that antiepileptic drugs can subtly – or not so subtly – affect a patient's personality. In F's case, two drugs, primidone (which is notorious for its negative affect on behavior) and valproate (which is not usually associated with behavior abnormalities) altered his personality for the worse. When he was not on either of these drugs, F usually had a very placid disposition.

Third, I learned that if an imaging study is more than a few years old and there is reason to believe the patient has a lesion, a MRI scan with state-of-the-art equipment should be performed. F's first MRI was "normal". A follow-up scan revealed clear-cut mesial temporal sclerosis. Many older MRI scans did not have the resolution of today's scans, and significant pathology can be missed.

How did this case alter my approach to the care and treatment of my epilepsy patients?

F's case reinforced the concept that one must always ask: "why does this patient have epilepsy?" I think that physicians tend to neglect this question because the answer in the past usually was "I don't know", as in F's case, even after a thorough evaluation. Now, with modern imaging, we can often answer that question and arrive at a more accurate diagnosis and prognosis. Learning why F had epilepsy permitted me to offer him the appropriate treatment.

FURTHER READING

Benbadis SR. Is the underlying cause of epilepsy a major prognostic factor for recurrence? *Neurology* 1999;**53**:440.

Engel J. Etiology as a risk factor for medically refractory epilepsy. *Neurology* 1998;**51**:1243–4.

Semah F, Picot MC, Adam C, *et al.* Is the underlying cause of epilepsy a major prognostic factor for recurrence? *Neurology* 1998;**51**:1256–62.

Mattson RH, Cramer JA, Collins JF. Prognosis for total control of complex partial and secondarily generalized tonic clonic seizures. *Neurology* 1996;**47**:68–76.

Why Antiepileptic Drugs Fail in Some Patients: A Preclinical Perspective

Heidrun Potschka

In more than 30% of patients with epilepsy, seizures are or will become refractory to pharmacotherapy.[1] As in Dr. Wilner's case, seizure control cannot be achieved in this subgroup of patients despite the use of different antiepileptic drugs with different mechanisms of action.

The elucidation of the mechanisms of pharmacoresistance may aid the prediction of responsiveness, which would avoid ongoing trials with a series of antiepileptic drugs in such patients in which failure is predetermined. This would render a basis for an early straightforward decision for alternative therapeutic strategies such as surgery. Patients will clearly benefit from a prediction of broad refractoriness. Repeated trials with alternative antiepileptic drugs generally imply the risk of a variety of side effects including the exacerbation of behavioral disturbances as reported for patient F.

Recent research has focused on two hypotheses of pharmacoresistance. First, changes in the pharmacodynamics may contribute to failure. Changes in the subunit composition of $GABA_A$ receptors as well as sodium channels have been described.[2] These changes proved to be associated with a reduced pharmacological response of these target sites, and may thus mediate refractoriness toward GABAergic compounds or sodium channel blockers. A limited electrophysiological response of sodium channels has been substantiated by investigations in tissue dissected from pharmacoresistant patients with epilepsy. Techniques for a clinical diagnosis of these molecular and functional changes in target sites have not been developed up to now. An intronic polymorphism in the SCN1A gene which encodes the alpha-subunit of sodium channels proved to be associated with maximum doses of phenytoin and carbamazepine.[3] However, these genetic studies have not been extended to a comparison between pharmacoresistant and pharmacosensitive patients. Thus, currently, pharmacogenetic knowledge does not render a basis for a clinical application.

Besides pharmacodynamics, the pharmacokinetics of antiepileptic drugs can also be affected in the epileptic brain.[4,5] An upregulation of blood–brain barrier multidrug transporters has been reported in a variety of acute and chronic epilepsy models in rodents. Studies in human epileptic tissue dissected from pharmacoresistant patients also revealed an overexpression of transporter molecules such as P-glycoprotein and members of the multidrug-resistance associated protein family. In models of pharmacoresistant epilepsy, a correlation was evident between transporter expression and pharmacosensitivity. Based on an efflux function directed toward the capillary lumen of brain capillaries, these transporters efficiently limit brain penetration of their substrates.

Although contradictory data exist for specific antiepileptic drugs, evidence has indicated that several antiepileptic drugs are substrates of blood–brain barrier efflux transporters. Based on their broad substrate spectrum, overexpression of multidrug transporters can also explain non-specific pharmacoresistance to a variety of antiepileptic drugs.

Recent data indicated that at least for phenytoin as well as the major active oxcarbazepine metabolite, 10(OH)-oxcarbazepine, these findings also apply to human transporter isoforms. Experimental proof-of-principle came from several studies in which it was possible to enhance the anticonvulsant efficacy of antiepileptic drugs by co-administration of multidrug transporter modulators. Most importantly, it proved to be possible to overcome resistance to phenobarbital in a chronic rat model with spontaneous seizures by co-administration of the highly specific P-glycoprotein inhibitor tariquidar.[6] One major open question remains with regard to the clinical relevance of the overexpression, especially as multidrug resistance of epilepsy is likely to constitute a multifactorial phenomenon.

Recently, Langer et al.[7] reported the first evidence for an increased Pgp efflux function at the blood–brain barrier of pharmacoresistant temporal lobe epilepsy patients as indicated by PET imaging. Further validation of PET imaging as a technique to image transporter function in patients will render a basis to determine the clinical relevance of transporter overexpression. Moreover, it may be a suitable approach to select patients who may benefit from new therapeutic strategies designed to overcome transporter-mediated resistance.

Modulation of transporter function by co-administration of inhibitors such as tariquidar is generally considered as a new treatment option. However, in view of the protective function of multidrug transporters, which limit access of xenobiotics to sensitive tissue throughout the body, putative long-term risks of such a strategy need to be carefully considered.

Non-pharmacological strategies such as surgery are well-established alternatives. Provided that thorough clinical investigations suggest that the patient is a candidate for surgery, this may transform pharmacoresistant into pharmacosensitive epilepsy as reported for patient F.

Pharmacogenetic analysis of the P-glycoprotein encoding gene MDR1 has revealed contradictory data.[8] Whereas some studies indicated an association between polymorphisms in the MDR1-coding sequence and pharmacosensitivity, other studies did not support a correlation. Clearly, analysis of polymorphisms in the MDR1-coding sequence will not allow one to predict individual pharmacoresponsiveness. This is not surprising, as the basis for high expression rates in pharmacoresistant individuals and lower expression rates in pharmacosensitive patients are rather caused by a different extent of transporter up-regulation in response to seizure activity in both subgroups. Thus, differences may rather exist in regulatory sequences of MDR1. Moreover, we recently demonstrated that a cascade of events seems to mediate seizure-induced transporter upregulation, and therefore genetic differences in a series of factors may contribute to the differences in expression rates[9]. Considering the complexity of the molecular events, further development of pharmacogenetic analyses may in fact render information about individual risk factors for refractoriness; however, it is unlikely to be suitable for a definite prediction in individual patients.

p0430 Thus, further development of imaging techniques needs to be awaited in order to establish an analysis of this putative resistance mechanism in patients. There is hope that at least in some patients these techniques may in the future help to avoid long-term subsequent pharmacotherapy trials that are doomed to failure.

REFERENCES

1. Kwan P, Brodie M. Refractory epilepsy: mechanisms and solutions. *Expert Rev Neurother* 2006;**6**:397–406.
2. Beck H. Plasticity of antiepileptic drug targets. *Epilepsia* 2007;**48(suppl.1)**:14–8.
3. Tate SK, Depondt C, Sisodiya SM, et al. Genetic predictors of the maximum doses patients receive during clinical use of the anti-epileptic drugs carbamazepine and phenytoin. *Proc Natl Acad Sci USA* 2005;**102**:5507–12.
4. Löscher W, Potschka H. Drug resistance in brain diseases and the role of drug efflux transporters. *Nat Rev Neurosci* 2005;**6**:591–602.
5. Löscher W. Drug transporters in the epileptic brain. *Epilepsia* 2007;**48(suppl 1)**:8–13.
6. Brandt C, Bethmann K, Gastens AM, Löscher W. The multidrug transporter hypothesis of drug resistance in epilepsy: proof-of-principle in a rat model of temporal lobe epilepsy. *Neurbiol Dis* 2006; **24**:202–11.
7. Langer O, Bauer M, Hammers A, et al. Pharmacoresistance in epilepsy: a pilot PET study with the P-glycoprotein substrate R-[(11C)] verapamil. *Epilepsia* 2007;**48**:1774–84.
8. Tate SK, Sisidiya SM. Multidrug resistance in epilepsy: a pharmcogenomic update. *Expert Opin Pharmacother* 2007;**8**:1441–9.
9. Bauer B, Hartz AM, Pekcec A, Toellner K, Miller DS, Potschka H. Seizure-induced upregulation of P-glycoprotein at the blood-brain barrier through glutamate and cyclooxygenase-2 signaling. *Mol Pharmacol* 2008;**73**:444–53.

The Continuing Conundrum of Reversible Drug-resistant Epilepsy: A Clinical Perspective

Dieter Schmidt

Antiepileptic drugs (AEDs) continue to be the first-line treatment of epilepsy. Two of three patients will eventually become seizure-free from treatment with AEDs. However, in one of three cases, the seizures of patients with epilepsy are drug-resistant, that is patients either do not become seizure-free or have intolerable side effects or, most commonly, both.[1] Although AEDs can be expected to reduce the frequency of seizures, if they work, the number of patients remaining seizure-free declines over time with prolonged treatment due to tolerance. While AED tolerance is not a serious issue for most patients becoming seizure-free, it is a significant aspect of treatment in some patients that requires evaluation in long-term clinical trials.[2] A further limitation of drug treatment of epilepsy is that AEDs do not seem to alter the underlying epileptic disease or prevent its progression.

A very influential study suggested that permanent, life-long drug resistance, defined as failure to reach 12-month remission during follow-up, can be identified from the initial response to the first AED.[3] Insightful case reports, controlled trials and long-term clinical observational trials suggest, however, that a number of patients with apparent drug-resistant seizures will eventually enter remission after a change of drug regimen. That apparently drug-resistant epilepsy can be attenuated, at least in part and transiently, is a well-known fact in a number of placebo-controlled randomized trials where add-on treatment with an investigational AED achieves significant seizure reduction in as many as 50% of patients with chronic previously refractory epilepsy with often weekly seizures prior to the introduction of the new drug.[1] Furthermore and most welcome, some patients – in the 5–8% range – will be seizure-free during the trial. This figure, however, does not represent the likelihood of patients remaining seizure-free over a long-term period. Long-term observations indicate that as many as 20–30% with apparent drug-resistant seizures will eventually enter remission after a change of drug regimen.[4,5] Our own study from patients with childhood-onset epilepsy who were tracked over an average of 37 years showed four distinct patterns of response over time.[6] Patients who were always in remission (16%), patients who started off in remission but subsequently could not maintain remission (14%), patients

TABLE 101.1   The Mechanisms of Drug Resistance

Disease-related mechanisms include
• Progression of disease
• Etiology of seizures/epilepsy
• Structural brain alterations
• Network changes
• Alteration of drug targets
• Alteration in drug uptake into the brain (transport)

Drug-related mechanisms include
• Loss of effect (tolerance)
• Ineffective mechanism of action
• Gene polymorphisms or mutations

Source: Modified from Ref. [1].

who started off with no remission but subsequently went into remission (52%) and patients who were never in remission (19%). Thus the case of Wilner belongs to the large group of patients who seem to become seizure-free only after several AED regimens failed to control seizures. One question of particular interest for clinicians is the mechanism(s) responsible for reversing apparent drug resistance. The mechanisms underlying tolerance and permanent drug resistance have been extensively discussed elsewhere (Refs. [1] and [2]; see also the comment by Potschka in this volume). In general, it is believed that AED resistance could arise from either disease-related mechanisms or drug-related mechanisms or both (Table 101.1).

p0460   Novel biological mechanisms have been postulated largely surrounding the "target and transporter" hypothesis. Genetic and structural defects may affect drug targets and drug transport or other AED-related mechanisms and result in drug resistance. In the former, for example, reduced drug-target sensitivity in epileptogenic tissue could give rise to drug resistance. The removal of AEDs from the epileptogenic tissue through excessive expression of multidrug transporters as suggested in the "transporter" hypothesis could also lead to pharmacoresistance.

p0470   For our discussion it is important to consider that neurobiological mechanisms of pharmacoresistance may be different in patients who have never responded to an AED versus those who progressed to pharmacoresistance after they responded initially to therapy. In addition, the mechanisms of reversing pharmacoresistance may differ from those generating pharmacoresistance. The critical question to be discussed here briefly is which of the many putative mechanisms of lifelong drug resistance may be operative in allowing patients to become seizure-free after several AED regimens failed. A number of hypotheses can be entertained (Table 101.2).

s0080   ## FLUCTUATION AND SPONTANEOUS REMISSION OF DISEASE

p0480   In their description of patterns of seizure remission, Shorvon and Sander[7] described an intermittent pattern in which active epilepsy is interrupted by periods of remission. They defined remission as a period of freedom from seizures for 2 years or more. In a group of 181 patients with chronic uncontrolled seizures attending a specialized hospital

TABLE 101.2   Putative Mechanisms of Reversible Drug Resistance

Disease-related mechanisms
• Fluctuation and spontaneous remission of disease • Genetic variation including polymorphisms or mutations
Drug-related mechanisms
• Target/network specific AED treatment • Adequate AED dosage • Adequate AED exposure at target • Effective mechanism of action
Surgery-related mechanism
• Resection transfers drug-resistant epilepsy into drug-responsive epilepsy with seizure freedom on AEDs • Resection transfers drug-resistant epilepsy into drug-responsive epilepsy with seizure freedom maintained after AED discontinuation

outpatient service, the intermittent pattern was found in 39 patients (22%). These data suggest that in some patients pharmacoresistance may be reversible, at least for a period of several years. Although no claim can be made or is intended that AEDs are involved in reversing pharmacoresistance, these data show that any theory for pharmacoresistance needs to take into account that pharmacoresistance may be reversible in some patients with partial epilepsy.

Seizure control may be achieved only after subsequent treatment with several AEDs. What is then the chance of a patient with new-onset epilepsy becoming seizure-free or achieving a 50% reduction of seizure frequency if the previous AED has failed to control the seizures? Is a failure to respond to an AED of prognostic value for long-term outcome? To that end, a study evaluated the likelihood that a patient who had become seizure-free at 6 months of single AED treatment will lose that response at 12 months, or vice versa.[8] The main findings in the population included in the analysis are that those patients who are seizure-free at 6 months have a 90% chance of being seizure-free at 12 months, while those not seizure-free at 6 months have only a 45% chance of being seizure-free at 12 months (Chi-Square $= 118.716, p < 0.000001$, odd ratio $= 11.23$ with 95% confidence limits 6.8 and 18.7). In a worst-case assessment, those not seizure-free at 6 months have only an 18% chance of being seizure-free at 12 months (Chi-Square $= 408.105, p < 0.000001$, odd ratio $= 41.23$ with 95% confidence limits 26.4–65.85). Failure to maintain the response in 10% of patients, including 4% with two or more seizures, was noted with all AEDs studied here and in patients with newly treated as well as chronic epilepsy. As could be expected, among patients with seizures at month 1–6, those with early epilepsy became seizure-free more often over time than those with chronic epilepsy. The main conclusion was that the response at 6 months is an excellent predictor of response at 12 months.[8]

PHARMACOGENETICS

Although the field of pharmacogenetics has existed for nearly 50 years, it has begun to enter mainstream clinical practice only recently. The ultimate goal of pharmacogenetics is to use the genetic makeup of an individual to predict drug response and efficacy, as well as potential adverse drug events. Drug treatment of epilepsy is characterized by unpredictability of efficacy, adverse drug reactions and optimal doses in individual patients, which, at least in part, is a consequence of genetic variation. Since genetic variability in drug metabolism was reported to affect treatment with phenytoin more than 25 years ago, numerous studies have explored how variation in genes alters the pharmacokinetics and, more recently, pharmacodynamic effects of AEDs, suggesting that a wide assortment of genetic variants influence how individuals respond to AEDs. For example, the US FDA recently informed healthcare professionals that dangerous or even fatal skin reactions (Stevens–Johnson syndrome and toxic epidermal necrolysis), which can be caused by carbamazepine therapy, are significantly more common in patients with a particular human leukocyte antigen (HLA) allele, HLA-B★1502. This allele occurs almost exclusively in patients with ancestry across broad areas of Asia, including South Asian Indians.

p0510   However, determining the practical relevance of pharmacogenetic variants remains difficult, in part because of problems with study design and replication. Although the current studies associating particular genes and their mutations with seizure control or adverse events have inherent weaknesses and have not provided unifying conclusions, several results such as the one outlined above are encouraging and helpful to increase our knowledge of how genetic variation affects the treatment of epilepsy. A better understanding of the genetic influences on epilepsy outcome is key to developing much needed new therapeutic strategies for individuals with epilepsy.

DRUG-RELATED MECHANISMS

p0520   Ideally, the successful AED that achieves seizure control reacts to the individual pharmacological profile of the seizure-generating process. However, our knowledge of key pharmacodynamic parameters such as the individual target or the effective mechanism of action are too limited to understand why the same AED works in some patients and not in others.[2,9]

SURGERY-RELATED MECHANISMS

As in the case of Wilner, seizure control may be achieved only after resective surgery. Adjunctive resective surgery is a standard of care for drug-resistant partial epilepsy, especially mesial temporal lobe epilepsy, based on compelling short-term evidence including the only randomized controlled trial comparing surgery plus AEDs versus AEDs alone.[10] The patients were randomized prior to presurgical evaluation, so the study allowed for an intent-to-treat analysis. At 12 months after surgery, 15/40 surgical (including four patients who were randomized to surgery but were not operated on) and 1 of 40 medical patients were free of seizures as defined by the authors. Several supportive studies employing non-randomized medical controls showed that surgical treatment of drug-refractory temporal lobe epilepsy in properly selected patients is superior to that of continued medical treatment.[11] The mechanism(s) by which the resection is able to transfer drug-resistant epilepsy in drug-responsive epilepsy (with seizure freedom on or off AEDs) is unclear.

REFERENCES

1. Schmidt D, Löscher W. Drug resistance in epilepsy: putative neurobiological and clinical mechanisms. *Epilepsia* 2005;**46**:858–77.
2. Löscher W, Schmidt D. Experimental and clinical evidence for loss of effect (tolerance) during prolonged treatment with antiepileptic drugs. *Epilepsia* 2006;**47(8)**:1253–84.
3. Kwan P, Brodie M. Early identification of refractory epilepsy. *N Engl J Med* 2000;**346**:314–9.
4. Callaghan BC, Anand K, Hesdorffer D, Hauser WA, French JA. Likelihood of seizure remission in an adult population with refractory epilepsy. *Ann Neurol* 2007;**62**:382–9.
5. Luciano AL, Shorvon SD. Results of treatment changes in patients with apparently drug-resistant chronic epilepsy. *Ann Neurol* 2007;**62(4)**:375–81.
6. Sillanpää M, Schmidt D. Natural history of treated childhood-onset epilepsy: prospective, long-term population-based study. *Brain* 2006;**129**:617–24.
7. Shorvon SD, Sander JWAS. Temporal patterns of remission and relapse in seizures of patients with epilepsy. In: Schmidt D, Morselli PL, eds. *Intractable epilepsy. Experimental and clinical aspects.* New York: Raven Press, 1986: 13–24.
8. Schmidt D. How reliable is early treatment response in predicting long-term seizure outcome? *Epilepsy Behav* 2007;**10(4)**:588–94.
9. Schmidt D, Rogawski MA. New strategies for the identification of drugs to prevent the development or progression of epilepsy. *Epilepsy Res* 2002;**50**:71–8.
10. Wiebe S, Blume WT, Girvin JP, Eliasziw M, et al. A randomized, controlled trial of surgery for temporal-lobe epilepsy. *N Engl J Med* 2001;**345**:311–8.
11. Bien CG, Schulze-Bonhage A, Soeder BM, et al. Assessment of the long-term effects of epilepsy surgery with three different reference groups. *Epilepsia* 2006;**47(11)**:1865–9.

c000102

Why Do Some Patients Have Seizures After Brain Surgery While Others Do Not?

Christine Bower, David Millett and Jerome Engel Jr

s0010

POST-OPERATIVE SEIZURE RECURRENCE AFTER A STANDARD ANTERIOR TEMPORAL LOBECTOMY

s0020

History

p0020

The patient is a 45-year-old right-handed male who had his first seizure at the age of 2 months in the context of a fever. The patient started having recurrent seizures as an adolescent. These seizures were characterized by an aura of *déjà vu* and then loss of awareness with lip smacking and hand automatisms lasting for approximately 1 min. Post-ictally he was confused and sometimes agitated and violent, occasionally causing injury to himself, or others. He had approximately six seizures per month, typically occurring in clusters every 2 weeks.

p0030

Over the years the patient was treated with multiple antiepileptic drug (AEDs) including phenobarbital, phenytoin, lamotrigine, primidone, valproic acid, and most recently levetiracetam and carbamazepine. He had a full presurgical evaluation over a 4-year period (1988–91) at another hospital, including bilateral temporal subdural strips. The patient was offered right anterior temporal lobectomy, but declined. Further medication trials were unhelpful. He had a vagal nerve stimulation (VNS) placed in 1997 that resulted in decreased intensity of seizures, but no change in frequency. In 2000, he had a repeat Phase I evaluation and subsequently underwent right anterior temporal lobectomy. VNS was removed a year later.

p0040

The patient was seizure-free for 2 years after surgery on lamotrigine and carbamazepine. Medications were lowered 1 year after surgery. Two years post-operatively, while on lamotrigine monotherapy, he began to have isolated auras. Six months later he began to have complex partial seizures again. These seizures were similar in semiology and frequency to those experienced prior to surgery. He is now on levetiracetam and carbamazepine therapy.

Examination and investigations

Neurological examinations have consistently been normal.

Initial non-invasive video electro-encephalography (EEG) monitoring in 1988 showed a focal right sphenoidal ictal onset. The patient subsequently underwent Phase II monitoring (bilateral medial and lateral temporal, medial and lateral frontal, and orbital frontal strips) in order to exclude a frontal onset. During this evaluation the patient had nine complex partial seizures, six of which were felt to be clearly originating in the right mesial temporal lobe, with one "suggestive" and two "suspicious" of onset in that region.

Interictal EEG in 2000 showed right greater than left temporal spikes. During non-invasive video EEG monitoring the patient had 14 complex partial seizures, the majority of which were of right anterior temporal onset with rapid spread to the left. The left temporal onset seizures occurred only after a cluster of right temporal onset seizures. Magnetic resonance imaging (MRI) showed right mesial temporal sclerosis (MTS) while fluoro-deoxy-glucose positron emission tomography (FDG-PET) showed mild right temporal hypometabolism. Neurocognitive testing revealed mild dysfunction in both hemispheres. Wada identified left hemispheric language dominance after left-sided injection and intact memory following right-sided injection. Pathological exam of the excised right anterior temporal tissue showed Chaslin's gliosis, rare neurons in the subcortical white matter, and a small focus of minimal neuronal disorganization. In addition, the hippocampus was unusual for the extensive degree of cell loss in all fields including dentate and subiculum.

Repeat MRI post-operatively showed residual hyperintense signal on T2/fluid attenuation inversion recovery (FLAIR) in the right body to tail of the residual hippocampus with a large amount of gliotic tissue in the right temporal stem and temporal white matter. Post-operative interictal EEG showed a right temporal breach artifact, right greater than left fronto-temporal intermittent slowing, and rare left midtemporal spikes. During post-operative Phase I video EEG monitoring the patient had three secondarily generalized seizures beginning with oral and manual automatisms followed by head version to the left, left arm tonic extension, and generalization. EEG showed an ictal rhythm in the right mid temporal region within 30s of clinical onset.

Treatment and outcome

Initially the patient was treated with AEDs. Multiple medication trials were unhelpful over the years. Although initially declining surgery in the early 1990s the patient had a VNS placed in 1997. VNS resulted in decreased intensity of seizures, but no change in frequency. In 2000, the patient underwent right anterior temporal lobectomy. VNS was removed a year later. Two years post-operatively, the patient began to have isolated auras and then 6 months later he began to have complex partial seizures. Now, on a combination of levetiracetam and carbamazepine, these seizures are similar in semiology and frequency to those experienced prior to surgery. The patient has been offered extension of prior surgical resection and is currently contemplating this option.

Diagnosis

This patient's history and evaluation is typical of mesial temporal lobe epilepsy with hippocampal sclerosis (MTLE with HS), a diagnosis that was confirmed on examination of the resected tissue. The seizure that occurred with fever at 2 months is a bit early for the febrile seizures that often precede the onset of MTLE, but not inconsistent with the diagnosis. The seizures that originated from the contralateral temporal lobe at the end of clusters during the video–EEG monitoring in 2001 is not unusual for unilateral HS, and does not preclude surgery.

POST-OPERATIVE SEIZURE FREEDOM AFTER CORTICAL RESECTION BASED ON EEG, AND NO CLEAR MRI LESION

History

The patient is a 24-year-old left-handed Caucasian woman whose seizures likely began at age 3 or 4 with nocturnal episodes of emesis but she was not diagnosed until age 6 when she suffered her first convulsive seizure. Carbamazepine was initiated but she continued to have a few complex partial seizures per month, beginning with an indescribable "weird" sensation and nausea, followed by oral automatisms and unresponsiveness for 1–3 min. These seizures increased in frequency during her teens and at the age 16 she was switched to gabapentin and felbamate due to weight gain and intractability. Seizure frequency improved on felbamate but occasional breakthrough seizures persisted and she experienced weight loss, insomnia, memory impairment, and nausea. Nausea worsened when felbamate was replaced by levetiracitam in the late 1990s, and she was eventually placed on a combination of lamotrigine and zonisamide at the age of 21. At the time of presentation to our center, her seizure frequency was 1–2 per week during sleep with additional auras in isolation consisting of a strange sensation beginning in her head and traveling down through her body.

Examination and investigations

General and neurological examinations were unremarkable. Video–EEG monitoring was completed in April 2004 and demonstrated frequent epileptiform discharges over the right posterior temporal and bilateral occipital electrodes as well as occasional discharges over the mid- and anterior-temporal regions on the right. Seizure semiology revealed no lateralizing features and ictal EEG was frequently obscured by muscle artifact at onset, but developed into a 6–7 Hz right basal anterior temporal rhythm within 6–7 s. Two seizures began with attenuation across the right hemisphere and polymorphic slowing across the left hemisphere for the first 6 s after electrographic change. (*Note*: prior video–EEG monitoring at another epilepsy center in 2002 included four similar seizures.) MRI revealed decreased FLAIR signal of the white matter within the right temporal lobe but no evidence of MTS; and PET revealed right temporal hypometabolism. Neurocognitive testing identified a mild abnormality of language processing suggesting dominant fronto-temporal neocortical dysfunction, as well as non-dominant mesial temporal dysfunction.

On review of these investigations and the clinical history, our multidisciplinary team concluded that the aura, ictal EEG, MRI, PET, and neurocognitive evaluations were all consistent with right mesial temporal epilepsy with two minor exceptions: bilateral occipital interictal discharges on the EEG and dominant frontotemporal dysfunction on neurocognitive evaluation raised the possibility of either dual pathology or bilateral temporal disease. In order to investigate these latter possibilities an magneto-encephalography (MEG) and additional MR studies (diffusion tensor imaging (DTI) and surface coil) of the occiput were requested. It was agreed, however, that while these ancillary tests might corroborate an extratemporal lesion, they probably would not alter the surgical plan for right anterior temporal resection. Accordingly, a Wada test and functional magnetic resonance imaging (fMRI) were scheduled for language lateralization and memory testing, and the patient was counseled regarding her sub-optimal chances of post-surgical seizure freedom.

The additional tests produced unexpected results. Intracarotid amytal injection of the right ICA revealed right hemispheric language and the patient failed memory testing on two separate injections (125 and 90 mg of amytal) of the right ICA. Right hemisphere language was subsequently corroborated with functional fMRI, which revealed increased activation in the right hemisphere equivalents of Broca's and Wernicke's areas. An interictal MEG revealed a dense, confluent cluster of dipoles across the right occiput with a few independent dipoles arising from the left occipital lobe and the right temporal lobe. Surface-coil and diffusion tensor imaging of the right occipital lobe suggested the presence of increased cellularity in the occipital white matter and an abnormal occipital gyrus. In combination, these studies supported the hypothesis of a subtle malformation of cortical development (MCD) within the right occipital lobe. In addition, they indicated that anterior right temporal resection with amygdahippocampectomy would result in substantial verbal memory deficits.

Treatment and outcome

After multiple discussions among the interdisciplinary team members, the patient, and her family, she was offered either an intracranial depth electrode study or a focal right occipital resection under the guidance of electrocorticography. Although the patient was informed that a right occipital resection may fail to produce complete seizure control, possibly leading to a subsequent intracranial study and right (dominant) temporal resection, she decided to pursue a focal occipital resection. Focal resection of a portion of tissue within the right occipital lobe was performed under the guidance of electrocorticography and introperative language mapping in January 2005. Pathological review of resected tissues demonstrated only unremarkable cerebral cortex. She has been followed for over 2 years since surgery and has surprisingly remained seizure-free on her prior medical regimen.

Diagnosis

The diagnosis in this patient is unclear. If she remains seizure-free it is highly likely, although not definite, that the epileptogenic region was in the area of resected occipital cortex. It is always possible that surgery was effective because it interrupted an essential pathway, leaving the epileptogenic region intact. A tentative diagnosis, based on surface coil and diffusion tensor imaging is focal cortical dysplasia, but this was not confirmed by pathological evaluation of the resected tissue. There remains a possibility of an epileptogenic region in the right mesial temporal lobe, as originally suspected, which became inactive as a result of surgery. This is not unheard of. Patients occasionally stop having seizures after depth electrode evaluation, and extracranial surgery such as appendectomy and thymectomy. Although well documented, the reasons for such results remain unknown.

s0110   **Commentary**

p0170   Despite the long history of medication- and VNS-resistant seizures, the first patient had MTLE with HS and an excellent prognosis for a seizure-free post-operative outcome. In fact, he was seizure-free for 2 years, but seizures ultimately returned and were as frequent and severe as they had been pre-operatively. Two years post-operative seizure freedom is usually taken to indicate a good outcome, although seizures can recur after that. In most cases, however, they are considerably less frequent or severe than pre-operatively and may be easily controlled on medication. This patient is unusual not only because of the recurrence of seizures, but because the surgery appeared to have provided no benefit at all. This most likely is attributable to the fact that his HS was extremely severe, involving all hippocampal fields, and extended posteriorly beyond the standard anteromesial temporal resection. Reoperation with a much more extensive resection is possible given that this is in the nondominant hemisphere, with a good likelihood of post-operative seizure freedom. The epileptogenic pathophysiology of MTLE with HS, however, is not limited to mesial temporal structures; many brain areas, bilaterally, can participate in the epileptogenic process, and occasionally patients who appear to have an excellent prognosis will continue to have residual seizures originating outside the mesial temporal area, or contralaterally.

p0180   The second patient, surprisingly, had a happier outcome in that there were many confounding features revealed by her detailed evaluation. Although she appeared to have right temporal lobe epilepsy, she was right hemisphere-dominant for language, suggesting left hemisphere dysfunction even though she was left-handed (most left-handers are left hemisphere-dominant for language). The presence of bilateral disturbances was further confirmed by the Wada test and bilateral occipital interictal spikes on EEG. Localization of the occipital epileptogenic tissue, which eventually was resected, derived primary from the interictal MEG study, which is a relatively new diagnostic technique and usually not sufficient grounds for moving directly to surgery. In this case, however, there was some evidence of a structural lesion in that area revealed by surface coil and diffusion tensor imaging. Neocortical resections based on electrographic localization of the epileptogenic region only, whether extraoperative or intraoperative, usually do not result in a seizure-free outcome; however, the subtle evidence of a structural lesion in that area permitted us to offer the patient an alternative to a depth electrode study. She opted for this even though the prognosis for complete seizure freedom was relatively poor. The failure to confirm cortical dysplasia on pathological evaluation of the resected tissue further reduced expectations for post-operative seizure freedom. Her outcome, therefore, was much better than expected although, as with the first patient, there remains a chance that seizures will recur several years later.

p0190   In summary, modern diagnostic techniques for localizing the epileptogenic region, and microsurgical procedures, have greatly improved the efficacy and safety of surgery for medically intractable seizures. Although MTLE with HS still has the best prognosis, not all patients are seizure-free post-operatively, and the reasons for this are variable and often unpredictable. On the other hand, whereas localized cortical resections in the absence of a clear structural lesion is associated with a relatively poor likelihood of post-operative seizure freedom, most patients experience a significant benefit and some do become seizure-free, although, again, for unpredictable and poorly understood reasons.

Why Do Some Patients Have Seizures After Brain Surgery While Others Do Not? A Comment on the Evidence

Samuel Wiebe

While these cases illustrate the principles that guide clinicians in selecting patients for epilepsy surgery and in estimating their prognosis, they also exemplify uncertainties surrounding these very issues. In the patient with unilateral mesial temporal lobe epilepsy (MTLE) who underwent adequate surgery at an experienced center, clinical wisdom would indicate a better than 50% chance of becoming seizure-free. Why did seizures recur? Why was the semiology identical to pre-operative seizures? Why did it take 2 years for seizures to recur? By contrast, in the patient with MRI-negative neocortical epilepsy, discordant results on presurgical evaluation and a limited neocortical resection based exclusively on intraoperative electro-corticography (ECoG), clinical judgment would point toward a lower chance of seizure freedom. Why did this patient remain seizure-free? Our current understanding of epileptogenesis and of mechanisms by which surgery disrupts epileptogenesis does not allow for firm answers, but basic research involving human data sheds some light on these uncertainties.

Less is known about the mechanisms of focal, surgically treatable epilepsies than about generalized epilepsies. Although patients with surgically remediable epilepsy syndromes like MTLE share important characteristics, there remains substantial heterogeneity between and within patients. The plethora of pathophysiological mechanisms and their variable relative contribution to epileptogenesis precludes the identification of a universal, single common pathway, and of a single common surgical target.

Multifocal abnormalities are more often the rule than the exception in focal epilepsy. Multiple abnormalities and epileptogenic areas often exist in individual patients with focal seizures. In MTLE, structural abnormalities are not limited to the hippocampus and amygdala, but also involve the entorhinal and piriform cortex, as well as the thalamus,[1,2] and they are often bilateral.[3] Areas demonstrating irritative properties produce epileptiform discharges that are not strictly correlated chronologically.[4] Although maximum at sites of seizure onset, multifocal spikes are common, and their topographical association with the epileptogenic zone is not perfect, reflecting the ability of many cortical areas to produce epileptiform discharges.[5] Different seizure types and propagation patterns occur in similar cortical areas and also within individual patients, reflecting different pathophysiological mechanisms and emphasizing the lack of a single common pathway or pattern.[6] There usually is not one, but several sites of seizure origin within one system, and seizure onset typically is not focal but regional or multifocal within that system.[7] The balance between excitation and inhibition also varies among patients. In some patients with MTLE, a predominantly inhibitory, hypersynchronous spike–wave ictal pattern occurs; whereas in others an excitatory, low-voltage fast rhythmic activity predominates.[8] In turn, each pattern is associated with different degrees of focality of seizure onset, rapidity of propagation, and histopathological abnormalities.[8]

p0240   Although the mechanisms are not clear, neuronal reorganization with cell loss, neurogenesis, and aberrant proliferation of excitatory and inhibitory fibers is thought to underlie aspects of epileptogenesis in mesial temporal sclerosis (MTS).[9] Accordingly, the atrophic hippocampus is the main target for surgical resection in MTLE. However, patients without these structural changes can have seizures that are clinically and electrographically identical to those occurring with MTS. This suggests that focusing surgery on a sclerotic hippocampus may ablate the epileptogenic zones only partially, because other areas remain that may develop epileptogenic properties sufficient to support seizure generation. Furthermore, specific components of an epileptogenic circuit (e.g., hippocampus, amygdala, entorhinal, and piriform cortex) may have varying proclivity for seizure production. Consequently, the same operation for the same syndrome yields different results, with poorer seizure control if the usual resection excludes areas of important epileptogenicity (e.g., entorhinal and piriform cortex).[10]

p0250   This raises the important aspect of brain plasticity and rearrangement of focal neuronal circuits as a mechanism of epileptogenesis. Conceivably, surgery is effective to the extent that it interrupts local seizure generators and circuits. However, partial removal or interruption can result in reassembly of the circuits, leading to seizure recurrence after a seizure-free period. Seizure semiology of recurrent seizures is often similar to pre-operative seizures and may reflect the reactivation of an insufficiently interrupted pathway. This concept underpins the notion that epileptogenesis develops gradually. This is supported by the observations that longer post-operative follow-up is associated with higher rates of seizure recurrence,[11] that some lesions only give rise to seizures after prolonged quiescent periods, and that epilepsy is progressive in many patients. By corollary, new epileptogenic zones and circuits can arise *de novo* or evolve following successful resection of another epileptogenic area.[12]

p0260   In malformations of cortical development, varied and complex mechanisms underpin epileptogenicity, including abnormal connectivity, excess excitation, and decreased inhibition. In addition, the full extent of the abnormality is often unclear, resulting in surgical resections that may be insufficient to interrupt epileptogenesis.[13]

p0270   An imperfect understanding of epileptogenicity in individual patients poses important barriers to the selection and stratification of patients for surgical studies. Clinical data deriving from numerous retrospective and some prospective surgical studies point to the prognostic value of a number of clinical variables. Published results vary; mirroring within and between-patient heterogeneity alluded to earlier. However, systematic reviews of prognostic variables[14] show that, in general, better seizure outcomes can be expected in patients with hippocampal sclerosis (HS) or foreign tissue, a lesion on MRI, history of febrile seizures, and imaging or macroscopic evidence of complete lesion resection.[14] Conversely, poorer surgical outcomes can be seen in patients who require intracranial EEG, and those exhibiting epileptiform discharges on post-operative scalp EEG.[14] Some studies suggest that early post-operative seizures are strong predictors of seizure relapse following surgery.[15,16,17]

In summary, the epileptogenic zone, the target in resective epilepsy surgery, is multifaceted, complex, and diverse even in seemingly simple cases. Our limited ability to understand the specific circuits and structures at play in individual patients underpins the variability of surgical results in groups of clinically similar patients. Research into methods that allow the identification of critical epileptogenic structures in individual patients is needed to fine tune patient selection, interventions, and prognosis in epilepsy surgery.

REFERENCES

1. Margerison JH, Corsellis JAN. Epilepsy and the temporal lobes: a clinical, electroencephalographic and neuropathological study of the brain in epilepsy, with particular reference to the temporal lobes. *Brain* 1966;**89**:499–530.
2. Mathieson G. Pathology of temporal lobe foci. *Adv Neurol* 1975;**11**:163–85.
3. Quigg M, Bertram EH, Jackson T, Laws E. Volumetric magnetic resonance imaging evidence of bilateral hippocampal atrophy in mesial temporal lobe epilepsy. *Epilepsia* 1997;**38(5)**:588–94.
4. Gotman J. Relationships between interictal spiking and seizures: human and experimental evidence. *Can J Neurol Sci* 1991;**18(4 Suppl)**:573–6.
5. Ma HT, Wu CH, Wu JY. Initiation of spontaneous epileptiform events in the rat neocortex in vivo. *J Neurophysiol* 2004;**91(2)**:934–45.
6. Schiller Y, Cascino GD, Busacker NE, Sharbrough FW. Characterization and comparison of local onset and remote propagated electrographic seizures recorded with intracranial electrodes. *Epilepsia* 1998;**39(4)**:380–8.
7. Spencer SS, Guimaraes P, Katz A, Kim J, Spencer D. Morphological patterns of seizures recorded intracranially. *Epilepsia* 1992;**33(3)**:537–45.
8. Velasco AL, Wilson CL, Babb TL, Engel J Jr. Functional and anatomic correlates of two frequently observed temporal lobe seizure-onset patterns. *Neural Plast* 2000;**7(1–2)**:49–63.
9. Parent JM, Lowenstein DH. Mossy fiber reorganization in the epileptic hippocampus. *Curr Opin Neurol* 1997;**10(2)**:103–9.
10. Bertram EH. Why does surgery fail to cure limbic epilepsy? Seizure functional anatomy may hold the answer. *Epilepsy Res* 2003;**56(2–3)**:93–9.
11. Tellez-Zenteno JF, Dhar R, Wiebe S. Long-term seizure outcomes following epilepsy surgery: a systematic review and meta-analysis. *Brain* 2005;**128(Pt 5)**:1188–98.
12. Chang BS, Lowenstein DH. Epilepsy. *N Engl J Med* 2003;**349(13)**:1257–66.
13. Jacobs KM, Kharazia VN, Prince DA. Mechanisms underlying epileptogenesis in cortical malformations. *Epilepsy Res* 1999;**36(2–3)**:165–88.
14. Tonini C, Beghi E, Berg AT, et al. Predictors of epilepsy surgery outcome: a meta-analysis. *Epilepsy Res* 2004;**62(1)**:75–87.
15. Berg AT, Vickrey BG, Langfitt JT. Reduction of AEDs in postsurgical patients who attain remission. *Epilepsia* 2006;**47**:64–71.
16. McIntosh AM, Kalnins RM, Mitchell LA, Berkovic SF. Early seizures after temporal lobectomy predict subsequent seizure recurrence. *Ann Neurol* 2005;**57(2)**:283–8.
17. Spencer SS, Berg AT, Vickrey BG, et al. Predicting long-term seizure outcome after resective epilepsy surgery: the multicenter study. *Neurology* 2005;**65**:912–8.

Why Do Some Patients Have Seizures After Brain Surgery While Others Do Not? A Clinical Perspective

József Janszky and Andras Fogarasi

In some difficult-to-treat epilepsies and especially in temporal lobe epilepsy along with hippocampal sclerosis (TLE–HS), surgical treatment is superior to pharmacotherapy[1]; most patients become seizure-free after temporal lobe resections.[2] Still, about one-third of the patients continue to have seizures. The reason for unsuccessful surgery is not completely known. Seizures after unsuccessful operation may arise not only from ipsilateral structures but also from the hemisphere contralateral to the surgery.[3] The retrospective identification of prognostic factors for surgical failure may improve general understanding of the pathophysiology of surgical failure and there are numerous studies investigating the predictive factors for epilepsy surgery.

The most frequently reported predictors for unfavorable outcome are the absence of an MRI detectable epileptogenic lesion, bilateral interictal epileptiform discharges (IED), long epilepsy duration, and contralateral spreading of ictal activity.[2, 4–6]

Despite many studies in this field, we still cannot adequately predict the outcome of epilepsy surgery: the conclusions of these studies are strikingly variable as many prognostic factors found in one study were not found to have predictive value in the other studies. This may be due to several reasons: (1) Epilepsy surgery centers have different surgical and presurgical protocols, diagnostic tools (type of MRI, EEG, using PET, single photon emission computer tomography (SPECT), or MEG) or even definitions for IED or for MRI abnormalities. (2) The post-operative follow-up is highly variable across these studies. (3) Due to methodological differences, the studies investigating predictors are performed in single surgical centers only; thus, the number of patients is relatively low.

Seizure outcome is typically assessed only after the first or second post-operative years; very little is known as to what occurs in the subsequent 5–20 years.[2] Some initially non-seizure-free patients may achieve long-term seizure freedom[7] while some patients may relapse after many years of seizure freedom[8]; thus, the long-term outcome is worse than the short-term and 48–58% of patients do not become seizure-free >5 years after the operation.[2,6] Worsening of the outcome typically occurs in TLE-HS compared to neocortical epilepsies. Spencer et al.[9] found that patients with TLE-HS who were seizure-free 1 year after the operation had a 24% relapse rate compared to neocortical epilepsy where the relapse rate in initially seizure-free patients was only 4%.

Concentrating on the 5-year outcome after TLE-HS surgery, epilepsy duration was found to be the most important factor: only 30% of patients became seizure-free who had an epilepsy illness for >30 years, while 90% of patients had a seizure-free outcome on whom the surgery was performed within 10 years of epilepsy onset. Interestingly, epilepsy duration seems to predict only the long-term outcome and does not predict the short-term outcome.[6,8] It was also found that >20 years duration of epilepsy predicted the late relapse.

Considering the uncertainty of predicting the outcome of TLE-HS surgery, the prognosis in a particular patient cannot be known with certainty. Thus, predicting the post-operative outcome in the first patient of Bower and colleagues has all the above-mentioned limitations. The failed long-term seizure freedom in this particular patient, however, can be the result of the summation of numerous negative predictors: (1) bilateral IED,[4] (2) contralateral propagation,[5] and (3) contralateral seizure onset.[5] The post-operatively persistent bilateral IED and incomplete resection also predicted an unfavorable surgical outcome.[10] In TLE-HS the long-term relapse is not surprising.[9] Moreover, the patient had an epilepsy duration of >30 years in which case the late relapse after initial seizure occurs very often.[6] Thus, considering the numerous negative predictors, the long-term surgical failure in the first patient is not surprising at all. This case demonstrates that an early operation is required in patients with drug-resistant TLE-HS not only due to the worsening surgical outcome over time but also to prevent increasing social burden, growing neuropsychological deficit, and psychiatric co-morbidity associated with longer epilepsy duration.[11]

The second patient presented by Bower et al. most probably had an occipital-lobe epilepsy (OLE) and became seizure-free after the excision of the presumed epileptogenic region. The prognostic factors for extratemporal epilepsies are even more uncertain than predictors for TLE-HS. This is because (1) studies included only small numbers of patients, (2) the extratemporal epilepsies are not homogenous epilepsy syndromes considering the variable clinical, EEG, and neuroimaging features, and (3) there is no standardized surgical procedure compared to TLE-HS surgery. There are no systematic studies investigating the prognostic factors in surgery of pure OLE. Concerning the particular patient of Bower et al. there were so many atypical features that a prediction of surgical outcome is impossible on the basis of the present scientific knowledge. Although this patient had complex partial seizures, this can frequently occur in OLE.[12,13] The suspected MRI lesion, EEG, and MEG data did not contradict the possibility of OLE. Additionally, sophisticated diagnostic methods (MEG, surface-coil and diffusion tensor imaging) supported the possibility of a subtle cortical dysgenesis in the right occipital lobe. Presurgical evaluation with intracranial electrodes might have improved the diagnostic accuracy, however, using invasive electrophysiology does not improve the surgical outcome in extratemporal epilepsy.[14] Conversely, the second case report addressed another interesting aspect of presurgical evaluation: can we suggest brain surgery if – because of the patient's wish – we could not complete all investigations we planned? We reported on a similar situation of a child with OLE whose parents declined invasive investigation with subdural electrodes.[15] Intraoperative electrocorticography was extremely useful in that case.

In conclusion, the prognosis of epilepsy surgery is quite uncertain and especially in extratemporal patients, the prediction is inaccurate on an individual level. However, these uncertain factors and the need to individualize the approach make epilepsy surgery an interesting and challenging art.

s0130
ACKNOWLEDGEMENTS

p0370
This work was supported by a grant from the Hungarian Research Council (ETT 219/2006) and the Hungarian Scientific Research Fund (OTKA T043045, D048517, F68720). J. Janszky and A. Fogarasi were supported by the Bolyai Scholarship.

REFERENCES

1. Wiebe S, Blume WT, Girvin JP, Eliasziw M: Effectiveness and Efficiency of Surgery for Temporal Lobe Epilepsy Study Group: a randomized, controlled trial of surgery for temporal-lobe epilepsy. *N Engl J Med* 2001;**345**:311–8.
2. McIntosh AM, Wilson SJ, Berkovic SF. Seizure outcome after temporal lobectomy: current research practice and findings. *Epilepsia* 2001;**42**:1288–307.
3. Hennessy MJ, Elwes RD, Binnie CD, Polkey CE. Failed surgery for epilepsy: a study of persistence and recurrence of seizures following temporal resection. *Brain* 2000;**123**:2445–66.
4. Radhakrishnan K, So EL, Silbert PL, *et al*. Predictors of outcome of anterior temporal lobectomy for intractable epilepsy – a multivariate study. *Neurology* 1998;**51**:465–71.
5. Schulz R, Lüder HO, Hoppe M, Tuxhorn I, May T, Ebner A. Interictal EEG and ictal scalp EEG propagation are highly predictive of surgical outcome in mesial temporal lobe epilepsy. *Epilepsia* 2000;**41**:564–70.
6. Janszky J, Janszky I, Schulz R, *et al*. Temporal lobe epilepsy with hippocampal sclerosis: predictors for long-term surgical outcome. *Brain* 2005;**128**:395–404.
7. Rasmussen T. The neurosurgical treatment of focal epilepsy. In: Niedermeyer E, ed. *Modern problems of pharmacopsychiatry: epilepsy*, vol 4. New York: Krager, 1970: 306–25.
8. Yoon HH, Kwon HL, Mattson RH, Spencer DD, Spencer SS. Long-term seizure outcome in patients initially seizure-free after resective epilepsy surgery. *Neurology* 2003;**61**:445–50.
9. Spencer SS, Berg AT, Vickrey BG, *et al*. Initial outcomes in the Multicenter Study of Epilepsy Surgery. *Neurology* 2003;**61**:1680–5.
10. Halász P, Janszky J, Rasonyi G, *et al*. Postoperative interictal spikes during sleep contralateral to the operated side is associated with unfavourable surgical outcome in patients with preoperative bitemporal spikes. *Seizure* 2004;**13**:460–6.
11. Engel J Jr. The timing of surgical intervention for mesial temporal lobe epilepsy. *Arch Neurol* 1999;**56**:1338–41.
12. Lee SK, Lee SY, Kim DW, Lee DS, Chung CK. Occipital lobe epilepsy: clinical characteristics, surgical outcome, and the role of diagnostic modalities. *Epilepsia* 2005;**46**:688–95.
13. Fogarasi A, Tuxhorn I, Hegyi M, Janszky J. Predictive clinical factors for the differential diagnosis of childhood extratemporal seizures. *Epilepsia* 2005;**46**:1280–5.
14. Janszky J, Jokeit H, Schulz R, Hoppe M, Ebner A. EEG predicts surgical outcome in lesional frontal lobe epilepsy. *Neurology* 2000;**54**:1470–6.
15. Fogarasi A, Neuwirth M, Hegyi M, *et al*. Bilateral epilepsy surgery in a 4-year-old child. *Neuropediatrics* 2004;**35**:360–3.